FOR REFERENCE

Do Not Take From This Room

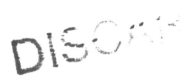

Evidence-Based Imaging

L. Santiago Medina, MD, MPH

Director, Health Outcomes, Policy and Economics (HOPE) Center, Co-Director Division of Neuroradiology, Department of Radiology, Miami Children's Hospital, Miami, Florida Former Lecturer in Radiology, Harvard Medical School, Boston, Massachusetts

C. Craig Blackmore, MD, MPH

Professor, Department of Radiology, Adjunct Professor, Health Services, University of Washington, Co-Director Radiology Health Services Research Section, Harborview Injury Prevention and Research Center, Seattle, Washington

Evidence-Based Imaging

Optimizing Imaging in Patient Care

With 183 Illustrations, 14 in Full Color
With a CD-ROM

Foreword by Bruce J. Hillman, MD

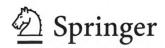 Springer

L. Santiago Medina, MD, MPH
Director
Health Outcomes
Policy and Economics (HOPE) Center
Co-Director Division of Neuroradiology
Department of Radiology
Miami Children's Hospital
Miami, FL 33155
Former Lecturer in Radiology
Harvard Medical School
Boston, MA 02114
USA

C. Craig Blackmore, MD, MPH
Professor
Department of Radiology
Adjunct Professor Health Services
University of Washington
Co-Director Radiology Health
Services Research Section
Harborview Injury Prevention
and Research Center
Seattle, WA 98104
USA

Library of Congress Control Number: 2005925501

ISBN 10: 0-387-25916-3
ISBN 13: 987-0387-25916-1

Printed on acid-free paper.

Printed in the United States of America.   (BS/EB)

9 8 7 6 5 4 3 2 1

springeronline.com

*To the many patients and researchers
who have made the evidence for this book possible.
To our families, friends, and mentors.*

Foreword

Despite our best intentions, most of what constitutes modern medical imaging practice is based on habit, anecdotes, and scientific writings that are too often fraught with biases. Best estimates suggest that only around 30% of what constitutes "imaging knowledge" is substantiated by reliable scientific inquiry. This poses problems for clinicians and radiologists, because inevitably, much of what we do for patients ends up being inefficient, inefficacious, or occasionally even harmful.

In recent years, recognition of how the unsubstantiated practice of medicine can result in poor-quality care and poorer health outcomes has led to a number of initiatives. Most significant in my mind is the evidence-based medicine movement that seeks to improve clinical research and research synthesis as a means of providing a more definitive knowledge basis for medical practice. Although the roots of evidence-based medicine are in fields other than radiology, in recent years, a number of radiologists have emerged to assume leadership roles. Many are represented among the authors and editors of this excellent book, the purpose of which is to enhance understanding of what constitutes the evidence basis for the practice of medical imaging and where that evidence basis is lacking.

It comes not a moment too soon, given how much is going on in the regulatory and payer worlds concerning health care quality. There is a general lack of awareness among radiologists about the insubstantiality of the foundations of our practices. Through years of teaching medical students, radiology residents and fellows, and practicing radiologists in various venues, it occurs to me that at the root of the problem is a lack of sophistication in reading the radiology literature. Many clinicians and radiologists are busy physicians, who, over time, have taken more to reading reviews and scanning abstracts than critically examining the source of practice pronouncements. Even in our most esteemed journals, literature reviews tend to be exhaustive regurgitations of everything that has been written, without providing much insight into which studies were performed more rigorously, and hence are more believable. Radiology training programs spend inordinate time cramming the best and brightest young minds with acronyms, imaging "signs," and unsubstantiated factoids while mostly ignoring teaching future radiologists how to think rigorously about what they are reading and hearing.

As I see it, the aim of this book is nothing less than to begin to reverse these conditions. This book is not a traditional radiology text. Rather, the editors and authors have provided first a framework for how to think about many of the most important imaging issues of our day, and then fleshed out each chapter with a critical review of the information available in the literature.

There are a number of very appealing things about the approach employed here. First, the chapter authors are a veritable "who's who" of the most thoughtful individuals in our field. Reading this book provides a window into how they think as they evaluate the literature and arrive at their conclusions, which we can use as models for our own improvement. Many of the chapters are coauthored by radiologists and practicing clinicians, allowing for more diverse perspectives. The editors have designed a uniform approach for each chapter and held the authors' feet to the fire to adhere to it. Chapters 3 to 30 provide, up front, a summary of the key points. The literature reviews that follow are selective and critical, rating the strength of the literature to provide insight for the critical reader into the degree of confidence he or she might have in reviewing the conclusions. At the end of each chapter, the authors present the imaging approaches that are best supported by the evidence and discuss the gaps that exist in the evidence that should cause us lingering uncertainty. Figures and tables help focus the reader on the most important information, while decision trees provide the potential for more active engagement. Case studies help actualize the main points brought home in each chapter. At the end of each chapter, bullets are used to highlight areas where there are important gaps in research.

The result is a highly approachable text that suits the needs of both the busy practitioner who wants a quick consultation on a patient with whom he or she is actively engaged or the radiologist who wishes a comprehensive, in-depth view of an important topic. Most importantly, from my perspective, the book goes counter to the current trend of "dumbing down" radiology that I abhor in many modern textbooks. To the contrary, this book is an intelligent effort that respects the reader's potential to think for him- or herself and gives substance to Plutarch's famous admonition, "The mind is not a vessel to be filled but a fire to be kindled."

Bruce J. Hillman, MD
Theodore E. Keats
Professor of Radiology
University of Virginia

Preface

All is flux, nothing stays still.
Nothing endures but change.
Heraclitus, 540–480 B.C.

Medical imaging has grown exponentially in the last three decades with the development of many promising and often noninvasive diagnostic studies and therapeutic modalities. The corresponding medical literature has also exploded in volume and can be overwhelming to physicians. In addition, the literature varies in scientific rigor and clinical applicability. The purpose of this book is to employ stringent evidence-based medicine criteria to systematically review the evidence defining the appropriate use of medical imaging, and to present to the reader a concise summary of the best medical imaging choices for patient care.

The 30 chapters cover the most prevalent diseases in developed countries including the four major causes of mortality and morbidity: injury, coronary artery disease, cancer, and cerebrovascular disease. Most of the chapters have been written by radiologists and imagers in close collaboration with clinical physicians and surgeons to provide a balanced and fair analysis of the different medical topics. In addition, we address in detail both the adult and pediatric sides of the issues. We cannot answer all questions—medical imaging is a delicate balance of science and art, often without data for guidance—but we can empower the reader with the current evidence behind medical imaging.

To make the book user-friendly and to enable fast access to pertinent information, we have organized all of the chapters in the same format. The chapters are framed around important and provocative clinical questions relevant to the daily physician's practice. A short table of contents at the beginning of each chapter helps three different tiers of users: (1) the busy physician searching for quick guidance, (2) the meticulous physician seeking deeper understanding, and (3) the medical-imaging researcher requiring a comprehensive resource. Key points and summarized answers to the important clinical issues are at the beginning of the chapters, so the busy clinician can understand the most important evidence-based imaging data in seconds. This fast bottom-line information is also available in a CD-ROM format, so an expeditious search can be done at the medical office or hospital, or at home. Each important question and summary is followed by a detailed discussion of the supporting evidence so that the meticulous physician can have a clear understanding of the science behind the evidence.

In each chapter the evidence discussed is presented in tables and figures that provide an easy review in the form of summary tables and flow charts. The imaging case series highlights the strengths and limitations of the different imaging studies with vivid examples. Toward the end of the chapters, the best imaging protocols are described to ensure that the imaging studies are well standardized and done with the highest available quality. The final section of the chapters is Future Research, in which provocative questions are raised for physicians and nonphysicians interested in advancing medical imaging.

Not all research and not all evidence are created equal. Accordingly, throughout the book, we use a four-level classification detailing the strength of the evidence: level I (strong evidence), level II (moderate evidence), level III (limited evidence), and level IV (insufficient evidence). The strength of the evidence is presented in parenthesis throughout the chapter so the reader gets immediate feedback on the weight of the evidence behind each topic.

Finally, we had the privilege of working with a group of outstanding contributors from major medical centers and universities in North America and the United Kingdom. We believe that the authors' expertise, breadth of knowledge, and thoroughness in writing the chapters provide a valuable source of information and can guide decision making for physicians and patients. In addition to guiding practice, the evidence summarized in the chapters may have policy-making and public health implications. Finally, we hope that the book highlights key points and generates discussion, promoting new ideas for future research.

L. Santiago Medina, MD, MPH
C. Craig Blackmore, MD, MPH

Contents

Contributors

Nolan Altman, MD
Director and Chair, Department of Radiology, Miami Children's Hospital,
Miami, FL 33155, USA

Yoshimi Anzai, MD, MPH
Associate Professor, Department of Radiology, University of Washington,
Seattle, WA 98195, USA

Kimberly E. Applegate, MD, MS
Associate Professor, Department of Radiology, Riley Hospital for Children,
Indianapolis, IN 46202, USA

Stephen Ashwal, MD
Chief, Division of Child Neurology, Department of Pediatrics, Loma Linda
University School of Medicine, Loma Linda, CA 92350, USA

Anil Kumar Attili, MBBS, (A)FRCS, FRCR
Lecturer II, Department of Thoracic Radiology, University of Michigan,
Ann Arbor, MI 48109, USA

Gregory David Avey, MD
Department of Radiology, Harborview Medical Center, Seattle, WA 98115,
USA

Martha Cecilia Ballesteros, MD
Staff Radiologist, Department of Radiology, Miami Children's Hospital,
Miami, FL 33155, USA

Alex M. Barrocas, MD, MS
Instructor, Mallinckrodt Institute of Radiology, Washington University in
St. Louis School of Medicine, St. Louis, MO 63110, USA

Wendie A. Berg, MD, PhD
Breast Imaging Consultant and Study Chair, American Radiology Services,
Johns Hopkins Greenspring, Lutherville, MD 21093, USA

Byron Bernal, MD
Neuroscientist, Department of Radiology, Miami Children's Hospital, Miami, FL 33155, USA

Andrew J. Bierhals, MD, MPH
Mallinckrodt Institute of Radiology, Washington University in St. Louis School of Medicine. St. Louis, MO 63110, USA

C. Craig Blackmore, MD, MPH
Professor, Department of Radiology, Adjunct Professor, Health Services, University of Washington, Co-Director Radiology Health Services Research Section, Harborview Injury Prevention and Research Center, Seattle, WA 98104, USA

Ruth C. Carlos, MD, MS
Assistant Professor, Department of Radiology, University of Michigan, Ann Arbor, MI 48109, USA

Soonmee Cha, MD
Assistant Professor, Department of Radiology and Neurological Surgery, University of California San Francisco Medical Center, San Francisco, CA 94143, USA

Tina A. Chang, MD
Clinical Faculty, Department of Medicine, Harborview Medical Center, University of Washington, Seattle WA 98104, USA

Colin P. Derdeyn, MD
Associate Professor, Mallinckrodt Institute of Radiology, Departments of Neurology and Neurological Surgery, Washington University in St. Louis School of Medicine, St. Louis, MO 63110, USA

Adrian K. Dixon, MD, FRCR, FRCP, FRCS, FMEDSci
Professor, Department of Radiology, University of Cambridge, Addenbrooke's Hospital, Cambridge CB2 2QQ, UK

John Eng, MD
Assistant Professor, Department of Radiology, The Johns Hopkins University, Baltimore, MD 21030, USA

Laurie L. Fajardo, MD, MBA, FACR
Professor and Chair, Department of Radiology, University of Iowa Hospital, Iowa City, IA 52242, USA

Julia R. Fielding, MD
Associate Professor, Department of Radiology, University of North Carolina at Chapel Hill, Chapel Hill, NC 27599, USA

Brian E. Grottkau MD
Chief, Department of Pediatric Orthopaedics, Harvard Medical School/ Massachusetts General Hospital for Children, Yawkey Center for Outpatient Care, Boston, MA 02114, USA

William Hollingworth, PhD
Research Assistant Professor, Department of Radiology, University of Washington, Seattle, WA 98104, USA

Barbara A. Holshouser, PhD
Associate Professor, Department of Radiology, Loma Linda University Medical Center, Loma Linda, CA 92354, USA

Clifford R. Jack, Jr., MD
Professor, Department of Radiology, Mayo Clinic, Rochester, MN 55905, USA

Diego Jaramillo, MD, MPH
Radiologist-in-Chief and Chairman, Department of Radiology, Children's Hospital of Philadelphia, Philadelphia, PA 19104, USA

Jeffrey G. Jarvik, MD, MPH
Professor, Department of Radiology and Neurosurgery, Adjunct Professor, Health Services; Chief, Neuroradiology; Associate Director, Multidisciplinary Clinical Research Center for Upper Extremity and Spinal Disorders; Co-Director, Health Services Research Section, Department of Radiology, Department of Radiology and Neurosurgery; Adjunct Health Services, University of Washington Medical Center, Seattle, WA 98195, USA

John R. Jenner, MD, FRCP
Consultant in Rheumatology and Rehabilitation, Division of Rheumatology, Department of Medicine, Addenbrooke's Hospital, Cambridge CB22QQ, UK

Krishna Juluru, MD
Department of Radiology, The Johns Hopkins University, Baltimore, MD 21287, USA

Kejal Kantarci, MD
Assistant Professor, Department of Radiology, Mayo Clinic, Rochester, MN 55905, USA

Ella A. Kazerooni, MD, MS
Professor and Director, Thoracic Radiology Division, Department of Radiology, University of Michigan Medical Center, Ann Arbor, MI 48109, USA

John Y. Kim, MD
Assistant Radiologist, Department of Radiology/Division of Pediatric Radiology, Harvard Medical School/Massachusetts General Hospital, Boston, MA 02114, USA

Jin-Moo Lee, MD, PhD
Assistant Professor, Department of Neurology and the Hope Center for Neurological Disease, Washington University in St. Louis School of Medicine, St Louis, MO 63130, USA

Weili Lin, PhD
Professor, Department of Radiology, University of North Carolina at Chapel Hill, Chapel Hill, NC 27599, USA

Brian C. Lucey, MB, BCh, BAO, MRCPI, FFR (RCSI)
Assistant Professor, Division of Body Imaging, Boston University and Boston Medical Center, Boston, MA 02118, USA

Frederick A. Mann, MD
Professor, Department of Radiology and Orthopaedics, Director and Chair, Department of Radiology, University of Washington, Harborview Medical Center, Seattle WA, 98104, USA

L. Santiago Medina, MD, MPH
Director, Health Outcomes, Policy and Economics (HOPE) Center, Co-Director Division of Neuroradiology, Department of Radiology, Miami Children's Hospital, Miami, FL 33155, USA, Former Lecturer in Radiology, Harvard Medical School, Boston, MA 02114, USA

Lucy E. Modahl, MD, PhD
Department of Radiology, Harvard Medical School/Massachusetts General Hospital, Boston, MA 02114, USA

William E. Neighbor Jr., MD
Associate Professor, Department of Family Medicine, University of Washington, Seattle, WA 98105, USA

Jeffrey H. Newhouse, MD
Professor, Department of Radiology and Urology; Vice-Chairman, Department of Radiology, Columbia University Medical Center, New York, NY 10032, USA

Udo Oyoyo, MPH
Department of Epidemiology and Biostatistics, Loma Linda University School of Public Health, Loma Linda, CA 92350, USA

Esperanza Pacheco-Jacome, MD
Co-Director, Division of Neuroradiology, Department of Radiology, Miami Children's Hospital, Miami, FL 33155, USA

Raj S. Pruthi, MD
Assistant Professor, Director of Urologic Oncology, Department of Surgery/Urology, University of North Carolina, Chapel Hill, NC 27599, USA

James G. Ravenel, MD
Assistant Professor, Department of Radiology, Medical University of South Carolina, Charleston, SC, 29425, USA

Max P. Rosen, MD, MPH
Associate Chief of Radiology for Community Network Services, Beth Israel Deaconess Medical Center, Associate Professor of Radiology, Harvard Medical School, Boston, MA 02215, USA

Marla B.K. Sammer, MD
Department of Radiology, University of Washington, Seattle, WA 98195, USA

Amisha Shah, MD
Instructor, Department of Radiology, Indiana University School of Medicine, Riley Hospital for Children, Indianapolis, IN 46202, USA

Gerard A. Silvestri, MD, MS
Associate Professor, Department of Medicine, Medical University of South Carolina, Charleston, SC 29425, USA

James M.A. Slattery, MRCPI, FFR RCSI, FRCR
Department of Radiology, Division of Abdominal Imaging and Intervention, Massachusetts General Hospital, Boston, MA 02114, USA

Robert A. Smith, PhD
Director of Cancer Screening, Department of Cancer Control Science, American Cancer Society, Atlanta, GA 30329, USA

Jorge A. Soto, MD
Associate Professor, Department of Radiology, Director, Division of Body Imaging, Boston University Medical Center, Boston, MA 02118, USA

Karen A. Tong, MD
Assistant Professor, Department of Radiology, Section of Neuroradiology, Loma Linda University Medical Center, Loma Linda, CA 92354, USA

Jose C. Varghese, MD
Associate Professor, Department of Radiology, Boston Medical Center, Boston, MA 02118, USA

Elza Vasconcellos, MD
Director, Headache Center, Department of Neurology, Miami Children's Hospital, Miami, FL 33155, USA

Katie D. Vo, MD
Assistant Professor, Department of Neuroradiology, Director of Neuromagnetic Resonance Imaging, Director of Advanced Stroke and Cerebrovascular Imaging, Mallinckrodt Institute of Radiology, Washington University in St. Louis School of Medicine, St. Louis, MO 63110, USA

Pamela K. Woodard, MD
Associate Professor, Cardiovascular Imaging Laboratory, Mallinckrodt Institute of Radiology, Washington University in St. Louis School of Medicine, St. Louis, MO 63110, USA

Michael E. Zalis, MD
Assistant Professor, Department of Radiology, Harvard Medical School, Massachusetts General Hospital, Boston, MA 02114, USA

Principles of Evidence-Based Imaging

L. Santiago Medina and C. Craig Blackmore

Medicine is a science of uncertainty and an art of probability.

Sir William Osler

Issues

I. What is evidence-based imaging?
II. The evidence-based imaging process
  A. Formulating the clinical question
  B. Identifying the medical literature
  C. Assessing the literature
    1. What are the types of clinical studies?
    2. What is the diagnostic performance of a test: sensitivity, specificity, and receiver operating characteristic (ROC) curve?
    3. What are cost-effectiveness and cost-utility studies?
  D. Types of economic analyses in medicine
  E. Summarizing the data
  F. Applying the evidence
III. How to use this book

I. What Is Evidence-Based Imaging?

The standard medical education in Western medicine has emphasized skills and knowledge learned from experts, particularly those encountered in the course of postgraduate medical education, and through national publications and meetings. This reliance on experts, referred to by Dr. Paul Gerber of Dartmouth Medical School as "eminence-based medicine" (1), is based on the construct that the individual practitioner, particularly a specialist devoting extensive time to a given discipline, can arrive at the best approach to a problem through his or her experience. The practitioner builds up an experience base over years and digests information from national experts who have a greater base of experience due to their focus in a particular area. The evidence-based imaging (EBI) paradigm, in contradistinction, is based on the precept that a single practitioner cannot through experience alone arrive at an unbiased assessment of the best course of action. Assessment of appropriate medical care should instead be derived through evidence-based research. The role of the practitioner, then, is not simply to accept information from an expert, but rather to assimilate and critically assess the research evidence that exists in the literature to guide a clinical decision (2–4).

Fundamental to the adoption of the principles of EBI is the understanding that medical care is not optimal. The life expectancy at birth in the United States for males and females in 2000 was 79.7 and 84.6 years, respectively (Table 1.1). This is comparable to the life expectancies in other industrialized nations such as the United Kingdom and Australia (Table 1.1). The United States spends 13.3% of the gross domestic product in order to achieve this life expectancy. This is significantly more than the United Kingdom and Australia, which spend less than 8.5% of their gross domestic product (Table 1.1). In addition, the U.S. per capita health expenditure is $4672, which is more than twice of these expenditures in the U.K. or Australia. In conclusion, the U.S. spends significantly more money and resources than other industrialized countries to achieve a similar outcome in life expectancy. This implies that significant amount of resources are wasted in the U.S. health care system. The U.S. in 2001 spent $1.4 trillion in health care. By 2011, the U.S. health percent of the gross domestic product is expected to grow to 17% and at $2.8 trillion double the health care expenditures in the decade since 2001 (5).

Simultaneous with the increase in health care costs has been an explosion in available medical information. The National Library of Medicine PubMed search engine now lists over 15 million citations. Practitioners cannot maintain familiarity with even a minute subset of this literature without a method of filtering out publications that lack appropriate methodological quality. Evidence-based imaging is a promising method of identifying appropriate information to guide practice and to improve the efficiency and effectiveness of imaging.

Evidence-based imaging is defined as medical decision making based on clinical integration of the best medical imaging research evidence with

Table 1.1. Life expectancy rates in three developed countries

	Life expectancy at birth (2000)		% GDP in health care (2000)[1,2]	Per capita health expenditure (2000)[1,2]
	Male	Female		
U.S.	79.7[3]	84.6[3]	13.3%	$4672
U.K.	75.2[4]	80.1[4]	7.3%	$1763
Australia	76.6[5]	82.1[5]	8.3%	$2211

GDP, gross domestic product.
[1] Organization for Economic Cooperation and Development Health Data File 2002. www.oecd.org/els/health.
[2] National Health Statistic Group, 2001. www.cms.hhs.gov/statistics/nhe.
[3] Solovy A, Towne J. 2003 Digest of Health Care's Future. American Hospital Association. 2003:1–48.
[4] United Kingdom Office of National Statistics.
[5] Australian Bureau of Statistics.

the physician's expertise and with patient's expectations (2–4). The best medical imaging research evidence often comes from the basic sciences of medicine. In EBI, however, the basic science knowledge has been translated into patient-centered clinical research, which determines the accuracy and role of diagnostic and therapeutic imaging in patient care (3). New evidence may both make current diagnostic tests obsolete and new ones more accurate, less invasive, safer, and less costly (3). The physician's expertise entails the ability to use the referring physician's clinical skills and past experience to rapidly identify high-risk individuals who will benefit from the diagnostic information of an imaging test (4). Patient's expectations are important because each individual has values and preferences that should be integrated into the clinical decision making in order to serve our patients' best interests (3). When these three components of medicine come together, clinicians and imagers form a diagnostic team, which will optimize clinical outcomes and quality of life for our patients.

II. The Evidence-Based Imaging Process

The evidence based imaging process involves a series of steps: (A) formulation of the clinical question, (B) identification of the medical literature, (C) assessment of the literature, (D) summary of the evidence, and (E) application of the evidence to derive an appropriate clinical action. This book is designed to bring the EBI process to the clinician and imager in a user-friendly way. This introductory chapter details each of the steps in the EBI process. Chapter 2 discusses how to critically assess the literature. The rest of the book makes available to practitioners the EBI approach to numerous key medical imaging issues. Each chapter addresses common medical disorders ranging from cancer to appendicitis. Relevant clinical questions are delineated, and then each chapter discusses the results of the critical analysis of the identified literature. The results of this analysis are presented with meta-analyses where appropriate. Finally, we provide simple recommendations for the various clinical questions, including the strength of the evidence that supports these recommendations.

A. Formulating the Clinical Question

The first step in the EBI process is formulation of the clinical question. The entire process of evidence-based imaging arises from a question that is asked in the context of clinical practice. However, often formulating a question for the EBI approach can be more challenging than one would believe intuitively. To be approachable by the EBI format, a question must be specific to a clinical situation, a patient group, and an outcome or action. For example, it would not be appropriate to simply ask which imaging technique is better—computed tomography (CT) or radiography. The question must be refined to include the particular patient population and the action that the imaging will be used to direct. One can refine the question to include a particular population (which imaging technique is better in adult victims of high-energy blunt trauma) and to guide a particular action or decision (to exclude the presence of unstable cervical spine fracture). The full EBI question then becomes: In adult victims of high-energy blunt trauma, which imaging modality is preferred, CT or radiography, to exclude the presence of unstable cervical spine fracture? This book addresses questions that commonly arise when employing an EBI approach. These questions and issues are detailed at the start of each chapter.

B. Identifying the Medical Literature

The process of EBI requires timely access to the relevant medical literature to answer the question. Fortunately, massive on-line bibliographical references such as PubMed are available. In general, titles, indexing terms, abstracts, and often the complete text of much of the world's medical literature are available through these on-line sources. Also, medical librarians are a potential resource to aid identification of the relevant imaging literature. A limitation of today's literature data sources is that often too much information is available and too many potential resources are identified in a literature search. There are currently over 50 radiology journals, and imaging research is also frequently published in journals from other medical subspecialties. We are often confronted with more literature and information than we can process. The greater challenge is to sift through the literature that is identified to select that which is appropriate.

C. Assessing the Literature

To incorporate evidence into practice, the clinician must be able to understand the published literature and to critically evaluate the strength of the evidence. In this introductory chapter on the process of EBI we focus on discussing types of research studies. Chapter 2 is a detailed discussion of the issues in determining the validity and reliability of the reported results.

1. What Are the Types of Clinical Studies?
An initial assessment of the literature begins with determination of the type of clinical study: descriptive, analytical, or experimental (6). *Descriptive* studies are the most rudimentary, as they only summarize disease processes as seen by imaging, or discuss how an imaging modality can be used to create images. Descriptive studies include case reports and case series. Although they may provide important information that leads to further investigation, descriptive studies are not usually the basis for EBI.

Analytic or *observational* studies include cohort, case-control, and cross-sectional studies (Table 1.2). Cohort studies are defined by risk factor status, and case-control studies consist of groups defined by disease status (7). Both case-control and cohort studies may be used to define the association between an intervention, such as an imaging test, and patient

Table 1.2. Study design

	Prospective follow-up	Randomization of subjects	Controls
Case report or series	No	No	No
Cross-sectional study	No	No	Yes
Case-control study	No	No	Yes
Cohort study	Yes/No	No	Yes
Randomized controlled trial	Yes	Yes	Yes

outcome (8). In a cross-sectional (prevalence) study, the researcher makes all of his measurements on a single occasion. The investigator draws a sample from the population (i.e., abdominal aorta aneurysms at age 50 to 80 years) and determines distribution of variables within that sample (6). The structure of a cross-sectional study is similar to that of a cohort study except that all pertinent measurements (i.e., abdominal aorta size) are made at once, without a follow-up period. Cross-sectional studies can be used as a major source for health and habits of different populations and countries, providing estimates of such parameters as the prevalence of abdominal aorta aneurysm, arterial hypertension and hyperlipidemia (6,9).

In *experimental studies* or *clinical trials*, a specific intervention is performed and the effect of the intervention is measured by using a control group (Table 1.2). The control group may be tested with a different diagnostic test, and treated with a placebo or an alternative mode of therapy (6,10). Clinical trials are epidemiologic designs that can provide data of high quality that resemble the controlled experiments done by basic science investigators (7). For example, clinical trials may be used to assess new diagnostic tests (e.g., contrast enhanced CT angiogram for carotid artery disease) or new interventional procedures (e.g., stenting for carotid artery disease).

Studies are also traditionally divided into retrospective and prospective (Table 1.2) (6,10). These terms refer more to the way the data are gathered than to the specific type of study design. In *retrospective studies*, the events of interest have occurred before study onset. Retrospective studies are usually done to assess rare disorders, for pilot studies, and when prospective investigations are not possible. If the disease process is considered rare, retrospective studies facilitate the collection of enough subjects to have meaningful data. For a pilot project, retrospective studies facilitate the collection of preliminary data that can be used to improve the study design in future prospective studies. The major drawback of a retrospective study is incomplete data acquisition (9). Case-control studies are usually retrospective. For example, in a case-control study, subjects in the case group (patients with hemorrhagic brain aneurysms) are compared with subjects in a control group (nonhemorrhagic brain aneurysms) to determine a possible cause of bleed (e.g., size and characteristics of the aneurysm) (9).

In *prospective studies*, the event of interest transpires after study onset. Prospective studies, therefore, are the preferred mode of study design, as they facilitate better control of the design and the quality of the data acquired (6). Prospective studies, even large studies, can be performed efficiently and in a timely fashion if done on common diseases at major institutions, as multicenter trials with adequate study populations (11). The major drawback of a prospective study is the need to make sure that the institution and personnel comply with strict rules concerning consents, protocols, and data acquisition (10). Persistence, to the point of irritation, is crucial to completing a prospective study. Cohort studies and clinical trials are usually prospective. For example, a cohort study could be performed in which the risk factor of brain aneurysm size is correlated with the outcome of intracranial hemorrhage morbidity and mortality, as the patients are followed prospectively over time (9).

The strongest study design is the prospective randomized, blinded clinical trial (Table 1.2) (6). The randomization process helps to distribute known and unknown confounding factors, and blinding helps to prevent observer bias from affecting the results (6,7). However, there are often circumstances in which it is not ethical or practical to randomize and follow patients prospectively. This is particularly true in rare conditions, and in studies to determine causes or predictors of a particular condition (8). Finally, randomized clinical trials are expensive and may require many years of follow-up. For example, the currently ongoing randomized clinical trial of lung cancer CT screening will require 10 years for completion, with costs estimated at $200 million. Not surprisingly, randomized clinical trials are uncommon in radiology. The evidence that supports much of radiology practice is derived from cohort and other observational studies. More randomized clinical trials are necessary in radiology to provide sound data to use for EBI practice (3).

2. What Is the Diagnostic Performance of a Test: Sensitivity, Specificity, and Receiver Operating Characteristic (ROC) Curve?

Defining the presence or absence of an outcome (i.e., disease and nondisease) is based on a standard of reference (Table 1.3). While a perfect standard of reference or so-called gold standard can never be obtained, careful attention should be paid to the selection of the standard that should be widely believed to offer the best approximation to the truth (12).

In evaluating diagnostic tests, we rely on the statistical calculations of sensitivity and specificity (see Appendix 1 at the end of this chapter). Sensitivity and specificity of a diagnostic test is based on the two-way (2×2) table (Table 1.3). Sensitivity refers to the proportion of subjects with the disease who have a positive test and is referred to as the true positive rate (Fig. 1.1). Sensitivity, therefore, indicates how well a test identifies the subjects with disease (6,13).

Specificity is defined as the proportion of subjects without the disease who have a negative index test (Fig. 1.1) and is referred to as the true negative rate. Specificity, therefore, indicates how well a test identifies the subjects with no disease (6,10). It is important to note that the sensitivity and specificity are characteristics of the test being evaluated and are therefore usually independent of the prevalence (proportion of individuals in a population who have disease at a specific instant) because the sensitivity only deals with the diseased subjects, whereas the specificity only deals with the nondiseased subjects. However, sensitivity and specificity both depend on a threshold point for considering a test positive, and hence may change according to which threshold is selected in the study (10,13,14) (Fig. 1.1A). Excellent diagnostic tests have high values (close to 1.0) for both sensitivity and specificity. Given exactly the same diagnostic test, and exactly the same subjects confirmed with the same reference test, the sensitivity with a low threshold is greater than the sensitivity with a high threshold. Conversely, the specificity with a low threshold is less than the specificity with a high threshold (Fig. 1.1B) (13,14).

Table 1.3. Two-way table of diagnostic testing

| Test result | Disease (standard of reference: gold standard) | |
	Present	Absent
Positive	a (TP)	b (FP)
Negative	c (FN)	d (TN)

FN, false negative; FP, false positive; TN, true negative; TP, true positive.

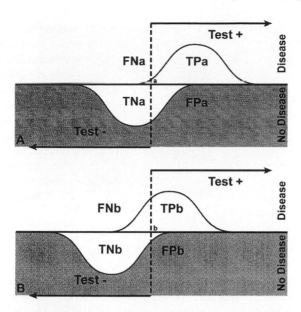

Figure 1.1. Test with a low (A) and high (B) threshold. The sensitivity and specificity of a test changes according to the threshold selected; hence, these diagnostic performance parameters are threshold dependent. Sensitivity with low threshold (TPa/diseased patients) is greater than sensitivity with a higher threshold (TPb/diseased patients). Specificity with a low threshold (TNa/nondiseased patients) is less than specificity with a high threshold (TNb/nondiseased patients). FN, false negative; FP, false positive; TN, true negative; TP, true positive. [*Source*: Medina (10), with permission from the American Society of Neuroradiology.]

The effect of threshold on the ability of a test to discriminate between disease and nondisease can be measured by a receiver operating characteristic (ROC) curve (10,14). The ROC curve is used to indicate the trade-offs between sensitivity and specificity for a particular diagnostic test, and hence describes the discrimination capacity of that test. An ROC graph shows the relationship between sensitivity (y-axis) and 1—specificity (x-axis) plotted for various cutoff points. If the threshold for sensitivity and specificity are varied, a ROC curve can be generated. The diagnostic performance of a test can be estimated by the area under the ROC curve. The steeper the ROC curve, the greater the area and the better the discrimination of the test (Fig. 1.2). A test with perfect discrimination has an area of 1.0, whereas a test with only random discrimination has an area of 0.5 (Fig. 1.2). The area under the ROC curve usually determines the overall diagnostic performance of the test independent of the threshold selected (10,14). The ROC curve is threshold independent because it is generated by using varied thresholds of sensitivity and specificity. Therefore, when evaluating a new imaging test, in addition to the sensitivity and specificity, a ROC curve analysis should be done so the threshold-dependent and -independent diagnostic performance can be fully determined (9).

3. What Are Cost-Effectiveness and Cost-Utility Studies?
Cost-effectiveness analysis (CEA) is an objective scientific technique used to assess alternative health care strategies on both cost and effectiveness (15–17). It can be used to develop clinical and imaging practice guidelines and to set health policy (18). However, it is not designed to be the final

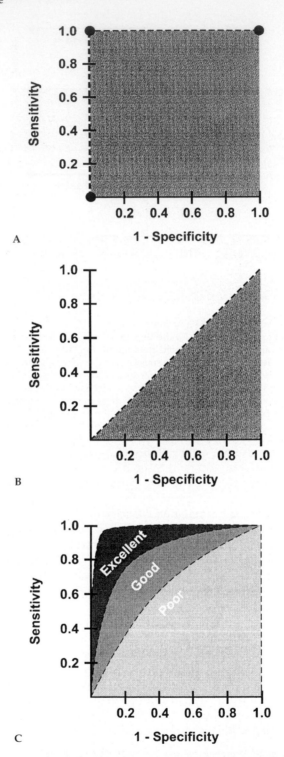

Figure 1.2. The perfect test (A) has an area under the curve (AUC) of 1. The useless test (B) has an AUC of 0.5. The typical test (C) has an AUC between 0.5 and 1. The greater the AUC (i.e., excellent > good > poor), the better the diagnostic performance. [*Source*: Medina (10), with permission from the American Society of Neuroradiology.]

answer to the decision-making process; rather, it provides a detailed analysis of the cost and outcome variables and how they are affected by competing medical and diagnostic choices.

Health dollars are limited regardless of the country's economic status. Hence, medical decision makers must weigh the benefits of a diagnostic test (or any intervention) in relation to its cost. Health care resources should be allocated so the maximum health care benefit for the entire population is achieved (9). Cost-effectiveness analysis is an important tool to address health cost-outcome issues in a cost-conscious society. Countries such as Australia usually require robust CEA before drugs are approved for national use (9).

Unfortunately, the term *cost-effectiveness* is often misused in the medical literature (19). To say that a diagnostic test is truly cost-effective, a comprehensive analysis of the entire short- and long-term outcomes and costs need to be considered. Cost-effectiveness analysis is an objective technique used to determine which of the available tests or treatments are worth the additional costs (20).

There are established guidelines for conducting robust CEA. The U.S. Public Health Service formed a panel of experts on cost-effectiveness in health and medicine to create detailed standards for cost-effectiveness analysis. The panel's recommendations were published as a book in 1996 (20).

D. Types of Economic Analyses in Medicine

There are four well-defined types of economic evaluations in medicine: cost-minimization studies, cost-benefit analyses, cost-effectiveness analyses, and cost-utility analyses. They are all commonly lumped under the term *cost-effectiveness analysis*. However, significant differences exist among these different studies.

Cost-minimization analysis is a comparison of the cost of different health care strategies that are assumed to have identical or similar effectiveness (15). In medical practice, few diagnostic tests or treatments have identical or similar effectiveness. Therefore, relatively few articles have been published in the literature with this type of study design (21). For example, a recent study demonstrated that functional magnetic resonance imaging (MRI) and the Wada test have similar effectiveness for language lateralization, but the later is 3.7 times more costly than the former (22).

Cost-benefit analysis (CBA) uses monetary units such as dollars or euros to compare the costs of a health intervention with its health benefits (15). It converts all benefits to a cost equivalent, and is commonly used in the financial world where the cost and benefits of multiple industries can be changed to only monetary values. One method of converting health outcomes into dollars is through a contingent valuation, or willingness-to-pay approach. Using this technique, subjects are asked how much money they would be willing to spend to obtain, or avoid, a health outcome. For example, a study by Appel and colleagues (23) found that individuals would be willing to pay $50 for low osmolar contrast agents to decrease the probability of side effects from intravenous contrast. However, in general, health outcomes and benefits are difficult to transform to monetary units; hence, CBA has had limited acceptance and use in medicine and diagnostic imaging (15,24).

Cost-effectiveness analysis (CEA) refers to analyses that study both the effectiveness and cost of competing diagnostic or treatment strategies, where effectiveness is an objective measure (e.g., intermediate outcome: number of strokes detected; or long-term outcome: life-years saved). Radiology CEAs often use intermediate outcomes, such as lesion identified, length of stay, and number of avoidable surgeries (15,17). However, ideally long-term outcomes such as life-years saved (LYS) should be used (20). By using LYS, different health care fields or interventions can be compared. For example, annual mammography for women age 55 to 64 years costs $110,000 per LYS (updated to 1993 U.S. dollars) (25), annual cervical cancer screening for women beginning at age 20 years costs $220,000 per LYS (updated to 1993 U.S. dollars) (25,26), and colonoscopy for colorectal cancer screening for people older than 40 years costs $90,000 per LYS (updated to 1993 U.S. dollars) (25,27).

Cost-utility analysis is similar to CEA except that the effectiveness also accounts for quality of life issues. Quality of life is measured as utilities that are based on patient preferences (15). The most commonly used utility measurement is the quality-adjusted life year (QALY). The rationale behind this concept is that the QALY of excellent health is more desirable than the same 1 year with substantial morbidity. The QALY model uses preferences with weight for each health state on a scale from 0 to 1, where 0 is death and 1 is perfect health. The utility score for each health state is multiplied by the length of time the patient spends in that specific health state (15,28). For example, let's assume that a patient with a moderate stroke has a utility of 0.7 and he spends 1 year in this health state. The patient with the moderate stroke would have a 0.7 QALY in comparison with his neighbor who has a perfect health and hence a 1 QALY.

Cost-utility analysis incorporates the patient's subjective value of the risk, discomfort, and pain into the effectiveness measurements of the different diagnostic or therapeutic alternatives. In the end, all medical decisions should reflect the patient's values and priorities (28). That is the explanation of why cost-utility analysis is becoming the preferred method for evaluation of economic issues in health (18,20). For example, in low-risk newborns with intergluteal dimple suspected of having occult spinal dysraphism, ultrasound was the most effective strategy with an incremented cost-effectiveness ratio of $55,100 per QALY. In intermediate-risk newborns with low anorectal malformation, however, MRI was more effective than ultrasound at an incremental cost-effectiveness of $1000 per QALY (29).

Assessment of Outcomes: The major challenge to cost-utility analysis is the quantification of health or quality of life. One way to quantify health is descriptively. By assessing what patients can and cannot do, how they feel, their mental state, their functional independence, their freedom from pain, and any number of other facets of health and well-being that are referred to as domains, one can summarize their overall health status. Instruments designed to measure these domains are called health status instruments. A large number of health status instruments exist, both general instruments such as the SF-36 (30), as well as instruments that are specific to particular disease states, such as the Roland scale for back pain. These various scales enable the quantification of health benefit. For example, Jarvik and colleagues (31) found no significant difference in the Roland score between patients randomized to MRI versus radiography for low back pain, suggesting that MRI was not worth the additional cost.

Assessment of Cost: All forms of economic analysis require assessment of cost. However, assessment of cost in medical care can be confusing, as the term *cost* is used to refer to many different things. The use of charges for any sort of cost estimation however, is inappropriate. Charges are arbitrary and have no meaningful use. Reimbursements, derived from Medicare and other fee schedules, are useful as an estimation of the amounts society pays for particular health care interventions. For an analysis taken from the societal perspective, such reimbursements may be most appropriate. For analyses from the institutional perspective or in situations where there are no meaningful Medicare reimbursements, assessment of actual direct and overhead costs may be appropriate (32).

Direct cost assessment centers on the determination of the resources that are consumed in the process of performing a given imaging study, including *fixed costs* such as equipment, and *variable costs* such as labor and supplies. Cost analysis often utilizes activity-based costing and time motion studies to determine the resources consumed for a single intervention in the context of the complex health care delivery system. *Overhead*, or *indirect cost*, assessment includes the costs of buildings, overall administration, taxes, and maintenance that cannot be easily assigned to one particular imaging study. Institutional cost accounting systems may be used to determine both the direct costs of an imaging study and the amount of institutional overhead costs that should be apportioned to that particular test. For example, Medina and colleagues (33) in a vesicoureteral reflux imaging study in children with urinary tract infection found a significant difference ($p < .0001$) between the mean total direct cost of voiding cystourethrography ($\$112.7 \pm \$10.33$) and radionuclide cystography ($\$64.58 \pm \$1.91$).

E. Summarizing the Data

The results of the EBI process are a summary of the literature on the topic, both quantitative and qualitative. *Quantitative analysis* involves at minimum, a descriptive summary of the data, and may include formal *meta-analysis* where there is sufficient reliably acquired data. *Qualitative analysis* requires an understanding of error, bias, and the subtleties of experimental design that can affect the reliability of study results. Qualitative assessment of the literature is covered in detail in Chapter 2; this section focuses on meta-analysis and the quantitative summary of data.

The goal of the EBI process is to produce a single summary of all of the data on a particular clinically relevant question. However, the underlying investigations on a particular topic may be too dissimilar in methods or study populations to allow for a simple summary. In such cases, the user of the EBI approach may have to rely on the single study that most closely resembles the clinical subjects upon whom the results are to be applied, or may be able only to reliably estimate a range of possible values for the data.

Often, there is abundant information available to answer an EBI question. Multiple studies may be identified that provide methodologically sound data. Therefore, some method must be used to combine the results of these studies in a summary statement. *Meta-analysis* is the method of combining results of multiple studies in a statistically valid manner to determine a summary measure of accuracy or effectiveness (34,35). For diagnostic studies, the summary estimate is generally a summary sensitivity and specificity, or a summary ROC curve.

The process of performing meta-analysis parallels that of performing primary research. However, instead of individual subjects, the meta-analysis is based on individual studies of a particular question. The process of selecting the studies for a meta-analysis is as important as unbiased selection of subjects for a primary investigation. Identification of studies for meta-analysis employs the same type of process as that for EBI described above, employing Medline and other literature search engines. Critical information from each of the selected studies is then abstracted usually by more than one investigator. For a meta-analysis of a diagnostic accuracy study, the numbers of true positives, false positives, true negatives, and false negatives would be determined for each of the eligible research publications. The results of a meta-analysis are derived not just by simply pooling the results of the individual studies, but instead by considering each individual study as a data point and determining a summary estimate for accuracy based on each of these individual investigations. There are sophisticated statistical methods of combining such results (36).

Like all research, the value of a meta-analysis is directly dependent on the validity of each of the data points. In other words, the quality of the meta-analysis can only be as good as the quality of the research studies that the meta-analysis summarizes. In general, meta-analysis cannot compensate for selection and other biases in primary data. If the studies included in a meta-analysis are different in some way, or are subject to some bias, then the results may be too heterogeneous to combine in a single summary measure. Exploration for such heterogeneity is an important component of meta-analysis.

The ideal for EBI is that all practice be based on the information from one or more well performed meta-analyses. However, there is often too little data or too much heterogeneity to support formal meta-analysis.

F. Applying the Evidence

The final step in the EBI process is to apply the summary results of the medical literature to the EBI question. Sometimes the answer to an EBI question is a simple yes or no, as for this question: Does a normal clinical exam exclude unstable cervical spine fracture in patients with minor trauma? Commonly, the answers to EBI questions are expressed as some measure of accuracy. For example, how good is CT for detecting appendicitis? The answer is that CT has an approximate sensitivity of 94% and specificity of 95% (37). However, to guide practice, EBI must be able to answer questions that go beyond simple accuracy, for example: Should CT scan then be used for appendicitis? To answer this question it is useful to divide the types of literature studies into a *hierarchical framework* (38) (Table 1.4). At the foundation in this hierarchy is assessment of *technical efficacy*: studies that are designed to determine if a particular proposed imaging method or application has the underlying ability to produce an image that contains useful information. Information for technical efficacy would include signal-to-noise ratios, image resolution, and freedom from artifacts. The second step in this hierarchy is to determine if the image predicts the truth. This is the *accuracy* of an imaging study and is generally studied by comparing the test results to a reference standard and defining the sensitivity and the specificity of the imaging test. The third step is to incorporate the physician into the evaluation of the imaging intervention

Table 1.4. Imaging Effectiveness Hierarchy

Technical efficacy: production of an image or information   Measures: signal-to-noise ratio, resolution, absence of artifacts

**Accuracy efficacy: ability of test to differentiate between disease and
        nondisease**
    Measures: sensitivity, specificity, receiver operator characteristic curves

**Diagnostic-thinking efficacy: impact of test on likelihood of diagnosis in a
        patient**
    Measures: pre- and posttest probability, diagnostic certainty

Treatment efficacy: potential of test to change therapy for a patient   Measures: treatment plan, operative or medical treatment frequency
Outcome efficacy: effect of use of test on patient health   Measures: mortality, quality adjusted life years, health status
Societal efficacy: appropriateness of test from perspective of society   Measures: cost-effectiveness analysis, cost-utility analysis

Source: Adapted from Fryback and Thornbury (38).

by evaluating the effect of the use of the particular imaging intervention on physician certainty of a given diagnosis (physician decision making) and on the actual management of the patient (*therapeutic efficacy*). Finally, to be of value to the patient, an imaging procedure must not only affect management but also improve outcome. *Patient outcome efficacy* is the determination of the effect of a given imaging intervention on the length and quality of life of a patient. A final efficacy level is that of society, which examines the question of not simply the health of a single patient, but that of the health of society as a whole, encompassing the effect of a given intervention on all patients and including the concepts of *cost* and *cost-effectiveness* (38).

Some additional research studies in imaging, such as clinical prediction rules, do not fit readily into this hierarchy. *Clinical prediction rules* are used to define a population in whom imaging is appropriate or can safely be avoided. Clinical prediction rules can also be used in combination with CEA as a way of deciding between competing imaging strategies (39).

Ideally, information would be available to address the effectiveness of a diagnostic test on all levels of the hierarchy. Commonly in imaging, however, the only reliable information that is available is that of diagnostic accuracy. It is incumbent upon the user of the imaging literature to determine if a test with a given sensitivity and specificity is appropriate for use in a given clinical situation. To address this issue, the concept of Bayes' theorem is critical. Bayes' theorem is based on the concept that the value of the diagnostic tests depends not only on the characteristics of the test (sensitivity and specificity), but also on the prevalence (pretest probability) of the disease in the test population. As the prevalence of a specific disease decreases, it becomes less likely that someone with a positive test will actually have the disease, and more likely that the positive test result is a false positive. The relationship between the sensitivity and specificity of the test and the prevalence (pretest probability), can be expressed through the use of Bayes' theorem (see Appendix 2) (10,13) and the likelihood ratio. The positive likelihood ratio (PLR) estimates the likelihood that a positive test result will raise or lower the pretest probability, resulting in estimation of the posttest probability [where PLR = sensitivity/(1 − specificity)]. The negative likelihood ratio (NLR) estimates the likelihood that a negative test result will raise or lower the pretest probability, resulting in estimation of the posttest probability [where NLR = (1 − sensitivity)/specificity] (40). The likelihood ratio (LR) is not a probability but a ratio of probabilities and as such is not intuitively interpretable. The positive predictive value (PPV) refers to the probability that a person with a positive test result actually has the disease. The negative predictive value (NPV) is the probability that a person with a negative test result does not have the disease. Since the predictive value is determined once the test results are known (i.e., sensitivity and specificity), it actually represents a posttest probability; hence, the posttest probability is determined by both the prevalence (pretest probability) and the test information (i.e., sensitivity and specificity). Thus, the predictive values are affected by the prevalence of disease in the study population.

A practical understanding of this concept is shown in examples 1 and 2 in Appendix 2. The example shows an increase in the PPV from 0.67 to 0.98 when the prevalence of carotid artery disease is increased from 0.16 to 0.82. Note that the sensitivity and specificity of 0.83 and 0.92, respectively, remain unchanged. If the test information is kept constant (same sensitivity and specificity), the pretest probability (prevalence) affects the posttest probability (predictive value) results.

The concept of diagnostic performance discussed above can be summarized by incorporating the data from Appendix 2 into a nomogram for interpreting diagnostic test results (Fig. 1.3). For example, two patients present to the emergency department complaining of left-sided weakness. The treating physician wants to determine if they have a stroke from carotid artery disease. The first patient is an 8-year-old boy complaining of chronic left-sided weakness. Because of the patient's young age and chronic history, he was determined clinically to be in a low-risk category for carotid artery disease–induced stroke and hence with a low pretest probability of 0.05 (5%). Conversely, the second patient is 65 years old and is complaining of acute onset of severe left-sided weakness. Because of the patients older age and acute history, he was determined clinically to be in a high-risk category for carotid artery disease–induced stroke and hence with a high pretest probability of 0.70 (70%). The available diagnostic imaging test was unenhanced head and neck CT followed by CT angiography. According to the radiologist's available literature, the sensitivity and specificity of these tests for carotid artery disease and stroke were each 0.90. The positive likelihood ratio (sensitivity/1 − specificity) calculation derived by the radiologist was 0.90/(1 − 0.90) = 9. The posttest probability for the 8-year-old patient is therefore 30% based on a pretest probability of 0.05 and a likelihood ratio of 9 (Fig. 1.3, dashed line A). Conversely, the posttest probability for the 65-year-old patient is greater than 0.95 based on a pretest probability of 0.70 and a positive likelihood ratio of 9 (Fig. 1.3, dashed line B). Clinicians and radiologists can use this scale to understand the probability of disease in different risk groups and for imaging studies with different diagnostic performance.

Jaeschke et al. (40) have proposed a rule of thumb regarding the interpretation of the LR. For PLR, tests with values greater than 10 have a large difference between pretest and posttest probability with conclusive diagnostic impact; values of 5 to 10 have a moderate difference in test proba-

Figure 1.3. Bayes' theorem nomogram for determining posttest probability of disease using the pretest probability of disease and the likelihood ratio from the imaging test. Clinical and imaging guidelines are aimed at increasing the pretest probability and likelihood ratio, respectively. Worked example is explained in the text. [*Source*: Medina (9), with permission from Elsevier.]

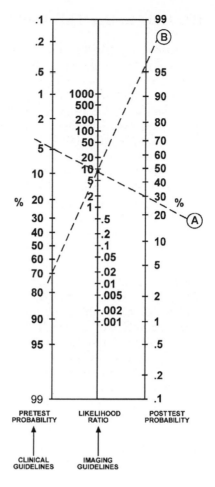

bilities and moderate diagnostic impact; values of 2 to 5 have a small difference in test probabilities and sometimes an important diagnostic impact; and values less than 2 have a small difference in test probabilities and seldom important diagnostic impact. For NLR, tests with values less than 0.1 have a large difference between pretest and posttest probability with conclusive diagnostic impact; values of 0.1 and less than 0.2 have a moderate difference in test probabilities and moderate diagnostic impact; values of 0.2 and less than 0.5 have a small difference in test probabilities and sometimes an important diagnostic impact; and values of 0.5 to 1 have small difference in test probabilities and seldom important diagnostic impact.

The role of the clinical guidelines is to increase the pretest probability by adequately distinguishing low-risk from high-risk groups. The role of imaging guidelines is to increase the likelihood ratio by recommending the diagnostic test with the highest sensitivity and specificity. Comprehensive use of clinical and imaging guidelines will improve the posttest probability, hence, increasing the diagnostic outcome (9).

III. How to Use This Book

As these examples illustrate, the EBI process can be lengthy. The literature is overwhelming in scope and somewhat frustrating in methodologic quality. The process of summarizing data can be challenging to the clinician not skilled in meta-analysis. The time demands on busy practitioners can limit their appropriate use of the EBI approach. This book can obviate these challenges in the use of EBI and make the EBI accessible to all imagers and users of medical imaging.

This book is organized by major diseases and injuries. In the table of contents within each chapter you will find a series of EBI issues provided as clinically relevant questions. Readers can quickly find the relevant clinical question and receive guidance as to the appropriate recommendation based on the literature. Where appropriate, these questions are further broken down by age, gender, or other clinically important circumstances. Following the chapter's table of contents is a summary of the key points determined from the critical literature review that forms the basis of EBI. Sections on pathophysiology, epidemiology, and cost are next, followed by the goals of imaging and the search methodology. The chapter is then broken down into the clinical issues. Discussion of each issue begins with a brief summary of the literature, including a quantification of the strength of the evidence, and then continues with detailed examination of the supporting evidence. At the end of the chapter, the reader will find the take-home tables and imaging case studies, which highlight key imaging recommendations and their supporting evidence. Finally, questions are included where further research is necessary to understand the role of imaging for each of the topics discussed.

Acknowledgment: We appreciate the contribution of Ruth Carlos, MD, MS, to the discussion of likelihood ratios in this chapter.

Take-Home Appendix 1: Equations

Nomenclature for two-way table (diagnostic testing)

Test Result	Present	Outcome	Absent
Positive	a (TP)		b (FP)
Negative	c (FN)		d (TN)

a. Sensitivity	a/(a + c)
b. Specificity	d/(b + d)
c. Prevalence	(a + c)/(a + b + c + d)
d. Accuracy	(a + d)/(a + b + c + d)
e. Positive predictive value*	a/(a + b)
f. Negative predictive value*	d/(c + d)
g. 95% confidence interval (CI)	$p \pm 1.96$ square root $(p(1 - p)/n)$
	p = proportion
	n = number of subjects
h. Likelihood ratio	Sensitivity/(1 − specificity) =
	a(b + d)/[b(a + c)]

* Only correct if the prevalence of the outcome is estimated from a random sample or based on an *a priori* estimate of prevalence in the general population; otherwise, use of Bayes' theorem must be used to calculate PPV and NPV. TP, true positive; FP, false positive; FN, false negative; TN, true negative.

Take-Home Appendix 2: Summary of Bayes' Theorem

A. Information before Test × Information from Test = Information after Test
B. Pretest Probability (Prevalence) × Sensitivity/1 − Specificity = Posttest Probability (Predictive Value)
C. Information from the test also known as the likelihood ratio, described by the Equation: Sensitivity/1 − Specificity
D. Examples 1 and 2
Predictive values: The predictive values (posttest probability) change according to the differences in prevalence (pretest probability), although the diagnostic performance of the test (i.e., sensitivity and specificity) is unchanged. The following examples illustrate how the prevalence (pretest probability) can affect the predictive values (posttest probability) having the same information in two different study groups.

Example 1: low prevalence of carotid artery disease

	Disease (Carotid artery disease)	No disease (no carotid artery disease)	Total
Test positive (positive CTA)	20	10	30
Test negative (negative CTA)	4	120	124
Total	24	130	154

Results: sensitivity = 20/24 = 0.83; specificity = 120/130 = 0.92; prevalence = 24/154 = 0.16; positive predictive value = 0.67; negative predictive value = 0.98.

Example 2: high prevalence of carotid artery disease

	Disease (Carotid artery disease)	No disease (no carotid artery disease)	Total
Test positive (positive CTA)	500	10	510
Test negative (negative CTA)	100	120	220
Total	600	130	730

Results: sensitivity = 500/600 = 0.83; specificity = 120/130 = 0.92; prevalence = 600/730 = 0.82; positive predictive value = 0.98; negative predictive value = 0.55.

Equations for calculating the results in the previous examples are listed in Appendix 1. As the prevalence of carotid artery disease increases from 0.16 (low) to 0.82 (high), the positive predictive value (PPV) of a positive contrast-enhanced CT increases from 0.67 to 0.98, respectively. The sensitivity and specificity remain unchanged at 0.83 and 0.92, respectively. These examples also illustrate that the diagnostic performance of the test (i.e., sensitivity and specificity) do not depend on the prevalence (pretest probability) of the disease. CTA, CT angiogram.

References

1. Levin A. Ann Intern Med 1998;128:334–336.
2. Evidence-Based Medicine Working Group. JAMA 1992;268:2420–2425.
3. The Evidence-Based Radiology Working Group. Radiology 2001;220:566–575.
4. Wood BP. Radiology 1999;213:635–637.
5. Solovy A, Towne J. Digest of Healthcare's Future: American Hospital Association, 2003.

6. Hulley SB, Cummings SR. Designing Clinical Research. Baltimore: Williams and Wilkins, 1998.
7. Kelsey J, Whittemore A, Evans A, Thompson W. Methods in Observational Epidemiology. New York: Oxford University Press, 1996.
8. Blackmore C, Cummings P. AJR 2004;183(5):1203–1208.
9. Medina L, Aguirre E, Zurakowski D. Neuroimag Clin North Am 2003;13:157–165.
10. Medina L. AJNR 1999;20:1584–1596.
11. Sunshine JH, McNeil BJ. Radiology 1997;205:549–557.
12. Black WC. AJR 1990;154:17–22.
13. Sox HC, Blatt MA, Higgins MC, Marton KI. Medical Decision Making. Boston: Butterworth, 1988.
14. Metz CE. Semin Nucl Med 1978;8:283–298.
15. Singer M, Applegate K. Radiology 2001;219:611–620.
16. Weinstein MC, Fineberg HV. Clinical Decision Analysis. Philadelphia: WB Saunders, 1980.
17. Carlos R. Acad Radiol 2004;11:141–148.
18. Detsky AS, Naglie IG. Ann Intern Med 1990;113:147–154.
19. Doubilet P, Weinstein MC, McNeil BJ. N Engl J Med 1986;314:253–256.
20. Gold MR, Siegel JE, Russell LB, Weinstein MC. Cost-Effectiveness in Health and Medicine. New York: Oxford University Press, 1996.
21. Hillemann D, Lucas B, Mohiuddin S, Holmberg M. Ann Pharmacother 1997:974–979.
22. Medina L, Aguirre E, Bernal B, Altman N. Radiology 2004;230:49–54.
23. Appel LJ, Steinberg EP, Powe NR, Anderson GF, Dwyer SA, Faden RR. Med Care 1990;28:324–337.
24. Evens RG. Cancer 1991;67:1245–1252.
25. Tengs T, Adams M, Pliskin J, Siegel J, Graham J. Risk Analysis 1995;13:369–390.
26. Eddy DM. Gynecol Oncol 1981;12:S168–187.
27. England W, Halls J, Hunt V. Med Decis Making 1989;9:3–13.
28. Yin D, Forman HP, Langlotz CP. AJR 1995;165:1323–1328.
29. Medina L, Crone K, Kuntz K. Pediatrics 2001;108:E101.
30. Ware JE, Sherbourne CD. Medical Care 1992;30:473–483.
31. Jarvik J, Hollingworth W, Martin B, et al. JAMA 2003:2810–2818.
32. Blackmore CC, Magid DJ. Radiology 1997;203:87–91.
33. Medina L, Aguirre E, Altman N. Acad Radiol 2003;10:139–144.
34. Zou K, Fielding J, Ondategui-Parra S. Acad Radiol 2004;11:127–133.
35. Langlotz C, Sonnad S. Acad Radiol 1998;5(suppl 2):S269–S273.
36. Littenberg B, Moses LE. Med Decis Making 1993;13:313–321.
37. Terasawa T, Blackmore C, Bent S, Kohlwes R. Ann Intern Med 2004;141(7):537–546.
38. Fryback DG, Thornbury JR. Med Decis Making 1991;11:88–94.
39. Blackmore C. Radiology 2005;235(2):371–374.
40. Jaeschke R, Guyatt GH, Sackett DL. JAMA 1994;271:703–707.

2

Critically Assessing the Literature: Understanding Error and Bias

C. Craig Blackmore, L. Santiago Medina, James G. Ravenel, and Gerard A. Silvestri

The keystone of the evidence-based imaging (EBI) approach is to critically assess the research data that are provided and to determine if the information is appropriate for use in answering the EBI question. Unfortunately, the published studies are often limited by bias, small sample size, and methodological inadequacy. Further, the information provided in published reports may be insufficient to allow estimation of the quality of the research. Two recent initiatives, the CONSORT (1) and STARD (2), aim to improve the reporting of clinical trials and studies of diagnostic accuracy, respectively. However, these guidelines are only now being implemented.

This chapter summarizes the common sources of error and bias in the imaging literature. Using the EBI approach requires an understanding of these issues.

I. What Are Error and Bias?

Errors in the medical literature can be divided into two main types. *Random error* occurs due to chance variation, causing a sample to be different from the underlying population. Random error is more likely to be problematic when the sample size is small. *Systematic error*, or *bias*, is an incorrect study result due to nonrandom distortion of the data. Systematic error is not

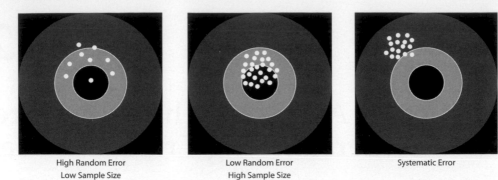

| High Random Error | Low Random Error | Systematic Error |
| Low Sample Size | High Sample Size | |

Figure 2.1. Random and systematic error. Using the bull's-eye analogy, the larger the sample size, the less the random error and the larger the chance of hitting the center of the target. In systematic error, regardless of the sample size, the bias would not allow the researcher to hit the center of the target.

affected by sample size, but rather is a function of flaws in the study design, data collection, or analysis. A second way to think about random and systematic error is in terms of precision and accuracy (3). Random error affects the precision of a result (Fig. 2.1). The larger the sample size, the more precision in the results and the more likely that two samples from truly different populations will be differentiated from each other. Using the bull's-eye analogy, the larger the sample size, the less the random error and the larger the chance of hitting the center of the target (Fig. 2.1). Systematic error, on the other hand, is a distortion in the accuracy of an estimate. Regardless of precision, the underlying estimate is flawed by some aspect of the research procedure. Using the bull's-eye analogy, in systematic error regardless of the sample size the bias would not allow the researcher to hit the center of the target (Fig. 2.1).

II. What Is Random Error?

Random error is divided into two main types: Type I, or alpha error, is when the investigator concludes that an effect or difference is present when in fact there is no true difference. Type II, or beta error, occurs when an investigator concludes that there is no effect or no difference when in fact a true difference exists in the underlying population (3). Quantification of the likelihood of alpha error is provided by the familiar p value. A p value of less than .05 indicates that there is a less than 5% chance that the observed difference in a sample would be seen if there was in fact no true difference in the population. In effect, the difference observed in a sample is due to chance variation rather than a true underlying difference in the population.

A. Type I Error

There are limitations to the ubiquitous p values seen in imaging research reports (4). The p values are a function of both sample size and magnitude of effect. In other words, there could be a very large difference between two groups under study, but the p value might not be significant if the sample sizes are small. Conversely, there could be a very small, clinically unimportant difference between two groups of subjects or between two imaging tests, but with a large enough sample size even this clinically unimportant result would be statistically significant. Because of these limitations, many journals are underemphasizing the use of p values and encouraging research results to be reported by way of confidence intervals.

B. Confidence Intervals

Confidence intervals are preferred because they provide much more information than p values. Confidence intervals provide information about the precision of an estimate (how wide are the confidence intervals), the size of an estimate (magnitude of the confidence intervals), and the statistical significance of an estimate (whether the intervals include the null) (5).

If you assume that your sample was randomly selected from some population (that follows a normal distribution), you can be 95% certain that the confidence interval (CI) includes the population mean. More precisely, if you generate many 95% CIs from many data sets, you can expect that the CI will include the true population mean in 95% of the cases and not include the true mean value in the other 5% (4). Therefore, the 95% CI is related to statistical significance at the $p = .05$ level, which means that the interval itself can be used to determine if an estimated change is statistically significant at the .05 level (6). Whereas the p value is often interpreted as being either statistically significant or not, the CI, by providing a range of values, allows the reader to interpret the implications of the results at either end (6,7). In addition, while p values have no units, CIs are presented in the units of the variable of interest, which helps readers to interpret the results. The CIs shift the interpretation from a qualitative judgment about the role of chance to a quantitative estimation of the biologic measure of effect (4,6,7).

Confidence intervals can be constructed for any desired level of confidence. There is nothing magical about the 95% that is traditionally used. If greater confidence is needed, then the intervals have to be wider. Consequently, 99% CIs are wider than 95%, and 90% CIs are narrower than 95%. Wider CIs are associated with greater confidence but less precision. This is the trade-off (4).

As an example, two hypothetical transcranial circle of Willis vascular ultrasound studies in patients with sickle cell disease describe mean peak systolic velocities of 200 cm/sec associated with 70% of vascular diameter stenosis and higher risk of stroke. Both articles reported the same standard deviation (SD) of 50 cm/sec. However, one study had 50 subjects while the other one had 500 subjects. At first glance, both studies appear to provide similar information. However, the narrower confidence intervals for the larger study reflect the greater precision, and indicate the value of the larger sample size. For a smaller sample:

$$95\% \, CI = 200 \pm 1.96\left(\frac{50}{\sqrt{50}}\right)$$

$$95\% \, CI = 200 \pm 14 = 186 - 214$$

For a larger sample:

$$95\% \, CI = 200 \pm 1.96\left(\frac{50}{\sqrt{500}}\right)$$

$$95\% \, CI = 200 \pm 4 = 196 - 204$$

In the smaller series, the 95% CI was 186 to 214 cm/sec while in the larger series the 95% CI was 196 to 204 cm/sec. Therefore, the larger series has a narrower 95% CI (4).

C. Type II Error

The familiar p value does not provide information as to the probability of a type II or beta error. A p value greater than .05 does not necessarily mean that there is no difference in the underlying population. The size of the sample studied may be too small to detect an important difference even if such a difference does exist. The ability of a study to detect an important difference, if that difference does in fact exist in the underlying population, is called the power of a study. Power analysis can be performed in advance of a research investigation to avoid type II error.

D. Power Analysis

Power analysis plays an important role in determining what an adequate sample size is, so that meaningful results can be obtained (8). Power analysis is the probability of observing an effect in a sample of patients if the specified effect size, or greater, is found in the population (3). Mathematically, power is defined as 1 minus beta $(1 - \beta)$, where β is the probability of having a type II error. Type II errors are commonly referred to as false negatives in a study population. The other type of error is type I or alpha (α), also known as false positives in a study population (7). For example, if β is set at 0.10, then the researchers acknowledge they are willing to accept a 10% chance of missing a correlation between abnormal computed tomography (CT) angiographic finding and the diagnosis of carotid artery disease. This represents a power of 1 minus 0.10, or 0.90, which represents a 90% probability of finding a correlation of this magnitude.

Ideally, the power should be 100% by setting β at 0. In addition, ideally α should also be 0. By accomplishing this, false-negative and false-positive results are eliminated, respectively. In practice, however, powers near 100% are rarely achievable, so, at best, a study should reduce the false negatives β and false positives α to a minimum (3,9). Achieving an acceptable reduction of false negatives and false positives requires a large subject sample size. Optimal power, α and β, settings are based on a balance between scientific rigorousness and the issues of feasibility and cost. For example, assuming an α error of 0.10, your sample size increases from 96 to 118 subjects per study arm (carotid and noncarotid artery disease arms) if you change your desired power from 85% to 90% (10). Studies with more complete reporting and better study design will often report the power of the study, for example, by stating that the study has 90% power to detect a difference in sensitivity of 10% between CT angiography and Doppler ultrasound in carotid artery disease.

III. What Is Bias?

The risk of an error from bias decreases as the rigorousness of the study design and analysis increases. Randomized controlled trials are considered the best design for minimizing the risk of bias because patients are randomly allocated. This random allocation allows for unbiased distribution of both known and unknown confounding variables between the study groups. In nonrandomized studies, appropriate study design and statistical analysis can only control for known or measurable bias.

Detection of and correction for bias, or systematic error, in research is a vexing challenge for both researchers and users of the medical literature alike. Maclure and Schneeweiss (11) have identified 10 different levels at which biases can distort the relationship between published study results and truth. Unfortunately, bias is common in published reports (12), and reports with identifiable biases often overestimate the accuracy of diagnostic tests (13). Careful surveillance for each of these individual bias phenomena is critical, but may be a challenge. Different study designs also are susceptible to different types of bias, as will be discussed below. Well-reported studies often include a section on limitations of the work, spelling out the potential sources of bias that the investigator acknowledges from a study as well as the likely direction of the bias and steps that may have been taken to overcome it. However, the final determination of whether a research study is sufficiently distorted by bias to be unusable is left to the discretion of the user of the imaging literature. The imaging practitioner must determine if results of a particular study are true, are relevant to a given clinical question, and are sufficient as a basis to change practice.

A common bias encountered in imaging research is that of *selection bias* (14). Because a research study cannot include all individuals in the world who have a particular clinical situation, research is conducted on samples. Selection bias can arise if the sample is not a true representation of the relevant underlying clinical population (Fig. 2.2). Numerous subtypes of selection bias have been identified, and it is a challenge to the researcher to avoid all of these biases when performing a study. One particularly severe form of selection bias occurs if the diagnostic test is applied to subjects with a spectrum of disease that differs from the clinically relevant group. The extreme form of this spectrum bias occurs when the diagnostic test is evaluated on subjects with severe disease and on normal controls. In an evaluation of the effect of bias on study results, Lijmer et al. (13) found the greatest overestimation of test accuracy with this type of spectrum bias.

A second frequently encountered bias in imaging literature is that of *observer bias* (15,16), also called test-review bias and diagnostic-review bias (17). Imaging tests are largely subjective. The radiologist interpreting an imaging study forms an impression based on the appearance of the image, not based on an objective number or measurement. This subjective impression can be biased by numerous factors including the radiologist's experience; the context of the interpretation (clinical vs. research setting); the information about the patient's history that is known by the radiologist; incentives that the radiologist may have, both monetary and otherwise, to produce a particular report; and the memory of a recent experience. But because of all these factors, it is critical that the interpreting physician be blinded to the outcome or gold standard when a diagnostic test or intervention is being assessed. Important distortions in research results have been found when observers are not blinded vs. blinded. For example, Schulz et al. (18) showed a 17% greater outcome improvement in studies with unblinded assessment of outcomes versus those with blinded assess-

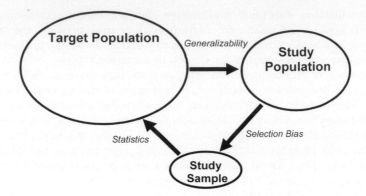

Figure 2.2. Population and sample. The target population represents the universe of subjects who are at risk for a particular disease or condition. In this example, all subjects with abdominal pain are at risk for appendicitis. The sample population is the group of eligible subjects available to the investigators. These may be at a single center, or group of centers. The sample is the group of subjects who are actually studied. Selection bias occurs when the sample is not truly representative of the study population. How closely the study population reflects the target population determines the generalizability of the research. Finally, statistics are used to determine what inference about the target population can be drawn from the sample data.

ment. To obtain objective scientific assessment of an imaging test, all readers should be blinded to other diagnostic tests and final diagnosis, and all patient-identifying marks on the test should be masked.

Bias can also be introduced by the *reference standard* used to confirm the final diagnosis. First, the interpretation of the reference standard must be made without knowledge of the test results. Reference standards, like the diagnostic tests themselves, may have a subjective component, and therefore may be affected by knowledge of the results of the diagnostic test. In addition, it is critical that all subjects undergo the same reference standard. The use of different reference standards (called differential reference standard bias) for subjects with different diagnostic test results may falsely elevate both sensitivity and specificity (13,16). Of course, sometimes it is not possible or ethical to perform the same reference standard procedure on all subjects. For example, in a recent meta-analysis of imaging for appendicitis, Terasawa et al. (19) found that all of the identified studies used a different reference standard for subjects with positive imaging (appendectomy and pathologic evaluation) than for those with negative imaging (clinical follow-up). It simply wouldn't be ethical to perform appendectomy on all subjects. Likely the sensitivity and specificity of imaging for appendicitis was overestimated as a result.

IV. What Are the Inherent Biases in Screening?

Investigations of screening tests are susceptible to an additional set of biases. Screening case-control trials are vulnerable to *screening selection bias*. For example, lung cancer case-control studies have been performed in

Japan where long-running tuberculosis control programs have been in place. This allowed for analysis of those who were screened to be matched with a database of matched unscreened controls to arrive at a relative risk of dying from lung cancer in screened and unscreened populations. Because screening is a choice in these studies, selection bias plays a prominent role. That is, people who present for elective screening tend to have better health habits (20). In assessing the exposure history of cases, the inclusion of the test on which the diagnosis is made, regardless of whether it is truly screen or symptom detected, can lead to an odds ratio greater than 1 even in the absence of benefit (21). Similarly, excluding the test on which the diagnosis is made may underestimate screening effectiveness. The magnitude of bias is further reflected in the disease preclinical phase; the longer the preclinical phase, the greater the magnitude of the bias.

Prospective nonrandomized screening trials perform an intervention on subjects, such as screening for lung cancer, and follow them for many years. These studies can give information of the stage distribution and survival of a screened population; however, these measures do not allow an accurate comparison to an unscreened group due to lead time, length time, and overdiagnosis bias (22) (Fig. 2.3). *Lead-time bias* results from the earlier detection of the disease, which leads to longer time from diagnosis and an apparent survival advantage but does not truly impact the date of death. *Length-time bias* relates to the virulence of tumors. More indolent tumors will be more likely to be detected by screening, whereas aggressive tumors

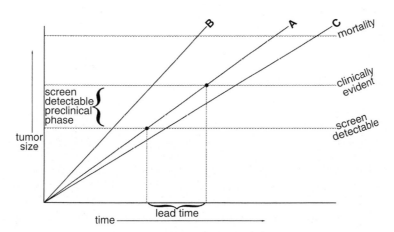

Figure 2.3. Screening biases. For this figure, cancers are assumed to grow at a continuous rate until they reach a size at which death of the subject occurs. At a small size, the cancers may be evident on screening, but not yet evident clinically. This is the preclinical screen detectable phase. Screening is potentially helpful if it detects cancer in this phase. After further growth, the cancer will be clinically evident. Even if the growth and outcome of the cancer is unaffected by screening, merely detecting the cancer earlier will increase apparent survival. This is the screening lead time. In addition, slower growing cancers (such as C) will exist in the preclinical screen detectable phase for longer than faster growing cancers (such as B). Therefore, screening is more likely to detect more indolent cancers, a phenomenon known as length bias.

are more likely to be detected by symptoms. This disproportionally assigns more indolent disease to the intervention group and results in the appearance of a benefit. *Overdiagnosis* is the most extreme form of length-time bias in which a disease is detected and "cured", but is so indolent it would never have caused symptoms during life. Thus, survival alone is not an appropriate measure of the effectiveness of screening (23).

For this reason a randomized controlled trial (RCT) with disease-specific mortality as an end point is the preferred methodology. Randomization should even out the selection process in both arms, eliminating the bias of case-control studies and allow direct comparison of groups that underwent the intervention and those that did not, to see if the intervention lowers deaths due to the target disease. The disadvantage of the RCT is that it takes many years and is expensive to perform. There are two biases that can occur in RCTs and are important to understand: *sticky diagnosis* and *slippery linkage* (24). Because the target disease is more likely to be detected in a screened population, it is more likely to be listed as a cause of death, even if not the true cause. As such, the diagnosis "sticks" and tends to underestimate the true value of the test. On the other hand, screening may set into motion a series of events in order to diagnose and treat the illness. If these procedures remotely lead to mortality, such as a myocardial infarction during surgery with death several months later, the linkage of the cause of death to the screening may no longer be obvious (slippery linkage). Because the death is not appropriately assigned to the target disease, the value of screening may be overestimated. For this reason, in addition to disease-specific mortality, all-cause mortality should also be evaluated in the context of screening trials (24). Ultimately, to show the effectiveness of screening, not only do more early-stage cancers need to be found in the screened group, but there must also be fewer late-stage cancers (stage shift) (22).

V. Qualitative Literature Summary

The potential for error and bias makes the process of critically assessing a journal article complex and challenging, and no investigation is perfect. Producing an overall summation of the quality of a research report is difficult. However, there are grading schemes that provide a useful estimation of the value of a research report for guiding clinical practice. The method used in this book is derived from that of Kent et al. (25) and is shown in Table 2.1. Use of such a grading scheme is by nature an oversimplification. However, such simple guidelines can provide a useful quick overview of the quality of a research report.

Conclusion

Critical analysis of a research publication can be a challenging task. The reader must consider the potential for type I and type II random error, as well as systematic error introduced by biases including selection bias, observer bias, and reference standard bias. Screening includes an additional set of challenges related to lead time, length bias, and overdiagnosis.

Table 2.1. Evidence classification for evaluation of a study

Level I: strong evidence
Studies with broad generalizability to most patients suspected of having the disease of concern: a prospective, blinded comparison of a diagnostic test result with a well-defined final diagnosis in an unbiased sample when assessing diagnostic accuracy or blinded randomized control trials or when assessing therapeutic impact or patient outcomes. Well-designed meta-analysis based on level I or II studies.

Level II: moderate evidence
Prospective or retrospective studies with narrower spectrum of generalizability, with only a few flaws that are well described so that their impact can be assessed, but still requiring a blinded study of diagnostic accuracy on an unbiased sample. This includes well-designed cohort or case-control studies, and randomized trials for therapeutic effects or patient outcomes.

Level III: limited evidence
Diagnostic accuracy studies with several flaws in research methods, small sample sizes, or incomplete reporting, or nonrandomized comparisons for therapeutic impact or patient outcomes.

Level IV: insufficient evidence
Studies with multiple flaws in research methods, case series, descriptive studies, or expert opinions without substantiating data.

References

1. Moher D, Schulz K, Altman D. JAMA 2001;285:1987–1991.
2. Bossuyt PM, Reitsma J, Bruns D, et al. Acad Radiol 2003;10:664–669.
3. Hulley SB, Cummings SR. Designing Clinical Research. Baltimore: Williams and Wilkins, 1998.
4. Medina L, Zurakowski D. Radiology 2003;226:297–301.
5. Gallagher E. Acad Emerg Med 1999;6:1084–1087.
6. Lang T, Secic M. How to Report Statistics in Medicine. Philadelphia: American College of Physicians, 1997.
7. Gardener M, Altman D. Br Med J 1986:746–750.
8. Medina L, Aguirre E, Zurakowski D. Neuroimag Clin North Am 2003; 13:157–165.
9. Medina L. AJNR 1999;20:1584–1596.
10. Donner A. Stat Med 1984;3:199–214.
11. Maclure M, Schneeweiss S. Epidemiology 2001;12:114–122.
12. Reid MC, Lachs MS, Feinstein AR. JAMA 1995;274:645–651.
13. Lijmer JG, Mol BW, Heisterkamp S, et al. JAMA 1999;282:1061–1066.
14. Blackmore C. Acad Radiol 2004;11:134–140.
15. Ransohoff DF, Feinstein AR. N Engl J Med 1978;299:926–930.
16. Black WC. AJR 1990;154:17–22.
17. Begg CB, McNeil BJ. Radiology 1988;167:565–569.
18. Schulz K, Chalmers I, Hayes R, Altman D. JAMA 1995;273:408–412.
19. Terasawa T, Blackmore C, Dent S, Kohlwes R. Ann Intern Med 2004;141:537–546.
20. Marcus P. Lung Cancer 2003;41:37–39.
21. Hosek R, Flanders W, Sasco A. Am J Epidemiol 1996;143:193–201.
22. Patz E, Goodman P, Bepler G. N Engl J Med 2000;343:1627–1633.
23. Black WC, Welch HG. AJR 1997;168:3–11.
24. Black W, Haggstrom D, Welch H. J Natl Cancer Inst 2002;94.
25. Kent DL, Haynor DR, Longstreth WT, Jr, Larson EB. Ann Intern Med 1994;120: 856–871.

3

Breast Imaging

Laurie L. Fajardo, Wendie A. Berg, and Robert A. Smith

Key Points

Mammography

- Prospective randomized controlled trials have demonstrated reduced breast cancer mortality of approximately 30% associated with mammography screening (strong evidence).

- Evaluations of mammography screening in community settings have shown greater mortality reductions associated with participating in screening (moderate evidence).
- Women aged 40 to 54 should be screened at intervals of 12 to 18 months in order to achieve similar mortality reductions compared with women 55 years of age and older due to faster tumor growth in younger women (moderate evidence).

Ultrasound

- Data from single center studies of screening ultrasound suggest that it has a detection benefit as a supplement to screening mammography in patients with dense (at least 50% of the breast is not fatty) breast parenchyma (moderate evidence).
- Reports from single-institution studies found a high percentage (91%) of breast cancers identified on supplemental screening sonography are stage I invasive cancers. Detecting this subset of breast cancers is most likely to reduce breast cancer mortality (moderate evidence).
- In patients with dense breast parenchyma, mammography and sonography appear complementary in that ductal carcinoma in situ (DCIS) is better depicted by mammography and small, <1 cm, invasive breast cancers are better detected sonographically (moderate evidence).
- Women with dense breast parenchyma on mammography, contemplating a supplemental sonographic screening examination, should consider the risk of a false-positive sonogram, possibly resulting in the recommendation for a breast biopsy (moderate evidence).
- Sonography is appropriate in the evaluation of palpable breast masses (moderate evidence).
- Sonography is appropriate in the evaluation of mammographically circumscribed, obscured, or indistinctly marginated masses and focal asymmetries (moderate evidence).
- The combination of mammography and sonography depicts 96% to 97% of palpable breast cancer and 92% of nonpalpable breast cancer (moderate evidence).
- Sonography can help identify the invasive component of mixed invasive and intraductal carcinoma and guide optimal percutaneous biopsy (limited evidence).
- Sonography is a useful supplement to mammography in depicting the extent of invasive carcinoma in dense breasts (moderate evidence).
- Sonography is useful in the evaluation of the patient with nipple discharge (limited evidence).

Biopsy

- Percutaneous image-guided breast biopsy is not indicated for nonpalpable lesions classified as BIRADS 3. For these lesions, short-term interval follow-up, generally at 6-month intervals, is recommended (strong evidence).
- For BIRADS 4 and 5 lesions, image-guided percutaneous biopsy is cost-effective as the initial strategy for diagnosing nonpalpable breast lesions (strong evidence).

Pathophysiology and Epidemiology

Breast cancer takes a tremendous toll in the United States. For 2004, the American Cancer Society predicted that 217,440 new cases of breast cancer would be diagnosed, and 40,580 individuals would die from the disease (1). Mammographic screening remains controversial, as reflected in greatly varying national policies. The specificity and positive predictive value of mammography are limited because of overlap in the appearance of benign and malignant breast lesions (2–4). However, until research uncovers a way to better cure or prevent breast cancer, early detection is viewed as the best hope for reducing the burden of this disease.

The risk of breast cancer increases with increasing age. A family history of breast cancer confers a variable degree of increased risk. The Gail (5–8), Claus (9), and other models have been developed to calculate a woman's risk of breast cancer primarily as a function of age and family history. The risk of developing breast cancer nearly doubles with a family history of breast cancer in a first-degree relative (10). Women with a personal history of breast cancer, and those with prior biopsies showing atypical ductal hyperplasia (ADH) or atypical lobular hyperplasia (ALH), are at a four- to fivefold increased risk of breast cancer (10). Women with prior lobular carcinoma in situ (LCIS) are also at high risk of breast cancer, with rates of eight- to 10-fold those of women without such risk (11). Such high-risk women are candidates for chemoprevention with agents such as tamoxifen. The National Surgical Adjuvant Breast and Bowel Project (NSABP) P-1 chemoprevention trial demonstrated that tamoxifen lowered the rate of invasive breast cancer by 49% in women at high risk (12).

Women with a history of prior axillary, chest, or mediastinal irradiation, usually for Hodgkin's disease, are another group at high risk of developing breast cancer. The relative risk of breast cancer is approximately sevenfold in women irradiated at 20 to 30 years of age and as high as 56-fold if exposure was after puberty and before age 20 (13–15).

The perception of cancer on mammography requires a difference in density compared to surrounding tissue, architectural distortion, or presence of microcalcifications. There are four grades of breast density: fatty (<25% dense), minimal scattered fibroglandular densities (25% to 50% dense), heterogeneously dense (51% to 75% dense), and extremely dense (>75% dense) (16). Identification of a mass against a background of equally dense tissue is problematic. In heterogeneously dense and extremely dense breasts, the sensitivity of mammography in several series is under 50% (17–19). Methods to supplement mammography, such as screening breast ultrasound, are being sought in women with dense breasts (>50% dense), and especially those women with higher rates of breast cancer (e.g., high-risk women) with dense breasts.

Ultrasound uses sound waves to penetrate tissue. Differences in the time to reflect the echo back to the transducer are used to create the image. With current high-frequency linear array transducers with a center frequency of 10 to 12 MHz, detailed images are produced at tissue depths of 0.2 to 4 cm, with lateral resolution (in effect, slice thickness) of 1 mm or less. The performance of ultrasound in dense breast tissue is equivalent (20) or superior to its performance in fatty breasts.

Biopsy remains the definitive method of confirming the diagnosis of breast cancer, and physicians perform millions of breast biopsies each year. Selecting the most appropriate method of biopsy for each patient has distinct health and economic benefits. Approximately 75% (range 65–86%) of breast abnormalities detected at mammography and referred for biopsy ultimately prove benign histopathologically (2,21–26). The fact that most breast biopsies are benign necessitates that the method of diagnosis be minimally invasive, have the best possible cosmetic outcome, and have high accuracy.

Overall Cost to Society

The cost of breast cancer to society can never fully be estimated because there are so many dimensions for which measurement in economic and social terms is indefinable. Nonetheless, a common approach to measuring the economic dimension of disease burden is cost-of-illness (COI) methodology, which encompasses direct costs (costs associated with procedures, therapy, and care), morbidity costs (work-related costs associated with disability and absenteeism), and mortality costs (lost income, including the value of household work, due to premature death) (27). Based on previous estimates of the proportion of the direct costs of cancer attributable to breast cancer (27) and current estimates from the National Heart Lung and Blood Institute for the direct costs of all neoplasms (28), in 2004 direct costs of breast cancer were approximately $9.85 billion. This estimate does not include the costs of oral medications, such as tamoxifen, which in 1995 were estimated to be $400 million per year (27), or the annual cost of screening and diagnostic evaluations of women. Since there are no current indirect cost estimates by cancer site, if we assume that indirect costs as a percentage of COI in 2004 are the same for all cancers, then in 2004 the indirect cost of breast cancer was $26.94 billion, for a total COI of approximately $37 billion. The COI for all cancers in 2004 was estimated to be $198.8 billion (28).

Goals

The next section of this chapter is a summary of the evidence supporting the use of mammography to screen for breast cancer. The following section is a compilation of the evidence regarding the use of ultrasound in imaging the breast. Available evidence on the use of ultrasound in a variety of clinical scenarios, including screening, is analyzed and is used to present criteria that physicians can apply to individual patients. The final section is a compilation of the evidence regarding the selection of the method of breast biopsy for patients who have a suspicious nonpalpable breast lesion that should be biopsied. The evidence analyzed addresses nonpalpable lesions only and is used to present criteria that physicians can apply to these individual patients. By incorporating the evidence into clinical decision making, practitioners can develop personal or organizational guidelines that will assist in choosing the biopsy method that is best for each patient.

Methodology

Medline searches were performed using PubMed (National Library of Medicine, Bethesda, Maryland) for original research publications discussing the diagnostic performance and effectiveness of mammography, breast ultrasound, and imaging-guided percutaneous biopsy of nonpalpable breast lesions. The searches covered the years 1980 to 2004 (1997 to 2004 for mammography, 1980 to 2004 for breast ultrasound, and 1980 to 2002 for breast biopsy) and were limited to human studies and the English-language literature. The search strategies employed different combinations of the following terms: (1) *breast biopsy,* (2) *stereotactic* OR *ultrasound* OR *imaging guided,* (3) *nonpalpable breast lesion,* (4) *mammography,* (5) *ultrasound* OR *sonography* AND *breast,* (6) *breast screening,* (7) *breast screening guidelines,* (8) *harms and anxiety,* and (9) *cost-effectiveness.* Additional articles were identified by reviewing the reference lists of relevant papers and by including recently published studies not yet indexed in Medline. The authors performed an initial review of the titles and abstracts of the identified articles followed by review of the full text in articles that were relevant.

I. How Effective Is Mammographic Screening?

Summary of Evidence: The fundamental goal of mammographic screening is to reduce the incidence rate of advanced breast cancer by detecting the disease early in its natural history (29). There is strong evidence for the benefit of mammography from a series of prospective randomized controlled trials (RCT) and meta-analyses (30–34) and moderate evidence of benefit from institutional-based case series studies (35) and recent evaluations of population-based service screening (36,37). Results from individual trials showed significant mortality reductions ranging from 22% to 32% (38). A smaller level of benefit is observed in meta-analysis results that combine all trials, due to variability in end results (38,39). Results from service screening with modern mammography have shown greater mortality reductions (40–50%) among women who participate in regular screening (37,40).

Supporting Evidence: There have been eight prospective RCTs of breast cancer screening. As can be seen in Table 3.1, the first of these studies, the Health Insurance Plan (HIP) of Greater New York Study, was initiated in the early 1960s, while the most recent RCTs were initiated in Canada in 1980 (31,34,41–50). Each RCT followed a somewhat different protocol, and the outcome in each has been influenced by a number of design and protocol factors that have important implications for the interpretation of study end results. These factors include the study methodology, the clinical protocol, adherence to the randomization assignment (compliance and contamination), and the number of screening rounds before an invitation was extended to the control group. Other factors that likely influenced end results include the quality of the screening process, thresholds for diagnosis, and follow-up mechanisms for women with an abnormality. Individual RCT results and meta-analysis results should be interpreted in the context of study methodology to demonstrate efficacy rather than a measure of the potential effectiveness of mammography, since the classic intention-to-treat analysis compares breast cancer mortality in a group invited to screening with breast cancer mortality in a group receiving usual care rather than a screened vs. unscreened group. Moreover, variability in RCT outcomes is consistent with the performance of each study's success at reducing the risk of being diagnosed with an advanced breast cancer compared with the control group. Specifically, those RCTs that significantly reduced the risk of being diagnosed with a node-positive breast cancer showed similar reductions in the risk of breast cancer death in the group invited to screening (38,51).

Table 3.1. The randomized controlled trials of breast cancer screening

Study (duration)	Screening protocol Invited vs. control group	Frequency No. rounds	Age	Subgroup	Invited	Control	Years of follow-up	RR (95% CI)
HIP Study (1963–69)	2 V MM + CBE[1] vs. usual care	Annually 4 rounds	40–64	40–49	14,432	14,701	18	0.77 (0.52–1.13)
				50–64	16,568	16,299		0.79 (0.58–1.08)
Edinburgh (1979–88)	1 or 2 V MM + Initial CBE vs. usual care	24 months 4 rounds	45–64	45–49	11,755*	10,641*	13	0.75* (0.48–1.18)
				50–64	11,245	12,359		0.79 (0.60–1.02)
Two County (1977–85)	1 V MM vs. usual care	40–49: 24 months 50–69: 33 months 4 rounds	40–74	40–49	9,650	5,009	20	0.93 (0.63–1.37)
				50–74	28,939	13,551		0.65 (0.55–0.77)
Malmo (1976–90)	1 or 2 V MM vs. usual care	18–24 months 5 rounds	45–69	45–49	13,528†	12,242†	16	0.70† (0.49–1.00)
				50–69	17,134	17,165		0.83 (0.66–1.04)
Stockholm (1981–85)	1 V MM vs. usual care	28 months 2 rounds	40–64	40–49	14,185	7,985	15	1.52 (0.8–2.88)
				50–64	25,815	12,015		0.70 (0.46–1.07)
Gothenburg (1982–88)	1 or 2 V MM vs. usual care	18 months 5 rounds	39–59	39–49	11,724	14,217	18	0.65‡ (0.40–1.05)
					50–59	9,276	16,394	0.91 (0.61–1.36)
CNBSS-1 (1980–87)	2 V MM + CBE + BSE vs. Initial CBE	12 months 4–5 rounds	40–49	40–49	25,214	25,216	12	0.97 (0.78–1.33)
CNBSS-2 (1980–87)	2 V MM + CBE + BSE vs. CBE + BSE	12 months 4–5 rounds	50–59	50–59	19,711	19,694	12	1.02 (0.74–1.27)

[1] V MM (one-view mammography of each breast; 2 V MM (two-view mammography of each breast); CBE (clinical breast examination); BSE (breast self-examination); CNBSS = Canadian National Breast Screening Study.

* The Edinburgh trial included three separate groups of women 45–49 at entry: the first had 5,949 women in the invited group and 5,818 in the control group (with 14 years' follow-up); the next had 2,545 in the invited group and 2,482 in the control group (12 years' follow-up); and the third had 3,261 in the invited group and 2,341 in the control group (10 years' follow-up) (6). Only the first group's results had been reported previously.

† The Malmo trial included two groups of women aged 45–49 at entry: one group (MMST-I) received first-round screening in 1977–8 and had 3,954 women in the invited group, 4,030 women in the control group; the second group (MMST-II) received first-round screening from 1978–90 and had 9,574 women in the invited group, 8,212 women in the control group (2). Only the first group's results had been reported previously.

Over the years, there have been numerous studies reporting the results from the individual RCTs and meta-analyses, although screening policy in the United States began to take shape based on initial findings from the HIP study. The trials now have a substantial amount of follow-up time ranging from 12 to 20 years. In a recent overview of the RCTs, a meta-analysis of the most current data showed an overall relative risk of breast cancer death associated with an invitation to screening of 0.80 [95% confidence interval (CI), 0.75–0.86], with corresponding relative risks of 0.85 (95% CI, 0.73–0.98) for women randomized to an invitation between ages 39 and 49, and 0.78 (95% CI, 0.70–0.85) for women aged 50 years and older at the time of randomization (38). These estimates are lower than some of the individual RCTs, due to RCT variability, and considerably lower than mortality reductions observed in service screening, in large part due to measuring the benefit of an invitation to screening rather than actually being screened.

The breast cancer RCT data have recently undergone several independent reevaluations for the purpose of updating screening guidelines (33,39,52), and several evidence-based reviews (42,53–56). A recent review by the Cochrane Collaboration was sharply critical of the RCTs that had shown a benefit from mammographic screening, and concluded that there was insufficient evidence to recommend screening with mammography (53). Representatives from the RCTs and others responded to these criticisms and showed them to be either incorrect, inconsequential, or, if true, previously and satisfactorily addressed by the authors in original publications (34,50,55,57–61). Although the RCTs of breast cancer screening had some shortcomings, there is widespread agreement that they have provided solid and valid evidence regarding the efficacy of early breast cancer detection with mammography (42).

As noted above, while the breast cancer screening RCTs demonstrated the efficacy of screening, they provide a less clear measure of the effectiveness of screening. There has been increasing interest in evaluating the impact of screening in the community setting, also referred to as *service screening*, and to measure the effectiveness of screening among women who participate in screening. The evaluation of screening outside of research studies poses a set of unique methodologic challenges, including identifying when screening is introduced, the duration of time required to invite the eligible population to screening, the rate of screening uptake in a population, and finally the importance of distinguishing between screened and unscreened cohorts in mortality analysis since deaths resulting from cases diagnosed before the introduction of screening may predominate for 10 years or longer (62). In three recent reports evaluating Swedish data, investigators were able to classify breast cancer cases before and after the introduction to screening on the basis of exposure to screening in order to measure the benefit of screening among those women who attended screening (37,40,62). In a recent report that expanded an earlier analysis of two Swedish counties to seven counties in the Uppsala region, Duffy and colleagues (62) compared breast cancer mortality in the prescreening and postscreening periods among women aged 40 to 69 in six counties, and 50 to 69 in one county. Overall, they observed a 44% mortality reduction in women who actually underwent screening, and a 39% reduction in overall breast cancer mortality after adjustment for selection bias, associated with the policy of offering screening to the population. Greater breast cancer mortality reductions were observed in those counties that had offered screening longer than 10 years (–32%) compared with counties that had offered screening less than 10 years (−18%). Finally, in a separate analysis the investigators examined the effectiveness of mammography based on age at diagnosis, comparing mortality reductions in women diagnosed between ages 40 and 49 with women diagnosed after age 50 (37). They observed a 48% mortality reduction in women ages 40 to 49 at diagnosis based on an 18-month screening interval, and a 44% mortality reduction in women aged 50 to 69 at diagnosis based on a 24-month screening interval. These data demonstrate that organized screening with high rates of attendance in a setting that achieves a high degree of programmatic quality assurance can achieve breast cancer mortality reductions equal to or greater than observed in the randomized trials.

II. Who Should Undergo Screening?

Summary of Evidence: It is generally accepted that women should begin regular screening mammography in their 40s, and continue regular screening as long as they are in good health (39,52).

Supporting Evidence: There is widespread acceptance of the value of regular breast cancer screening with mammography as the single most important public health strategy to reduce mortality from breast cancer. For many years, breast cancer screening in women aged 40 to 49 was controversial based on the absence of a statistically significant mortality breast cancer reduction compared with women aged 50+ (63–66). Further, the benefit that was evident appeared much later in younger women, leading some to argue that the appearance of benefit was attributable to cases diagnosed after age 50 in the women who were randomized in their 40s (67). This argument persisted despite contrary evidence (40), and the eventual observation of statistically significant mortality reductions for this age group in two individual trials (Malmo II and Gothenburg) (44,47) and favorable meta-analysis results (32). Further, Tabar and colleagues (68,69) showed that the 24- to 33-month interval between screening exams in the Two County Study had been sufficient to reduce the incidence rate of advanced ductal grade 3 cancers in women aged 50+, but not in women aged 40 to 49. The appearance of a delayed benefit was due to the similar performance of mammography in younger and older women to reduce breast cancer deaths among women diagnosed with less aggressive tumors. These and other findings showing higher interval cancer rates in younger women (70) led the Swedish Board of Health and Welfare to set shorter screening intervals for younger women (18 months) compared with older women (24 months). As noted above, when the screening interval is tailored to women's age, similar benefits are evident. Recent analysis of service screening data also has shown similar mortality reductions in women aged 40 to 49 at diagnosis compared with women aged 50 years and older (37).

Setting an age to begin and end screening is admittedly arbitrary, although the HIP investigators were led to include women in their 40s because they observed that more than a third of all premature mortality associated with breast cancer deaths was attributable to women diagnosed between age 35 and 50 (30). This is less of an issue for guidelines today than the fact that the evidence base from RCTs is for average-risk women aged 39 and older. The American Cancer Society recommends that women at higher risk for diagnosis of breast cancer at a younger age due to family history could begin screening as early as age 25 depending on their risk profile, and also consider additional imaging modalities (52). An age at which screening could be stopped, for instance age 70, based on risk or potential benefit also has been proposed (71), although several observations argue against setting an specific age at which all women would no longer be invited to screening. First, risk of developing and dying of breast cancer is significant in older women. The age-specific incidence of breast cancer rises until age 70 to 74, and then declines somewhat, but not below the average risk of women aged 60 to 64 (72,73). Approximately 45% of new breast cancer cases and deaths occur in women aged 65 and older (1,46). Second, although tumor growth rate is slower (31), and breast cancers tend to be less aggressive in older women (31,74), it is important to emphasize that breast cancer is a potentially lethal disease at any age, and these tumor characteristics combined with declining breast density with age mean screening is somewhat less of a challenge in older women compared with younger women. Third, although only one RCT included women over age 69, observational studies have concluded that the effectiveness and performance of mammography in women over age 70 is equivalent to, if not better than, the screening of women under age 70 (75,76). Finally, although rates of significant comorbidity increase with increasing age (77) and longevity declines, the average 70-year-old woman is in good health with an *average* life expectancy to age 85 (78). Thus, a significant percentage of the population of women age 70 and older have the potential to still benefit from early breast cancer detection.

The American Cancer Society (ACS) recommends that chronological age alone should not be the reason for the cessation of regular screening, but rather screening decisions in older women should be individualized by considering the potential benefits and risks of mammography in the context of current health status and estimated life expectancy (52). If a woman has severe functional limitations or comorbidities, with estimated life expectancy of less than 3 to 5 years, it may be appropriate to consider cessation of screening. However, if an older woman is in reasonably good health and would tolerate treatment, she should continue to be screened with mammography.

III. How Frequently Should Women Be Screened?

Summary of Evidence: Current guidelines for breast cancer screening recommend breast cancer screening intervals of either 1 year (52) or 1 to 2 years (39). Current evidence suggests that adherence to annual screening has greater importance in premenopausal women compared with postmenopausal women.

Supporting Evidence: Current recommendations for the interval between screens are influenced by different approaches to evidence-based medicine. Insofar as there has not been a trial directly comparing annual vs. biannual screening in women of different age groups, some guideline groups recommend intervals of 1 to 2 years based on favorable results from trials that screened at intervals of 12 or 24 months. Other guideline groups have drawn inferential guidance from the RCTs, including the proportional incidence of interval cancers in the period after a normal screening, and estimates of the duration of the detectable preclinical phase, or *sojourn time*, to define screening intervals. Tabar and colleagues (31) used data from the Swedish Two County study and estimated the mean sojourn time for women by age as follows: 40 to 49, 2.4 years; 50 to 59, 3.7 years; 60 to 69, 4.2 years; and 70 to 79, 4 years. Since the average sojourn time properly should define the upper boundary of the screening interval, it becomes clear that annual screening is more important for younger women. Data from two trials (44,47) and inferential evidence used to estimate sojourn time (29,79) have provided persuasive evidence that younger women likely will benefit more from annual screening compared with screening at 2-year intervals. The evidence review accompanying the most current U.S. Preventive Services Task Force reached a similar conclusion (33). Recent data from the National Cancer Institute's (NCI) Breast Cancer Screening Consortium also concluded that women under age 50 derive greater benefit from annual screening compared with biannual screening, as measured by lower rates of detection of advanced disease (80). White and colleagues (80) concluded that annual screening offered no measurable advantage to women over age 77, but other studies support an advantage with shorter screening intervals for postmenopausal women. Estimating tumor characteristics associated with screening intervals of 24, 12, and 6 months, Michaelson et al. (81) showed that shorter screening intervals were associated with greater reductions in the proportion of cases diagnosed with distant metastases. Similar findings were reported by Hunt et al. (82) comparing tumor outcomes among women aged 40+ undergoing screening at intervals of 10 to 14 months vs. 22 to 26 months.

IV. How Cost-Effective Is Mammographic Screening?

Summary of Evidence: Mammography screening in women aged 40 to 79 years of age has been shown to meet conventional criteria for cost-effectiveness (55). The marginal cost per year of live saved (MCYLS) varies with age, with greater MCYLS in age groups between ages 40 and 79 with lower incidence or lower longevity.

Supporting Evidence: Cost-effectiveness studies in screening are focused on the net cost of achieving a particular health-related outcome, typically years of life gained expressed as the MCYLS, or the cost of a death avoided. Costs may be expressed in monetary terms, or in terms of the number of women needed to screen once or over some number of years, or number of screening exams conducted, to save one life. Although most cost-effectiveness analyses have concluded that screening for breast cancer is cost-effective, results have been highly variable overall and within age-specific subgroups due to differences in the underlying methodology (83–87), different assumptions about costs, amount and timing of benefits from screening, whether costs and benefits are discounted against future value, and whether or not benefits are quality adjusted. Even though there have been formal efforts to create some common guidelines for conducting cost-effectiveness analysis (88), the current literature estimating MCYLS shares little in common with respect to methodology, model inputs, and end results beyond the finding that screening is somewhat less cost-effective in women under age 50 and older than age 70 compared with women aged 50 to 69. There also has been variability in estimates of the number needed to screen to save one life, but here the explanation for wide differences in estimates has been due to the manner in which RCT data have been applied to estimate the fraction. It has been common to confuse the number invited to screening with the number of women actually screened, and to confuse the period of time women underwent screening with the tumor follow-up period, which usually is considerably longer. For example, a recent evidence review concluded that with 14 years of observation, the number needed to screen to save one life was 1224.5. However, when the number needed to screen is calculated on the basis of women actually attending screening, and the duration of the screening period, Tabar and colleagues (89) estimated that the number of women needed to screen for 7 years to save one life over 20 years is 465 (95% CI, 324–819). The number of mammographic examinations needed to save one life was 1499 (95% CI, 1046–2642). Put another way, on average 465 women needed just over three rounds of screening to prevent one death from breast cancer. With annual screening over a longer duration, say 10 years, the number needed to screen to save one life would be even lower.

V. How Should Ultrasound Be Applied To Breast Cancer Screening?

Summary of Evidence: Moderate evidence exists to support sonographic screening for breast cancer, though its efficacy is incompletely demonstrated by existing single-center studies (18,20,90–93). The studies to date have been limited to women with mammographic or clinical abnormalities (90), negative mammography and clinical examination (92,93), a combination of the two (20,91), or women presenting for screening (18,94). The results of mammography were known to the individual performing the sonogram in every case (not blinded). This creates potential bias in that areas of vague asymmetry may be unintentionally targeted sonographically, or there may be a tendency to dismiss otherwise subtle mammographic findings as negative.

Women with nonfatty breast parenchyma and average risk for breast cancer comprised the study populations with the exception of the Taiwan study of first-degree relatives of women with breast cancer invited to screening (94). Studies have focused on the application of ultrasound (US) as an adjunct or supplemental test to screening mammography. Supplemental screening with sonography (or magnetic resonance imaging), after mammography, increases the rate of early detection of breast cancer in women with dense breast parenchyma. The degree to which this additional testing adversely affects women is being studied (95). Whether or not additional detection of breast cancer by supplemental sonographic screening alters the outcome of the disease has not been established directly. Advocates hypothesize that surrogate end points, such as tumor size and presence of metastases to local lymph nodes, will inform future discussions and guidelines. Such end points have been shown to closely parallel survival outcomes (96).

Supporting Evidence: Across six series of average risk women, totaling 42,838 exams, 150 (0.35%) additional cancers have been identified only on sonography in 126 women (18,20,90–93) (Table 3.2). Of the 150 cancers seen

Table 3.2. Breast cancers detected by sonography and mammography

| Study | No. of examinations | No. of cancers | No. of cancers detected | | Ultrasound-induced biopsy | |
			Mammography	Ultrasound	Number of biopsies	Number of cancers (%)
Gordon and Goldenberg (90)	12,706	n/a	n/a	44	279	44 (16)
Buchberger et al. (91)	8,970	182	142	160	405	40 (10)
Kaplan (92)	1,862	n/a	n/a	6	57	6 (11)
Kolb et al. (18) (all women)	13,547	246[a]	191	110	358	37 (10)
Crystal et al. (93)	1,517	n/a	n/a	7	38	7 (18)
LeConte et al. (20)	4,236	50	34	44	n/a	n/a
Overall	42,838	478	367 (76.8%)	371, with 314/478 (65.7%) where mammography also reported	1,137	134 (12)

n/a, not available, not reported [Gordon and Goldenberg (90)], or not applicable as patients selected because of negative mammogram [Kaplan et al. (92), Crystal et al. (93)].
[a] Includes four invasive cancers detected only on clinical breast examination. In 5826 examinations in women <50 years of age, 42 cancers were identified including 21 seen on mammography and 33 on ultrasound.

only on sonography, 141 (94%) were invasive and nine (6%) ductal carcinoma in situ (DCIS) (Table 3.3). Of the 141 invasive cancers, 99 (70%) were 1 cm or smaller. The detection benefit of supplemental sonography increased with increasing grades of breast density. Indeed, of the 126 women with sonographically detected cancers, 114 (90.5%) had either heterogeneously dense or extremely dense parenchyma. When results of mammography were also reported across 26,753 examinations (Table 3.3), another 56 cancers were seen only mammographically, of which 42 (75%)

Table 3.3. Histopathology of breast cancer seen only on ultrasound[a]

| Study | No. of cancers | Invasive | | | DCIS | Size (range), mm |
		Total	Ductal	Lobular		
Gordon and Goldenberg (90)	44	44[b]	n/a[a]	n/a	0	Mean 11, median 10 (4–25)
Buchberger et al. (91)	40	35	26	9	5	Mean 9.1 (4–20)
Kaplan (92)	6	5	3	2	1	Mean 9 (6–14) —US size
Kolb et al. (18)	37	36[b]	n/a	n/a	1	Mean 9.9
Crystal et al. (93)	7	7	6	1	0	Median 10 (4–12)
Leconte et al. (20)	16	14	9	5	2	Mean 11, median 9 (2–30)
Overall	150	141 (94%)	44 (29%)	17 (11%)	9 (6%)	

n/a = not available.
[a] Women had both whole breast ultrasound and mammography.
[b] Cancers are listed only as invasive with no further details available; 26 of 37 cancers were 1 cm or smaller with range not available.

were DCIS and 14 (25%) invasive. Women at higher risk of breast cancer were two- to threefold more likely to have a cancer seen only sonographically. Overall sensitivity of US was slightly lower than mammography, at 66% compared to 77% where both exams were performed.

Biopsy of benign lesions seen only sonographically and induced short interval follow-up are the risks of undergoing screening ultrasound. Across the five series where specifics are detailed (Table 3.2), after 38,602 screening sonograms, 1137 (2.9%) resulted in biopsy and 134 (11.8%) biopsies showed malignancy. In the four series with details (18,90,92,93), short interval follow-up was recommended in another 6.6% of women. It should be noted that in all but one series (18), only a single prevalence screen was performed; these rates of false positives are likely higher than would be seen on annual incidence screens.

A prospective multicenter trial funded by the Avon Foundation and the NCI, Screening Breast Ultrasound in High-Risk Women, opened April 19, 2004, through the American College of Radiology Imaging Network (ACRIN) (95). Importantly, sonography will be performed blinded to the results of mammography. Tumor size, grade, and nodal status will be determined.

Another point of controversy in sonographic screening is generalizability across investigators. For a sonogram to depict a cancer, the sonographer must perceive it as an abnormality while scanning. No amount of subsequent review of images will correct for lack of real-time detection. Optimal technique requires appropriate real-time adjustments of pressure, angle of insonation, focal zones, dynamic range, time-gain compensation, and depth. Methods to automate scanning may facilitate standardization of technique and documentation. Consistent interpretation is another area of concern as with any imaging technique (97). To assure high standards of performance in both detection and interpretation, investigator qualification tasks have been developed for ACRIN Protocol 6666, including a phantom lesion detection task, and interpretive skills tests for proven sonographic and mammographic lesions. Materials to complete these tasks are available to interested individuals through ACRIN (www.acrin.org).

In the screening series (Table 3.2) as above, mammography showed better overall performance than ultrasound, with invasive cancer overrepresented among cancers seen only sonographically and DCIS overrepresented among cancers seen only mammographically (Table 3.3). Among invasive cancers, 17 (28%) of the 61 seen only sonographically were invasive lobular type, which is often especially subtle mammographically. Where detailed, supplemental US the greatest detection benefit in dense parenchyma (19,98). Ductal carcinoma in situ is most often manifest mammographically as microcalcifications (99) and is therefore problematic for US. In the reported US series, 62% of DCIS was detected sonographically, compared to 78% for mammography.

VI. How Accurate Is Ultrasound in Evaluating Palpable Breast Masses?

Summary of Evidence: Moderate evidence supports the use of US in addition to mammography in the evaluation of women with palpable masses or thickening.

Supporting Evidence: In addition to its potential use in screening, US can also be used to evaluate palpable breast masses. Ultrasound is the initial test of choice in evaluating a lump in a young woman (under 30 years old) (100). The most common cause of a palpable mass in a woman under age 30 is a fibroadenoma (101). A palpable, circumscribed, oval mass with no posterior features or minimal posterior enhancement is most likely a fibroadenoma. If the mass has clinically been known to the patient and stable for a period of months, then follow-up is a reasonable alternative to biopsy. Since 15% of fibroadenomas are multiple, bilateral whole breast US is reasonable as part of the initial evaluation. Many women prefer excision of a palpable lump, and direct excision of a probable fibroadenoma is reasonable in a young woman. The finding of a sonographically suspicious mass, or a clinically suspicious mass without a sonographic correlate, should prompt bilateral mammographic evaluation to better define the extent of malignancy if any. At age 30 and over, breast cancer is increasingly common, and mammography is the initial test of choice for symptomatic women.

Moderate evidence supports the use of US in addition to mammography in the evaluation of women with palpable masses or thickening. The combination of US and mammography is especially effective in evaluating women with palpable masses (Table 3.4). In the multiinstitutional study of Georgian-Smith et al. (102), 616 palpable lesions were evaluated sonographically and all 293 palpable cancers were depicted sonographically. Across several series, of 545 cancers in women with symptoms, 529 (97.1%)

Table 3.4. Sensitivity and negative predictive value of combined mammography and US in symptomatic women

	No. of cancers	Sensitivity (%)	NPV (%)	Purpose of study/patient population	Detection of misses	Cancers missed
Georgian-Smith et al. (101)	293	293 (100)	n/a	Palpable, sensitivity of US to cancers	Biopsy	None
Dennis et al. 2001 (102)	0	n/a	600/600 (100)	Palpable, Biopsy avoidance	Biopsy or 2-year follow-up	None
Moy et al. 2002 (103)	6	0	227/233 (97.4)	Palpable	Tumor registry, 2-year follow-up	2 DCIS, 1 ILC, 3 IDC
Kaiser et al. 2002 (104)	6	6 (100)	117/117 (100)	Thickening	Biopsy or 14-month follow-up	n/a
Houssami et al. 2003 (105)	240	230 (95.8)[a]	174/184 (94.6)	Symptoms[a]	Tumor registry, 2-year follow-up	n/a
Overall	545	529 (97.1)	1118/1134 (98.6)			

NPV, negative predictive value; n/a, not applicable; DCIS, ductal carcinoma in situ; ILC, invasive lobular carcinoma; IDC, invasive ductal carcinoma.

[a] In the series of Houssami et al. (106), 157 women with cancer had a lump and 114 without cancer had a lump.

were depicted. A negative result after both mammography and US is highly predictive of benign outcome with 98.6% negative predictive value across these series (102–106). Nevertheless, final management of a clinically suspicious mass must be based on clinical grounds.

VII. How Accurate Is Ultrasound in Evaluating Nipple Discharge?

Summary of Evidence: Bloody nipple discharge and spontaneous unilateral clear nipple discharge merit imaging and clinical evaluation, with malignancy found in 13% of patients on average (range 1–23%) across multiple series (reviewed in ref. 107).

Supporting Evidence: Papilloma is the most common cause of nipple discharge, found in 44% to 45% of patients (107,108), with fibrocystic changes accounting for the rest. Milky discharge is almost always physiologic or due to hyperprolactinemia (107) and does not warrant imaging workup. Injection of contrast into the discharging duct, followed by magnification craniocaudal and true lateral mammographic views (galactography), has been the standard for imaging evaluation of nipple discharge (109). Ultrasound has the advantage of being noninvasive. A few studies have compared US and galactography, with promising but limited evidence for the utility of US in this setting (110,111). The visualization of intraductal masses on US is facilitated by distention of the duct. Whether or not the full extent of multiple intraductal lesions is well depicted on US has not been systematically studied (insufficient evidence).

VIII. How Accurate Is Ultrasound in Determining Local Extent of Disease?

Summary of Evidence: Sonography may aid in determining the local extent of breast cancer when used in conjunction with mammography and clinical exam (moderate evidence).

Supporting Evidence: Moderate evidence from several unblinded prospective series supports a detection benefit of sonography after mammography and clinical examination in evaluating the preoperative extent of breast cancer (Table 3.5). When magnetic resonance imaging (MRI) was used in addition, the limitations of combined US, mammography, and clinical examination became evident. In particular, an extensive intraductal component was often underestimated without MRI in one series (19). On average, 48% of breasts with cancer will have additional tumor foci not depicted on mammography or clinical examination (112). If US is being used to guide biopsy, there is an advantage to at least scanning the quadrant containing the cancer as 89% to 93% of additional tumor foci are within the same quadrant as the index lesion (19,112,113), and over 90% of malignant foci will be detected by combined mammography and US in this setting.

Ultrasound is not particularly sensitive to lesions manifest solely as calcifications due to their small size and speckle artifact present in tissue (114).

Table 3.5. Use of combined mammography and US in evaluating local extent of breast cancer

	No. of cancers	Sensitivity (%)	Detection of misses	Cancers missed
Fischer et al. 1999 (158)	405	366[a] (90.4)	MRI	4 DCIS, 3 ILC, 32 IDC
Berg and Gilbreath 2000 (159)[b]	64	62 (97)	Some surgery, details not specified	2 ILC
Hlawatsch et al. 2002 (98)	105 breasts with cancer	94/105 (90%) accurate extent	MRI	7 invasive NOS, 1 DCIS
Moon et al. 2002 (116)	289	276 (95.5)[a]	Some surgery, details not specified	5 IDC, 1 ILC, 7 DCIS
Berg et al. 2004 (19)[b]	96 breasts with cancer	81 (84%)[a]	MRI, 2-year follow-up	7 DCIS, 6 IDC, 2 ILC
Berg et al. 2004 (19)	177	162 (91.5)	MRI, 2-year follow-up	8 DCIS, 4 ILC, 3 IDC

MRI, magnetic resonance imaging; DCIS, ductal carcinoma in situ; ILC, invasive lobular carcinoma; IDC, invasive ductal carcinoma.
[a] Includes clinical breast examination.
[b] References (157) and (19) are nonoverlapping series.

Nevertheless, US can help identify the invasive component of malignant calcifications. Soo et al. (115) evaluated 111 cases of suspicious calcifications and only 26 (23%) could be seen sonographically. Of those seen on US, 69% were malignant compared to only 21% of those not seen on US (115). Those cancers seen on US were more likely invasive (72% vs. 28%), and underestimation of disease was less common when biopsies were performed with US guidance than stereotactic guidance. Similarly, Moon et al. (116) showed that 45 (45%) of 100 suspicious microcalcifications were sonographically visible, including 31 (82%) of 38 malignant calcifications and 14 (23%) of 62 benign calcifications.

IX. Which Lesions (BIRADS 1-6) Should Undergo Biopsy?

Summary of Evidence: The widespread use of screening mammography has resulted in the detection of clinically occult and probably benign lesions in up to 11% of patients (117). One concern regarding the dissemination and utilization of image-guided percutaneous biopsy was that unnecessary sampling of probably benign lesions would result in an unacceptably low positive predictive value. There has also been concern that it might replace the short-interval, 6-month imaging follow-up that has been demonstrated as effective management of probably benign [Breast Imaging and Reporting and Data Systems (BIRADS) category 3] masses and microcalcifications. The positive biopsy rate of mammography is improved when the procedure is performed primarily on lesions categorized by BIRADS (16) as category 4 (suspicious) or 5 (highly suspicious) and when short-interval, 6-month follow-up mammography is judiciously used in place of biopsy for the majority or probably benign (BIRADS category 3) lesions (117–121).

Supporting Evidence: Early studies reporting the low yield of breast cancer in BIRADS category 3, probably benign, nonpalpable lesions were largely level II (moderate evidence) investigations, both prospective and retrospective from single institutions (122–124) that were limited by small patient populations, incomplete mammographic follow-up, and short durations of follow-up (6 to 20 months).

A single level I (strong evidence) report was published by Sickles (125) in 1991. This prospective trial included 3.5 years of mammographic follow-up in a population of 3184 probably benign breast lesions, of which 17 (positive predictive value for cancer, 0.5%) were found to be malignant. These results established the validity of managing mammographically depicted, probably benign (BIRADS category 3) lesions with periodic mammographic surveillance (125).

A. Special Case: Radial Sclerosing Lesions (Radial Scars)

The reported incidence of radial scar is 0.1 to 2.0 per 1000 screening mammograms and 1.7% to 14% of autopsy specimens (126) (Fig. 3.1). Their major significance pertains to an association with atypical ductal hyperplasia and carcinoma that is seen in up to 50% of cases (Table 3.6) (127). However, multiinstitutional studies of larger patient populations evaluating percutaneous biopsy find a much lower incidence of cancer associated with radial scar than previously reported (128–130). Although the largest published studies are retrospective level II (moderate evidence), excisional biopsy is recommended when percutaneous biopsy results show radial scar, especially when associated with atypical hyperplasia.

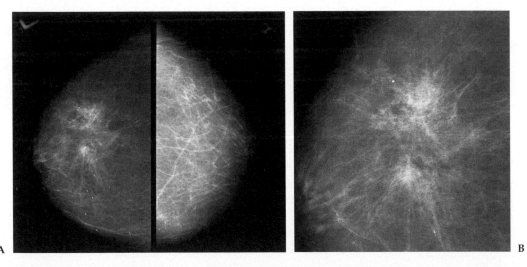

Figure 3.1. Radial scar. Right and left cranial-caudal (CC) (A) and coned right CC (B) mammography images demonstrate an ill-defined mass associated with architectural distortion in the left breast (right). Image-guided percutaneous biopsy demonstrated sclerosing radial lesion associated with sclerosing adenosis, atypical ductal hyperplasia, and fibrosis histopathologically. Surgical excision demonstrated a 7-mm tubular carcinoma in addition to the aforementioned findings.

Table 3.6. Published reports and evidence classification of radial scar (RS): association with malignancy and diagnostic accuracy by percutaneous biopsy (PB)

Authors, year	No. of RS diagnosed by PB	No. of gold standard correlation	Incidence of cancer	Cancer missed by PB	Study characteristics	Evidence classification
Brenner et al. 2002 (128)	198	Surgical excision: 102 mammography: 55	8.2% cancer 28% ADH	3% overall 5% for spring loaded 0% for vacuum device	2, 3, 4, 6	Level II
Philpotts et al. 2000 (129)	9	8	0% cancer 50% ADH		2, 3, 5, 7	Level II
Alleva et al. 1999 (127)	N/A	Surgical excision: 22	41%	N/A	2, 5	Level II
Orel et al. 1992 (130)	4	Surgical excision: 4	0% cancer 0% ADH	N/A	2, 5, 7	Level II

Study characteristics: 1, prospective; 2, retrospective; 3, nonpalpable lesions only; 4, multiinstitutional; 5, single institution; 6, lack of follow-up in some cases; 7, small population; ADH, atypical ductal hyperplasia.

X. What Is the Performance of Percutaneous Image-Guided Breast Biopsy Compared with Standard Surgical Excisional Biopsy?

Summary of Evidence: Percutaneous, image-guided breast biopsy has been found to be an accurate, safe, well-accepted, reliable method for diagnosing nonpalpable breast abnormalities. When a carcinoma is initially diagnosed by percutaneous biopsy significantly fewer surgical procedures are required to achieve clear margins when breast conservation is the therapeutic goal (131).

Supporting Evidence: There have been several studies evaluating percutaneous breast biopsy guided by both stereotactic (Fig. 3.2) or ultrasound (Fig. 3.3) imaging guidance (Table 3.7) (132–146). The majority were prospective, single-institution studies, but three were multiinstitutional (132,141,145). Several studies were limited by small study populations (defined as less than 200 subjects). All studies having a pathologic gold standard (i.e., all patients went to surgical biopsy after percutaneous image-guided biopsy) were less than 200 patients in size. In all studies over 200 patients in size, those with a benign percutaneous biopsy result were followed with either mammography or US. No study had complete imaging follow-up on this category of patients, and delayed cancers were diagnosed in the follow-up groups. For six studies evaluated as level II (moderate evidence) and two studies evaluated as level I (strong evidence), percutaneous imaging-guided biopsy diagnosed cancer in 72% to 98% of malignant lesions.

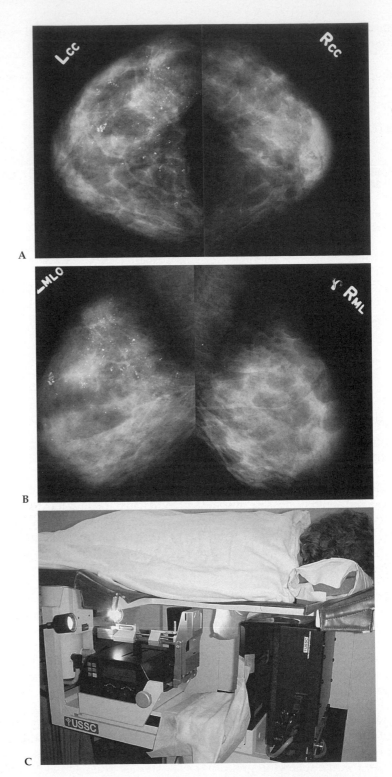

Figure 3.2. Stereotactic biopsy of microcalcifications. Right and left craniocaudal (A) and medial-lateral oblique (B) mammography images demonstrate suspicious microcalcifications in the upper outer and upper inner quadrants of the left breast. C: Patient positioning for stereotactic biopsy. X-ray and biopsy equipment are located beneath the table.

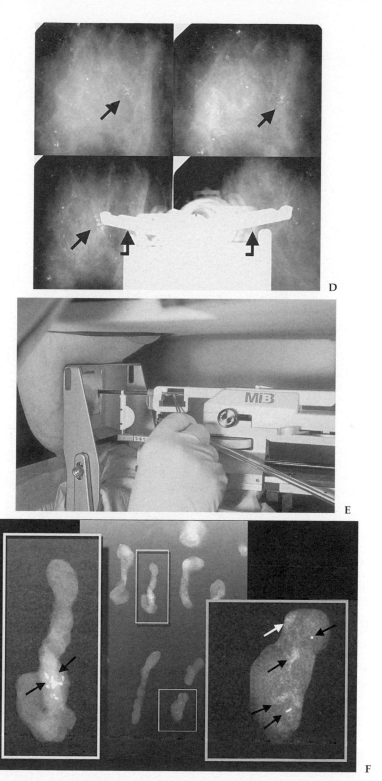

Figure 3.2. D: Stereotactic images of calcifications (arrows) performed for targeting (upper row of images) of a microcalcification cluster are shown above and images performed after placement of the biopsy probe (curved arrows in lower images) are shown below (biopsy probe obscured the cluster of interest in lower right image). E: Biopsy probe positioned within breast for retrieval of tissues samples from microcalcifications that were targeted with computer assistance from stereotactic images acquired digitally. F: Radiographs of the biopsy specimens document presence of microcalcifications (arrows) within the tissue. Ductal carcinoma in situ was diagnosed histopathologically. (For part E, see color insert.)

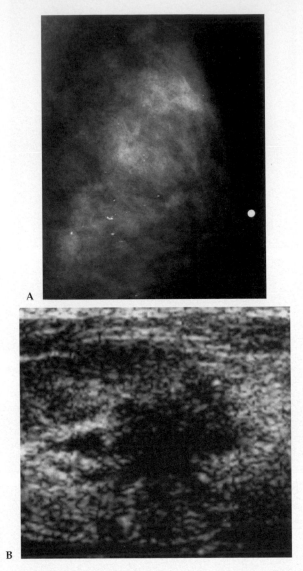

Figure 3.3. Ultrasound of mammographically occult malignancy. A: Mediolateral oblique mammogram with dense parenchyma in a 53-year-old with a palpable mass (marked with radiopaque marker). No discrete mammographic correlate is seen. B: Transverse sonogram over the palpable abnormality demonstrates a spiculated hypoechoic mass highly suggestive of malignancy. Sonographically guided core biopsy showed infiltrating and intraductal carcinoma.

Table 3.7. Published reports and evidence classification: image-guided breast biopsy compared to surgical biopsy

Authors, year	Method	Needle size (gauge)	No. of patients	No. of PB	Gold standard (GS)		% of cancers diagnosed on PB compared with GS	Other	Evidence classification
					F/U M or US	Surgical Biopsy			
Parker et al. 1990 (133)	S	14, 16, 18	103	102	102	102	14/16 (88%)	1, 3, 5, 7	III
Parker et al. 1991 (134)	S	14	102	102	102	102	22/23 (96%)	1, 5, 7	III
Parker et al. 1993 (135)	US	14	164	181	112	49	48/49 (98%)	1, 5, 6, 7	III
Elvecrog et al. 1993 (136)	S	14	100	100	N/A	100	34/36 (94%)	1, 3, 5, 7	III
Brendlinger et al. 1994 (137)	S	14	75	75	65	15	13/15 (87%)	1, 3, 5, 7	III
Burbank et al. 1994 (138)	US/S	14	105	105	NG	24	13/13 (100%)	1, 5, 6, 7	III
Gisvold, 1994 (139)	S	14	158	160	N/A	160	55/67 (82%)	1, 3, 7	III
Jackman et al. 1994 (140)	S	14	379	450	NG	116	99/116 (85%)	1, 3, 5	II
Parker et al. 1994 (141)	US/S	14	6152	6152	3765	1363	910/925 (98%)	1, 4, 6	II
Meyer et al. 1998 (142)	S	14	1032	1032	706	214	196/214 (96%)	1, 3, 5, 6	II
Jackman et al. 1999 (143)	S	14	483	483	259	221	55/76 (72%)	1, 3, 5, 6	II
Meyer et al. 1999 (144)	S	14, 14V, 11V	1643	1836	855	614	412/444 (93%)	1, 3, 5, 6	II
Brenner et al. 2001 (145)	S	14	1003	1003	596	307	242/254 (95%)	1, 3, 4	I
Margolin et al. 2001 (146)	S/US	16	1183	1333	963	175	135/147 (92%)	1, 3, 5, 6	II
Fajardo et al. 2004 (132)	US/S	14, 14V, 11V	2403	1174	1051	631	410/452 (91%)	1, 3, 4, 6, 8	I

S, stereotactic; M, mammography; US, ultrasound; V, vacuum-assisted; PB, percutaneous biopsy; NA, not applicable; NG, not given.

Other: 1, prospective; 2, retrospective; 3, nonpalpable lesions only or could separate data for nonpalpable lesions from palpable; 4, multiinstitutional; 5, single institution; 6, follow-up incomplete in some cases; 7, small population; 8, randomized.

XI. What Type of Imaging Guidance Is Best Suited for Breast Lesions Manifest as Masses or as Microcalcifications?

Summary of Evidence: Any lesion that is adequately visualized by US is best biopsied using this guidance method. Ultrasound biopsy is less costly than stereotactic biopsy and more comfortable for the patient. However, most microcalcification clusters are not visualized with US and require stereotactic guidance for tissue acquisition. Radiography of the core biopsy specimens should be performed whenever microcalcifications are biopsied to document adequate retrieval of calcifications in the biopsy specimens (132).

Supporting Evidence: The only major prospective randomized study that attempted to study which type of imaging guidance was best suited for percutaneous breast biopsy was the Radiology Diagnostic Oncology Group (RDOG) trial (132). In this study, 1103 subjects were assigned to stereotactic core biopsy and 578 were assigned to US core biopsy. However, 86 (8%) of subjects assigned to stereotactic biopsy were changed to US-guided biopsy by the physician performing the procedure, and 415 (72%) of subjects assigned to US biopsy were changed to stereotactic biopsy. All patients changed from stereotactic to US biopsy had a solid breast mass, and the most frequent reasons for change were lesion inaccessibility by the stereotactic system or a breast that was very thin on compression in the stereotactic biopsy device. Among patients where the breast lesion was calcifications, none were switched from stereotactic to US biopsy, while 99% (255 of 257) of subjects with calcifications assigned to US biopsy were switched to stereotactic biopsy because the calcifications were not well seen with US.

The RDOG5 trial reported summary measures for sensitivity, specificity, and predictive values for image-guided biopsy by the type of lesion biopsied (masses or calcifications) and imaging guidance used (US or stereotactic) (132). The overall sensitivity, specificity, and accuracy for all breast lesions by either imaging guidance method in this trial were 0.91, 1.00, and 0.98 respectively. The combined sensitivity, negative predictive value, and accuracy for US and stereotactic biopsy for diagnosing masses (0.96, 0.99, and 0.99, respectively) were significantly greater ($p < .001$, Chi-square) than for calcifications (0.84, 0.94, and 0.96, respectively) (132). The sensitivity (0.89) of stereotactic biopsy for diagnosing all lesions was significantly lower ($p = .029$, Fisher's exact) than that of US biopsy (0.97) because of the preponderance of calcifications biopsied by stereotactic versus US guidance (718 versus two) (131). There was no difference between US and stereotactic guidance in sensitivity, specificity, or accuracy for the diagnosis of masses (0.97, 1.00, 0.99, respectively, for ultrasound core biopsy (USCB) and 0.96, 100, and 0.99, respectively, for stereotactic core biopsy [SCB]) (133). The calculated overall false negative-rate for percutaneous image-guided biopsy in this trial was 0.093 (132). Figure 3.4 is an algorithm of decision support regarding the use of imaging-guided biopsy for diagnosing nonpalpable breast lesions.

A. Special Case: Biopsy of Breast Lesions Detected on Breast Magnetic Resonance Imaging

With increasing use of magnetic resonance to image the breast, investigators are reporting that MRI finds lesions that are not detected by mam-

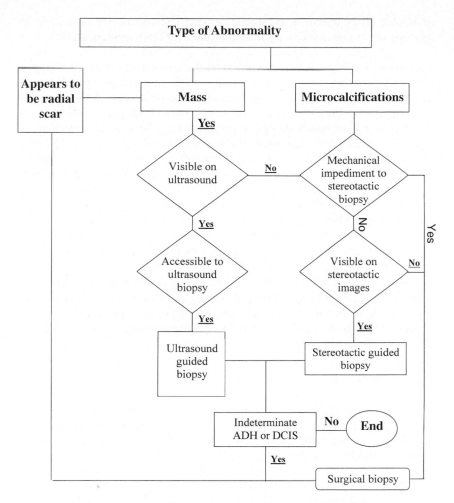

Figure 3.4. Decision support: determining the method of diagnostic breast biopsy for nonpalpable abnormalities.

mography or physical examination (50). Although MRI has a high sensitivity in detecting breast cancer, approaching 100% in some series, the reported specificity has ranged from 37% to 97% (147–151). Biopsying the lesions seen by MRI has gained attention in recent years. In some cases, a focused breast ultrasound examination, guided by the MRI findings, permits biopsy using US guidance. Some investigators report limited, single-institution experience with different approaches to performing percutaneous biopsy guided by MRI (147–151); however, there is insufficient evidence to substantiate its use. The cost-effectiveness of using MRI for the breast poses additional concerns. At present, there is insufficient evidence and there are currently are no level I, II, or III studies to guide which patient populations should undergo breast MRI.

XII. How Cost-Effective Is Image-Guided Biopsy?

Summary of Evidence: Percutaneous biopsy of a nonpalpable breast lesion using either stereotactic of US guidance is less expensive than surgical biopsy. The cost savings are greater if the biopsy is performed with US guidance (152); however, most calcification lesions are not visualized by US and are better evaluated with stereotactic biopsy guidance (132).

Supporting Evidence: Previous studies of the cost-effectiveness of imaging-guided biopsy have involved analysis of both stereotactic and US biopsy (132,152–157). Lindfors and Rosenquist (154) reported that the marginal cost per year of life saved with screening was reduced by 23% with the use of stereotactic rather than open surgical breast biopsy. Liberman et al. (152,153) found that stereotactic biopsy decreased the cost of diagnosis by more than 50%; if these results were generalized to the national level, annual savings in the United States would approach $200 million. Liberman et al. (153) and Lee et al. (155) found that the savings were greater with breast masses than with calcifications, probably due underestimation of pathology when atypical ductal hyperplasia and DCIS are associated with microcalcifications. When a lesion is visible by US—and many micro-calcification clusters are not—biopsy is least expensive using this imaging guided modality. This is in part due to the fact that US equipment is less costly than stereotactic systems and US can be used for imaging purposes other than guiding biopsy. When data by Liberman et al. (152) were used to estimate what the annual national cost savings would be if US rather than open surgical biopsy was used to diagnose breast masses, a figure of $59,523,000 was derived.

Future Research

- Data evaluating the performance of digital mammography relative to conventional screen film mammography for breast cancer screening are currently be analyzed from the recently completed ACRIN Digital Mammography Imaging Screening Trial (DMIST). Information from this trial, which recruited approximately 49,520 women, should be reported in mid- to late 2005 (http://www.acrin.org/6652_protocol.html).
- The efficacy of whole breast US imaging as a screening tool or adjunct to screening mammography in currently undergoing evaluation in the ACRIN 6666 trial, Breast Cancer Screening in High-Risk Women (http://www.acrin.org/6666_protocol.html). Results may be reported in early 2006.
- Data evaluating the efficacy of breast MRI to screen women at high risk for breast cancer are also undergoing analysis and may be reported in mid- to late 2005 (ACRIN 6667 trial, Breast Cancer: Screening of Contralateral Breast with MRI, http://www.acrin.org/6667_protocol.html).

References

1. American Cancer Society Surveillance Program. Estimated new cancer cases by sex and age. Atlanta: American Cancer Society, 2003.
2. Elmore JG, Barton MB, Moceri VM, Polk S, Arena PJ, Fletcher SW. N Engl J Med 1998;16:1089–1096.
3. Kerlikowske K. J Natl Cancer Inst Monogr 1997;22:79–86.
4. Kerlikowske K, Grady D, Barclay J, Sickles EA, Eaton A, Ernster V. JAMA 1993;270:2444–2450.
5. Gail MH, Costantino JP. J Natl Cancer Inst 2001;93(5):334–355.
6. Gail MH, Brinton LA, Byar DP, et al. J Natl Cancer Inst 1989;81(24):1879–1886.

7. Gail MH. Ann N Y Acad Sci 2001;949:286–291.
8. Gail MH, Benichou J. J Natl Cancer Inst 1994;86(8):573–575.
9. Claus EB, Risch N, Thompson WD. Breast Cancer Res Treat 1993;28(2):115–120.
10. Page DL, Dupont WD, Rogers LW, Rados MS. Cancer 1985;55(11):2698–2708.
11. Page DL, Kidd TE Jr, Dupont WD, Simpson JF, Rogers LW. Hum Pathol 1991;22(12):1232–1239.
12. Fisher B, Costantino JP, Wickerham DL, et al. J Natl Cancer Inst 1998;90(18):1371–1388.
13. Hancock SL, Tucker MA, Hoppe RT. J Natl Cancer Inst 1993;85(1):25–31.
14. Aisenberg AC, Finkelstein DM, Doppke KP, Koerner FC, Boivin JF, Willett CG. Cancer 1997;79(6):1203–1210.
15. Clemons M, Loijens L, Goss P. Cancer Treat Rev 2000;26(4):291–302.
16. American College of Radiology. Illustrated Breast Imaging Reporting and Data System (BI-RADS): Mammography, 4th ed. Reston, VA: ACR, 2003.
17. Mandelson MT, Oestreicher N, Porter PL, et al. J Natl Cancer Inst 2000;92(13):1081–1087.
18. Kolb TM, Lichy J, Newhouse JH. Radiology 2002;225(1):165–175.
19. Berg WA, Gutierrez L, NessAiver M, et al. Radiology 2004;233(3):830–849.
20. Leconte I, Feger C, Galant C, et al. AJR 2003;180(6):1675–1679.
21. Ciatto S, Cataliotti L, Distante V. Radiology 1987;165:99–102.
22. Hall FM, Storella JM, Silverstone DZ, Wyshak G. Radiology 1988;167:353–358.
23. Sickles EA, Ominsky SH, Sollitto RA, Galvin HB, Monticciolo DL. Radiology 1990;175:323–327.
24. Skinner MA, Swain M, Simmons R, McCarty KS, Jr, Sullivan DC, Iglehart JD. Ann Surg 1988;208:203–208.
25. Spivey GH, Perry BW, Clark VA, Coulson AH, Coulson WF. Am Surg 1982;48:326–332.
26. Molloy M, Azarow K, Garcia VF, Daniel JR. J Surg Oncol 1989;40:152–154.
27. Brown ML, Lipscomb J, Snyder C. Annu Rev Public Health 2001;22:91–113.
28. National Heart Lung and Blood Institute. NHLBI Year 2003 Fact Book. Washington, DC: National Institutes of Health, 2003.
29. Tabar L, Duffy SW, Vitak B, Chen HH, Prevost TC. Cancer 1999;86(3):449–462.
30. Shapiro S, Venet W, Strax P, Venet L. Periodic Screening for Breast Cancer: The Health Insurance Plan Project and Its Sequelae. Baltimore: Johns Hopkins Press, 1988.
31. Tabar L, Vitak B, Chen HH, et al. Radiol Clin North Am 2000;38(4):625–651.
32. Hendrick RE, Smith RA, Rutledge JH 3rd, Smart CR. J Natl Cancer Inst Monogr 1997;22:87–92.
33. Humphrey LL, Helfand M, Chan BK, Woolf SH. Ann Intern Med 2002;137 (5 pt 1):347–360.
34. Nystrom L, Andersson I, Bjurstam N, Frisell J, Nordenskjold B, Rutqvist LE. Lancet 2002;359(9310):909–919.
35. Michaelson J, Satija S, Moore R, et al. Cancer 2002;94(1):37–43.
36. Paci E, Duffy SW, Giorgi D, et al. Br J Cancer 2002;87(1):65–69.
37. Tabar L, Yen MF, Vitak B, Chen HH, Smith RA, Duffy SW. Lancet 2003; 361(9367):1405–1410.
38. Smith RA, Duffy SW, Gabe R, Tabar L, Yen AM, Chen TH. Radiol Clin North Am 2004;42(5):793–806, v.
39. U.S. Preventive Services Task Force. Ann Intern Med 2002;137(5 pt 1):344–346.
40. Tabar L, Vitak B, Tony HH, Yen MF, Duffy SW, Smith RA. Cancer 2001; 91(9):1724–1731.
41. Shapiro S. Health Insurance Plan. J Natl Cancer Inst Monogr 1997;22:27–30.
42. IARC Working Group on the Evaluation of Cancer-Preventive Strategies. Breast Cancer Screening, vol. 7. Lyon: IARC Press, 2002.
43. Alexander FE, Anderson TJ, Brown HK, et al. Lancet 1999;353(9168):1903–1908.
44. Andersson I, Janzon L. J Natl Cancer Inst Monogr 1997;22:63–67.
45. Frisell J, Lidbrink E. J Natl Cancer Inst Monogr 1997;22:49–51.

46. Frisell J, Lidbrink E, Hellstrom L, Rutqvist LE. Breast Cancer Res Treat 1997;45(3):263–270.
47. Bjurstam N, Bjorneld L, Duffy SW, et al. Cancer 1997;80(11):2091–2099.
48. Bjurstam N, Bjorneld L, Warwick J, et al. Cancer 2003;97(10):2387–2396.
49. Miller AB, To T, Baines CJ, Wall C. J Natl Cancer Inst 2000;92(18):1490–1499.
50. Miller AB, To T, Baines CJ, Wall C. Ann Intern Med 2002;137(5 pt 1):305–312.
51. Organizing Committee and Collaborators. Int J Cancer 1996;68:693–699.
52. Smith RA, Saslow D, Sawyer KA, et al. CA Cancer J Clin 2003;53(3):141–169.
53. Olsen O, Gotzsche P. Lancet 2001;358:1340.
54. Swedish Board of Health and Welfare. Vilka Effekter Har Mammografiscreening? Referat av ett expertmöte anordnat av Socialstyrelsen och Cancerfonden. Stockholm: 2002.
55. Health Council of the Netherlands. The benefit of population screening for breast cancer with mammography. Health Council of the Netherlands, 2002.
56. Veronese U, Forrest P, Wood W, Boyle P. Statement from the chair: Global Summit on Mammographic Screening, June 3–5, 2002. European Institute of Oncology, 2002.
57. Duffy SW, Tabar L, Vitak B, et al. Ann Oncol 2003;14(8):1196–1198.
58. Tabar L, Smith RA, Duffy SW. Lancet 2002;360(9329):337, discussion 39–40.
59. Duffy SW, Tabar L, Vitak B, et al. Eur J Cancer 2003;39(12):1755–1760.
60. Smith RA, Cokkinides V, Eyre HJ. CA Cancer J Clin 2003;53(1):27–43.
61. Freedman DA, Petitti DB, Robins JM. Int J Epidemiol 2004;33(1):43–55.
62. Duffy S, Tabar L, Chen HH, et al. Cancer 2002;95:458–469.
63. U.S. Preventive Services Task Force. Ann Intern Med 2002;137(5 pt 1):I47.
64. Fletcher SW, Black W, Harris R, Rimer BK, Shapiro S. J Natl Cancer Inst 1993;85(20):1644–1656.
65. U.S. Preventive Services Task Force. Guide to Clinical Preventive Services, 2nd ed. Baltimore: Williams & Wilkins, 1996.
66. National Institutes of Health Consensus Development Panel. J Natl Cancer Inst 1997;89(14):1015–1026.
67. de Koning HJ, Boer R, Warmerdam PG, Beemsterboer PM, van der Maas PJ. J Natl Cancer Inst 1995;87(16):1217–1223.
68. Tabar L, Duffy SW, Chen HH. J Natl Cancer Inst 1996;88(1):52–55.
69. Tabar L, Chen HH, Fagerberg G, Duffy SW, Smith TC. J Natl Cancer Inst Monogr 1997;22:43–47.
70. Tabar L, Faberberg G, Day NE, Holmberg L. Br J Cancer 1987;55(5):547–551.
71. Kerlikowske K, Salzmann P, Phillips KA, Cauley JA, Cummings SR. JAMA 1999;282(22):2156–2163.
72. Ries L, Eisner M, Kosary C, et al, SEER Cancer Statistics Review, 1975–2001. National Cancer Institute, 2004.
73. National Cancer Institute. SEER*Stat 4/2, ed. 4.2. Bethesda: National Cancer Institute, 2002.
74. Nixon AJ, Neuberg D, Hayes DF, et al. J Clin Oncol 1994;12(5):888–894.
75. McCarthy EP, Burns RB, Freund KM, et al. J Am Geriatr Soc 2000;48(10):1226–1233.
76. McPherson CP, Swenson KK, Lee MW. J Am Geriatr Soc 2002;50(6):1061–1068.
77. Walter LC, Covinsky KE. JAMA 2001;285(21):2750–2756.
78. Arias E. United States life tables, 2002. Center for Health Statistics, 2004.
79. Duffy SW, Day NE, Tabar L, Chen HH, Smith TC. J Natl Cancer Inst Monogr 1997;22:93–97.
80. White E, Miglioretti DL, Yankaskas BC, et al. J Natl Cancer Inst 2004;96(24):1832–1839.
81. Michaelson JS, Halpern E, Kopans DB. Radiology 1999;212(2):551–560.
82. Hunt KA, Rosen EL, Sickles EA. Outcome analysis for women undergoing annual versus biennial screening mammography: a review of 24,211 examinations. Am J Roentgenol 1999;173(2):285–289.

83. Rosenquist CJ, Lindfors KK. Cancer 1998;82(11):2235–2240.

84. Rosenquist CJ, Lindfors KK. Radiology 1994;191(3):647–650.

85. Lindfors KK, Rosenquist CJ. JAMA 1995;274(11):881–884.

86. Salzmann P, Kerlikowske K, Phillips K. Ann Intern Med 1997;127(11):955–965.

87. Mandelblatt J, Saha S, Teutsch S, et al. Ann Intern Med 2003;139(10):835–842.

88. Gold M. JAMA 1996;276:1253–1258.

89. Tabar L, Tony Chen HH, Amy Yen MF, et al. Cancer 2004;101(8):1745–1759.

90. Gordon PB, Goldenberg SL. Cancer 1995;76(4):626–630.

91. Buchberger W, Niehoff A, Obrist P, DeKoekkoek-Doll P, Dunser M. Semin Ultrasound CT MR 2000;21(4):325–336.

92. Kaplan SS. Radiology 2001;221(3):641–649.

93. Crystal P, Strano SD, Shcharynski S, Koretz MJ. AJR 2003;181(1):177–182.

94. Hou MF, Chuang HY, Ou-Yang F, et al. Ultrasound Med Biol 2002;28(4): 415–420.

95. Berg WA. AJR 2003;180:1225–1228.

96. Michaelson JS, Silverstein M, Wyatt J, et al. Cancer 2002;95(4):713–723.

97. Baker JA, Kornguth PJ, Soo MS, Walsh R, Mengoni P. AJR 1999;172(6): 1621–1625.

98. Hlawatsch A, Teifke A, Schmidt M, Thelen M. AJR 2002;179(6):1493–1501.

99. Dershaw DD, Abramson A, Kinne DW. Radiology 1989;170(2):411–415.

100. Bassett LW. Radiol Clin North Am 2000;38(4):669–691.

101. Bartow SA, Pathak DR, Black WC, Key CR, Teaf SR. Cancer 1987;60(11): 2751–2760.

102. Georgian-Smith D, Taylor KJ, Madjar H, et al. J Clin Ultrasound 2000;28(5): 211–216.

103. Dennis MA, Parker SH, Klaus AJ, Stavros AT, Kaske TI, Clark SB. Radiology 2001;219(1):186–191.

104. Moy L, Slanetz PJ, Moore R, et al. Radiology 2002;225(1):176–181.

105. Kaiser JS, Helvie MA, Blacklaw RL, Roubidoux MA. Radiology 2002;223(3): 839–844.

106. Houssami N, Irwig L, Simpson JM, McKessar M, Blome S, Noakes J. AJR 2003;180(4):935–940.

107. Paterok EM, Rosenthal H, Sabel M. Eur J Obstet Gynecol Reprod Biol 1993; 50(3):227–234.

108. Leis HP, Jr, Greene FL, Cammarata A, Hilfer SE. South Med J 1988;81(1):20–26.

109. Cardenosa G, Doudna C, Eklund GW. AJR 1994;162(5):1081–1087.

110. Yang WT, Tse GM. AJR 2004;182(1):101–110.

111. Hild F, Duda VF, Albert U, Schulz KD. Eur J Cancer Prev 1998;7(suppl 1): S57–56.

112. Liberman L, Morris EA, Dershaw DD, Abramson AF, Tan LK. AJR 2003;180(4): 901–910.

113. Holland R, Veling SH, Mravunac M, Hendriks JH. Cancer 1985;56(5):979–990.

114. Anderson ME, Soo MS, Bentley RC, Trahey GE. J Acoust Soc Am 1997;101(1): 29–39.

115. Soo MS, Baker JA, Rosen EL. AJR 2003;180(4):941–948.

116. Moon WK, Noh DY, Im JG. Radiology 2002;224(2):569–576.

117. Sickles EA. Radiology 1991;179:463–468.

118. Varas X, Leborgne F, Leborgne JH. Radiology 1992;184:409–414.

119. Sickles EA. Radiology 1994;192:439–442.

120. Sickles EA. Radiology 1998;208:471–475.

121. Vizcaino I, Gadea L, Andreo L, et al. Radiology 2001;219:475–483.

122. Hall FM. Arch Surg 1990;125:298–299.

123. Wolfe JN, Buck KA, Salane M, Parekh NJ. Radiology 1987;165:305–311.

124. Helvie MA, Pennes DR, Rebner M, Adler DD. Radiology 1991;178:155–158.

125. Sickles, EA. Radiology 1991;179:463–468.

126. Rosen PP. Rosen's breast pathology. Philadelphia: Lippincott-Raven, 1997:76–82.

127. Alleva DQ, Smetherman DH, Farr GH Jr, Cederbom GJ. Radiographics 1999;19:S27–S35.
128. Brenner RJ, Jackman RJ, Parker SH, et al. AJR 2002;179(5):1179–1184.
129. Philpotts LE, Shaheen NA, Jain KS, Carter D, Lee CH. Radiology 2000; 216:831–837.
130. Orel SG, Evers K, Yeh IT, Troupin RH. Radiology 1992;183:479–482.
131. Smith DN, Christian RL, Meyer JE. Arch Surg 1997;132:256–259.
132. Fajardo LL, Pisano ED, Caudry DJ, et al. Acad Radiol 2004;11:293–308.
133. Parker SH, Lovin JD, Jobe WE, et al. Radiology 1990;76:741–747.
134. Parker SH, Lovin JD, Jobe WE, Burke BJ, Hopper KD, Yakes WF. Radiology 1991;180:403–407.
135. Parker SH, Jobe WE, Dennis MA, et al. Radiology 1993;187:507–511.
136. Elvecrog EL, Lechner MC, Nelson MT. Radiology 1993;188:453–455.
137. Brendlinger DL, Robinson R, Sylvest V, Burton S. Va Med Q 1994;121(3): 179–184.
138. Burbank F, Kaye K, Belville J, Blumenfeld M. Radiology 1994;191:165–171.
139. Gisvold JJ, Goellner JR, Grant CS, et al. AJR 1994;162:815–820.
140. Jackman RJ, Nowels KS, Shepard NJ, Finkelstein SI, Marzoni FA. Radiology 1994;193:91–95.
141. Parker SH, Burbank F, Jackman RJ, et al. Radiology 1994;193:359–364.
142. Meyer JE, Smith DN, Lester SC, et al. Radiology 1998;206:717–720.
143. Jackman RJ, Nowels KW, Rodriquez-Soto J, Marzoni FA Jr, Finkelstein SI, Shepard MJ. Radiology 1999;210:799–805.
144. Meyer JE, Smith DN, Lester SC, et al. JAMA 1999;281:1638–1641.
145. Brenner RJ, Bassett LW, Fajardo LL, et al. Radiology 2001;218:866–872.
146. Margolin FR, Leung JWT, Jacobs RP, Denny SR. AJR 2001;177:559–564.
147. Orel SG, Schnall MD, Newman RW, Powell CM, Torosian MH, Rosato EF. Radiology 1994;193:97–102.
148. Orel SG, Schnall MD, Powell CM, et al. Radiology 1995;196:115–112.
149. Doler W, Fisher U, Metzger I, Harder D, Grabbe E. Radiology 1996;200: 863–864.
150. Daniel BL, Birdwell RL, Black JW, Ikeda DM, Glover GH, Herfkens RJ. Acad Radiol 1997;4:508–512.
151. Kuhl CK, Elevelt A, Leutner CC, Gieseke J, Pakos E, Schild HH. Radiology 1997;204:667–675.
152. Liberman L, Feng TL, Dershaw DD, Morris EA, Abramson, AF. Radiology 1998;208:717–723.
153. Liberman L, Fahs MC, Dershaw DD, et al. Radiology 1995;195:633–637.
154. Lindfors KK, Rosenquist CJ. Radiology 1994;190:217–222.
155. Lee CH, Egglin TK, Philpotts L, Mainiero MB, Tocino I. Radiology 1997;202: 849–854.
156. Fajardo LL. Acad Radiol 1996;3:521–523.
157. Hillner BE, Bear HD, Fajardo LL. Estimating the cost-effectiveness of stereotaxic biopsy for nonpalpable breast abnormalities: a decision analysis model. Acad Radiol 1996;3:351–360.
158. Fischer U, Kopka L, Grabbe E. Breast carcinoma: effect of preoperative contrast-enhanced MR imaging on the therapeutic approach. Radiology 1999; 213(3):881–888.
159. Berg WA, Gilbreath PL. Multicentric and multifocal cancer: whole-breast US in preoperative evaluation. Radiology 2000;214(1):59–66.

4

Imaging of Lung Cancer

James G. Ravenel and Gerard A. Silvestri

I. Is there a role for imaging in lung cancer screening?
   A. What is the role of chest x-ray?
   B. What is the role of computed tomography?
II. How should lung cancer be staged?
   A. How is the primary tumor evaluated?
   B. How is the mediastinum evaluated?
   C. How are distant metastases evaluated?
   D. Special case: how is small cell lung cancer evaluated?
   E. Special case: what is the appropriate radiologic follow-up?

Issues

- Screening with chest radiographs does not decrease disease specific lung cancer mortality (moderate evidence).
- CT scan is able to detect lung cancers at a smaller size. There is not adequate data to determine if CT screening is effective in reducing lung cancer deaths (insufficient evidence).
- CT and PET should be the primary tools for staging non–small cell lung cancer and guiding invasive studies (strong evidence).

Key Points

Definition and Pathophysiology

Malignant neoplasms of the pulmonary parenchyma can be loosely categorized as lung cancer. Simplistically stated, cancer in the lung occurs through a complex interaction of DNA damage, repair, and mutation (1,2). Lung cancer includes a variety of histologic cell types. Squamous cell, large cell, and adenocarcinoma are categorized as non–small cell carcinoma based on their common staging and treatment regimens. Small cell carcinoma is distinctly more aggressive and is treated differently from the other cell types.

Epidemiology

Lung cancer remains a preeminent public health concern, with over 170,000 cases diagnosed annually and over 150,000 deaths per year in the United States (3). Perhaps even more daunting is the fact that over 1 million people worldwide will succumb to the disease (4). Lung cancer is the leading cause of cancer-specific mortality, outpacing breast, prostate, colon, and ovarian cancer combined. Regardless of histologic subtype, smoking is the presumed causative agent in over 85% of cases (5). Although smoking cessation reduces the risk of developing lung cancer, up to 50% of newly diagnosed lung cancers occur in former smokers (6). Other occupational and environmental exposures can contribute to the risk and development of lung cancer, including arsenic, nickel, chromium, and asbestos (1). Radiation makes up the primary environmental source of lung cancer. Radon, of primary concern to uranium miners, is an ubiquitous environmental source (50 to 100 times lower than uranium mines) of high-LET (linear energy transfer) radiation (7,8). The relationship with low-level radiation is less clear. Intermittent lower dose radiation given to tuberculosis patients showed that the risk, if any, was small (9).

Overall Cost to Society

Tobacco smoke, the major risk for development of lung cancer, is estimated to result in costs over $157 billion in health related economic losses (10) and constitutes approximately 6% to 8% of personal health care expenditures in the United States (11). The estimated annual cost for the treatment of lung cancer is approximately $21,000 per patient but rises to approximately $47,000 for those who do not survive 1 year (12,13). Conservatively, this results in an annual cost of treating lung cancer in the United States of $3.6 billion per year.

Goals

The goal of screening is to detect serious disease at a preclinical stage where treatment for the disease is more effective when administered early (14). At this level, lung cancer appears to be an ideal candidate for screening. There is a well-defined high-risk population, and when detected by symptoms the disease is advanced in over 80% of cases. Furthermore, treatment is more efficacious at an earlier stage as measured by 5-year survival (15). The goal of staging is to define the extent of disease and help select the optimum course of treatment. As such, staging has both therapeutic and prognostic implications.

Methodology

A Medline search was performed using PubMed (National Library of Medicine, Bethesda, Maryland) for original research publications discussing the diagnostic performance and effectiveness of imaging strategies in lung cancer screening. The search covered the years 1966 to 2003 and included the following search terms: (1) *lung cancer screening*, (2) *lung cancer* and *computed tomography*, and (3) *lung cancer* and *chest x-ray*. Additional articles were identified by reviewing the reference lists of relevant papers. This review was limited to human studies and the English-language literature. For lung cancer staging, the authors built on a recent meta-analysis of the literature authored by one of the chapter's coauthors (G.A.S.) (16,17). This study included a full review of the literature from January 1991 to July 2001. Articles prior to 1991 were excluded due to marked improvements in imaging technology. To ensure that more recent articles were included, a search was performed using PubMed using the following terms: (1) *lung cancer* and *computed tomography*, (2) *lung cancer* and *positron emission tomography* (PET), (3) *lung cancer* and *magnetic resonance imaging* (MRI), and (4) *lung cancer staging* for the period July 1, 2001, to December 2003. The authors performed an initial review of the titles and abstracts of the identified articles followed by review of the full text in articles that were relevant.

I. Is There a Role for Imaging in Lung Cancer Screening?

Summary of Evidence: Screening for lung cancer with chest radiographs has not been shown to reduce lung cancer mortality. The addition of sputum cytology does not increase the yield of screening. Studies on CT are currently limited to nonrandomized trials and therefore the ability of CT to reduce lung cancer mortality has not been adequately assessed.

Supporting Evidence

A. What Is the Role of Chest X-Ray?

Radiographic screening for lung cancer dates back to the 1950s (Table 4.1). The Philadelphia Pulmonary Neoplasm Research Project performed

Table 4.1. Results of chest x-ray randomized control trials

Study site	Study arm	Sample size	No. of baseline screening cancers	No. of repeat screening cancers	Lung cancer mortality per 10,000 person-years
London 1960–1964	All	55,034	51	177	2.2
	Intervention	29,723	31	101	2.1
	Control	25,311	20	76	2.4
Mayo 1971–1983	All	10,933	91	366	NR
	Intervention	4,618[†]	NA	206	3.2
	Control	4,593[†]	NA	160	3.0
Czechoslovakia 1976–1980	All	6,364	18	66	NR
	Intervention	3,172[†]	NA	39	3.6
	Control	3,174[†]	NA	27	2.6
Memorial Sloan-Kettering Cancer Center 1974–1982	All	10,040	53	235	NR
	Intervention	4,968	30	114	2.7[‡]
	Control	5,072	23	121	2.7[‡]
Johns Hopkins 1973–1982	All	10,386	79	396[§]	
	Intervention	5,226	39	194	3.4[‡]
	Control	5,161	40	202	3.8[‡]

NA, not available; NR, not reported.
[†] Randomization subsequent to baseline screen. Sample size of the study arms do not equal number of total enrollees.
[‡] Randomization prior to baseline screen. Total number of deaths may include prevalence cases.
[§] Includes 379 cancer detected during screening period and 17 cancers detected after the end of screening.

periodic photofluorogram screening on over 6000 male volunteers, with disappointing results. Although survival was slightly better in the screen-detected cancers versus symptom-detected cancers, screen-detected cancers had the same outcome regardless of the time from the previous negative study (Fig. 4.1) (18). At about the same time, the North London study randomized over 50,000 men, ages 40 to 64, to biannual chest x-rays over 3 years or chest x-rays at the beginning and end of the 3-year period. More cancers were detected in the study group (101 vs. 77), and the 5-year survival rate was better (15% vs. 6%), although this was not statistically significant (19). The study also suffered from problems with randomization, as there were statistically more ex-smokers in the screened group and more participants aged 60 to 64 in the control group (20).

Case-control series of chest radiographs for lung cancer screening have been performed in Japan owing to the large amount of available data from tuberculosis control programs. The first trial reported from Osaka estimated a 28% reduction in mortality and better survival for those in the screen-detected group compared to those in the Osaka Cancer Registry (21). Four more recent case control series show an estimated mortality reduction between 30% and 60% (22–25). Pooling the data of these four Prefectures resulted in an estimated mortality reduction of 44% (26).

Two European nonrandomized trials of chest radiograph screening have been performed. In Varese, Italy, 2444 heavy smokers were screened annually for 3 years; 16 cancers were detected during the prevalence screen, 31% stage I, and seven cancers were detected during the two incidence screens, 71% stage I (27). The Turku Study in Finland studied 93 men out of 33,000 who had lung cancer detected on a one-time screen and compared them to those detected by symptoms or serendipitously noted on chest radiograph performed for other purposes. Screen-detected cases tended to be of an earlier stage and thus resectable (37% vs. 19%), and 5-year survival was better in the screen-detected group (19% vs. 10%) (28).

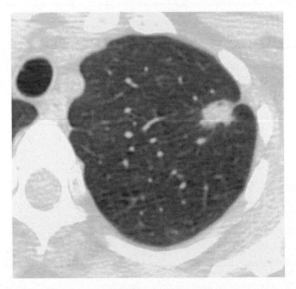

Figure 4.1. Typical CT screen detected lung cancer. Spiculated nodule present in left upper lobe measuring just over 1 cm. Surgery revealed T1N0 adenocarcinoma.

Taken all together, the nonrandomized studies performed in Europe and Japan would seemingly give credence to an advantage for screened populations. As pointed out previously, however, the biases present in the design of these studies make it impossible to definitively attribute the apparent benefit to screening. Furthermore, there are likely differences in the populations studied when compared to the U.S. population. In Japan, lung cancer in females is a disease of nonsmokers, and female smoking-related cases were excluded to facilitate matching controls (22,25). A high proportion of male never-smokers were present in the Miyagi screening study. Furthermore, peripheral adenocarcinoma occurs in a higher percentage of cases in Japan, and thus the efficacy of screening seen in Japan may not translate to U.S. populations (25).

Including the previously mentioned North London study, a total of six randomized controlled trials and one nonrandomized trial of chest radiograph lung cancer screening have been performed. In all of these studies, the control group underwent some form of screening, though less frequently than the intervention arm. The Kaiser Foundation trial, though not specifically performed for lung cancer, randomized over 10,000 participants ages 35 to 54 into an intervention group that was encouraged to participate in a multiphasic health checkup, including chest x-ray, and a control group that was not. Seventeen percent of participants in both groups were smokers. All-cause mortality was not significantly different between groups (29). The Erfurt, Germany, study was a nonrandomized trial with 41,000 males in the intervention group, who underwent biannual chest x-rays and 102,000 males in the control group, who had chest x-rays every 18 months. The intervention group had a higher rate of cancers detected (9% vs. 6.5%), a higher resection rate (28% vs. 19%), and better 5- and 10-year survival. However, there was no difference in lung cancer or all-cause mortality (30).

Under the auspices of the National Cancer Institute (NCI), three separate screening trials were performed in the U.S. during the 1970s (31). Two of these studies, the Johns Hopkins study (32) and the Memorial Sloan-Kettering (33) study, enrolled over 10,000 males each into an intervention group that received annual chest x-rays and sputum cytology every 4 months, and a control group that received only an annual chest x-ray. While there was a slight benefit to sputum cytology at the prevalence screen, all-cause mortality was the same in both groups (34–36). The results led to the conclusion that sputum cytology does not significantly improve the yield of chest x-ray screening.

The Czech Study on Lung Cancer Screening had a rather unique design. At the initial screen, all participants received a chest x-ray and sputum analysis. After 19 prevalence cases were excluded, 6345 were randomized to either semiannual chest x-rays and sputum analysis for 3 years or a chest x-ray and sputum analysis at the end of the 3-year period. Both groups then received annual chest x-rays at 1-year intervals from years 4 through 6. The first reported results were promising, with 48% diagnosed at stage I or II and 27% undergoing curative resections in the intervention arm (37). The number of stage III cancers in each arm was similar (17 vs. 15). At follow-up, however, despite the fact that the lung cancer in the screened group was of earlier stage, almost three times as likely to be resectable, and had a better 5-year survival from time of diagnosis, there were more lung cancer deaths in the intervention arm, all-cause mortality was greater in the intervention arm, and smoking-related deaths were greater in the interventional arm (38). Conclusions did not change at extended follow-up (39).

The Mayo Lung Project randomized 10,933 participants into an intervention arm of chest x-ray and sputum cytology every 4 months and a control arm of "usual care" for 6 years (40). Ninety-one prevalence cancers were detected with over 50% postsurgical stage I or II and 5-year survival of 40%. Prevalence cases tended to be of a more well-differentiated histology (41) and complete resection could be performed in twice as many screening participants compared to a previous cohort of over 1700 patients. By the end of the trial, 206 lung cancers had been detected in the screening arm and 160 in the control arm. Although screen-detected cancers were more resectable (54% vs. 30%), there was no stage shift and no statistically significant difference between the groups in lung cancer mortality (42,43). With follow-up out to 20 years, no benefit could be detected in the screened group (44).

The results of the Mayo Lung Project remain controversial. Contamination of the control group was considered substantial. Over 73% of subjects received a chest radiograph in the last 2 years of the study, and 30% of the cancers in the control group were discovered on chest radiographs performed for reasons other than suspicion of lung cancer (43). The majority of these ostensibly "screen" cancers in the control group were resectable. Overdiagnosis bias is one of the proposed reasons for the excess cancers in the screen group, although this hypothesis, particularly as it applies to lung cancer, remains controversial (45–47). It has also been suggested that the Mayo Lung Project was underpowered and thus had only a 20% chance of showing a mortality benefit should it have existed (48). Although it was also suggested that there was heterogeneity between the groups that affected mortality (49), reappraisal of the populations in the study showed no difference in age at entry, cigarette smoking history, exposure to nontobacco lung carcinogens, and comorbid pulmonary diseases (50). Regardless of the controversy, it is important to realize that to date, lung cancer screening with chest radiographs has not been shown to reduce lung cancer mortality. There is one ongoing larger randomized control trial of lung cancer screening with chest radiograph as part of the Prostate, Lung, Colorectal, and Ovarian Cancer Screening Trial (51).

B. What Is the Role of Computed Tomography?

The literature review revealed a total of nine trials of nonrandomized screening, three in Japan, three in Europe, and three in the United States, enrolling a total of 20,116 individuals for prevalence screens (52–60). Several of these studies have reported annual incidence data, and thus far 25,406 incidence screens have been reported (55,57,61–63) (Table 4.2). It is important to realize that the superiority of CT for the detection of abnormalities is not in question; however, CT identifies many smaller, "indeterminate" nodules, the majority of which will eventually turn out to be benign, but represent a diagnostic dilemma at the time of screening. The rate of false-positive exams must be taken into consideration in the context of lung cancer screening.

The most extensive experience has been seen in Japan where the three trials, Anti-Lung Cancer Association (ALCA) (55), Hitachi Employee's Health Insurance Group(Hitachi) (57), and Matsumoto Research Centre

Table 4.2. Results of CT screening trials

Study site	Date of publication	Baseline screen				Annual repeat screening			
		No. of patients screened	No. of abnormal results (% of total)	No. of malignancies detected (% of total)	Detected malignancies, stage 1 (%)	No. of patients screened	No. of newly identified abnormal results	No. of detected malignancies (% of total)	Detected malignancies, stage 1 (%)
Cornell University, United States (ELCAP)	1999, 2001	1000	233 (23)	27 (2.70)	81	1184	63 (5)	7 (0.59)	85
Muenster University, Germany	2001	919	NR	17 (1.85)	76	NR	NR	2 (NR)	100
Matsumoto Research Center	2001	5483	676 (12)	22 (0.40)	100	8303	518 (6)	34 (0.41)	86
Hitachi Health Care Center	2001	8546	NR	35 (0.41)	97	7434	NR	7 (0.09)	100
Mayo Clinic, United States	2002	1520	782 (51)	22 (1.4)	59	1464	191 (13)	3 (0.20)	0
Anti–Lung Cancer Association	2002	1611	186 (11.5)	14 (0.87)	77	7891	721 (9.1)	22 (0.28)	82
Helsinki, Finland	2002	602	111 (18)	5 (0.8)	0	NR	NR	NR	NR
Milan, Italy	2003	1035	199 (19)	11 (1.1)	55	996	99 (10)	11	91

NR, not reported.

(Matsumoto) (52,61), have reported on 15,050 participants. These studies utilized 10-mm collimation for the computed tomography (CT) scans. Two studies, ALCA and Matsumoto, included sputum cytology in the screening regimen and screening was performed at 6-month intervals in ALCA. A total of 72 lung cancers were detected during the prevalence screen (0.5%), 57 of which were stage IA (79.2%). At the same time, non-calcified nodules were present in 2564 (17%, range 5–26%) individuals. A total of 7891 follow-up examinations have been reported in the ALCA study with 19 additional cancers detected, 15 of which were stage IA (78.9%). One incidence screen has been reported in the Hitachi study in 5568 individuals with four additional detected lung cancers, three stage IA. In total, 8303 incidence screens have been reported over 2 years in the Matsumoto study with a total of 37 cancers detected, 32 of which were stage IA (86.5%). A major consideration in the Japanese trials is that screening was made available at a younger age, usually 40, and that smoking history was not a requirement for participation (nonsmokers accounted for 14% of the ALCA study, 38% of the Hitachi study, and 53% of the Matsumoto study). Thus it is unclear that these results can be generalized to usual screening cohorts.

Three European trials have been reported in the literature. In Germany, 817 asymptomatic volunteers over the age of 40 with at least a 20-pack-a-year smoking history underwent screening. At the prevalence screen 43% were found to have at least one noncalcified nodule, and 11 patients had malignancy including seven stage IA (one participant had two squamous cell carcinomas considered to be synchronous primary lesion) (60). One video-assisted thoracotomy surgery (VATS) was performed for benign disease. In Finland, 602 workers with asbestos exposure (mean 26 years) and smoking history underwent screening. The prevalence screen detected 111 cases with at least one nodule by consensus review (18%) and five lung cancers (all at least stage IIA). The authors also provided the number of follow-up procedures required; 54 repeat CT, 15 bronchoscopy, six image-guided fine-needle aspiration (FNA) and nine thoracotomy/thoracoscopy (only one for malignant disease) (53). Finally, the first 2 years of screening of 1035 subjects in Italy have been reported. All were 50 years old or older and had at least a 20-pack-a-year smoking history. The study is scheduled to perform annual screening for 5 years. Twenty percent had indeterminate nodules at baseline screening. Twenty-two lung cancers have been detected, 11 during the prevalence screen (six stage IA) and 11 during the incidence screen (10 stage IA) (56).

Three studies in the U.S. have published results. A small study designed to test the feasibility of a randomized controlled trial showed that almost 80% of subjects would be willing to be randomized to either observation or chest CT (59). Of the initial 92 randomized to CT, 30 had noncalcified nodules (32.6%). One stage I and one stage IV lung cancer were detected. The Mayo Clinic evaluated 1520 individuals 50 and older with at least a 20-pack-a-year smoking history (54,62). Sputum cytology was also performed. Noncalcified nodules were found in 69% of participants. Over 3 years, 40 cancers were detected in the population: 26 prevalence, 10 incidence, two interval (symptom detected between screening exams), and two by sputum cytology alone. Twenty-two cancers were stage 1A, 17 prevalence and five incidence. There were four limited-stage small cell carcinomas. The first U.S. CT screening study, the Early Lung Cancer Action Project (ELCAP), enrolled 1000 symptom-free individuals 60 and older with at least a 10-pack-a-year smoking history (64). The prevalence screen revealed 233 noncalcified nodules and 27 lung cancers, 23 stage I. During incidence screens, seven additional lung cancers were identified by screening, five stage I, and two by symptoms, both advanced (63).

Several trends become evident when all the trials are grouped together. The average yield for lung cancer on the prevalence screen ranges from 0.3% to 2.3%, and depends greatly on the characteristics of the screened population; in general, the yield drops off two to three times with incidence screens. The rate of detection of stage I cancers ranges from 50% to 80% at prevalence screen or 71% by pooling all screens at prevalence. During follow-up screens 75% of detected cancers are stage I; however, in the U.S. only 10 of 22 cancers (45%) detected following the prevalence screen were stage I. While this represents an improvement over chest radiograph, it is not clear that this will be enough to give a large mortality advantage. The lower percentage of stage I cancers at incidence also raises the question of overdiagnosis, particularly for prevalence cases.

Prevalence data from the Lung Screening Study, a randomized-controlled feasibility study, suggests that the stage shift needed to show an advantage of CT over chest x-ray may not be present (65). There were 3318 participants randomized to either posteroanterior (PA) radiograph or low-dose CT. Nodules or other suspicious findings were present in 20% of the CT group and 9% of the chest x-ray group. A lung cancer diagnosis was established in 30 participants in the CT arm; 16 were stage I (53%). Seven lung cancers were diagnosed in the chest x-ray arm; 6 were stage I (86%). Thus CT detected more cancers overall and more stage I cancers, but also detected more late-stage cancers. The difference in proportions, however, was not statistically significant ($p = 0.2$). The NCI-sponsored National Lung Screening Trial randomized over 50,000 male and female heavy smokers to annual chest x-ray or annual low-dose helical CT for 3 years and finished the accrual phase in early 2004. Final results are not expected until 2010.

Will Computed Tomography Screening Be Cost-Effective?
The ultimate fate of CT screening for lung cancer rests with the presence or absence of mortality benefit as well as the magnitude of benefit. Even if a benefit is detected, screening may be cost-prohibitive for the population as a whole. In the absence of long-term results, particularly as it relates to efficacy and morbidity associated with evaluation of nodules eventually deemed benign, cost-effectiveness is largely speculative as determined by cost-efficacy analysis. Two analyses have been wildly optimistic, suggesting that lung cancer screening may cost less than $10,000 per life year saved (66,67). This becomes more apparent when compared with other well-accepted intervention screening strategies such as mammography, hypertension screening in 60 year olds, and screening donated blood for HIV, which all result in a cost per life year saved of approximately $20,000 (68). In general, these studies have not accounted well for follow-up of indeterminate nodules and the possible harms of the diagnostic algorithms on benign disease. Two studies try to account for these factors. In one study, assuming 50% of cancers detected were localized and accounting for a full range of diagnostic workup and scenarios presumes a cost per life year saved ranging from $33,000 to $48,000 (69). The least optimistic model, assuming a stage-shift of 50%, used data from previous trials to account for follow-up procedures, benign biopsies, and nonadherence. Under these circumstances the cost per life year saved was calculated as $116,000 for

current smokers, $558,600 for quitting smokers, and $2,322,700 for former smokers (70). Thus, the cost-effectiveness of lung cancer screening will have a great effect on its implementation.

II. How Should Lung Cancer Be Staged?

Summary of Evidence: Current staging of lung cancer usually consists of complementary anatomic and physiologic imaging by CT and PET (Fig. 4.2). Magnetic resonance imaging is useful for evaluating local extension of superior sulcus tumors into the brachial plexus. It may also be used for

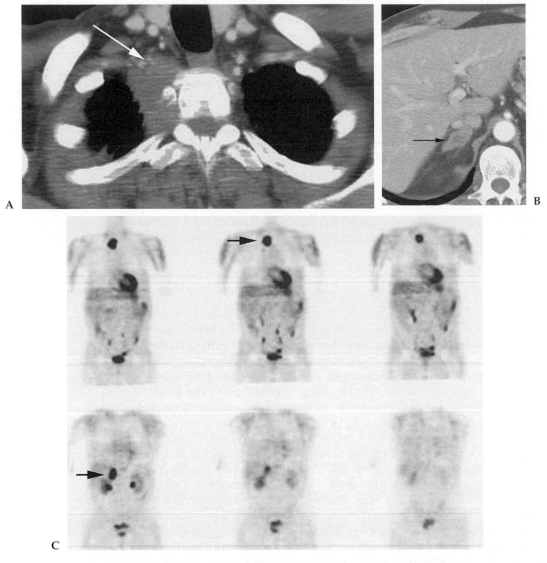

Figure 4.2. Staging lung cancer with CT and positron emission tomography (PET). A: Contrast-enhanced CT reveals right apical mass with invasion of chest wall (arrow), T3 tumor. B: Abnormal thickening of right adrenal gland (arrow) with lobular contours and central low attenuation suspicious for metastasis. C: Fluorodeoxyglucose (FDG)-PET confirms primary neoplasm and adrenal metastasis (arrow).

Table 4.3. Staging of lung cancer: tumor, node, metastasis (TNM) descriptors

Site	Name	Comment
Primary lesion	T0	No evidence of primary tumor
	Tis	Carcinoma in situ
	T1	Tumor <3 cm or less surrounded by lung or visceral pleura without invasion proximal to lobar bronchus
	T2	Tumors >3 cm; any tumor invading main bronchi but >2 cm from the carina; invasion of visceral pleura; obstructive pneumonitis extending to hila but does not involve entire lung
	T3	Tumor of any size that directly invades chest wall, diaphragm, mediastinal pleura, or parietal pericardium; or involves main bronchus within 2 cm of carina, but does not involve carina; or results in obstructive atelectasis or pneumonitis of entire lung
	T4	Tumor invades any of the following: mediastinum, heart great vessels, trachea, esophagus, vertebral body or carina; malignant ipsilateral pleural or peri cardial effusion; satellite tumor nodule within primary tumor lobe
Lymph nodes	N0	No regional lymph node metastases
	N1	Spread to ipsilateral peribronchial or hilar nodes
	N2	Spread to ipsilateral mediastinal or subcarinal nodes
	N3	Spread to contralateral mediastinal or hilar nodes; scalene nodes; supraclavicular nodes
Distant disease	M0	No distant metastases
	M1	Distant metastases present

Data from Mountain[15] and Mountain.[71]

imaging the central nervous system and occasionally to image the liver and adrenal glands. Bone scintigraphy may be used to assess for osseous metastases. Histologic subtypes including squamous cell, adenocarcinoma, and large cell carcinoma are categorized as non–small-cell lung cancer (NSCLC) due to the similar treatment and prognosis based on stage. Small cell carcinoma, the fourth major subtype, is staged separately.

Supporting Evidence: Staging of lung cancer is critical for choosing the appropriate treatment and for assessing overall prognosis. Staging is categorized by the tumor, node, metastasis (TNM) system as set forth by the American Joint Committee on Cancer and takes into account features of the primary tumor as well as dissemination to the mediastinum and distant organs (Tables 4.3 and 4.4).

A. How Is the Primary Tumor Evaluated?

Computed tomography is the preferred modality for initially establishing the diagnosis of lung cancer and providing initial staging information, as it is widely available, more sensitive than chest radiograph, rapid to perform, and guides further workup. The use of intravenous contrast is largely based on physician preference, as few studies have been performed to assess interpretive difference. Those that have been performed do not show clear superiority of enhanced over unenhanced scans (72–74). The

Table 4.4. Stage of non–small-cell lung cancer (NSCLC) based on TNM classification

0	Carcinoma in situ
1A	T1N0M0
1B	T2N0M0
2A	T1N1M0
2B	T2N1M0
	T3N0M0
3A	T3N1M0
	T1–3N2M0
3B	Any T4
	Any T3
4	Any M1

Data from Mountain[15] and Mountain.[71]

evaluation of T stage is often straightforward with CT. Difficulty may arise in the evaluation of invasion into the chest wall and mediastinum. Rib erosion, bone destruction, or tumor adjacent to mediastinal structures provides reliable evidence of invasion. Without these features, proximity and secondary signs (greater than 3 cm of contact with the pleural surface, pleural thickening, absent fat planes, and obtuse angle of tumor with the chest wall) are only moderately helpful in predicting invasion (75–78), and localized chest pain is a more specific finding (75). Magnetic resonance imaging is slightly more successful at detecting chest wall invasion (79–81) owing to better spatial resolution particularly in the lung apex (Table 4.5). Using dynamic cine evaluation of the tumor during breathing provides reliable exclusion of parietal pleura invasion, although false-positive results still occur (82–84).

B. How Is the Mediastinum Evaluated?

Because size is the determining factor for the interpretation of mediastinal adenopathy, usually 1 cm in short axis, CT is an imperfect tool for categorization of mediastinal disease. Twenty studies performed between 1991 and 2001 showed sensitivity ranges from 26% to 86% and specificity from 57% to 93% (85–104). Pooling the 3438 patients among these studies (prevalence of adenopathy 28%) gives a sensitivity, specificity, positive predictive value (PPV), and negative predictive value (NPV) of 57%, 82%, 56%, and 83%, respectively, for mediastinal disease (17). Despite advances in CT technology, there does not appear to be a significant improvement in the ability to stage the mediastinum. Few studies continue to look at CT as a staging tool, and those that do are generally studies devoted to PET imaging; thus CT technique and interpretive information is relatively spotty. The range of sensitivity (43–83%), specificity (52–94%), and accuracy (63–86%) all overlap with previous studies (105–108).

Table 4.5. Suggested imaging studies for staging lung cancer

Non–small-cell lung cancer	Small-cell lung cancer
CT of chest	CT of chest/abdomen
Whole-body PET	MRI brain
Bone scintigraphy (optional; see text)	Bone scintigraphy
MRI brain (optional; see text)	

PET, positron emission tomography.

While MRI staging is feasible, it is not widely utilized due to cost and availability. It has been suggested that MR is better at detecting hilar lymph nodes, although the clinical utility of this is unclear (109,110). The few studies performed suggest that unenhanced MRI is at best equivalent to CT (111,112), although gadolinium or new iron oxide contrast agents may ultimately increase the utility of MRI (111–113).

Fluorodeoxyglucose (FDG)-PET was initially hoped to provide definitive noninvasive staging of the mediastinum. Rather than using size as a criterion, metabolism of glucose is used as a marker of malignancy. Early studies fostered extreme optimism and it was not uncommon to see sensitivity or specificity quoted at 100% (97,114–118). In studies without either perfect sensitivity or specificity, sensitivity ranged from 52% to 93% and specificity 43% to 93% (87–89,92,94,95,119–124). Pooling the aforementioned studies resulted in sensitivity, specificity, PPV, and NPV of 84%, 89%, 79%, and 93%, respectively, in 1045 patients with a prevalence of mediastinal disease of 32% (17). A similar sensitivity and specificity (85% and 90%) were found in a second meta-analysis (125). This study also showed that the value of PET was dependent on CT findings. In the setting of a positive CT scan, sensitivity approached 100%, whereas specificity fell to 78%. When the CT did not reveal adenopathy, PET was 82% sensitive and 93% specific (125). Most recently, five studies, each with over 100 patients, have presented a less optimistic view of PET for staging the mediastinum, with sensitivity ranging from 61% to 94% and specificity from 77% to 84% (105,126–129). More importantly, in two of these studies the false-negative rate of PET in the mediastinum was over 10% (126,127). While PET clearly has better test characteristics than CT for staging the mediastinum, it is far from perfect. However, it may not be fair to judge the value of PET in staging lung cancer based on the accuracy in the mediastinum alone. The utility of PET lies in its ability to upstage or downstage patients with lung cancer based on its ability to detect previously unsuspected disease in the lung, mediastinum, or extrathoracic disease. Two studies have now shown that PET avoids unnecessary thoracotomy in approximately 20% of cases (126,130).

Most studies show incremental benefit when the combination of CT and PET is used. Newer technology allowing fusion of images either obtained at different times or on a dedicated PET/CT scanner has helped to streamline this process with promising results, increasing the sensitivity of PET alone by 5% to 8% without a change in specificity for lymph nodes and more accurate overall stage evaluation (131–133).

C. How Are Distant Metastases Evaluated?

Liver Metastasis
In the setting of negative clinical exam including normal liver function tests, the yield of CT for liver metastasis is less than 5% (17,134). Furthermore, the liver is rarely the sole site of metastatic disease at the time of diagnosis, occurring in approximately 3% of cases (135,136). Therefore, the majority of isolated liver lesions encountered during the workup of NSCLC will be benign hemangiomas or cysts. As most chest CT scans cover the majority of the liver, dedicated hepatic imaging is generally not indicated. In equivocal cases ultrasound, MRI, technetium 99m (Tc-99m)-tagged red blood cell scan, and PET may have a role and can be appro-

priately selected based on the pretest probability and the characteristics at CT. No formal studies have evaluated the merits of these imaging techniques in lung cancer.

Adrenal Metastasis

Incidental adrenal lesions are frequently encountered in the general population and thus encountered in up to 10% of lung cancer patients (137). The likelihood of metastasis is to some extent related to cancer stage, with benign adenomas predominating in stage I disease and metastases predominating in late-stage disease (134,138–140). With CT, lesions can be assumed to be benign if <10 Hounsfield units (HU) on unenhanced images (141), or <60% washout of contrast is observed with 15-minute delayed contrast-enhanced images (142–144). Signal dropout with MR chemical shift imaging (145) and a negative PET scan (146,147) can also be used to reliably confirm the benign nature of an incidental adrenal lesion. In rare cases, biopsy or adrenalectomy may be necessary.

Bone Metastasis

The majority of patients with bone metastases are either symptomatic or have an elevated alkaline phosphatase (148). Since fewer than 5% of lung cancer patients have occult bone metastases at presentation (149), routine radiologic evaluation is not warranted in asymptomatic individuals. The sensitivity of a thorough clinical exam ranges from 79% to 100% (17,148,150,151). While bone scintigraphy is quite sensitive for the detection of osseous metastases, the false-positive rate approaches 40%. Positron emission tomography also has the ability to detect bone metastases with a similar sensitivity to scintigraphy, but with a much higher specificity and negative predictive value (152–154).

Cerebral Metastasis

In the setting of a normal central nervous system exam, the yield of cerebral imaging ranges from 0% to 10% (155–161). Asymptomatic cerebral metastases are most frequently associated with adenocarcinoma and large-cell carcinoma histologic subtypes (161,162). Potentially operable tumors >3 cm in size are those most likely to benefit from routine cerebral imaging (163), but cerebral imaging is not routinely necessary for T1 tumors (160,164). Both CT and MRI with contrast are accurate for the detection of cerebral lesions. Although MRI is slightly more sensitive (165), this may not be clinically meaningful and thus far has not been shown to more accurately stage lung cancer than CT alone. Positron emission tomography has rather poor sensitivity and is not suitable for excluding cerebral metastases (166) because the brain utilizes glucose at a high rate, thus obscuring metastatic uptake if present.

D. Special Case: How Is Small Cell Lung Cancer Evaluated?

Summary of Evidence: Small cell lung cancer (SCLC) is an aggressive neoplasm of neuroendocrine cell origin with a distinct biologic behavior and is therefore grouped separately from NSCLC. Staging is determined by a two-stage system developed by the Veterans Administration Lung Cancer Study Group (167). Limited-stage disease includes disease confined to the chest and supraclavicular nodes that can be contained within a single, tolerable radiation port. For example, small cell carcinoma with bilateral paratracheal and unilateral supraclavicular adenopathy could be contained within a reasonable, single radiation port. On the other hand, a pleural effusion would require, in theory, including the entire hemithorax within a radiation port and would encompass too large a field. Extensive-stage disease includes all lesions not characterized as limited stage and those with distant metastases. Staging strategies for SCLC are similar to NSCLC. Due to the high incidence of brain metastases, routine imaging of the central nervous system is warranted.

Supporting Evidence: Bone is considered to be the most common site of metastatic disease overall (35% of cases), and therefore bone scintigraphy should be part of the initial staging evaluation (168). In patients with extensive-stage disease, up to 60% have metastatic disease in the abdomen at the time of diagnosis (169,170). This frequency warrants routine staging of the abdomen with CT scan or MRI. Cerebral metastases may be present in up to 10% of individuals at the time of diagnosis (171,172). One small study looked at the efficacy of whole-body MRI as an alternative to CT and bone scintigraphy and found it to be equivalent (173). Fluorodeoxyglucose-PET has the potential to provide definitive whole-body staging in SCLC; however, experience at this time is limited. Three studies with a total of 59 exams in 53 patients showed agreement of PET with conventional staging in 43 of 59 cases and resulted in upstaging from limited to extensive disease in nine cases (15%) (174–176).

E. Special Case: What Is the Appropriate Radiologic Follow-Up?

Summary of Evidence: Two issues arise during the follow-up of lung cancer: measurement of tumors to document response to therapy and what routine follow-up tests are warranted after the completion of first-line therapy. Long-axis unidimensional measurements are appropriate for following lesions with CT or MRI. To the extent possible, the same scanning technique and interpreter should follow an individual case. Fluorodeoxyglucose-PET may eventually provide additional data by following metabolic response via standard uptake value (SUV) determination. After definitive therapy, routine imaging evaluations are not necessary.

Supporting Evidence: Originally, tumor response in clinical trials was guided by the World Health Organization (WHO) and required bidimensional measurements. Several studies have looked at the use of unidimensional long axis measurements [Response Evaluation Criteria in Solid Tumors (RECIST) Group] compared to bidimensional and volumetric measures of response. The RECIST criteria have been shown to be equivalent to WHO criteria and volumetric measurements in the classification of response to therapy (177–181). Evaluating 1221 lung cancer patients in clinical trials, a 31% response rate was documented by using both RECIST and WHO criteria with only one disagreement between stable disease and partial response (180). While the criterion used does not seem to have an impact on response evaluation, two studies have looked at the effect of reader variability. Inter- and intraobserver variation for initial tumor size is 10% to 15% and 5%, respectively (182,183). The impact on disease progression and response is affected to a greater degree. Using RECIST criteria, inter- and intraobserver variability for progressive disease ranged from 21% to 48% (average, 30%) and 3% to 15% (average, 9%), respectively.

Response was affected to a lesser degree, interobserver 3% to 27% (average, 15%) and intraobserver 0% to 6% (average, 4%) (182).

Induction chemotherapy may be employed in selected patients with mediastinal disease in order to render patients resectable for cure. Because of the inherent difficulties of repeat mediastinoscopy, PET has been evaluated as a means of re-staging the mediastinum in 130 patients in four separate studies (184–187). Two reports, which included a total of 49 patients, had a combined accuracy of 95% (184,187). This experience, however, has not been reproducible, with two other studies showing an accuracy of 50%. When compared directly to CT for all lymph nodes, accuracy was better for PET in one (185) and CT in the other (186). Positron emission tomography response, however, does correlate to some degree with survival as those with follow-up SUV less than 2.5 or decreased over 20% have improved time to disease progression and overall survival (188,189).

Imaging following treatment with curative intent is of unclear value. Although the major professional societies include surveillance chest radiograph as part of follow-up recommendations (190–192), the hard evidence for this practice is difficult to find (193,194). One prospective study of 192 patients with aggressive follow-up showed better 3-year survival for asymptomatic recurrence detection (31% vs. 13%) and that 43% of asymptomatic recurrences could be treated surgically (195). Similar to the screened population setting, lead and length time bias make the relevance of the survival data unclear. Two retrospective studies separately came to the conclusion that strict follow-up had little effect on mortality (196,197).

Suggested Imaging Protocols

Low-Dose Screening Computed Tomography

Collimation: 1.25–2.5 mm
Reconstruction interval: 2 mm
Technique: 120 kVp/20–50 milliampere-second (mAs)
Extent: Scan from lung apices through posterior costophrenic sulcus
Breath hold: full inspiration
Reconstruction algorithm: standard or detail
Contrast: none

Chest Computed Tomography for Lung Cancer Staging

Collimation: 5 mm
Technique: 120 kVp/100–150 mAs
Extent: scan from lung apices through adrenal glands
Breath hold: full inspiration
Reconstruction algorithm: standard
Contrast (optional): ~100 cc nonionic contrast; injection rate = 2.5 cc/sec; 30 second prescan delay

Future Research

1. Can biomarker analysis provide a better target population for screening?
2. Does PET with SUV provide better or improved prognostic information than the current staging system?

3. Can imaging be utilized noninvasively to detect microscopic metastases?
4. Can imaging of biomarkers be utilized to select the most appropriate treatment regimen and aid in the delivery of novel treatments?

References

1. Alberg AJ, Samet JM. Chest 2003;123(1 suppl):21S–49S.
2. Hecht SS. J Natl Cancer Inst 1999;91(14):1194–1210.
3. Jemal A, Murray T, Samuels A, Ghafoor A, Ward E, Thun MJ. CA Cancer J Clin 2003;53(1):5–26.
4. Carney DN. N Engl J Med 2002;346(2):126–128.
5. Wingo PA, Ries LA, Giovino GA, et al. J Natl Cancer Inst 1999;91(8):675–690.
6. Tong L, Spitz MR, Fueger JJ, Amos CA. Cancer. 1996;78(5):1004–1010.
7. Lubin JH, Boice JD Jr, Edling C, et al. J Natl Cancer Inst 1995;87(11):817–827.
8. Lubin JH, Boice JD Jr. J Natl Cancer Inst 1997;89(1):49–57.
9. Howe GR. Radiat Res 1995;142(3):295–304.
10. MMWR 2002;51(14):300–303.
11. Warner KE, Hodgson TA, Carroll CE. Tob Control 1999;8(3):290–300.
12. Penberthy L, Retchin SM, McDonald MK, et al. Health Care Manag Sci 1999;2(3):149–160.
13. Hillner BE, McDonald MK, Desch CE, et al. J Clin Oncol 1998;16(4):1420–1424.
14. Herman CR, Gill HK, Eng J, Fajardo LL. AJR Am J Roentgenol 2002; 179(4):825–831.
15. Mountain C. Chest 1997;111:1710–1717.
16. Silvestri GA, Tanoue LT, Margolis ML, Barker J, Detterbeck F. Chest 2003;123 (1 suppl):147S–156S.
17. Toloza EM, Harpole L, McCrory DC. Chest 2003;123(1 suppl):137S–146S.
18. Boucot KR, Weiss W. JAMA 1973;224(10):1361–1365.
19. Brett GZ. Br Med J 1969;4:260–262.
20. Manser RL, Irving LB, Stone C, Byrnes G, Abramson M, Campbell D. Cochrane Database Syst Rev 2001;3.
21. Sobue T, Suzuki T, Naruke T. Jpn J Cancer Res 1992;83(5):424–430.
22. Tsukada H, Kurita Y, Yokoyama A, et al. Br J Cancer 2001;85(9):1326–1331.
23. Sagawa M, Tsubono Y, Saito Y, et al. Cancer 2001;92(3):588–594.
24. Nishii K, Ueoka H, Kiura K, et al. Lung Cancer 2001;34(3):325–332.
25. Nakayama T, Baba T, Suzuki T, Sagawa M, Kaneko M. Eur J Cancer 2002;38(10):1380–1387.
26. Sagawa M, Nakayama T, Tsukada H, et al. Lung Cancer 2003;41(1):29–36.
27. Dominioni L, Imperatori A, Rovera F, Ochetti A, Paolucci M, Dionigi G. Cancer 2000;89(11 suppl):2345–2348.
28. Salomaa ER. Cancer 2000;89(11 suppl):2387–2391.
29. Friedman GD, Collen MF, Fireman BH. J Chronic Dis 1986;39(6):453–463.
30. Wilde J. Eur Respir J 1989;2(7):656–662.
31. Berlin NI, Buncher CR, Fontana RS, Frost JK, Melamed MR. Am Rev Respir Dis 1984;130(4):545–549.
32. Frost JK, Ball WC Jr, Levin ML, et al. Am Rev Respir Dis 1984;130(4):549–554.
33. Flehinger BJ, Melamed MR, Zaman MB, Heelan RT, Perchick WB, Martini N. Am Rev Respir Dis 1984;130(4):555–560.
34. Melamed MR, Flehinger BJ, Zaman MB, Heelan RT, Perchick WA, Martini N. Chest 1984;86(1):44–53.
35. Melamed MR. Cancer 2000;89(11 suppl):2356–2362.
36. Berlin NI. Cancer 2000;89(11 suppl):2349–2351.
37. Kubik A, Polak J. Cancer 1986;57(12):2427–2437.
38. Kubik A, Parkin D, Khlat M, Erban J, Polak J, Adamec M. Int J Cancer 1990;45:26–33.

39. Kubik AK, Parkin DM, Zatloukal P. Cancer 2000;89(11 suppl):2363–2368.
40. Fontana RS, Sanderson DR, Woolner LB, et al. Clin Notes Respir Dis 1976; 15(3):13–14.
41. Fontana R, Sanderson D, Taylor W, et al. Am Rev Respir Dis 1984;130:561–565.
42. Fontana RS. Cancer 2000;89(11 suppl):2352–2355.
43. Fontana RS, Sanderson DR, Woolner LB, et al. Cancer 1991;67(4 suppl):1 155–1164.
44. Marcus P, Bergstralh E, Fagerstrom R, et al. J Natl Cancer Inst 2000;92: 1308–1316.
45. Grannis FW Jr. Chest 2001;119(2):322–323.
46. Strauss G. J Clin Oncol 2002;20:1973–1983.
47. Strauss GM, Gleason RE, Sugarbaker DJ. Chest 1995;107(6 suppl):270S– 279S.
48. Flehinger BJ, Kimmel M, Polyak T, Melamed MR. Cancer 1993;72(5):1573–1580.
49. Strauss GM, Gleason RE, Sugarbaker DJ. Chest 1997;111(3):754–768.
50. Marcus PM, Prorok PC. J Med Screen 1999;6(1):47–49.
51. Prorok PC, Andriole GL, Bresalier RS, et al. Control Clin Trials 2000;21 (6 suppl):273S–309S.
52. Sone S, Takashima S, Li F, et al. Lancet 1998;351(9111):1242–1245.
53. Tiitola M, Kivisaari L, Huuskonen MS, et al. Lung Cancer 2002;35(1):17–22.
54. Swensen S, Jett J, Sloan J, et al. Am J Respir Crit Care Med 2002;165:508–513.
55. Sobue T, Moriyama N, Kaneko M, et al. J Clin Oncol 2002;20(4):911–920.
56. Pastorino U, Bellomi M, Landoni C, et al. Lancet 2003;362(9384):593–597.
57. Nawa T, Nakagawa T, Kusano S, Kawasaki Y, Sugawara Y, Nakata H. Chest 2002;122(1):15–20.
58. Henschke CI. Cancer 1 2000;89(11 suppl):2474–2482.
59. Garg K, Keith RL, Byers T, et al. Radiology 2002;225(2):506–510.
60. Diederich S, Wormanns D, Semik M, et al. Radiology 2002;222:773–781.
61. Sone S, Li F, Yang ZG, et al. Br J Cancer 2001;84(1):25–32.
62. Swensen S, Jett J, Hartman T, et al. Radiology 2003;226:756–761.
63. Henschke CI, Naidich DP, Yankelevitz DF, et al. Cancer 2001;92(1):153–159.
64. Henschke C, McCauley D, Yankelevitz D, et al. Lancet 1999;354:99–105.
65. Gohagan J, Marcus P, Fagerstrom R, Pinsky P, Kramer B, Prorok P. Chest 2004;126(1):114–121.
66. Miettinen OS. Can Med Assoc J 2000;162(10):1431–1436.
67. Wisnivesky JP, Mushlin AI, Sicherman N, Henschke C. Chest 2003;124(2): 614–621.
68. Tengs TO, Adams ME, Pliskin JS, et al. Risk Anal 1995;15(3):369–390.
69. Chirikos T, Hazelton T, Tockman M, Clark R. Chest 2002;121:1507–1514.
70. Mahadevia PJ, Fleisher LA, Frick KD, Eng J, Goodman SN, Powe NR. JAMA 2003;289(3):313–322.
71. Mountain C, Dresler C. Chest 1997;111:1718–1723.
72. Haramati LB, Cartagena AM, Austin JH. J Comput Assist Tomogr 1995; 19(3):375–378.
73. Cascade PN, Gross BH, Kazerooni EA, et al. AJR 1998;170(4):927–931.
74. Patz EJ, Erasmus J, McAdams H, et al. Radiology 1999;212:56–60.
75. Glazer HS, Duncan-Meyer J, Aronberg DJ, Moran JF, Levitt RG, Sagel SS. Radiology 1985;157(1):191–194.
76. Glazer HS, Kaiser LR, Anderson DJ, et al. Radiology 1989;173(1):37–42.
77. Pearlberg JL, Sandler MA, Beute GH, Lewis JW Jr, Madrazo BL. J Comput Assist Tomogr 1987;11(2):290–293.
78. Pennes DR, Glazer GM, Wimbish KJ, Gross BH, Long RW, Orringer MB. AJR 1985;144(3):507–511.
79. Heelan R, Demas B, Caravelli J, et al. Radiology 1989;170:637–641.
80. Padovani B, Mouroux J, Seksik L, et al. Radiology 1993;187(1):33–38.
81. Haggar AM, Pearlberg JL, Froelich JW, et al. AJR 1987;148(6):1075–1078.
82. Kodalli N, Erzen C, Yuksel M. Clin Imaging 1999;23(4):227–235.

83. Sakai S, Murayama S, Murakami J, Hashiguchi N, Masuda K. J Comput Assist Tomogr 1997;21(4):595–600.
84. Shiotani S, Sugimura K, Sugihara M, et al. Radiat Med 2000;20:697–713.
85. Suzuki K, Nagai K, Yoshida J, Nishimura M, Takahashi K, Nishiwaki Y. J Thorac Cardiovasc Surg 1999;117(3):593–598.
86. Takamochi K, Nagai K, Yoshida J, et al. J Thorac Cardiovasc Surg 2000;119: 1135–1140.
87. Vansteenkiste JF, Stroobants SG, De Leyn PR, et al. J Clin Oncol 1998;16: 2142–2149.
88. Vansteenkiste JF, Stroobants SG, Dupont PJ, et al. Eur J Nucl Med 1998;25: 1495–1501.
89. Dunagan DP, Chin R, McCain TW, et al. Chest 2001;119:333–339.
90. Kamiyoshihara M, Kawashima O, Ishikawa S, Morishita Y. J Cardiovasc Surg 2001;42:119–124.
91. Osada H, Kojima K, Tsukada H, Nakajima Y, Imamura K, Matsumoto J. Jpn J Thorac Cardiovasc Surg 2001;49:1–10.
92. Pieterman R, van Putten J, Meuzelaar J, et al. N Engl J Med 2000;343:254–261.
93. Primack SL, Lee KS, Logan PM, Miller RR, Muller NL. Radiology 1994;193: 795–800.
94. Marom EM, McAdams HP, Erasmus JJ, et al. Radiology 1999;212(3):803–809.
95. Saunders CAB, Dussek JE, O'Doherty MJ, et al. Ann Thorac Surg 1999;67: 790–797.
96. Gdeedo A, Van Schil P, Corthouts B, Van Mieghem F, Van Meerbeeck J, Van Marck E. Eur Respir J 1997;10:1547–1551.
97. Bury T, Paulus P, Dowlati A, et al. Eur Respir J 1996;9:2560–2564.
98. Bury T, Dowlati A, Paulus P, et al. Eur Respir J 1997;10:2529–2534.
99. Buccheri G, Biggi A, Ferrigno D, et al. Thorax 1996;51(4):359–363.
100. Aaby C, Kristensen S, Nielsen S. ORL J Otorhinolaryngol Relat Spec 1995; 57:279–285.
101. Yokoi K, Okuyama A, Mori K, et al. Radiology 1994;192(3):813–817.
102. McLoud T, Bourgouin P, Greenberg R, et al. Radiology 1992;182:319–323.
103. Jolly PC, Hutchinson CH, Detterbeck F, Guyton SW, Hofer B, Anderson RP. J Thorac Cardiovasc Surg 1991;102:266–270.
104. Cole PH, Roszkowski A, Firouz-Abadi A, Dare A. Aust N Z J Med 1993;23(6): 688–691.
105. Cerfolio RJ, Ojha B, Bryant AS, Bass CS, Bartalucci AA, Mountz JM. Ann Thorac Surg 2003;76(3):861–866.
106. Kiernan PD, Sheridan MJ, Lamberti J, et al. South Med J 2002;95(10):1168–1172.
107. Luketich JD, Friedman DM, Meltzer CC, et al. Clin Lung Cancer 2001; 2(3):229–233.
108. Zimny M, Hochstenbag M, Lamers R, et al. Eur Radiol 2003;13(4):740–747.
109. Hasegawa I, Eguchi K, Kohda E, et al. Eur J Radiol 2003;45(2):129–134.
110. Boiselle PM, Patz EF Jr, Vining DJ, Weissleder R, Shepard JA, McLoud TC. Radiographics 1998;18(5):1061–1069.
111. Crisci R, Di Cesare E, Lupattelli L, Coloni GF. Eur J Cardiothorac Surg 1997; 11:214–217.
112. Glazer GM. Chest 1989;96(1 suppl):44S–47S.
113. Kernstine KH, Stanford W, Mullan BF, et al. Ann Thorac Surg 1999;68(3): 1022–1028.
114. Bury T, Dowlati A, Paulus P, et al. Eur Respir J 1997;10:2529–2534.
115. Farrell M, McAdams H, Herndon J, Patz E Jr. Radiology 2000;215:886–890.
116. Guhlmann A, Storck M, Kotzerke J, Moog F, Sunder-Plassmann L, Reske SN. Thorax 1997;52:438–441.
117. Sazon DA, Santiago SM, Soo Hoo GW, et al. Am J Respir Crit Care Med 1996;153:417–421.
118. Scott WJ, Gobar LS, Terry JD, Dewan NA, Sunderland JJ. J Thorac Cardiovasc Surg 1996;111:642–648.

119. Wahl RL, Quint LE, Greenough RL, Meyer CR, White RJ, Orringer MB. Radiology 1994;191:371–377.
120. Chin R, Jr., Ward R, Keyes JW, et al. Am J Respir Crit Care Med 1995; 152:2090–2096.
121. Steinert HC, Hauser M, Allemann F, et al. Radiology 1997;202:441–446.
122. Magnani P, Carretta A, Rizzo G, et al. J Cardiovasc Surg 1999;40:741–748.
123. Liewald F, Grosse S, Storck M, et al. Thorac Cardiovasac Surg 2000;48:93–96.
124. Roberts PF, Follette DM, von Haag D, et al. Ann Thorac Surg 2000; 70:1154–1160.
125. Gould MK, Kuschner WG, Rydzak CE, et al. Ann Intern Med 2003; 139(11):879–892.
126. Reed CE, Harpole DH, Posther KE, et al. J Thorac Cardiovasc Surg 2003; 126(6):1943–1951.
127. Gonzalez-Stawinski GV, Lemaire A, Merchant F, et al. J Thorac Cardiovasc Surg 2003;126(6):1900–1905.
128. Graeter TP, Hellwig D, Hoffmann K, Ukena D, Kirsch CM, Schafers HJ. Ann Thorac Surg 2003;75(1):231–235, discussion 235–236.
129. Kernstine KH, McLaughlin KA, Menda Y, et al. Ann Thorac Surg 2002; 73(2):394–401; discussion 401–392.
130. van Tinteren H, Hoekstra OS, Smit EF, et al. Lancet 2002;359(9315):1388–1393.
131. Antoch G, Stattaus J, Nemat AT, et al. Non-small cell lung cancer: dual-modality PET/CT in preoperative staging. Radiology 2003;229(2):526–533.
132. Hany TF, Steinert HC, Goerres GW, Buck A, von Schulthess GK. Radiology 2002;225(2):575–581.
133. Lardinois D, Weder W, Hany TF, et al. N Engl J Med 2003;348(25):2500–2507.
134. Silvestri G, Littenberg B, Colice G. Am J Respir Crit Care Med 1995; 152:225–230.
135. Kagohashi K, Satoh H, Ishikawa H, Ohtsuka M, Sekizawa K. Med Oncol 2003;20(1):25–28.
136. Hillers T, Sauve M, Guyatt G. Thorax 1994;49:14–19.
137. Oliver T Jr, Bernardino M, Miller J, Mansour K, Greene D, Davis W. Radiology 1984;153:217–218.
138. Pearlberg JL, Sandler MA, Beute GH, et al. Radiology 1985;157:187–190.
139. Heavey LR, Glazer GM, Gross BH, Francis IR, Orringer MB. AJR 1986; 146(2):285–290.
140. Eggesbo HB, Hansen G. Acta Radiol 1996;37:343–347.
141. Boland GW, Lee MJ, Gazelle GS, Halpern EF, McNicholas MM, Mueller PR. AJR 1998;171(1):201–204.
142. Caoili EM, Korobkin M, Francis IR, Cohan RH, Dunnick NR. AJR 2000; 175(5):1411–1415.
143. Caoili EM, Korobkin M, Francis IR, et al. Radiology 2002;222(3):629–633.
144. Korobkin M, Brodeur FJ, Francis IR, Quint LE, Dunnick NR, Londy F. AJR 1998;170(3):747–752.
145. Heinz-Peer G, Honigschnabi S, Schneider B, et al. AJR 1999;173:15–22.
146. Gupta NC, Graeber GM, Tamim WJ, Rogers JS, Irisari L, Bishop HA. Clin Lung Cancer 2001;3(1):59–64.
147. Erasmus JJ, Patz EF Jr, McAdams HP, et al. AJR 1997;168(5):1357–1360.
148. Salvatierra A, Baamonde C, Llamas JM, et al. Chest 1990;97:1052–1058.
149. Little AG, Stitik FP. Chest 1990;97(6):1431–1438.
150. Tornyos K, Garcia O, Karr B, et al. Clin Nucl Med 1991;16:107–109.
151. Michel F, Soler M, Imhof E, et al. Thorax 1991;46:469–473.
152. Hsia TC, Shen YY, Yen RF, Kao CH, Changlai SP. Neoplasma 2002; 49(4):267–271.
153. Bury T, Barreto A, Daenen F, Barthelemy N, Ghaye B, Rigo P. Eur J Nucl Med 1998;25(9):1244–1247.
154. Gayed I, Vu T, Johnson M, Macapinlac H, Podoloff D. Mol Imaging Biol 2003;5(1):26–31.

155. Cole FH Jr, Thomas JE, Wilcox AB, Halford HH 3rd. Ann Thorac Surg 1994;57(4):838–840.
156. Colice G, Birkmeyer J, Black W, Littenberg B, Silvestri G. Chest 1995;108: 1264–1271.
157. Butler AR, Leo JS, Lin JP, et al. Radiology 1979;131:339–401.
158. Ferrigno D, Buccheri G. Chest 1994;106:1025–1029.
159. Jacobs L, Kinkel WR, Vincent RG. Arch Neurol 1977;77:690–693.
160. Kormas P, Bradshaw J, Jeyasingham K. Thorax 1992;47:106–108.
161. Mintz BJ, Turhim S, Alexander S, et al. Chest 1984;86:850–853.
162. Hooper RG, Tenholder MF, Underwood, et al. Chest 1984;85:774–777.
163. Earnest F, Ryu J, Miller G, et al. Radiology 1999;211:137–145.
164. Cole JFH, Thomas JE, Wilcox AB, et al. Ann Thorac Surg 1994;57:838–840.
165. Davis PC, Hudgins PA, Peterman SB, et al. AJR 1991;156:1039–1046.
166. Rohren EM, Provenzale JM, Barboriak DP, Coleman RE. Radiology 2003; 226(1):181–187.
167. Osterlind K, Ihde DC, Ettinger DS, et al. Cancer Treat Rep 1983;67(1):3–9.
168. Adjei AA, Marks RS, Bonner JA. Mayo Clin Proc 1999;74(8):809–816.
169. Whitley NO, Mirvis SE. Crit Rev Diagn Imaging 1989;29(2):103–116.
170. Mirvis SE, Whitley NO, Aisner J, Moody M, Whitacre M, Whitley JE. AJR 1987; 148(5):845–847.
171. Hirsch FR, Paulson OB, Hansen HH, Larsen SO. Cancer 1983;51(3):529–533.
172. Giannone L, Johnson DH, Hande KR, Greco FA. Ann Intern Med 1987; 106(3):386–389.
173. Jelinek JS, Redmond J 3rd, Perry JJ, et al. Radiology 1990;177(3):837–842.
174. Hauber HP, Bohuslavizki KH, Lund CH, Fritscher-Ravens A, Meyer A, Pforte A. Chest 2001;119(3):950–954.
175. Chin R Jr, McCain TW, Miller AA, et al. Lung Cancer 2002;37(1):1–6.
176. Schumacher T, Brink I, Mix M, et al. Eur J Nucl Med 2001;28(4):483–488.
177. Sohaib SA, Turner B, Hanson JA, Farquharson M, Oliver RT, Reznek RH. Br J Radiol 2000;73(875):1178–1184.
178. Watanabe H, Yamamoto S, Kunitoh H, et al. Cancer Sci 2003;94(11):1015–1020.
179. Werner-Wasik M, Xiao Y, Pequignot E, Curran WJ, Hauck W. Int J Radiat Oncol Biol Phys 2001;51(1):56–61.
180. Therasse P, Arbuck SG, Eisenhauer EA, et al. J Natl Cancer Inst 2000; 92(3):205–216.
181. James K, Eisenhauer E, Christian M, et al. J Natl Cancer Inst 1999;91(6):523–528.
182. Erasmus JJ, Gladish GW, Broemeling L, et al. J Clin Oncol 2003; 21(13):2574–2582.
183. Hopper KD, Kasales CJ, Van Slyke MA, Schwartz TA, TenHave TR, Jozefiak JA. AJR 1996;167(4):851–854.
184. Cerfolio RJ, Ojha B, Mukherjee S, Pask AH, Bass CS, Katholi CR. J Thorac Cardiovasc Surg 2003;125(4):938–944.
185. Akhurst T, Downey RJ, Ginsberg MS, et al. Ann Thorac Surg 2002; 73(1):259–264; discussion 264–256.
186. Port JL, Kent MS, Korst RJ, Keresztes R, Levin MA, Altorki NK. Ann Thorac Surg 2004;77(1):254–259.
187. Vansteenkiste JF, Stroobants SG, De Leyn PR, Dupont PJ, Verbeken EK. Ann Oncol 1998;9(11):1193–1198.
188. Patz EF Jr, Connolly J, Herndon J. AJR 2000;174(3):769–774.
189. Weber WA, Petersen V, Schmidt B, et al. J Clin Oncol 2003;21(14):2651–2657.
190. Association of Community Cancer Centers. Oncology patient management guidelines, version 3.0. Rockville, MD: Association of Community Cancer Centers, 2000.
191. National Comprehensive Cancer Network. Practice guidelines for non-small-cell lung cancer. Rockledge, PA: National Comprehensive Cancer Network, 2000.

192. American College of Radiology. Follow-up of non-small cell lung cancer: appropriateness criteria. Reston, VA: American College of Radiology, 1999.
193. Smith TJ. Semin Oncol 2003;30(3):361–368.
194. Colice GL, Rubins J, Unger M. Chest 2003;123(1 suppl):272S–283S.
195. Westeel V, Choma D, Clement F, et al. Ann Thorac Surg 2000;70(4):1185–1190.
196. Walsh GL, O'Connor M, Willis KM, et al. Ann Thorac Surg 1995;60(6): 1563–1570, discussion 1570–1562.
197. Younes RN, Gross JL, Deheinzelin D. Chest 1999;115(6):1494–1499.

5

Imaging-Based Screening for Colorectal Cancer

James M.A. Slattery, Lucy E. Modahl, and Michael E. Zalis

Key Points

- Screening reduces colorectal cancer (CRC) incidence and mortality (strong evidence).
- All major strategies for CRC screening have favorable cost-effectiveness ratios compared to no screening (moderate evidence).
- Available evidence does not support choosing one test over another (moderate evidence).
- Increased compliance with CRC screening is critical to reduce CRC incidence and mortality (moderate evidence).

Definition and Pathophysiology

The consensus now holds that in the vast majority of sporadic cases, colorectal cancer (CRC) arises within a precursor lesion, the adenomatous polyp (1,2). The adenoma–carcinoma sequence hypothesis is supported by indirect evidence from several sources. Both CRC and polyps have a similar anatomic distribution. The mean age of onset of polyps predates the mean age of onset of carcinoma by several years, and cancer rarely develops in the absence of polyps (3). Patients with one or more large adenomatous polyps ($\geq$1 cm) are at increased risk of developing CRC (4,5), most of which develop at the site of the polyp, if left in place (5). In addition, patients with genetic predisposition to colonic polyp formation are at greatly increased risk of CRC (6). Finally, several studies have shown that polypectomy significantly reduces the incidence of CRC (7–9). Importantly for imaging-based screening, the risk of a polyp harboring a carcinoma is related directly to the size of the lesion: in polyps less than 1 cm in size, the risk is estimated to be <1%; in polyps measuring 1 to 2 cm, the risk increases to 10%; and in polyps larger than 2 cm, the risk is 25% or more (10).

Initiation of CRC is thought to require only two mutations in the adenomatous polyposis coli (*APC*) gene (a tumor suppressor gene). *APC* mutations are seen in about 60% of sporadic CRC (11). The germline *APC* gene is mutated in familial adenomatous polyposis (FAP) coli (12). Progression from premalignant polyp to invasive carcinoma is the result of further mutations in other genes, including *K-ras*, *DCC*, and *p53*.

Epidemiology

Colorectal cancer remains the second most common cause of cancer-related death in the United States, with an estimated annual incidence of 150,000 (13). Mortality rates from CRC are equal in both sexes, with approximately 60,000 individuals in the U.S. succumbing to this disease annually, which accounts for approximately 10% of cancer deaths. The lifetime risk of developing CRC is approximately 6%, while the estimated lifetime risk of CRC-related death is approximately 2.6%. The 5-year survival rate is 90% for early-stage CRC localized to the colon or rectum, 66% if there is regional spread, and 10% if there are distant metastases (13). Only 38% of CRC is diagnosed before it has spread beyond the bowel (13). The overall 5-year survival has increased from 50% in 1974 to 62% in 1999 (13). Risk factors for CRC include FAP, hereditary nonpolyposis colorectal cancer (HNPCC), family history of CRC in a first-degree relative before age 60, personal history of CRC, age, diet high in animal fat, chronic inflammatory bowel disease, obesity, physical inactivity, diabetes, smoking, and alcohol.

Overall Cost to Society

Treatment of colorectal carcinoma is estimated to cost between $5.5 and $6.5 billion per year in the U.S., and between $14 and $22 billion worldwide. All currently available screening strategies are estimated to cost less than $40,000 per year of life saved, comparable to other screening programs utilized in the U.S., such as screening mammography in women over age 50 (14).

Goals

In general, screening for any disease can be justified in the following circumstances: (a) the disease is prevalent and is associated with clinically significant morbidity and mortality; (b) screening tests are available, acceptable, feasible, and sufficiently accurate for the detection of early disease; (c) earlier diagnosis and treatment is associated with improved prognosis; and (d) the sum of the benefits associated with screening outweighs the sum of the potential harms and costs. Colorectal cancer screening fulfills each of these criteria. The goal of image-based screening is to detect premalignant adenomatous polyps in an average risk population, thereby enabling removal prior to the development of invasive CRC. There is growing consensus that the target lesion is the advanced adenoma, a polyp containing high-grade cellular dysplasia, the vast majority of which are >1 cm in size (15).

Methodology

We reviewed listings and articles available by Medline (PubMed, National Library of Medicine, Bethesda, Maryland) related to colorectal cancer, colon cancer screening strategies, and cost-effectiveness of colon cancer screening. The search covered the period 1966 to January 2004, and employed search strategies including the terms *colon cancer*, *colon cancer screening*, *barium enema*, *CT colonography*, *virtual colonoscopy*, and *colonoscopy*. The authors performed preliminary evaluation of abstracts resulting from the on-line search and followed this with analysis of full articles; analysis was limited to articles and material relating to human subjects and published in English.

I. Who Should Undergo Colorectal Screening?

Summary of Evidence: In a person with average risk for CRC, the most significant risk factor for developing CRC is age. Over 90% of CRC occurs over the age of 50. Average-risk individuals are those who are deemed not to have an increased or high risk for colorectal carcinoma. Individuals at increased or high risk are those who have a personal or family history of FAP syndrome, hereditary nonpolyposis colorectal cancer, adenomatous polyps, or colorectal cancer, or a personal history of inflammatory bowel disease, colonic polyps, or CRC. Methods to detect polyps and colon cancer include fecal occult blood testing (FOBT), flexible sigmoidoscopy, and colonoscopy. Imaging-based screening methods are double-contrast barium enema (DCBE), and more recently computed tomographic colonography (CTC). Published randomized controlled trials (RCTs) and case-control studies have demonstrated that FOBT and sigmoidoscopy can reduce CRC incidence and mortality. To date, there are no RCTs evaluating sigmoidoscopy, DCBE, or colonoscopy in average risk screening populations. Recent data suggest that CTC has performance characteristics equivalent to conventional colonoscopy for detection of polyps, when adequately trained radiologists employing state-of-the-art technique perform it. The American Cancer Society currently recommends that all adults aged 50 or older with average risk of CRC follow one of the following screening schedules: FOBT every year; flexible sigmoidoscopy every 5 years; annual FOBT and flexible sigmoidoscopy every 5 years (preferred to either alone); DCBE every 5 years; colonoscopy every 10 years. In persons with increased risk of CRC, screening may be more frequent and start at an earlier age (see Special Case: Patients with Increased Risk of Colorectal Cancer, below).

Supporting Evidence

A. Fecal Occult Blood Testing (FOBT)

The strongest evidence for CRC screening efficacy comes from trials using FOBTs. The FOBT is used to detect blood in the stool and is a guaiac-based test for peroxidase activity. Three RCTs have demonstrated that FOBT when followed by colonoscopy can reduce CRC mortality (7,16,17) (strong evidence). The largest of these is the Minnesota Trial (7), which has reported a mortality reduction of 33% at 13 years of follow-up, based on annual FOBT with hydration and 21% at 18 years of follow-up based on biennial testing. The two European studies have examined biennial testing without rehydration and have reported mortality reductions at 7.8 (16) and 10 years (17) of 15% and 18%, respectively. Fecal occult blood testing, while inexpensive and well tolerated, has limitations. One-time testing has sensitivity for cancer detection of only 33% to 50% (7,18). Specificity ranges from 90% to 98% (7,16,17). This means that up to 10% of all patients screening will have a false-positive result. In fact, only 5% to 10% of positive reactions are due to cancer (19). The diagnostic performance for detection of asymptomatic polyps is poor, the majority of patients with adenomas testing negative (20,21). Furthermore, FOBT offers no precise anatomic localization of lesions. Current guidelines suggest yearly FOBT testing with colonoscopic follow-up for patients with a positive test.

B. Sigmoidoscopy

Evidence of mortality reduction for sigmoidoscopy is derived from case-control studies (8,22,23) and a cohort study (24). One study estimated that sigmoidoscopy reduced rectal cancer mortality by approximately 70% (22). However, a rigid sigmoidoscope was used and therefore, on the basis of strict technique-linked criterion, the results are not applicable to flexible sigmoidoscopy (moderate evidence). In another case-control study (23), approximately two thirds of the procedures were performed with a flexible sigmoidoscope. However, only 27 patients had fatal distal cancer and some were at higher risk for CRC (limited evidence). In a case-control study by Muller and Sonnenberg (8), the study population was symptomatic (moderate evidence). A cohort study of 25,000 asymptomatic men and women followed from 1986 to 1994 showed that sigmoidoscopy reduced the overall risk of colorectal carcinoma by 40% (24) (moderate evidence). Sigmoidoscopy has several limitations. Total colon exam recommended by several expert panels, including the American Cancer Society (25), is not accomplished. Flexible sigmoidoscopy allows examination of only about 60 cm of the colon and detects only 60% of colon cancers, while lesions in the transverse and right colon are not at all detected by this technique (26). Approximately 30% of patients with colon cancer have disease proximal to the splenic flexure without evidence of neoplasia distal to the splenic flexure, which will not be detected at sigmoidoscopy (27). A screening study of 2000 patients (28), demonstrated that 62% of patients with advanced proximal neoplasia had either no distal lesions or only hyperplastic polyps, which currently do not warrant colonoscopy. Clearly, sigmoidoscopy is inadequate in this setting.

C. Combined Sigmoidoscopy and FOBT

The evidence base for combining FOBT with sigmoidoscopy is limited, but it is likely that the combination of both screening methods is more effective than either method of screening alone for several reasons. Both strategies have been demonstrated to reduce deaths from CRC individually. A study of biennial FOBT (29) reported a reduction in mortality from CRC of 8% when lesions were located in the sigmoid/rectum and 28% when located elsewhere in the colon. This suggests that FOBT is less sensitive for the detection of distal colorectal lesions. Based on this evidence, the authors recommended a prospective RCT to evaluate the possible benefit of combining FOBT with sigmoidoscopy by increasing cancer detection in the distal colon (limited evidence). A recent study (30) demonstrated that by combining a one-time FOBT with sigmoidoscopy, the detection rate for advanced neoplasia increased to 76% from 70% with sigmoidoscopy alone (limited evidence).

D. Colonoscopy

At present, video-assisted colonoscopy is the clinical gold standard for polyp detection. Current recommendations suggest colonoscopy once every 10 years. To date, there are no studies evaluating whether screening colonoscopy alone reduces the incidence or mortality from CRC in patients at average risk. However, colonoscopy was the primary method of diagnostic follow-up used in three fecal occult blood trials (7,16,17). Direct identification of cancer was actually responsible for the mortality reduction (moderate evidence). Two cohort studies have demonstrated the efficacy of colonoscopy and polypectomy in reducing the incidence of colorectal cancer (9,31) (moderate evidence). In the National Polyp Study (9) in which the screening population underwent colonoscopic polypectomy at the time of entry and during surveillance, researchers determined a 76% to 90% decrease in cancer incidence compared with that expected on the basis of historical controls, suggesting a strong correlation between adenoma removal and cancer reduction (moderate evidence). The Italian multicenter study (31) reported a two-thirds risk reduction for colorectal carcinoma following colonoscopic removal of an adenoma (moderate evidence). In addition, indirect evidence from studies demonstrating that sigmoidoscopy reduces CRC mortality points toward the effectiveness of colonoscopy. A recent randomized trial examining screening sigmoidoscopy with follow-up colonoscopy for those patients with polyps versus no screening has demonstrated a significant reduction in CRC incidence in the screened group (32) (moderate evidence). Despite being widely accepted as the gold standard for interrogation of the large bowel, colonoscopy has limitations. There is a risk of approximately 0.2% for serious bleeding or perforation during the screening exam, the risk being greatest if polypectomy is performed (33). In addition, it has been estimated that the cost of colonoscopic screening in adults over age 50 could reach $3.5 billion per year, in part due to the conscious sedation required to perform the exam (34). The diagnostic performance of colonoscopy has been estimated by evaluation of interobserver variability for detection of polyps (35). The overall miss rate for adenomas was 24%. The miss rate was 27% for adenomas ≥5mm, 13% for adenomas 6 to 9mm, and 6% for adenomas ≥10mm. Right colon adenomas were missed more often (27%) than left colon adenomas (21%), but the difference was not significant.

II. What Imaging-Based Screening Methods Are Available, and How Do They Compare with FOBT, Sigmoidoscopy, and Colonoscopy?

Summary of Evidence

Until recently the DCBE was the only imaging-based study for CRC screening. Evidence for the use of DCBE in the average-risk screening population is limited. Over the past decade computed tomographic colonography (CTC) has rapidly developed and is becoming a realistic option for CRC screening. Recent data suggest that properly performed CTC rivals colonoscopy for lesion detection in the average-risk screening population.

Supporting Evidence

A. Double Contrast Barium Enema (DCBE)

The efficacy of DCBE as a screening test has not been evaluated in a randomized trial. The strongest support for DCBE is based on the observation that treatment of early cancer in asymptomatic individuals lowers disease-specific mortality, and the removal of adenomatous polyps reduces cancer incidence. The National Polyp Study reported a reduction in cancer incidence after adenoma removal (9). The relative contribution of initial polypectomy and surveillance to this effect cannot be determined. However, initial polypectomy is likely to have been the major contributing factor in incidence reduction given the size and nature of lesions at entry and the relatively short follow-up time in this study. Approximately one third of patients with polyps entered the study after receiving positive results on barium enema (36) (limited evidence). Several studies have looked at the sensitivity of DCBE in polyp detection. A meta-analysis (37) demonstrated a sensitivity of 70% or greater for polyps of 5mm or more in size (range 30% to 96%). A retrospective review (38) of 2193 consecutive colorectal cancers demonstrated DCBE sensitivity for cancer detection to be 85% versus 95% for colonoscopy. More recently, as part of the National Polyp study, Winawer and colleagues (39) undertook colonic surveillance of patients postpolypectomy using both colonoscopy and DCBE. The DCBE was performed first and the endoscopist was blinded to its result. Detection rates of DCBE for polyps of 1.0cm and greater was 48%, with an overall detection rate for adenomas of only 39%. Although this study has raised doubts about the justification of using DCBE for CRC screening, the results relate to a symptomatic population and are therefore not applicable to the average risk population. In addition, only 23 patients with polyps greater than 1.0cm were included, which seems a small number on which to base conclusions regarding the effectiveness of DCBE in polyp detection (limited evidence). DCBE is currently not recommended by the American College of Gastroenterologists as a primary screening strategy in average-risk patients.

B. Computed Tomographic Colonography (CTC)

Computed tomographic colonography is a rapidly evolving technique for total colon examination and is the only imaging alternative developed since the barium enema with the potential for CRC screening. First described in 1994, CTC utilizes high-resolution helical CT data in combination with advanced graphical software to generate two-dimensional (2D) and three-dimensional (3D) endoluminal views of the colon. The endoluminal images, which may be viewed dynamically and interactively, simulate what is seen at conventional colonoscopy. Volumetric data are acquired with the patient in both the prone and supine positions. While limited only to detection, CTC offers several potential advantages: it presents minimal risk to patients, has a short procedure time of approximately 15 minutes, can be performed in patients with distal occluding lesions, and affords more precise lesion localization than colonoscopy. It is performed using a low x-ray dose technique that results in approximately 15% absorbed dose reduction compared to DCBE (40). It also is well tolerated, with less discomfort reported for the exam than for either colonoscopy or DCBE (41,42). With over 2000 cases reported in the literature, there are no reports of serious morbidity or mortality associated with CTC. Conscious sedation is not required, limiting cost and time for the patient. In addition, as the entire abdomen and pelvis are visualized, this method has the potential to simultaneously detect and stage malignant lesions in a single sitting; however, this capability has not yet been fully validated in a clinical trial. The diagnosis of extracolonic pathology is also possible (43,44). Moderately significant findings such as gallstones, as well as highly significant findings such as renal cell carcinoma, large abdominal aortic aneurysms, and liver and adrenal masses can be identified. This may prove advantageous if the cost-effectiveness of CTC is not affected by the diagnostic workup of these lesions.

The performance characteristics of CT colonography in polyp detection have been assessed in several published studies. Results have been encouraging in symptomatic cohorts and in populations with an increased incidence of polyps (45–47) (limited evidence). The sensitivity of CTC for detection of polyps measuring 10 mm or more compares favorably with the gold standard of colonoscopy, ranging from 90% to 93%. Reported sensitivity in populations with a lower prevalence of polyps has until recently been relatively poor (48,49). However, at least one of these studies (48) was performed with essentially naive CTC readers and limited evaluation software. Recently the first large cohort evaluation (50) in 1200 individuals from an average-risk population comparing CTC to colonoscopy has been completed (moderate evidence). Using a combination of digital subtraction bowel cleansing (see below) and traditional cathartic preparation, CTC was performed prior to colonoscopy. The results of the CTC were disclosed when colonoscopic examination of a colon segment was complete, thereby allowing unblinded colonoscopic reevaluation of each bowel segment. The final unblinded colonoscopy was used as the reference standard. The sensitivity of CTC for adenomatous polyps was 93.8% for polyps at least 10 mm in diameter, 93.9% for polyps at least 8 mm in diameter, and 88.7% for polyps at least 6 mm in diameter. The sensitivity of optical colonoscopy for detection of adenomatous polyps was 87.5%, 91.5%, and 92.3% for the three sizes of polyps, respectively. The specificity of CTC for adenomatous polyps was 96.0% for polyps at least 10mm in diameter and 92.2% for polyps at least 8mm in diameter. Setting the threshold polyp size for colonoscopic referral at 8mm results in 13.5% of patients who undergo screening being referred for colonoscopic evaluation. This reduces to 7.5% if a threshold polyp size of 10mm is chosen. Interestingly, the frequency of extracolonic findings was less than half that reported in higher-risk populations, which may have implications for cost-effectiveness in the future.

The excellent performance data for CTC reported in this trial are at odds with other published series (48,49). The authors suggest that the discrepancy in results, while probably multifactorial, is primarily attributable to the use of 3D display, which aids polyp conspicuity and duration of visualization. Previous studies have primarily used 2D image interpretation. Further studies are required to clarify the factors that contributed to the high performance observed in this study and to ensure reproducibility of these data. Despite great advances in CTC, however, the current implementation of the technique is subject to three important limitations. First, the cost of CTC remains a significant hurdle to its implementation as a mainstream screening modality. If the cost of CTC reflects standard contrast-enhanced abdominal and pelvic CT rather than a special reduced cost for CTC, then it is doubtful that it will be adopted as a first-line screening tool. Second, in its current form, CTC requires full cathartic bowel preparation. This has been identified as a barrier to improved screening compliance. Future developments in fecal tagging techniques (see below) may help to address this problem. Finally, although the interpretation time for a CTC study has decreased as better technology and more expertise become available, the mean time required in the Bethesda study was still almost 20 minutes. Strategies to streamline study interpretation need to be addressed if CTC is to cope with the huge population eligible for CRC screening.

C. Special Case: Patients with Increased Risk of Colorectal Cancer

Summary of Evidence: People at increased risk of CRC include those with a family history of CRC or adenomatous polyps, and those with a personal history of adenomatous polyps, CTC, or inflammatory bowel disease.

Supporting Evidence

Family History of Colorectal Cancer or Adenomatous Polyps

Colon cancer screening recommendations based on familial risk are derived from the known effectiveness of available screening strategies and the observed colon cancer risk in relatives of patients with large-bowel malignancy and relatives of patients diagnosed with adenomas at a young age (≤60 years). The lifetime risk for CRC in the general population is 6%. Estimates of risk of CRC in close relatives of individuals with adenomatous polyps are still evolving. A meta-analysis (51) examined all studies that assessed familial risk of colon cancers and adenomatous polyps (27 studies) since 1966 (moderate evidence). The relative risk of colon cancer when a first-degree relative was affected with large-bowel malignancy was 2.4. Increased risk was found when the relative was affected with either colon or rectal cancers, but was greater for colon. If more than one relative was affected, the risk increased to 4.2. The risk was 3.8 for relatives if colon cancer was diagnosed before age 45 years, 2.2 if it was diagnosed between ages 45 and 59 years, and 1.8 if the cancer was diagnosed at >59 years. The relative risk for colon cancer if the first-degree relative had an adenomatous polyp was 1.9. People with a first-degree relative (parent, sibling, or child) with colon cancer or adenomatous polyps diagnosed at age >60 years or two first-degree relatives diagnosed with CRC at any age are recommended to have screening colonoscopy starting at age 40 years or 10 years younger than the earliest diagnosis in their family, whichever comes first, and repeated every 5 years (52). People with a first-degree relative with colon cancer or adenomatous polyp diagnosed at age ≥60 years or two second-degree relatives (grandparent, aunt, or uncle) with CRC are recommended to undergo screening as average risk persons, but beginning at age 40 years. People with one second-degree relative or third-degree relative (great-grandparent or cousin) with CRC should be screened as average risk persons.

History of Adenomatous Polyps: Several studies have demonstrated that colonoscopic polypectomy and surveillance reduces subsequent CRC incidence (9,31). The rate of developing advanced adenomas after polypectomy is low after several years of follow-up, suggesting that the initial colonoscopy and polypectomy offers the major benefit and that surveillance may only benefit those at highest risk. The National Polyp Study (53) found that the rate of adenoma detection 3 years after the initial adenoma resection was 32% to 42%. Recurrent adenomas were mostly small, tubular adenomas with low-grade dysplasia and therefore were of negligible immediate clinical significance. Only 3.3% of patients in each follow-up group had advanced adenomas (>1 cm, or with villous tissue or high-grade dysplasia) after 3 years of follow-up (moderate evidence). Another long-term follow-up study (4) of 1618 postpolypectomy patients also found no increased risk for cancer in patients undergoing resection of single small (<1 cm) tubular adenomas, but an increased risk of 3.6 times in those with index adenomas that were large (≥1 cm) or contained villous tissue, and 6.6 times in patients with multiple adenomas on their original examinations compared with the known rates in the local community. In patients found to have a colorectal adenoma, the prevalence of synchronous polyps is 30% to 50% (54–56). Some of these polyps, especially those measuring <1 cm in diameter, will be missed on the initial colonoscopy (57,58). Metachronous adenomas are reported in 20% to 50% of patients, depending on the follow-up surveillance interval used (59–63). Thus, the purpose of postpolypectomy colonoscopic surveillance is twofold. First, previously missed adenomas can be detected and removed. Second, the patient's tendency to form new adenomas with advanced pathology can be assessed.

In the National Polyp Study, colonoscopy performed 3 years after initial colonoscopic removal of adenomatous polyps detected advanced adenomas as effectively as follow-up colonoscopy performed after both 1 and 3 years. At 3 years, only 3.3% of patients in each group had advanced adenomas. On this basis, an interval of at least 3 years before follow-up colonoscopy after resection of newly diagnosed adenomatous polyps was recommended. Further analysis of these data as well as data from more recent studies suggest that it is possible to further stratify risk of recurrent advanced adenomas based on baseline features of each case (63–65). Patients with a relatively high risk of developing advanced adenomas during follow-up include those with multiple adenomas (more than two), large adenomas (≥1 cm), or a first-degree relative with CRC. Patients with a low risk of metachronous advanced adenomas include those with only one or two small adenomas (<1 cm) and no family history of colorectal cancer. Surveillance should be of greatest intensity in those most likely to benefit and reduced in those least likely to benefit so as to avoid complications associated with unnecessary removal of small polyps. Surveillance can be accomplished by well-performed CTC or colonoscopy.

History of Colorectal Cancer: Aside from recurrence of the original cancer, the incidence of CRC is increased after the first occurrence (66). Adenomatous polyps again precede these subsequent cancers. Although colonoscopy can detect recurrent colon cancer, anastomotic recurrences occur in only about 2% of colon cancers and are generally accompanied by surgically incurable disease (67). In an RCT performed in 325 patients with curative resections of colorectal cancer (68), the value of colonoscopy was confined to detection of metachronous adenomas and not recurrent intraluminal cancer (moderate evidence). Patients with a colon cancer that has been resected with curative intent should have a complete structural colon examination around the time of initial diagnosis to rule out synchronous neoplasms. This exam can be performed by either colonoscopy or CTC; CTC has proven especially effective in the setting of a colorectal mass that prevents passage of the colonoscope, as only air insufflation is required for evaluation (69). Thus, if the colon is obstructed preoperatively, CTC should be performed. It offers the advantage that extracolonic structures can be assessed simultaneously. If this does not reveal synchronous lesions, subsequent surveillance by colonoscopy or CTC should be offered after 3 years, and then, if normal, every 5 years.

Inflammatory Bowel Disease: There is extensive experience with DCBE for evaluation of inflammatory bowel disease and its complications, including CRC (70,71). Inflammatory polyps project above the level of the surrounding mucosa. Pseudopolyposis is seen when extensive ulceration of the mucosa down to the submucosa results in scattered circumscribed islands of relatively normal mucosal remnants. Postinflammatory polyps reflect a nonspecific healing of undermined mucosal and submucosal remnants and ulcers, and are mostly multiple. They have no malignant potential. Patients with extensive long-standing ulcerative colitis or Crohn's disease have an increased risk for the development of CRC (72). Importantly, cancers that develop in patients with inflammatory bowel disease differ from more typical colorectal cancers in that they generally develop not from adenomatous polyps but rather from areas of high-grade dysplasia (73). Dysplasia is a precancerous histologic finding, and the risk of colon cancer increases with the degree of mucosal dysplasia. Dysplasia may be found in a radiographically normal-appearing mucosa, or it may be accompanied by a slightly raised mucosal lesion, a so-called dysplasia-associated lesion or mass and as a consequence radiographically detectable. Because differentiation of adenocarcinoma and dysplasia from inflammatory or postinflammatory polyps is sometimes difficult or impossible on double-contrast enema, endoscopy and biopsy are necessary for making a final diagnosis. Therefore, regular colonoscopy and mucosal biopsy is recommended for both. There are no RCTs of surveillance colonoscopy in patients with chronic ulcerative colitis or Crohn's colitis. A case-control study has found better survival in ulcerative colitis patients in surveillance programs (74) (moderate evidence). Commonly colonoscopy is performed every 1 to 2 years after 8 years of disease. Patients with high-grade dysplasia or multifocal low-grade dysplasia in flat mucosa should be advised to undergo colectomy. While CTC could potentially permit evaluation of the colon, it has not been formally evaluated in this setting.

D. Special Case: Patients with High Risk of Colorectal Cancer

Summary of Evidence: Essentially, there are two broad categories of hereditary CRC–distal or proximal–based on the predominant location of disease. Colorectal cancers involving the distal colon are more likely to have mutations in the adenomatous polyposis coli (*APC*), *p53*, and *K-ras* genes, and behave more aggressively (75); proximal colorectal cancers are more likely to possess microsatellite instability (genomic regions in which short DNA sequences or a single nucleotide is repeated), harbor mutations in the mismatch-repair genes, and behave less aggressively, as in HNPCC (75). Familial adenomatous polyposis (FAP) and most sporadic cases may be considered a paradigm for the first, or distal, class of colorectal cancers, whereas hereditary nonpolyposis CRC more clearly represents the second, or proximal, class (75). Familial CRC is a major public health problem by virtue of its relatively high frequency. Some 15% to 20% of all CRCs are familial. Among these, FAP accounts for less than 1%; HNPCC, also called Lynch syndrome, accounts for approximately 5% to 8% of all CRC patients.

Supporting Evidence

Familial Adenomatous Polyposis
Familial adenomatous polyposis is an autosomal-dominant disease caused by mutations in the adenomatous polyposis coli (*APC*) gene. The associated risk of CRC approaches 100%. The average age of adenoma development in FAP is 16 years, and the average age of colon cancer is 39 years. Most affected patients develop >100 colorectal adenomas, and persons with more than 100 adenomas have FAP by definition. Attenuated APC (AAPC) is a variant of FAP and is associated with a variable number of adenomas, usually 20 to 100, a tendency toward right-sided colonic adenomas, and an age onset of CRC that is approximately 10 years later than for FAP. The CRC mortality rate is lower in FAP patients who choose to be screened compared with those who present with symptoms (76) (moderate evidence). Colonoscopy should be used in those with AAPC, beginning in the late teens or early 20s, depending on the age of polyp expression in the family, while sigmoidoscopy is adequate screening for most FAP patients as numerous polyps almost invariably involve the sigmoid and rectum. People who have a genetic diagnosis of FAP, or are at risk of having FAP but genetic testing has not been performed or is not feasible, should have annual sigmoidoscopy, beginning at age 10 to 12 years, to determine if they are expressing the genetic abnormality.

Hereditary Nonpolyposis Colorectal Cancer (HNPCC): Hereditary nonpolyposis colorectal cancer, also referred to as the Lynch syndrome, is the most common form of hereditary colorectal cancer. Multiple generations are affected with CRC at an early age (mean, approximately 45 years) with a predominance of right-sided CRC (approximately 70% proximal to the splenic flexure). There is an excess of synchronous CRC (multiple colorectal cancers at or within 6 months after surgical resection for CRC) and metachronous CRC (CRC occurring more than 6 months after surgery). In addition, there is an excess of extracolonic cancers, namely carcinoma of the endometrium (second only to CRC in frequency), ovary, stomach small bowel, pancreas, hepatobiliary tract, brain, and upper uroepithelial tract (77). A recent study suggests that HNPCC accounts for between 0.86% and 2.0% of colon cancer cases (78). Criteria for the diagnosis of HNPCC (the Amsterdam criteria) have been devised (79). The criteria are as follows: at least three relatives with an HNPCC-associated cancer (CRC and cancer of the endometrium, small bowel, ureter, or renal pelvis) plus all of the following: (a) one affected patient is a first-degree relative of the other two; (b) two or more successive generations affected; (c) one or more affected relative received CRC diagnosis at age <50 years; (d) FAP excluded in any case of colorectal cancer; and (e) tumors verified by pathologic examination.

The efficacy of surveillance for CRC in families with HNPCC was evaluated in a controlled clinical trial extending over a 15-year period (80). The study concluded that screening for CRC at 3-year intervals more than halves the risk of colorectal cancer, prevents deaths from colorectal cancer, and decreases the overall mortality rate by about 65% in such families (moderate evidence). The incidence of CRC in the screened group was 6%, suggesting that a shorter screening interval may be appropriate. The age to begin screening in HNPCC is based on the observation that the average age of colon cancer diagnosis is 44 years, and cancers before the age of 25 years are very unusual.

III. What Is the Role of Imaging in Staging Colorectal Carcinoma?

Depth of invasion (T stage) and nodal involvement (N stage) are both important features for prognosis. A reliable preoperative test that can accurately stage tumor invasion into the colorectal wall (T) and regional lymph involvement (N) is essential to assess these prognostic indicators and to correctly assign patients to an appropriate treatment strategy. Both transrectal ultrasonography (US) and magnetic resonance imaging (MRI) with endorectal coils are considered superior to conventional CT in the preoperative assessment of tumor depth in the rectal wall. In a meta-analysis of 90 published series, comparing endorectal US, CT, and MRI (81), MRI and US demonstrated equal sensitivity for detection of muscularis propria invasion. However, US specificity (86%) was significantly higher than that of MRI (69%). For perirectal tissue invasion, sensitivity of US (90%) was significantly higher than that of CT (79%) and MRI (82%); specificities were comparable. For adjacent organ invasion and lymph node involvement, estimates for US, CT, and MRI were comparable. Ultrasonography showed better diagnostic accuracy than that of CT and MRI for perirectal tissue invasion. Analysis of lymph node involvement showed no differences in accuracy (moderate evidence). Although endorectal US is very accurate for staging of superficial rectal cancer, it has several limitations including operator dependency, limitation to tumors located 8 to 10 cm from the anal verge when using a rigid probe, and inability to assess stenosing lesions. In addition, endorectal US fails to detect lymph nodes that are outside the range of the transducer and cannot discriminate between lymph nodes inside or outside the mesorectal fascia, since the fascia is not depicted at endorectal US—an important factor in determining the spread of T3 tumors considered for total mesorectal excision. This limitation does not apply to MRI with external coils, as the mesorectal fascia is clearly depicted. To improve the sensitivity values of MRI for lymph node detection, newer techniques, such as use of new lymph node–specific MRI contrast agents, may provide a more sensitive MRI method to detect lymph node involvement (82,83).

In the past, CT has been limited in differentiating and distinguishing the different layers of the rectal wall, demonstrating the mesorectal fascia, and depicting tumor invasion in surrounding pelvic structures due to poor spatial and contrast resolution. A recent study evaluated the role of CTC in local staging of CRC (84). The imaging protocol included contrast enhancement with 1-mm reconstruction intervals for arterial phase imaging. Overall accuracy for T and N staging was 73% and 59%, respectively. In this study the N staging accuracy increased to 80% with the use of multiplanar reconstruction. Improving CT spatial and contrast resolution combined with the use of arterial phase imaging and multiplanar reconstruction for bowel wall assessment may lead to increased diagnostic accuracy of local CRC staging.

IV. Applicability to Children

In general, CRC screening does not apply to children. However, if there is a family history of FAP, then screening beginning at puberty is recommended. Colectomy is advocated if genetic testing is positive.

V. Cost-Effectiveness

Evidence from several studies suggests that screening for, detecting, and removing CRC and precancerous polyps can reduce CRC incidence and related mortality. Accordingly, analyses have demonstrated that screening for CRC by any method is cost-effective when compared with no screening. The incremental cost-effectiveness ratio (ICER) for commonly considered strategies lies between $10,000 and $25,000 per life-year saved (85), which compares favorably with other cancer screening strategies such as annual mammography for women ages 55 to 64 years ($132,000 per life-year saved, in 1998 dollars) (86). However, because different models and modeling assumptions were used and because different strategies were compared, the studies vary widely in their recommended strategies and in their estimates of cost-effectiveness ratios. Some studies advocate annual

FOBT combined with a sigmoidoscopy every 5 years (87,88), while others advocate a colonoscopy every 10 years (89,90). McMahon and colleagues (91) compared and reanalyzed the results of three often-cited cost-effectiveness analyses of CRC screening in average-risk populations. The study found that in average-risk individuals, screening with double-contrast barium enema examination every 3 years, or every 5 years with annual fecal occult blood testing, had an ICER of less than $55,600 per life-year saved. However, double-contrast barium enema examination screening every 3 years plus annual fecal occult blood testing had an ICER of more than $100,000 per life-year saved. Colonoscopic screening had an ICER of more than $100,000 per life-year saved, was dominated by other screening strategies, and offered less benefit than did double-contrast barium enema examination screening. However, this analysis assumed a greater sensitivity for DCBE for polyp detection than that determined by Winawer and colleagues (39), thereby introducing a possible bias into their competitive choice analysis; CTC was not included in the analysis.

A further study compared cost-effectiveness of CTC to colonoscopy and to no screening, and CTC was found to be cost-effective compared to no screening but not cost-effective compared to colonoscopy (92). The author concluded that CTC must be 54% less expensive than conventional colonoscopy and be performed at 10-year intervals to have equal cost-effectiveness to conventional colonoscopy. This analysis was based on preliminary CTC results and may be overly pessimistic, especially given the more recent evidence from Pickhardt and colleagues (50). Clearly, these data demonstrated that sensitivity of CTC for clinically significant lesions is equal to if not better than colonoscopy. In addition, the competitive choice analysis of Sonnenberg (92) did not include the use of CTC for surveillance postpolypectomy. Given the performance of CTC for detection of polyps and relatively low likelihood of average risk individuals developing significant adenomas following colonoscopic resection (39), this omission may have biased the results of their analysis.

VI. What Imaging-Based Screening Developments Are on the Horizon that May Improve Compliance with Colorectal Screening?

Despite the observed prevalence of polyps and the modification of risk obtained through screening, by current estimates only 15% to 19% of individuals eligible for screening actually undergo colon evaluation of any kind (93). A recent study found that although 80% of the doctors advised screening for CRC to their patients over the age of 50, only about 50% of eligible patients studied had their stool tested for blood and about 30% had a sigmoidoscopy or colonoscopy (94). The perceived discomfort and inconvenience associated with bowel purgation has been identified as a barrier to screening (95,96). Hence, methods to improve patient tolerance may lead to improved compliance with colon cancer screening. Currently, CTC requires a full cathartic bowel preparation, as do sigmoidoscopy and colonoscopy. At present, electronic bowel cleansing using a digital subtraction technique is being developed (97–101). This "prepless" colonography requires the patient to ingest a tagging agent such as barium sulfate or nonionic iodinated contrast to tag solid stool and luminal fluid. The bowel contents are thus uniformly opacified allowing subsequent digital subtraction from the image; soft tissue elements such as polyps are unaffected. This method potentially obviates bowel catharsis, a major factor in poor compliance with CRC screening. Fecal tagging was successfully used in conjunction with catharsis in a screening setting by Pickhardt and coworkers (98). Data, beyond pilot data, to validate this noncathartic technique is not yet available, but this technique may lead to better patient compliance in the future (102).

Computer-assisted detection (CAD) algorithms are also being developed to aid lesion detection (103,104). Yoshida and colleagues (103) detected 89% of polyps (16 of 18) with 2.5 false-positive findings per patient. Such a CAD system has the potential to reduce the time of interpretation and may improve render performance. These developments, if rigorously validated in clinical trials, may make CT colonography a more easily tolerated, cost-effective alternative for CRC screening.

Take-Home Tables

Table 5.1. Computed tomographic colonography (CTC) results to date: sensitivity

Hospital (reference)	Polyp size: >10 mm	>5 to 10 mm	0 to 5 mm
University of California at San Francisco (46)	72% (all sizes)		
Boston University (47)	97%	97%	92%
Mayo Clinic (48)	98% (387/394)	95% (358/378)	
New York University (45)	98% (all sizes)		
Bethesda Naval (50)	96% (1137/1185)	92% (1061/1151)	n/a

n/a, not available.

Table 5.2. CTC results to date: specificity

Hospital (reference)	Polyp size: >10 mm	>5 to 10 mm	0 to 5 mm	No. of patients
University of California at San Francisco (46)	94% (64/68)	82% (72/78)	66% (95/142)	300
Boston University (47)	91% (20/22)	82% (33/40)	55% (29/53)	100
Mayo Clinic (48)	73% (27/37)	57% (36/63)	n/a	703
New York University (45)	93% (13/14)	70% (19/27)	12% (11/91)	105
Bethesda Naval (50)	92% (47/51)	92% (88/95)	n/a	1233

n/a, not available.

Table 5.3. Sensitivity and specificity of other modalities

Modality	Sensitivity (reference)	Specificity (reference)
FOBT	30–50% (one-time testing) (7,18)	90–98% (7)
DCBE	30–96% (all lesions) (37)	85–90%
Colonoscopy	94% (lesions ≥1 cm) (35)	100%

FOBT, fecal occult blood testing; DCBE, double contrast barium enema.

Imaging Case Studies

The following cases highlight the advantages and limitations of colonoscopy and CTC.

Case 1: False-Negative CTC

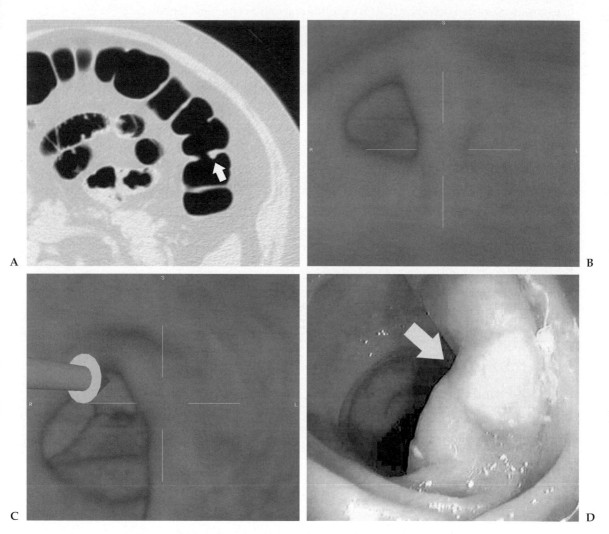

Figure 5.1. A: Axial supine computed tomographic colonography (CTC) image (viewed on lung settings) demonstrates a prominent haustral fold in the transverse colon. This was interpreted as being within normal limits. B, C: Three-dimensional (3D) reconstruction does not reveal a significant lesion. D: Endoscopic view of the transverse colon in the same region (arrow) reveals a 20-mm sessile lesion. Biopsy confirmed a tubular adenoma. (For parts B, C, and D, see color insert)

Case 2: False-Positive CTC

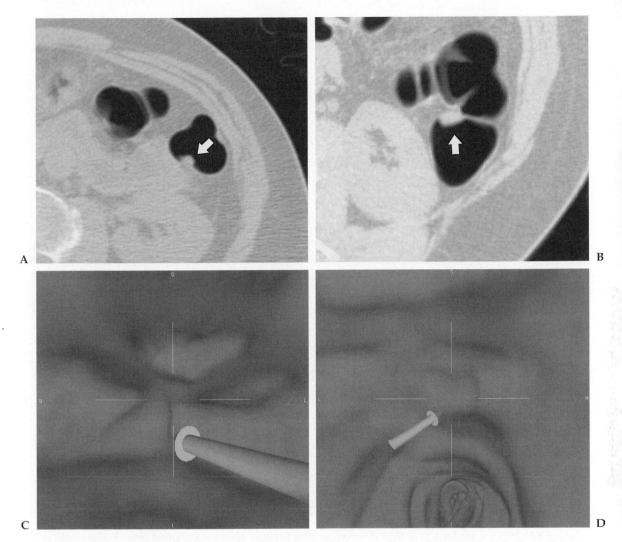

Figure 5.2. A, B: Axial supine and prone CTC images (viewed on lung settings) reveal a polypoid lesion (arrow) in the region of the splenic flexure. C, D: Three-dimensional (3D) reconstruction of region in A and B support the presence of a polypoid mass in the splenic flexure. Subsequent colonscopy was normal. (For parts C and D, see color insert)

Case 3: True-Positive CTC and Colonoscopy

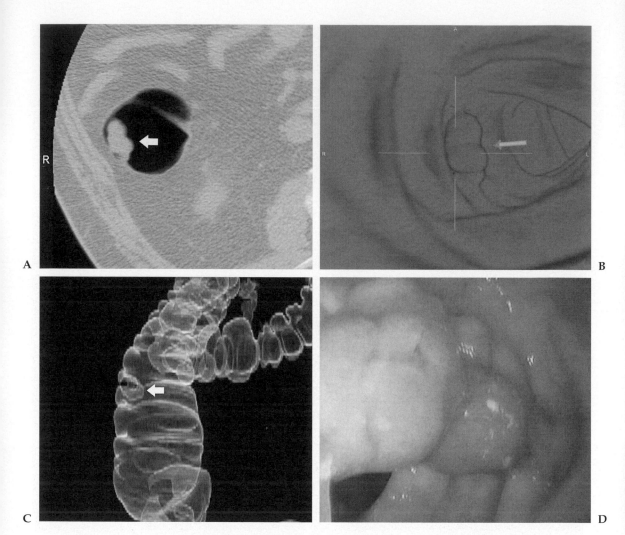

Figure 5.3. A: Axial supine CTC image (viewed on lung settings) reveals a polypoid mass in the ascending colon. B, C: Three-dimensional (3D) reconstruction of the region renders an endolumial view of the lesion (B). Digitally subtracted 3D image of the ascending colon provides a lesion projection similar to double contrast barium enema (DCBE) (C). D: Endoscopy reveals a 15-mm polyp. Biopsy confirmed a tubulovillous adenoma. (For parts B and D, see color insert)

Case 4: True-Positive CTC and False-Negative Colonoscopy

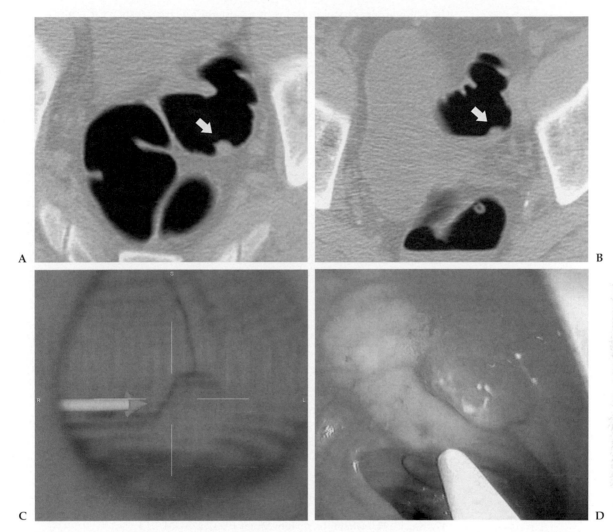

Figure 5.4. Axial supine (A) and prone (B) CTC images (viewed on lung settings) reveals a polypoid mass in the sigmoid colon. C: Three-dimensional (3D) endoluminal reconstruction supports the findings on axial imaging. D: Colonoscopy performed on the same day as the CTC in a trial protocol was negative. Repeat sigmoidoscopy was advised based on the CTC findings. This revealed a 10-mm invasive carcinoma in the sigmoid colon. (For parts C and D, see color insert)

Suggested Imaging Protocol for Asymptomatic Screening Patients

The following protocol pertains to a General Electric 16-slice CT scanner:

- Indication: structural evaluation of the colon in patients without colon symptoms or completion CTC if the patient presented to colonoscopy for asymptomatic screening, and no polyps, strictures, or masses found
- Bowel preparation: standard catharsis and air insufflation (patient or technician controlled)
- Collimation 2.5 mm, kVp 140, mA 70, sec 0.6
- Pitch 1.3, table speed 13.75 mm/rotation, reconstruction interval 1.25 mm
- Prone and supine series
- No intravenous contrast

Future Areas of Research

- Further clinical trials of CTC in average-risk populations
- CTC using digital subtraction bowel cleansing
- Computer-assisted polyp detection

References

1. Hill MJ, Morson BC, Bussey HJ. Lancet 1978;1:245–247.
2. Morson BC. Clin Radiol 1984;35:425–431.
3. Winawer SJ, Zauber AG, Diaz B. Gastrointest Endosc 1987;33:167–167.
4. Atkin WS, Morson BC, Cuzick J. N Engl J Med 1992;326:658–662.
5. Stryker SJ, Wolff BG, Culp CE, Libbe SD, Ilstrup DM, MacCarty RL. Gastroenterology 1987;93:1009–1013.
6. Burt RW, Bishop DT, Cannon LA, Dowdle MA, Lee RG, Skolnick MH. N Engl J Med 1985;312:1540–1544.
7. Mandel JS, Bond JH, Church TR, et al. N Engl J Med 1993;328:1365–1371.
8. Muller AD, Sonnenberg A. Ann Intern Med 1995;123:904–910.
9. Winawer SJ, Zauber AG, Ho MN, et al. N Engl J Med 1993;329:1977–1981.
10. Muto T, Bussey HJ, Morson BC. Cancer 1975;36:2251–2270.
11. Powell SM, Zilz N, Beazer-Barclay Y, et al. Nature 1992;359:235–237.
12. Nagase H, Nakamura Y. Hum Mutat 1993;2:425–434.
13. Jemal A, Tiwari RC, Murray T, et al. CA Cancer J Clin 2004;54:8–29.
14. Redaelli A, Cranor CW, Okano GJ, Reese PR. Pharmacoeconomics 2003; 21:1213–1238.
15. Bond JH. Semin Gastrointest Dis 2000;11:176–184.
16. Hardcastle JD, Chamberlain JO, Robinson MH, et al. Lancet 1996; 348:1472–1477.
17. Kronborg O, Fenger C, Olsen J, Jorgensen OD, Sondergaard O. Lancet 1996;348:1467–1471.
18. Ahlquist DA, Wieand HS, Moertel CG, et al. JAMA 1993;269:1262–1267.
19. Simon JB. Gastroenterologist 1998;6:66–78.
20. Rex DK, Lehman GA, Ulbright TM, et al. Am J Gastroenterol 1993;88:825–831.
21. Lieberman DA, Smith FW. Am J Gastroenterol 1991;86:946–951.
22. Selby JV, Friedman GD, Quesenberry CP Jr, Weiss NS. N Engl J Med 1992;326:653–657.
23. Newcomb PA, Norfleet RG, Storer BE, Surawicz TS, Marcus PM. J Natl Cancer Inst 1992;84:1572–1575.

24. Kavanagh AM, Giovannucci EL, Fuchs CS, Colditz GA. Cancer Causes Control 1998;9:455–462.

25. Dachman AH, Kuniyoshi JK, Boyle CM, et al. AJR 1998;171:989–995.

26. Maglinte DD, Keller KJ, Miller RE, Chernish SM. Radiology 1983;147:669–672.

27. Rex DK, Chak A, Vasudeva R, et al. Gastrointest Endosc 1999;49:727–730.

28. Imperiale TF, Wagner DR, Lin CY, Larkin GN, Rogge JD. N Engl J Med 2000;343:169–174.

29. Jorgensen OD, Kronborg O, Fenger C. Gut 2002;50:29–32.

30. Lieberman DA, Weiss DG, Veterans Affairs Cooperative Study Group 380. N Engl J Med 2001;345:555–560.

31. Citarda F, Tomaselli G, Capocaccia R, Barcherini S, Crespi M, Italian Multi-centre Study Group. Gut 2001;48:812–815.

32. Thiis-Evensen E, Hoff GS, Sauar J, Langmark F, Majak BM, Vatn MH. Scand J Gastroenterol 1999;34:414–420.

33. Winawer SJ, Fletcher RH, Miller L, et al. Gastroenterology 1997;112:594–642.

34. Ransohoff DF, Lang CA. N Engl J Med 1991;325:37–41.

35. Rex DK, Cutler CS, Lemmel GT, et al. Gastroenterology 1997;112:24–28.

36. Winawer SJ, Zauber AG, O'Brien MJ, et al. Cancer 1992;70:1236–1245.

37. Glick S, Wagner JL, Johnson CD. AJR 1998;170:629–636.

38. Rex DK, Rahmani EY, Haseman JH, Lemmel GT, Kaster S, Buckley JS. Gastroenterology 1997;112:17–23.

39. Winawer SJ, Stewart ET, Zauber AG, et al. N Engl J Med 2000;342:1766–1772.

40. Johnson CD, Dachman AH. Radiology 2000;216:331–341.

41. Taylor SA, Halligan S, Saunders BP, Bassett P, Vance M, Bartram CI. AJR 2003;181:913–921.

42. Svensson MH, Svensson E, Lasson A, Hellstrom M. Radiology 2002;222:337–345.

43. Hara AK, Johnson CD, MacCarty RL, Welch TJ. Radiology 2000;215:353–357.

44. Gluecker TM, Johnson CD, Wilson LA, et al. Gastroenterology 2003;124:911–916.

45. Macari M, Bini EJ, Xue X, et al. Radiology 2002;224:383–392.

46. Yee J, Akerkar GA, Hung RK, Steinauer-Gebauer AM, Wall SD, McQuaid KR. Radiology 2001;219:685–692.

47. Fenlon HM, Nunes DP, Schroy PC 3rd, Barish MA, Clarke PD, Ferrucci JT. N Engl J Med 1999;341:1496–1503.

48. Johnson CD, Harmsen WS, Wilson LA, et al. Gastroenterology 2003;125:311–319.

49. Cotton PB, Durkalski VL, Pineau BC, et al. JAMA 2004;291:1713–1719.

50. Pickhardt PJ, Choi JR, Hwang I, et al. N Engl J Med 2003;349:2191–2200.

51. Johns LE, Houlston RS. Am J Gastroenterol 2001;96:2992–3003.

52. Fuchs CS, Giovannucci EL, Colditz GA, Hunter DJ, Speizer FE, Willett WC. N Engl J Med 1994;331:1669–1674.

53. Winawer SJ, Zauber AG, O'Brien MJ, et al. N Engl J Med 1993;328:901–906.

54. Winawer SJ, O'Brien MJ, Waye JD, et al. Bull WHO 1990;68:789–795.

55. Rex DK, Smith JJ, Ulbright TM, Lehman GA. Gastroenterology 1992;102:317–319.

56. Morson BC, Konishi F. Gastrointest Radiol 1982;7:275–281.

57. Gilbertsen VA, Williams SE, Schuman L, McHugh R. Surg Gynecol Obstet 1979;149:877–878.

58. de Roos A, Hermans J, Shaw PC, Kroon H. Radiology 1985;154:11–13.

59. Henry LG, Condon RE, Schulte WJ, Aprahamian C, DeCosse JJ. Ann Surg 1975;182:511–515.

60. Kirsner JB, Rider JA, Moeller HC, Palmer WL, Gold SS. Gastroenterology 1960;39:178–182.

61. Waye JD, Braunfeld S. Endoscopy 1982;14:79–81.

62. Matek W, Guggenmoos-Holzmann I, Demling L. Endoscopy 1985;17:175–181.

63. Winawer SJ. Gastrointest Endosc 1999;49:S63–S66.

64. Noshirwani KC, van Stolk RU, Rybicki LA, Beck GJ. Gastrointest Endosc 2000;51:433–437.
65. van Stolk RU, Beck GJ, Baron JA, Haile R, Summers R. Gastroenterology 1998;115:13–18.
66. Cali RL, Pitsch RM, Thorson AG, et al. Dis Colon Rectum 1993;36:388–393.
67. Jahn H, Joergensen OD, Kronborg O, Fenger C. Dis Colon Rectum 1992; 35:253–256.
68. Schoemaker D, Black R, Giles L, Toouli J. Gastroenterology 1998;114:7–14.
69. Morrin MM, Farrell RJ, Raptopoulos V, McGee JB, Bleday R, Kruskal JB. Dis Colon Rectum 2000;43:303–311.
70. Carucci LR, Levine MS. Gastroenterol Clin North Am 2002;31:93–117, ix.
71. Hooyman JR, MacCarty RL, Carpenter HA, Schroeder KW, Carlson HC. AJR 1987;149:47–51.
72. Gillen CD, Walmsley RS, Prior P, Andrews HA, Allan RN. Gut 1994; 35:1590–1592.
73. Lennard-Jones JE, Melville DM, Morson BC, Ritchie JK, Williams CB. Gut 1990;31:800–806.
74. Choi PM, Nugent FW, Schoetz DJ Jr, Silverman ML, Haggitt RC. Gastroenterology 1993;105:418–424.
75. Lynch HT, de la Chapelle A. J Med Genet 1999;36:801–818.
76. Heiskanen I, Luostarinen T, Jarvinen HJ. Scand J Gastroenterol 2000; 35:1284–1287.
77. Lynch HT, de la Chapelle A. N Engl J Med 2003;348:919–932.
78. Samowitz WS, Curtin K, Lin HH, et al. Gastroenterology 2001;121:830–838.
79. Vasen HF, Watson P, Mecklin JP, Lynch HT. Gastroenterology 1999; 116:1453–1456.
80. Jarvinen HJ, Aarnio M, Mustonen H, et al. Gastroenterology 2000;118:829–834.
81. Bipat S, Glas AS, Slors FJ, Zwinderman AH, Bossuyt PM, Stoker J. Radiology 2004;232:773–783.
82. Harisinghani MG, Saini S, Weissleder R, et al. AJR 1999;172:1347–1351.
83. McCauley TR, Rifkin MD, Ledet CA. J Magn Reson Imaging 2002;15:492–497.
84. Filippone A, Ambrosini R, Fuschi M, Marinelli T, Genovesi D, Bonomo L. Radiology 2004;231:83–90.
85. Pignone M, Saha S, Hoerger T, Mandelblatt J. Ann Intern Med 2002;137:96–104.
86. Tengs TO, Adams ME, Pliskin JS, et al. Risk Anal 1995;15:369–390.
87. Vijan S, Hwang EW, Hofer TP, Hayward RA. Am J Med 2001;111:593–601.
88. Frazier AL, Colditz GA, Fuchs CS, Kuntz KM. JAMA 2000;284:1954–1961.
89. Khandker RK, Dulski JD, Kilpatrick JB, Ellis RP, Mitchell JB, Baine WB. Int J Technol Assess Health Care 2000;16:799–810.
90. Sonnenberg A, Delco F, Inadomi JM. Ann Intern Med 2000;133:573–584.
91. McMahon PM, Bosch JL, Gleason S, Halpern EF, Lester JS, Gazelle GS. Radiology 2001;219:44–50.
92. Sonnenberg A, Delco F, Bauerfeind P. Am J Gastroenterol 1999;94:2268–2274.
93. Brown ML, Potosky AL, Thompson GB, Kessler LG. Prev Med 1990; 19:562–574.
94. Hawley ST, Vernon SW, Levin B, Vallejo B. Cancer Epidemiol Biomarkers Prev 2004;13:314–319.
95. Wardle J, Sutton S, Williamson S, et al. Prev Med 2000;31:323–334.
96. Ristvedt SL, McFarland EG, Weinstock LB, Thyssen EP. Am J Gastroenterol 2003;98:578–585.
97. Zalis ME, Hahn PF. AJR 2001;176:646–648.
98. Pickhardt PJ, Choi JH. AJR 2003;181:799–805.
99. Lefere PA, Gryspeerdt SS, Dewyspelaere J, Baekelandt M, Van Holsbeeck BG. Radiology 2002;224:393–403.
100. Chen D, Liang Z, Wax MR, Li L, Li B, Kaufman AE. IEEE Trans Med Imaging 2000;19:1220–1226.
101. Callstrom MR, Johnson CD, Fletcher JG, et al. Radiology 2001;219:693–698.

102. Zalis ME, Perumpillichira J, Del Frate C, Hahn PF. Radiology 2003;226:911–917.
103. Yoshida H, Masutani Y, MacEneaney P, Rubin DT, Dachman AH. Radiology
     2002;222:327–336.
104. Summers RM, Johnson CD, Pusanik LM, Malley JD, Youssef AM, Reed JE.
     Radiology 2001;219:51–59.

6

Imaging of Brain Cancer

Soonmee Cha

Key Points

- Brain imaging is necessary for optimal localization, characterization, and management of brain cancer prior to surgery in patients with suspected or confirmed brain tumors (strong evidence).
- Due to its superior soft tissue contrast, multiplanar capability, and biosafety, magnetic resonance imaging (MRI) with and without gadolinium-based intravenous contrast material is the preferred method for brain cancer imaging when compared to computed tomography (moderate evidence).
- No adequate data exist on the role of imaging in monitoring brain cancer response to therapy and differentiating between tumor recurrence and therapy related changes (insufficient evidence).
- No adequate data exist on the role of nonanatomic, physiology-based imaging, such as proton magnetic resonance spectroscopy (MRS), perfusion and diffusion MRI, and nuclear medicine imaging [single photon emission computed tomography (SPECT) and positron emission tomography (PET)] in monitoring treatment response or in pre-

dicting prognosis and outcome in patients with brain cancer (insufficient evidence).

- Human studies conducted on the use of MRS for brain tumors demonstrate that this noninvasive method is technically feasible, and suggest potential benefits for some of the proposed indications. However, there is a paucity of high-quality direct evidence demonstrating the impact on diagnostic thinking and therapeutic decision making.

Definition and Pathophysiology

The term *brain cancer*, which is more commonly referred to as brain tumor, is used here to describe all primary and secondary neoplasms of the brain and its covering, including the leptomeninges, dura, skull, and scalp. Brain cancer comprises a variety of central nervous system tumors with a wide range of histopathology, molecular/genetic profile, clinical spectrum, treatment possibilities, and patient prognosis and outcome. The pathophysiology of brain cancer is complex and dependent on various factors, such as histology, molecular and chromosomal aberration, tumor-related protein expression, primary versus secondary origin, and host factors (1–4).

Unique Challenges of Brain Cancer

When compared to systemic cancers (e.g., lung, breast, colon), brain cancer is unique in several ways. First, the brain is covered by a tough, fibrous tissue, the dura matter, and a bony skull that protects the inner contents. This rigid covering allows very little, if any, increase in volume of the inner content, and therefore brain tumor cells adapt to grow in a more infiltrative rather than expansive pattern. This growth pattern limits the disruption to the underlying cytoarchitecture. Second, the brain capillaries have a unique barrier known as the blood—brain barrier (BBB), which limits the entrance of systemic circulation into the central nervous system. Cancer cells can hide behind the protective barrier of the BBB, migrate with minimal disruption to the structural and physiologic milieu of the brain, and escape imaging detection since an intravenous contrast agent becomes visible when there is BBB disruption, allowing the agent to leak into the interstitial space (5–9).

Epidemiology

Primary malignant or benign brain cancers were estimated to be newly diagnosed in about 35,519 Americans in 2001 [Central Brain Tumor Registry of the United States (10). Primary brain cancers are among the top 10 causes of cancer-related deaths (11). Nearly 13,000 people die from these cancers each year in the United States (CBTRUS, 2000). About 11 to 12 per 100,000 persons in the U.S. are diagnosed with a primary brain cancer each year, and 6 to 7 per 100,000 are diagnosed with a primary malignant brain cancer. Almost one in every 1300 children will develop some form of primary brain cancer before age 20 years (11). Between 1991 and 1995, 23%

of childhood cancers were brain cancers, and about one fourth of child-hood cancers deaths were from a malignant brain tumor.

The epidemiologic study of brain cancer is challenging and complex due to a number of factors unique to this disease. First, primary and secondary brain cancers are vastly different diseases that clearly need to be differentiated and categorized, which is an inherently difficult task. Second, histopathologic classification of brain cancer is complicated due to the heterogeneity of the tumors at virtually all levels of structural and functional organization such as differential growth rate, metastatic potential, sensitivity irradiation and chemotherapy, and genetic lability. Third, several brain cancer types have benign and malignant variants with a continuous spectrum of biologic aggressiveness. It is therefore difficult to assess the full spectrum of the disease at presentation (12).

The most common primary brain cancers are tumors of neuroepithelial origin, which include astrocytomas, oligodendrogliomas, mixed gliomas (oligoastrocytomas), ependymomas, choroids plexus tumors, neuroepithelial tumors of uncertain origin, neuronal and mixed neuronal-glial tumors, pineal tumors, and embryonal tumors. The most common type of primary brain tumor that involves the covering of the brain (as opposed to the substance) is meningioma, which accounts for more than 20% of all brain tumors (13). The most common type of primary brain cancer in adults is glioblastoma multiforme. In adults, brain metastases far outnumber primary neoplasms owing to the high incidence of systemic cancer (e.g., lung and breast carcinoma).

The incidence rate of all primary benign and malignant brain tumors based on CBTRUS is 14.0 cases per 100,000 person-years (5.7 per 100,000 person-years for benign tumors and 7.7 person-years for malignant tumors). The rate is higher in males (14.2 per 100,000 person-years) than in females (13.9 per 100,000 person-years). According to the Surveillance, Epidemiology, and End Results (SEER) program, the 5-year relative survival rate following the diagnosis of a primary malignant brain tumor (excluding lymphoma) is 32.7% for males and 31.6% for females. The prevalence rate for all primary brain tumors based on CBTRUS (11) is 130.8 per 100,000, and the estimated number of people living with a diagnosis of primary brain tumors was 359,000 persons. Two-, 5-, and 10-year observed and relative survival rates for each specific type of malignant brain tumor, according to the SEER report from 1973 to 1996, showed that glioblastoma multiforme (GBM) has the poorest prognosis. More detailed information on the brain cancer survival data is available at the CBTRUS Web site (http://www.cbtrus.org/2001/table2001_12.htm).

In terms of brain metastases, the exact annual incidence remains unknown due to a lack of a dedicated national cancer registry but is estimated to be 97,800 to 170,000 new cases each year in the U.S. The most common types of primary cancer causing brain metastasis are cancers of the lung, breast, unknown primary, melanoma, and colon.

Overall Cost to Society

Brain cancer is a rare neoplasm but affects people of all ages (11). It is more common in the pediatric population and tends to cause high morbidity and mortality (14). The overall cost to society in dollar amount is difficult to estimate and may not be as high as other, more common systemic cancers. The cost of treating brain cancer in the U.S. is difficult to determine but can be estimated to be far greater than $4 billion per year based on the estimated number of people living with brain cancer (359,000, as cited above; CBTRUS) and $11,365.23 per patient for initial cost of surgical treatment. There are very few articles in the literature that address the cost-effectiveness or overall cost to society in relation to imaging of brain cancer. One of the few articles that discusses the actual monetary cost to society is by Latif et al. (15) from Great Britain. They assessed the mean costs of medical care for 157 patients with brain cancer. Based on this study, the average cost of imaging was less than 3% of the total, whereas radiotherapy was responsible for greater than 50% of the total cost. The relative contribution of imaging in this study appears low, however, and what is not known from this report is what kind of imaging was done in these patients with brain cancer during their hospital stay and as outpatients, and how often it was done. In addition, the vastly different health care reimbursement structure in Britain and the U.S. makes interpretation difficult.

Goals of Neuroimaging

The goals of imaging in patients with suspected brain cancer are (1) diagnosis at acute presentation, (2) preoperative or treatment planning to further characterize brain abnormality, and (3) posttreatment evaluation for residual disease and therapy-related changes. The role of imaging is critical dependent on the clinical context that the study is being ordered (16). The initial diagnosis of brain cancer is often made based on a computed tomography (CT) scan in an emergency room setting when a patient presents with an acute clinical symptom such as seizure or focal neurologic deficit. Once a brain abnormality is detected on the initial scan, MRI with contrast agent is obtained to further characterize the lesion and the remainder of the brain and to serve as a part of preoperative planning for a definitive histologic diagnosis. If the nature of the brain lesion is still in question after comprehensive imaging, further imaging with advanced techniques such as diffusion, perfusion, or proton spectroscopic imaging may be warranted to differentiate brain cancer from tumor-mimicking lesions such as infarcts, abscesses, or demyelinating lesions (17–19). In the immediate postoperative imaging, the most important imaging objectives are to (1) determine the amount of residual or recurrent disease; (2) assess early postoperative complications such as hemorrhage, contusion, or other brain injury; and (3) determine delay treatment complications such as radiation necrosis and treatment leukoencephalopathy.

Methodology

A Medline search was performed using PubMed (National Library of Medicine, Bethesda, Maryland) for original research publications discussing the diagnostic performance and effectiveness of imaging strategies in brain cancer. Systematic literature review was performed from 1966 through August 2003. Key words included are (1) *brain cancer*, (2) *brain tumor*, (3) *glioma*, (4) *diagnostic imaging*, and (5) *neurosurgery*. In addition, the following three cancer databases were reviewed:

1. The SEER program maintained by the National Cancer Institute (www.seer.cancer.gov) for incidence, survival, and mortality rates, classified by tumor histology, brain topography, age, race, and gender. The SEER is a population-based reference standard for cancer data, and it collects incidence and follow-up data on malignant brain cancer only.

2. The CBTRUS (www.cbtrus.org) collects incidence data on all primary brain tumors from 11 collaborating state registries; however, follow-up data are not available.

3. The National Cancer Data Base (NCDB) (www.facs.org/cancer/ncdb) serves as a comprehensive clinical surveillance resource for cancer care in the U.S. While not population-based, the NCDB identifies newly diagnosed cases and conducts follow-up on all primary brain tumors from hospitals accredited by the American College of Surgeons. The NCDB is the largest of the three databases and also contains more complete information regarding treatment of tumors than either the SEER or CBTRUS databases.

I. Who Should Undergo Imaging to Exclude Brain Cancer?

Summary of Evidence: The scientific evidence on this topic is limited. No strong evidence studies are available. Most of the available literature is classified as limited and moderate evidence. The three most common clinical symptoms of brain cancer are headache, seizure, and focal weakness—all of which are neither unique nor specific for the presence of brain cancer (see Chapters 10 and 11). The clinical manifestation of brain cancer is heavily dependent on the topography of the lesion. For example, lesions in the motor cortex may have more acute presentation, whereas more insidious onset of cognitive or personality changes are commonly associated with prefrontal cortex tumors (20,21).

Despite the aforementioned nonspecific clinical presentation of subjects with brain cancer, Table 6.1 lists the clinical symptoms suggestive of brain

Table 6.1. Clinical symptoms suggestive of a brain cancer

Nonmigraine, nonchronic headache of moderate to severe degree (see Chapter 10)
Partial complex seizure (see Chapter 11)
Focal neurologic deficit
Speech disturbance
Cognitive or personality change
Visual disturbance
Altered consciousness
Sensory abnormalities
Gait problem or ataxia
Nausea and vomiting without other gastrointestinal illness
Papilledema
Cranial nerve palsy

cancer. A relatively acute onset of any one of these symptoms that progresses over time should strongly warrant brain imaging.

Supporting Evidence: It remains difficult, however, to narrow down the criteria for the "suspected" clinical symptomatology of brain cancer. In a retrospective study of 653 patients with supratentorial brain cancer, Salcman (22) found that the most common clinical features of brain cancer were headache (70%), seizure (54%), cognitive or personality change (52%), focal weakness (43%), nausea or vomiting (31%), speech disturbances (27%), alteration of consciousness (25%), sensory abnormalities (14%), and visual disturbances (8%) (moderate evidence). Similarly, Snyder et al. (23) studied 101 patients who were admitted to the emergency department and discharged with a diagnosis of brain cancer (moderate evidence). They found that the most frequent clinical features were headache (55%), cognitive or personality changes (50%), ataxia (40%), focal weakness (36%), nausea or vomiting (36%), papilledema (27%), cranial nerve palsy (25%), seizure (24%), visual disturbance (20%), speech disturbance (20%), sensory abnormalities (18%), and positive Babinski sign (17%). No combination of these factors has been shown to reliably differentiate brain cancer from other benign causes.

A. Applicability to Children

Brain cancers in childhood differ significantly from adult lesions in their sites of origin, histological features, clinical presentations, and likelihood to disseminate throughout the nervous system early in the course of disease. As succinctly summarized by Hutter et al. (24), there are vast differences in epidemiology, topography, histology, and prognosis of brain cancer between adults and children. Whereas the great majority of adult tumors arise in the cerebral cortex, about half of childhood brain cancers originate infratentorially—in the cerebellum, brainstem, or fourth ventricular region. Brain metastasis from systemic cancer is rare in children, whereas it is common in adults owing to the preponderance of systemic cancer (lung and breast being the two most common). Metastatic cancers in childhood mainly represent leptomeningeal dissemination from a primary brain lesion (25) such as medulloblastoma, pineoblastoma, or germinoma—hence the importance of imaging the entire neuroaxis in these patients (i.e., brain and entire spine). The incidence of primary brain cancer in children is most common from birth to age 4 years; the vast majority of histologic types are medulloblastomas and juvenile pilocytic astrocytomas (JPAs). Headache, posterior fossa symptoms (such as nausea and vomiting), ataxia, and cranial nerve symptoms predominate in children due to the fact that about half of pediatric brain cancer occurs infratentorially (12,25,26). Nonmigraine, nonchronic headache in a child should raise a high suspicion for an intracranial mass lesion, especially if there are any additional posterior fossa symptoms, and imaging should be conducted without delay (see Chapter 10).

II. What Is the Appropriate Imaging in Subjects at Risk for Brain Cancer?

Summary of Evidence: The sensitivity and specificity of MRI is higher than that of CT for brain neoplasms (moderate evidence). Therefore, in high-risk subjects suspected of having brain cancer, MRI with and without gadolinium-based contrast agent is the imaging modality of choice to further characterize the lesion. Table 6.2 lists the advantages and limitations of CT and MRI in the evaluation of subjects with suspected brain cancer.

There is no strong evidence to suggest that the addition of other diagnostic tests, such as MRS, perfusion MR, PET, or SPECT, improves either the cost-effectiveness or the outcome in the high-risk group at initial presentation.

Supporting Evidence: Medina et al. (27) found in a retrospective study of 315 pediatric patients that overall, MRI was more sensitive and specific than CT in detecting intracranial space-occupying lesions (92% and 99%, respectively, for MRI versus 81% and 92%, respectively, for CT). However, no difference in sensitivity and specificity was found in the surgical space-occupying lesions (27). Table 6.3 lists the sensitivity and specificity of MRI and CT for brain cancer as outlined by Hutter et al. (24).

There has been a tremendous progress in research involving various brain radiotracers, which provide the valuable functional and metabolic pathophysiology of brain cancer. Yet the question remains as to how best to incorporate radiotracer imaging methods into diagnosis and management of patients with brain cancer. The most widely used radiotracer imaging method in brain cancer imaging is [201]thalium SPECT. Although very purposeful, it has a limited role in initial diagnosis or predicting the degree of brain cancer malignancy. Positron emission tomography using ^{18}F-2-fluoro-2-deoxy-d-glucose (FDG) radiotracer can be useful in differentiating recurrent brain cancer from radiation necrosis, but similarly to SPECT its ability as an independent diagnostic and prognostic value above that of MRI and histology is debatable (28). There is limited evidence per-

Table 6.2. Advantages and limitations of computed tomography (CT) and magnetic resonance imaging (MRI)

	Advantages	Limitations
CT	Widely available Short imaging time Lower cost Excellent for detection of acute hemorrhage or bony abnormality	Inferior soft tissue resolution Prone to artifact in posterior fossa Ionizing radiation Risk of allergy to iodinated contrast agent
MRI	Multiplanar capability Superior soft tissue resolution No ionizing radiation Safer contrast agent (gadolinium-based) profile	Higher cost Not as widely available Suboptimal for detection of acute hemorrhage or bony/calcific abnormality

Table 6.3. Sensitivity and specificity of brain tumor imaging

Type of brain cancer	Imaging modality	Sensitivity (%)	Specificity (%)
Primary brain cancer	MRI with contrast	Gold standard	—
	CT with contrast	87	79
Primary brain cancer in children (27)	MRI	92	99
	CT	81	92
Brain metastasis	MRI with single dose contrast	93–100	—
	MRI without contrast	36	—
	^{201}Tl SPECT	70	—
	^{18}FDG PET	82	38
Recurrent tumor vs. treatment related necrosis	^{201}Tl SPECT	92	88
	^{18}FDG PET		
	MRI with co-registration	86	80
	MRI without co-registration	65	80

Source: Adapted from Hutter et al. (24), with permission from Elsevier.

taining to perfusion MRI in tumor diagnosis and grading despite several articles proposing its useful role. Similar to proton MRS (see issue III, below), perfusion MRI remains an investigational tool at this time pending stronger evidence proving its effect on health outcomes of patients with brain cancer.

A. Applicability to Children

In children with aggressive brain cancer such as medulloblastoma or ependymoma, special attention should be paid to the entire craniospinal axis to evaluate drop metastasis. Neuroimaging of the entire craniospinal axis should be done prior to the initial surgery in order to avoid postsurgical changes complicating the evaluation. Magnetic resonance imaging with gadolinium-based contrast agent is the modality of choice to look for enhancement along the leptomeningeal surface of the spinal cord (29,30).

B. Special Case: Can Imaging Be Used to Differentiate Posttreatment Necrosis from Residual Tumor?

Imaging differentiation of treatment necrosis and residual/recurrent tumor is challenging because they can appear similar and can coexist in a single given lesion. Hence the traditional anatomy-based imaging methods have a limited role in the accurate differentiation of the two entities. Nuclear medicine imaging techniques such as SPECT and PET provide functional information on tissue metabolism and oxygen consumption and thus offer a theoretical advantage over anatomic imaging in differentiation tissue necrosis and active tumor. Multiple studies demonstrate that SPECT is more sensitive and specific than is PET in differentiating tumor recurrence from radiation necrosis (24) (Table 6.2). There is also insufficient evidence of the role of MRS for this tumor type (see issue III, below).

C. Special Case: Neuroimaging Modality in Patients with Suspected Brain Metastatic Disease

Brain metastases are far more common than primary brain cancer in adults owing to the higher prevalence of systemic cancers and their propensity to metastasize (31–33). Focal neurologic symptoms in a patient with a history of systemic cancer should raise high suspicion for intracranial metastasis and prompt imaging. The preferred neuroimaging modality in patients with suspected brain metastatic disease is MRI with a single dose (0.1 mmol/kg body weight) of gadolinium-based contrast agent. Most studies described in the literature suggest that contrast-enhanced MRI is superior to contrast-enhanced CT in the detection of brain metastatic disease, especially if the lesions are less than 2 cm (moderate evidence).

Davis and colleagues (34) assessed imaging studies in 23 patients, comparing contrast-enhanced MRI with double dose-delayed CT (moderate evidence). Contrast-enhanced MRI demonstrated more than 67 definite or typical brain metastases. The double dose-delayed CT revealed only 37 metastatic lesions. The authors concluded that MRI with enhancement is superior to double dose-delayed CT scan for detecting brain metastasis, anatomic localization, and number of lesions. Golfieri and colleagues (35) reported similar findings (moderate evidence). They studied 44 patients with small-cell carcinoma to detect cerebral metastases. All patients were studied with contrast-enhanced CT scan and gadolinium-enhanced MRI; 43% had cerebral metastases. Both contrast-enhanced CT and gadolinium-enhanced MRI detected lesions greater than 2 cm. For lesions smaller than 2 cm, 9% were detected only by gadolinium-enhanced T1-weighted images. The authors concluded that gadolinium-enhanced T1-weighted images remain the most accurate technique in the assessment of cerebral metastases. Sze and colleagues (36) performed prospective and retrospective studies in 75 patients (moderate evidence). In 49 patients, MRI and contrast-enhanced CT were equivalent. In 26 patients, however, the results were discordant, with neither CT nor MRI being consistently superior; MRI demonstrated more metastases in 9 of these 26 patients. Contrast-enhanced CT, however, better depicted lesions in eight of 26 patients.

There are several reports on using a triple dose of contrast agent to increase the sensitivity of lesion detection (37,38). Another study by Sze et al. (39), however, found that routine triple-dose contrast agent administration in all cases of suspected brain metastasis was not helpful, and could lead to an increasing number of false-positive results. The authors concluded that the use of triple-dose contrast material is beneficial in selected cases with equivocal findings or solitary metastasis. Their study was based on 92 consecutive patients with negative or equivocal findings or a solitary metastasis on single-dose contrast-enhanced MRI who underwent triple-dose studies.

D. Special Case: How Can Tumor Be Differentiated from Tumor-Mimicking Lesions?

There are several intracranial disease processes that can mimic brain cancer and pose a diagnostic dilemma on both clinical presentation and conventional MRI (16,40–44), such as infarcts, radiation necrosis, demyelinating plaques, abscesses, hematomas, and encephalitis. On imaging, any one of these lesions and brain cancer can both demonstrate contrast enhancement, perilesional edema, varying degrees of mass effect, and central necrosis.

There are numerous reports in the literature of misdiagnosis and mismanagement of these subjects who were erroneously thought to have brain cancer and, in some cases, went on to surgical resection for histopathologic confirmation (15,43,45). Surgery is clearly contraindicated in these subjects and can lead to an unnecessary increase in morbidity and mortality. A large acute demyelinating plaque, in particular, is notorious for mimicking an aggressive brain cancer (43,46–49). Due to the presence of mitotic figures and atypical astrocytes, this uncertainty occurs not only on clinical presentation and imaging but also on histopathologic examination (44). The consequence of unnecessary surgery in subjects with tumor-mimicking lesions can be quite grave, and hence every effort should be made to differentiate these lesions from brain cancer.

Anatomic imaging of the brain suffers from nonspecificity and its inability to differentiate tumor from tumor-mimicking lesions (15). Recent developments in nonanatomic, physiology-based MRI methods, such as diffusion/perfusion MRI and proton spectroscopic imaging, promise to provide information not readily available from structural MRI and thus improve diagnostic accuracy (50,51).

Diffusion-weighted MRI has been shown to be particularly helpful in differentiating cystic/necrotic neoplasm from brain abscess by demonstrating marked reduced diffusion within an abscess. Chang et al. (52) compared diffusion-weighted imaging (DWI) and conventional anatomic MRI to distinguish brain abscesses from cystic or necrotic brain tumors in 11 patients with brain abscesses and 15 with cystic or necrotic brain gliomas or metastases. They found that postcontrast T1-weighted imaging yielded a sensitivity of 60%, a specificity of 27%, a positive predictive value (PPV) of 53%, and a negative predictive value (NPV) of 33% in the diagnosis of necrotic tumors. Diffusion-weighted imaging yielded a sensitivity of 93%, a specificity of 91%, a PPV of 93%, and a NPV of 91%. Based on the analysis of receiver operating characteristic (ROC) curves, they found a clear advantage for DWI as a diagnostic tool in detecting abscesses when compared to postcontrast T1-weighted imaging.

Table 6.4 lists lesions that can mimic brain cancer both on clinical grounds and on imaging. By using diffusion-weighted imaging, acute infarct and abscess could readily be distinguished from brain cancer because of the reduced diffusion seen with the first two entities (52–56). Highly cellular brain cancer can have reduced diffusion but not to the same degree as acute infarct or abscess (57).

Table 6.4. Brain cancer mimicking lesions

Infarct
Radiation necrosis
Abscess
Demyelinating plaque
Subacute hematoma
Encephalitis

III. What Is the Role of Proton Magnetic Resonance Spectroscopy (MRS) in the Diagnosis and Follow-Up of Brain Neoplasms?

Summary of Evidence: The Blue Cross–Blue Shield Association (BCBSA) Medical Advisory Panel concluded that the MRS in the evaluation of suspected brain cancer did not meet the Technology Evaluation Center (TEC) criteria as a diagnostic test, hence further studies in a prospectively defined population are needed.

Supporting Evidence: Recently, BCBSA Medical Advisory Panel made the following judgments about whether ^{1}H MRS for evaluation of suspected brain tumors meets the BCBSA TEC criteria based on the available evidence (58). The advisory panel reviewed seven published studies that included up to 271 subjects (59–65). These seven studies were selected for inclusion in the review of evidence because (1) the sample size was at least 10; (2) the criteria for a positive test were specified; (3) there was a method to confirm ^{1}H MRS diagnosis; and (4) the report provided sufficient data to calculate diagnostic test performance (sensitivity and specificity). The reviewers specifically addressed whether ^{1}H MRS for evaluation of suspected brain tumors meets the following five TEC criteria:

1. The technology must have approval from the appropriate governmental regulatory bodies.
2. The scientific evidence must permit conclusions concerning the effect of the technology on health outcomes.
3. The technology must improve the net health outcomes.
4. The technology must be as beneficial as any established alternatives.
5. The improvement must be attainable outside the investigational settings.

With the exception of the first criterion, the reviewers concluded that the available evidence on ^{1}H MRS in the evaluation of brain neoplasm was insufficient. The TEC also concluded that the overall body of evidence does not provide strong and consistent evidence regarding the diagnostic test characteristics of MRS in determining the presence or absence of brain neoplasm, both for differentiation of recurrent/residual tumor vs. delayed radiation necrosis (65) and for diagnosis of brain tumor versus other non-tumor diagnosis (59,60,62,64). Assessment of the health benefit of MRS in avoiding brain biopsy was evaluated in two studies (59,64), but the studies had limitations. However, other human studies conducted on the use of MRS for brain tumors demonstrate that this noninvasive method is technically feasible and suggest potential benefits for some of the proposed indications. But there is a paucity of high-quality direct evidence demonstrating the impact on diagnostic thinking and therapeutic decision making.

IV. What Is the Cost-Effectiveness of Imaging in Patients with Suspected Primary Brain Neoplasms or Brain Metastatic Disease?

Summary of Evidence: Routine brain CT in all patients with lung cancer has a cost-effectiveness ratio of $69,815 per quality-adjusted life year (QALY). However, the cost per QALY is highly sensitive to variations in the negative predictive value of a clinical evaluation, as well as to the cost of CT.

Cost-effectiveness analysis (CEA) of patients with headache suspected of having a brain neoplasm are presented in Chapter 10.

Supporting Evidence: In a study in the surgical literature, Colice et al. (64) compared the cost-effectiveness of two strategies for detecting brain metastases by CT in lung cancer patients: (1) routine CT for all patients irrespective of clinical (neurologic, hematologic) evidence of metastases (CT first); and (2) CT for only those patients in whom clinical symptoms developed (CT deferred). For a hypothetical cohort of patients, it was assumed that all primary lung carcinomas were potentially resectable. If no brain metastasis were detected by CT, the primary lung tumor would be resected. Brain metastasis as detected by CT would disqualify the patient for resection of the primary lung tumor. Costs were taken from the payer's perspective and based on prevailing Medicare payments. The rates of false-positive and false-negative findings were also considered in the calculation of the effectiveness of CT. The cost of the CT-first strategy was $11,108 and the cost for the CT-deferred strategy $10,915; however, the CT-first strategy increased life expectancy by merely 1.1 days. Its cost-effectiveness ratio was calculated to be $69,815 per QALY. The cost per QALY is highly sensitive to variations in the negative predictive value of a clinical evaluation, as well as to the cost of CT. This study is instructive because it highlights the importance of considering false-positive and false-negative findings and performing sensitivity analysis. For a detailed discussion of the specifics of the decision-analytic model and sensitivity analysis, the reader is referred to the articles by Colice et al. (66) and Hutter et al. (24).

Take-Home Figure

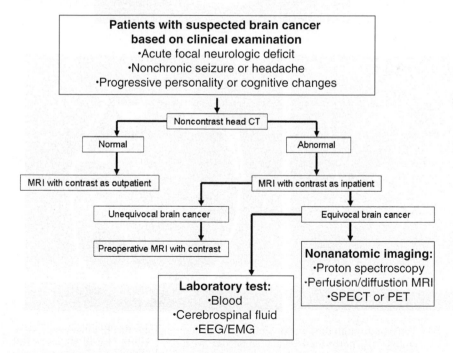

Figure 6.1. Decision flow chart to study patients with suspected brain cancer. In patients with presenting with an acute neurologic event such as seizure or focal deficit, noncontrast head CT examination should be done expeditiously to exclude any life-threatening conditions such as hemorrhage or herniation.

Imaging Case Studies

Several cases are shown to illustrate the pros and cons of different neuroimaging modalities differentiating true neoplasms from lesion mimicking neoplasms.

Case 1

A 54-year-old man with headache and seizures and a pathologic diagnosis of glioblastoma multiforme (GBM) (Figure 6.2 A and B).

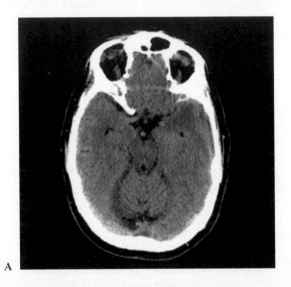

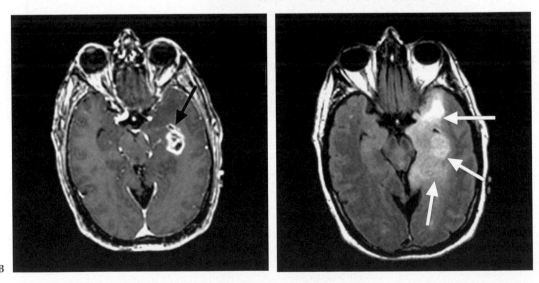

Figure 6.2. A: Unenhanced CT image through the level of temporal lobe demonstrates no obvious mass lesion. B: Contrast-enhanced T1-weighted MRI performed on the same day as the CT study clearly shows a rim enhancing centrally necrotic mass (black arrow) in the left temporal lobe. C: Fluid-attenuated inversion recovery (FLAIR) MRI better demonstrates the large extent of abnormality (white arrows) involving most of the left temporal lobe.

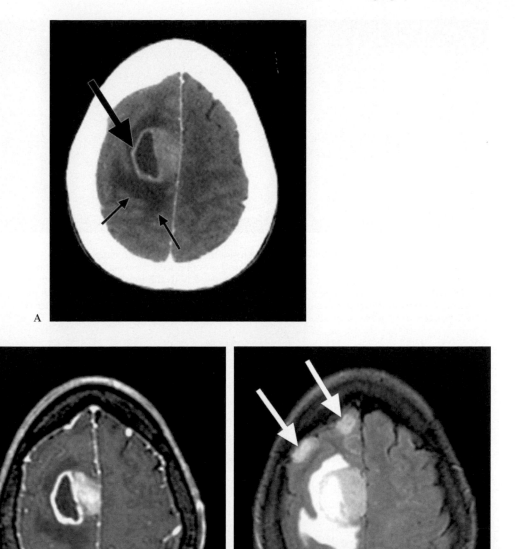

Figure 6.3. A: Contrast-enhanced CT image demonstrates an enhancing solid and necrotic mass (large black arrow) within the right superior frontal gyrus associated with surrounding low density (small arrows). B: Contrast-enhanced T1-weighted MRI performed on the same day as the CT study shows similar finding. C: FLAIR MRI clearly demonstrates two additional foci of cortically based signal abnormality (white arrows) that were found to be infiltrating glioma on histopathology.

Case 2

A 42-year old woman with difficulty in balancing, left-sided weakness, and a pathologic diagnosis of GBM (Fig 6.3).

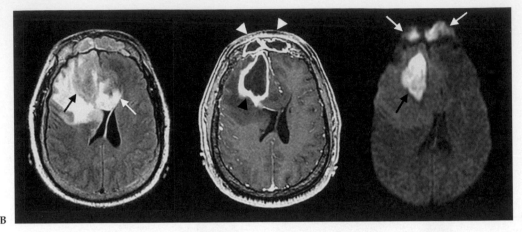

A,B   C

Figure 6.4. A: FLAIR MRI demonstrates a large mass lesion (black arrow) with extensive surrounding edema that crosses the corpus callosum (white arrow). B: Contrast-enhanced T1-weighted MRI shows thick rim enhancement (black arrowhead) and central necrosis associated with the mass. Similar pattern of abnormality is noted within the frontal sinuses (white arrowheads). C: Diffusion-weighted MRI depicts marked reduced diffusion within the frontal lesion (black arrow) and the frontal sinus lesion (white arrows), both of which were proven to be a bacterial abscess at histopathology.

Case 3

A 53-year-old man with frontal abscess with irregular enhancement with central necrosis simulating a brain cancer.

Suggested Imaging Protocol

In patient with suspected primary brain neoplasm or metastasis, this is the MRI protocol recommended (Table 6.5).

Future Research

- Rigorous technology assessment of noninvasive imaging modalities such as MRS, diffusion and perfusion MRI, functional MRI, PET, and SPECT

Table 6.5. MR imaging protocol for a subject with suspected brain cancer or metastasis

3D-localizer
Axial and sagittal precontrast T1-weighted imaging
Diffusion-weighted imaging
Axial fluid-attenuated inversion recovery (FLAIR)
Axial T2-weighted imaging
Axial, coronal, and sagittal postcontrast T1-weighted imaging
Optional: dynamic contrast-enhanced perfusion MRI
   Proton MR spectroscopic imaging
Consider doing gadolinium enhanced MRI of entire spine to rule out
   metastatic disease

- Assessment of the effects of imaging on the patient outcome and costs of diagnosis and management
- Rigorous cost-effectiveness analysis of competing imaging modalities

References

1. Burger PC, Vogel FS. The brain: tumors. In: Burger PC, Vogel FS, eds. Surgical Pathology of the Central Nervous System and Its Coverings. New York: Wiley, 1982:223–266.
2. Burger PC, Vogel FS, Green SB, Strike TA. Cancer 1985;56:1106–1111.
3. Kleihues P, Sobin LH. Cancer 2000;88:2887.
4. Kleihues P, Ohgaki H. Toxicol Pathol 2000;28:164–170.
5. Go KG. Adv Tech Stand Neurosurg 1997;23:47–142.
6. Sato S, Suga S, Yunoki K, Mihara B. Acta Neurochir Suppl 1994;60:116–118.
7. Stewart PA, Hayakawa K, Farrell CL, Del Maestro RF. J Neurosurg 1987;67:697–705.
8. Stewart PA, Magliocco M, Hayakawa K, et al. Microvasc Res 1987;33:270–282.
9. Abbott NJ, Chugani DC, Zaharchuk G, Rosen BR, Lo EH. Adv Drug Deliv Rev 1999;37:253–277.
10. Surawicz TS, McCarthy BJ, Kupelian V, Jukich PJ, Bruner JM, Davis FG. Descriptive epidemiology of primary brain and CNS tumors: results from the Central Brain Tumor Registry of the United States, 1990–1994. Neuro-oncol 1999;1:14–25.
11. Landis SH, Murray T, Bolden S, Wingo PA. Cancer statistics, 1998. CA Cancer J Clin 1998;48:6–29.
12. DeAngelis LM. N Engl J Med 2001;344:114–123.
13. Longstreth WT Jr, Dennis LK, McGuire VM, Drangsholt MT, Koepsell TD. Cancer 1993;72:639–648.
14. Pollack IF. Semin Surg Oncol 1999;16:73–90.
15. Latif AZ, Signorini D, Gregor A, Whittle IR. Br J Neurosurg 1998;12:118–122.
16. Ricci PE. Imaging of adult brain tumors. Neuroimaging Clin North Am 1999;9:651–669.
17. Cha S, Pierce S, Knopp EA, et al. AJNR 2001;22:1109–1116.
18. Kepes JJ. Ann Neurol 1993;33:18–27.
19. De Stefano N, Caramanos Z, Preul MC, Francis G, Antel JP, Arnold DL. Ann Neurol 1998;44:273–278.
20. Porter RJ, Gallagher P, Thompson JM, Young AH. Br J Psychiatry 2003;182:214–220.
21. Meyers CA. Oncology (Huntingt) 2000;14:75–79; discussion 79,81–72,85.
22. Salcman M. Supratentorial gliomas: clinical features and surgical therapy. In: Wilkins R, Rengachary S, eds. Neurosurgery. New York: McGraw-Hill, 1985:579–590.
23. Snyder H, Robinson K, Shah D, Brennan R, Handrigan M. J Emerg Med 1993;11:253–258.
24. Hutter A, Schwetye KE, Bierhals AJ, McKinstry RC. Neuroimaging Clin North Am 2003;13:237–250,x–xi.
25. Miltenburg D, Louw DF, Sutherland GR. Can J Neurol Sci 1996;23:118–122.
26. Becker LE. Neuroimaging Clin North Am 1999;9:671–690.
27. Medina LS, Pinter JD, Zurakowski D, Davis RG, Kuban K, Barnes PD. Radiology 1997;202:819–824.
28. Benard F, Romsa J, Hustinx R. Semin Nucl Med 2003;33:148–162.
29. Parizel PM, Baleriaux D, Rodesch G, et al. AJR 1989;152:1087–1096.
30. Blaser SI, Harwood-Nash DC. J Neurooncol 1996;29:23–34.
31. Walker AE, Robins M, Weinfeld FD. Neurology 1985;35:219–226.
32. Wingo PA, Tong T, Bolden S. CA Cancer J Clin 1995;45:8–30.

33. Patchell RA. Neurol Clin 1991;9:817–827.
34. Davis PC, Hudgins PA, Peterman SB, Hoffman JC Jr. AJNR 1991;12:293–300.
35. Golfieri R, Cherryman GR, Olliff JF, Husband JE. Radiol Med (Torino) 1991;82:27–34.
36. Sze G, Shin J, Krol G, Johnson C, Liu D, Deck MD. Radiology 1988;168:187–194.
37. Kuhn MJ, Hammer GM, Swenson LC, Youssef HT, Gleason TJ. Comput Med Imaging Graph 1994;18:391–399.
38. Yuh WT, Tali ET, Nguyen HD, Simonson TM, Mayr NA, Fisher DJ. AJNR 1995;16:373–380.
39. Sze G, Johnson C, Kawamura Y, et al. AJNR 1998;19:821–828.
40. Morgenstern LB, Frankowski RF. J Neurooncol 1999;44:47–52.
41. Barcikowska M, Chodakowska M, Klimowicz I, Liberski PP. Folia Neuropathol 1995;33:55–57.
42. Kim YJ, Chang KH, Song IC, et al. AJR 1998;171:1487–1490.
43. Zagzag D, Miller DC, Kleinman GM, Abati A, Donnenfeld H, Budzilovich GN. Am J Surg Pathol 1993;17:537–545.
44. Itto H, Yamano K, Mizukoshi H, Yamamoto S. No To Shinkei 1972;24:455–458.
45. Babu R, Huang PP, Epstein F, Budzilovich GN. J Neurooncol 1993;17:37–42.
46. Dagher AP, Smirniotopoulos J. Neuroradiology 1996;38:560–565.
47. Giang DW, Poduri KR, Eskin TA, et al. Neuroradiology 1992;34:150–154.
48. Kurihara N, Takahashi S, Furuta A, et al. Clin Imaging 1996;20:171–177.
49. Prockop LD, Heinz ER. Arch Neurol 1965;13:559–564.
50. Schaefer PW, Grant PE, Gonzalez RG. Radiology 2000;217:331–345.
51. Cha S, Knopp EA, Johnson G, Wetzel SG, Litt AW, Zagzag D. Radiology 2002;223:11–29.
52. Chang SC, Lai PH, Chen WL, et al. Clin Imaging 2002;26:227–236.
53. Castillo M, Mukherji SK. Semin Ultrasound CT MR 2000;21:405–416.
54. Ebisu T, Tanaka C, Umeda M, et al. Magn Reson Imaging 1996;14:1113–1116.
55. Laing AD, Mitchell PJ, Wallace D. Australas Radiol 1999;43:16–19.
56. Tsuruda JS, Chew WM, Moseley ME, Norman D. AJNR 1990;11:925–931; discussion 932–924.
57. Okamoto K, Ito J, Ishikawa K, Sakai K, Tokiguchi S. Eur Radiol 2000;10:1342–1350.
58. TEC Bull (Online) 2003;20:23–26.
59. Adamson AJ, Rand SD, Prost RW, Kim TA, Schultz C, Haughton VM. Radiology 1998;209:73–78.
60. Rand SD, Prost R, Haughton V, et al. AJNR 1997;18:1695–1704.
61. Shukla-Dave A, Gupta RK, Roy R, et al. Magn Reson Imaging 2001;19:103–110.
62. Kimura T, Sako K, Gotoh T, Tanaka K, Tanaka T. NMR Biomed 2001;14:339–349.
63. Wilken B, Dechent P, Herms J, et al. Pediatr Neurol 2000;23:22–31.
64. Lin A, Bluml S, Mamelak AN. J Neurooncol 1999;45:69–81.
65. Taylor JS, Langston JW, Reddick WE, et al. Int J Radiat Oncol Biol Phys 1996;36:1251–1261.
66. Colice GL, Birkmeyer JD, Black WC, Littenberg B, Silvestri G. Chest 1995; 108:1264–1271.

7

Imaging in the Evaluation of Patients with Prostate Cancer

Jeffrey H. Newhouse

Issues

I. Is transrectal ultrasound valuable as a prostate cancer screening tool?
II. Is transrectal ultrasound useful to guide prostate biopsy?
III. Is imaging accurate for staging prostate cancer?
   A. Ultrasound
   B. Computed tomography scan
   C. Magnetic resonance imaging
   D. Magnetic resonance spectroscopic imaging
   E. Positron emission tomography
IV. How accurate is bone scan for detecting metastatic prostate cancer?
   A. Special case: which patients should undergo imaging after initial treatment to look for metastatic disease?

Key Points

- Ultrasound probably aids in the effectiveness of biopsy for diagnosis, although imaging is not of proven value in screening (moderate evidence).
- Skeletal scintigraphy and computed tomography (CT) play a crucial role in assessing metastatic disease; they can be eliminated, however, in patients whose tumor volume, Gleason score, and prostate-specific antigen (PSA) are relatively low (strong evidence).
- Magnetic resonance imaging (MRI) is the most accurate of the imaging techniques in local staging, but its relative expense and persistent false-positive and false-negative rates for locally invasive disease suggest that it should be interpreted along with all additional available data, and reserved for patients in whom other data leave treatment choices ambiguous (strong evidence).
- Assessment of metastatic tumor burden by bone scan and CT are of prognostic value. After initial therapy, monitoring disease is primarily done with serial PSA determinations; imaging for recurrence should be limited to patients whose PSA levels clearly indicate recurrent or progressive disease and in whom imaging results have the potential to affect treatment (limited evidence).

Definition and Pathophysiology

Although there are a number of histologic varieties of prostate malignancies, overwhelmingly the most common is adenocarcinoma. Etiologic factors are not known in detail, but it is clearly an androgen-dependent disease in most cases; it is almost unheard of in chronically anorchid patients. Age is the most important risk factor; the disease is very rare in men under 40, but in men over 70, histologic evidence of intraprostatic adenocarcinoma can be found in at least half. A family history of the disease is a risk factor. Black men are more prone to develop the tumor, and it is more likely to be biologically malignant among them. There are probably environmental factors as well, but these are less well established.

Epidemiology

Prostate cancer is the most common internal malignancy of American men, and the second most common cause of death. In 2004, 230,110 new cases and 29,900 deaths were expected (1).

Overall Cost to Society

Although the low ratio of annual deaths to new cases reflects the fact that most histologic cases are not of clinical importance, the high absolute numbers of deaths and the 9-year average loss of life that each prostate cancer death causes suggest that the cost to society is huge. Most patients who die of prostate cancer are under treatment for years, and patients whose cancer is cured usually require major surgery or radiotherapy. The exact cost to society in the United States of prostate cancer is not clear, but if the cost of screening and treatment are added to the indirect cost of income loss and diversion of other resources, a very approximate figure of $10 billion a year would not be an excessive estimate.

Goals

The goals of imaging in prostate cancer are (1) to guide biopsy of the peripheral zone, (2) to stage prostate cancer accurately, and (3) to detect metastatic or recurrent cancer.

Methodology

The Ovid search engine was used to query the Medline database from 1966 to May 2004 for all searches. In all cases, the searches were limited to human investigations. No language limitations were imposed, but for articles published in languages other than English only the abstracts were reviewed. Multiple individual searches were conducted. In each, the phrase *prostate and (cancer or carcinoma)* limited the basic scope. Each search was also limited to the radiologic literature by the phrase *radiology or radiography or ultrasound or sonography or ct or (computed tomography) or MRI or (magnetic resonance imaging) or scan or scintigraphy or PET or (positron emission tomography)*. Individual searches were then limited by using the phrases *screen or screening, diagnosis, stage or staging,* or *recurrence or (monitor or monitoring)* as appropriate.

I. Is Transrectal Ultrasound Valuable as a Prostate Cancer Screening Tool?

Summary of Evidence: Transrectal ultrasound (TRUS) lacks the sensitivity and specificity that would be required to recommend it as a stand-alone screen. If it is used in combination with digital rectal examination (DRE) and prostate-specific antigen (PSA), the additionally discovered tumors are very few and a normal TRUS cannot obviate biopsy, which might otherwise be indicated by an abnormal DRE or PSA (insufficient evidence for using TRUS alone).

Supporting Evidence: Transabdominal sonography of the prostate gland provides insufficient resolution of prostatic tissue to be of value in searching for prostate cancer. High-frequency transrectal probes provide better spatial resolution, and since their introduction, there has been continued interest in the role of sonography in screening for prostate cancer (2–7).

The peripheral zone for most prostate glands appears relatively uniform in echogenicity, and the classic appearance of a focus of tumor in it is a relatively hypoechoic region (7). The central portions of the gland are more heterogeneous in appearance, especially in patients with benign prostatic hypertrophy; for this reason, and because only a minority of tumors are initially found in the central gland, tumors are primarily sought in the peripheral zone. Unfortunately, not all tumors are relatively hypoechoic; some are hyperechoic, some are isoechoic and some are of mixed echogenicity (8,9). Focal benign abnormalities of the peripheral zone of the prostate, including prostatitis, focal hypertrophy, hemorrhage, and even prostatic intraepithelial neoplasia (PIN) make differential diagnosis a problem. In some cases, the echogenicity of the tumor cannot be distinguished from that of the background tissue and only distortion of the prostatic capsule may provide a clue that a neoplasm exists. Given all of this, it has become apparent that TRUS is neither highly sensitive nor highly specific in the detection of prostate cancer (10–15).

Although current practice in the United States is not to employ TRUS frequently as a stand-alone screen for prostate cancer, finding a consensus in the literature is not easy. When the technique was introduced, investigators were enthusiastic about it, citing relatively high sensitivity and specificity values, and even a few relatively modern series purport to show high accuracy (2,6,7). But most current literature suggests relatively low sensitivity and specificity and does not recommend use of TRUS as a screen (1,8,9,13–16). The reasons for diminishing enthusiasm are probably several: In the earliest years of TRUS investigation, the only competing screening modality was DRE, with which TRUS compared relatively favorably (5,17), but nearly two decades ago PSA was introduced, which in most series proved to be more accurate and cheaper than TRUS (8,16,18,19). At the same time, the criteria for defining screening populations and statistics for assessing the efficacy of the test have become more stringent. There are probably several reasons for the widely varying claims regarding the efficacy of

TRUS as well, including the considerable subjectivity of analysis of findings on the TRUS images, varying practices with regard to blinding TRUS practitioners to results of other screening modalities, and the considerable lack of standardization and characterization of tested populations.

As recently as 2002, some authors claimed sensitivities of TRUS ranging from 74% to 94% (2). But other studies have looked more closely at the sensitivity of TRUS and found considerably lower numbers. For example, a series of patients with prostate cancer diagnosed only on one side of the prostate, in whom TRUS was followed by prostatectomy and careful pathologic examination of the entire prostate, found a sensitivity of 52%, specificity of 68%, positive predictive values (PPV) of 54%, and negative predictive value (NPV) of 66% (15). Another group found that among patients with normal PSA and DRE, if TRUS was positive only 9% of biopsied patients had tumor (8). Another investigator found that under the same circumstances the PPV for TRUS was 7% and that biopsies would have to be performed on 18 TRUS-positive patients to detect one tumor (11). Flanigan et al. (13) found a PPV for TRUS of 18% in patients with abnormal PSA or DRE; Cooner et al. (20) found that when DRE and PSA were normal, the PPV of TRUS was 9% (21). Babaian et al. (18) found that using a combination of DRE and PSA, a significantly higher PPV could be found than with a combination of TRUS and PSA. If TRUS is performed in addition to DRE, slightly more tumors are found than if DRE is used alone (3,17,21).

There have been technical advantages that have been applied in hopes of improving the performance of TRUS. Color Doppler imaging (22) improves the sensitivity from that of conventional gray-scale imaging, as does Doppler flow imaging using intravascular ultrasound contrast agent (23). Still, these techniques have not made the quantum leap that would be necessary to propel TRUS into a widely used screening role. Also, TRUS costs considerably more than DRE or PSA, which diminishes its cost-effectiveness further (17,18,24), as does the lower patient compliance with TRUS than with DRE and PSA (17).

Ultrasound does play a limited role in screening for prostate cancer by refining the use of serum PSA, which is another test with less-than-ideal sensitivity and specificity (23). The ratio of PSA to prostate volume, usually determined by TRUS and termed PSA density, has been found in some series to be a more accurate test than a single PSA determination (24–30). Transrectal ultrasound facilitates volume assessment of the peripheral zone, where most prostate cancer arises; using this volume to calculate PSA density may increase accuracy (31). The PSA density may help predict whether extracapsular disease will be found at surgery and longer-term prognosis (32,33).

II. Is Transrectal Ultrasound Useful to Guide Prostate Biopsy?

Summary of Evidence: Transrectal ultrasound appears to be useful to guide systematic biopsies into the peripheral zone, and increase diagnostic yield if focal abnormalities (especially those demonstrated by flow-sensitive techniques) are biopsied, hence justifying its continued use as a biopsy guide (limited evidence).

Supporting Evidence: Intraprostatic carcinoma can be diagnosed only histologically, and, as screening becomes more widespread and as fewer prostate resections are performed for voiding symptoms, an ever-higher percentage of prostate cancers are diagnosed by prostate biopsy. Originally, prostate biopsy was performed using digital guidance, but with the advent of TRUS an increasing number of biopsies have been performed using this method as guidance. Early after the invention of TRUS, it became apparent that certain prostates contained local abnormalities in echogenicity, which, at least sometimes, indicated foci of carcinoma. The commonest appearance was that of a local region of diminished echogenicity; with time, it became apparent that some prostate carcinomas presented as hyperechoic regions, some as discrete areas with echogenicity roughly equal to the surrounding tissue, and many were not visible at all (34). The last observation led to the realization that to biopsy only sonographically abnormal regions of the prostate would cause many cancers to be missed; with experience, it also became apparent that many focally abnormal regions were found by biopsy not to harbor neoplasm (35,36).

Given these findings, systematic biopsy of specific regions of the prostate, whether or not they were seen to obtain focal abnormalities, became commonplace. Originally, relatively few biopsies were performed: four or six biopsies, equally divided between the right and left sides and at different zones in the craniocaudad direction, were used. Since then, a number of studies have shown that increasing the number of biopsies to six, eight, 10, or even 12 cores leads to an increased likelihood of recovering cancer (37–42). Since many cancers could not be visualized, and their locations not be exactly predicted, the phenomenon appeared stochastic: that is, assuming random distribution of prostate cancers, the more biopsies were done the more likely cancer was to be found. This observation could call into question the necessity for performing TRUS during biopsy at all; indeed, at least one publication suggested that the performance of multiple segmental biopsies in a systematic pattern was more important than the method used to guide the biopsy needle (43).

Nevertheless, many authors continue to feel that visualization of the prostate by TRUS during biopsy leads to an increased yield. Several studies have shown that if, in addition to systematic biopsies, foci of ultrasound abnormality are also biopsied, an increased number of carcinomas are detected (44–46). These papers tend not to be controlled for the possibility that the extra biopsies might yield an increased number of prostate cancers simply because they involved a greater number of needle passes (the stochastic model) rather than because specific areas were biopsied. But there appears to be evidence that TRUS really can maximize the number of prostate cancers detected. First of all, since most carcinomas appear in the peripheral zone of the prostate, and since the peripheral zone can more accurately be localized with TRUS, using TRUS to biopsy the peripheral zone has led to an increased yield of carcinoma (39). In addition, statistical analysis of the likelihood of finding tumor with any given needle track has found that a sample from a region seen to be abnormal by TRUS is more likely to contain tumor than a sample obtained elsewhere. Technical enhancements of ultrasound also appear to be of assistance. The use of power Doppler ultrasound to assess the level of local tissue blood flow has shown that biopsies from sites of high blood flow are more likely to contain carcinoma than are biopsies from other sites (47). Enhanced visualization of flow permitted by simultaneous use of Doppler ultrasound and the intravenous infusion of an ultrasound contrast agent has also led to an increased yield (48).

In summary, the initial hopes that TRUS-guided biopsy of regions in the prostate that demonstrate focal ultrasound abnormality would be a technique of high sensitivity and specificity and that might permit a small number of biopsies have not been supported; to fail to biopsy systematically the various parts of the prostate leads to an unacceptable number of false-negative biopsy sessions. Nevertheless, TRUS still appears to be useful: its ability to guide systematic biopsies into the peripheral zone and the increase in diagnostic yield if focal abnormalities (especially those demonstrated by flow-sensitive techniques) are biopsied justify its continued use as a biopsy guide.

III. Is Imaging Accurate for Staging Prostate Cancer?

Summary of Evidence: Magnetic resonance imaging (MRI) is the most accurate of the imaging techniques in local staging, but its relative expense and persistent false-positive and false-negative rates for locally invasive disease suggest that it should be interpreted along with all additional available data, and reserved for patients in whom other data leave treatment choices ambiguous. Due to the higher accuracy of MRI in revealing the local extent of disease, computed tomography (CT) has been largely abandoned as an initial test for evaluating local disease (strong evidence).

Supporting Evidence

A. Ultrasound

The early literature regarding ultrasound of the prostate claimed a startlingly high accuracy for local staging (49), despite the fact that the images were transabdominal rather than transrectal, fine detail could not be observed, and that later investigation (50) showed that the ultrasound features identified as the capsule of the prostate correlated poorly with the anatomic capsule. Currently, transabdominal probes are not used for local staging of prostate cancer. It is not surprising that ultrasound was found to be relatively poor in evaluating lymph node metastases (51), given the technical difficulties in visualizing normal or slightly enlarged nodes, and the frequency with which tumor-bearing nodes are not enlarged.

The development of high-frequency TRUS probes was expected to produce more accurate results with regard to whether the tumor had transgressed the capsule or invaded the neurovascular bundles or seminal vesicles. But even the best probes produce images that turn out to be much less than 100% accurate in evaluating these features. The last decade and a half has seen continued controversy with regard to whether even transrectal probe images are sufficiently accurate to be used in stage-dependent therapeutic decisions.

A number of investigators remain relatively enthusiastic, stating that the sensitivity, specificity, PPV, NPV, and accuracy for identifying locally invasive disease are sufficiently high to be trustworthy for local staging (52–54). Others, realizing that very high accuracy is necessary to choose among therapies with significantly different side effects, have investigated ultrasound-guided biopsy of seminal vesicles and regions near the neurovascular bundles to confirm or help to exclude tumor invasion (55,56). Other investigators, citing a variety of figures, are convinced that TRUS is simply too inaccurate to trust for therapeutic planning (57–64).

Prior to the advent of imaging, only DRE provided direct information regarding local stage, and the inability to palpate all parts of the prostate and seminal vesicles, or to feel microscopic disease, limited the accuracy of this examination. The combination of stage estimation by both DRE and TRUS, however, with appropriate weighting for each, may lead to an overall increase in accuracy of staging (54,65). All other things being equal, the higher the PSA level, the higher the local stage is likely to be, but this single parameter does not permit exact establishment of local stage any more than DRE or TRUS can; but the combination of PSA levels and TRUS findings permits a more accurate determination of local stage.

The modality that continues to be used for the local staging of prostate cancer is MRI, which, when performed using an intrarectal coil, has the potential for high spatial resolution images of the prostate and adjacent structures. An early comparison of TRUS and MRI purported to demonstrate that TRUS was more accurate than MRI in evaluating capsular invasion but that MRI outperformed TRUS for invasion of the seminal vesicles (52). Later publications comparing the two suggest that MRI may be more sensitive but less specific in evaluating capsular invasion (66).

There are characteristics of intraprostatic tumor other than direct visualization of sites of extraglandular invasion that are correlated with the likelihood of invasive disease; in general, the larger the intraprostatic tumor is, the more likely it is to have escaped the bounds of the gland and the more likely it is to be histologically undifferentiated. These features can be used during TRUS analysis to predict likelihood of invasion; in particular, tumor volume, tumor diameter, and the area of the surface of the tumor that directly abuts the capsule are directly correlated with likelihood of invasion (67,68). Even the degree to which the tumor is visible at all may be important in this regard (69). Other publications, however, fail to find any correlation between sonographic visibility of the tumors and stage (70,71).

In keeping with the general tendency of many neoplasms to have high blood flow and vessel density correlate positively with degree of biologic malignancy, power Doppler assessment of the amount of flow within the tumor and visibility of the supplying vessels have been found, at least by a few investigators, to correlate with invasiveness, stage, grade, and tendency to recur after initial therapy (72–74). Reconstructed three-dimensional images of multiplanar data have also been found to increase slightly the likelihood that ultrasound will correctly predict stage (75).

In summary, it is probably fair to say that the literature to date does not support the capacity of TRUS to perform local staging of prostate cancer with great accuracy. The inability to detect microscopic portions of tumor, discrepancies between real anatomic and ultrasound findings, and the invisibility of certain tumors all suggest that the few publications that claim high accuracy for ultrasound are not likely to stand up to rigorous scrutiny or reproducibility. The main roles of staging ultrasound in prostate cancer are likely to be complementary in some cases in which other staging data are conflicting, and as a guide for biopsy of juxtaprostatic structures.

B. Computed Tomography Scan

In patients with newly diagnosed prostate cancer, management decisions depend critically on anatomic stage. In brief, among patients for whom treatment is necessary at all, those in whom disease is confined within the prostatic capsule may be treated with surgery or radiotherapy, those whose tumor remains local but has transgressed the capsule or invaded the seminal vesicle can be treated with radiotherapy, and those who have demonstrated metastatic disease or whose local stage and grade strongly suggest that metastases are present are treated with orchiectomy or anti-androgen therapy.

Early in the development of CT, when it became apparent that the prostate, seminal vesicle, and bladder could be demonstrated, there was considerable hope that local tumor extent could be established by this technique. Asymmetry in prostate shape, invasion of periprostatic fat, and obliteration of the angle between the seminal vesicle and bladder were signs thought to hold promise for indicating local extracapsular tumor extension. Early investigations involving a comparatively small series concluded that these signs were indeed reliable and that CT was quite accurate in detecting and excluding local extracapsular disease (76). It might be expected that, as scanning technology improved and anatomic detail could be seen better, accuracy of demonstrating disease extent should improve. Unfortunately, microscopic invasion of structures immediately outside the capsule is crucial, and microscopic changes cannot be detected by CT at all; high accuracy has never been possible (77). A careful study with appropriate blinding of observers yielded a sensitivity of only 50% in predicting intracapsular disease; errors were found in analysis of seminal vesicle images and other regions immediately surrounding the prostate (78). Since CT can demonstrate only morphologic changes of the seminal vesicles, and since tumor may invade these structures without changing their gross configuration, CT frequently misses such invasion; MRI, which is discussed later, may demonstrate similar abnormalities and thus be more sensitive (79). A larger study of CT, in which CT interpretation results were compared with surgical-pathologic findings, showed the accuracy of CT was only 24% for capsular extension and 59% for seminal vesicle invasion (80). Due to these discouraging results, and to the higher accuracy of MRI in revealing the local extent of disease, CT has been largely abandoned as an initial test for evaluating local disease.

Computed tomography may still have a role, however, in evaluating lymphatic metastases. Metastases may enlarge nodes, and since CT can evaluate nodal size well, it has become the primary modality for searching for nodal disease. It is well recognized that patients may have metastatic nodal disease from prostate cancer in which individual nodal deposits are sufficiently small that the overall node size is not enlarged, so that the sensitivity of the CT is considerably less than 100%. The studies of false-negative rates for CT in detecting nodal metastasis have reported sensitivities of only 0% to 7% (76,81,82). Careful dissection studies (83) have confirmed that this is due to the relatively small size of many tumor-bearing nodes. Large nodes are felt to be a more accurate CT sign of metastatic disease than small ones are of disease without metastases; still, enlarged nodes (77,83) may occasionally be found in patients without metastatic disease. The occasional false-positive case notwithstanding, definitely enlarged nodes seen on CT are usually regarded as reliable evidence of metastatic disease, especially if local tumor volume and grade suggest that metastases are likely, and if the location of the enlarged nodes is compatible with metastatic prostate cancer. This disease tends to spread to and enlarge nodes in the pelvic retroperitoneum before causing enlargement of nodes in the abdomen or elsewhere (84).

It has been well known for a long time that clinical stage, PSA, and Gleason score are independent predictors of the likelihood that metastases will be found in surgically resected lymph nodes. It seemed logical that these factors might be useful in predicting which CT scans are likely to show enlarged nodes, and, indeed, all three factors have been found to be independent predictors of CT-demonstrated lymphadenopathy (85). Of these, a high Gleason score seems to confer the highest risk (85). These findings have been substantiated by another study (86), and still others (87,88) corroborate the importance of PSA; all studies suggest that in patients with an initial PSA below 20, a positive CT scan is extremely unlikely. These findings have primarily been interpreted as indicators that for these patients at low risk, CT need not be performed; they may also be useful for radiologists confronted with CT scans with marginal nodal findings; in these cases, investigation of the PSA and Gleason score may aid in reaching radiologic decisions.

C. Magnetic Resonance Imaging

Early in the development of body MRI it became apparent that the prostate could be visualized, and even that the zones within it could be distinguished. Although little success was met in screening for prostate cancer, a series of publications investigated the technique as a staging technique for recently diagnosed prostate cancer. Most of these relied on external coils (89–93), which continued to be used in a later series as well (94). Staging of the local extent of disease, rather than detecting metastatic disease, was the task at hand, and the external coil was not highly accurate. Accuracy percents tended to be in the low 60's, and many studies found no improvement over simply using PSA or DRE. A few investigators managed to achieve higher accuracy with body coil MRI (95,96), finding that MRI was superior to sonography and CT for evaluating seminal vesicle invasion (95) and achieving high specificities in predicting capsular penetration (80%) and seminal vesicle invasion (86%) with a moderately high sensitivity for capsular penetration (62%) (96).

With the introduction of the intrarectal surface coil, the higher spatial resolution that the technique permitted improved accuracy of staging (92,97–102). Various levels of sensitivity, specificity, PPV, and NPV have been reported; overall staging accuracy ranges from 62% to 84%. Even with the rectal coil techniques, however, not all authors were enthusiastic (103,104). Ekici et al. (103) found endorectal coil MRI no better than TRUS for staging.

Detection of metastatic disease in pelvic and abdominal lymph nodes by body coil MRI suffers from the same problem as CT, which is that size is the only parameter that can be accurately measured, and that tumor is often found in nonenlarged nodes. In one study, sensitivity of MRI for tumor in nodes was only 27% (105). In attempts to continue to use endorectal MRI to improve staging, many authors have developed staging schemes that combine the results of PSA, PSA density, Gleason score, percentage of tumor-bearing cores in a biopsy series, and age, along with MRI, and have found various combinations that work better than individual ones. Statistics presented in support of the combinations use a variety of outcome parameters but do not permit gross comparisons of the studies, however (106–112). A combination of using highly trained observers and a computer system, without addition of non-MRI data, achieved an accuracy of 87% (113).

Most studies reporting interpretation of MRI rely most heavily on T2-weighted images. In these images, the peripheral zone of the prostate, where most tumors appear and from which extracapsular extension occurs, appears bright, and tumor tissue is relatively low intensity. A line felt to represent the prostatic capsule can usually be identified, and the seminal vesicles are visible by virtue of having comparatively dark walls and bright luminal fluid. When there is gross invasion of a large segment of tumor from the confines of the capsule, the low-intensity tumor can be seen to extend directly into periprostatic fat or the seminal vesicles; signs of more subtle invasion have included bulges of various configurations in the capsule, irregularity of the capsule, and thickening of the walls of the seminal vesicles. In T1-weighted images, all the portions of the prostate and seminal vesicles are of approximately the same medium-low intensity, and the capsule is not clearly visualized, so these images are less helpful in staging; they may be valuable, however, when looking for extracapsular tumor that invades the neurovascular bundles. Several publications describe evaluation of enhanced T1-weighted images using gadolinium chelates (114–117), some of which (113–117) use a dynamic technique. This technique has failed to improve consistently the accuracy of staging, but it is claimed to show enhanced delineation of the prostate capsule (114,115), a weak correlation between tumor permeability and MR stage (116), and accuracies of 84% to 97% in detecting specific features of extracapsular extension (117). A novel use of an MR contrast agent was reported for investigating nodes (30); administration of nanoparticles permitted identification of nonenlarged nodes (118) with focal regions of tumor and permitted 100% sensitivity in identifying patients with nodal metastases.

Investigators have also presented data regarding the ability of MRI findings to predict posttherapy PSA failures (106,109,111,119,120) and positive margins in surgical specimens (121). MRI in combination with other data permitted improvements of these prediction rates, but, as in evaluations of its ability to predict exact stage, did not achieve accuracies of 100%. Given the inability of MRI to achieve very high degrees of accuracy among all patients undergoing initial evaluation for prostate cancer, attempts have been made to find some groups in which MRI might be particularly useful. One of these investigations found that if MRI were limited to a subgroup of those with a Gleason score of 5 to 7 and a PSA higher than 10 to 20 ng/mL, increased accuracy for both extracapsular extension and seminal vesicle invasion could be achieved (107). Another study investigated only the ability of MRI to detect enlarged nodes, and suggested that the examination could be withheld from patients with a serum PSA of less than 20 ng/mL (122).

In summary, MRI probably permits better local staging than older techniques in certain subgroups of patients but with considerably less than 100% accuracy; the inability to detect microscopic invasion remains an important limitation, as does the inability to detect disease in nonenlarged lymph nodes with standard techniques. These facts have led to only cautious and scattered acceptance of the technique. Currently, it is probably wise to restrict its use to a subgroup of patients—those whose physical examination, PSA, Gleason score, results of standard workup for metastatic disease, and personal preferences leave them on the cusp of choosing surgery or local radiotherapy. When interpreting examinations in these patients, it should be remembered that diagnosis or exclusion of microscopic invasion cannot be performed with accuracy, but that visualization of gross tumor extension beyond the capsule or into the seminal vesicle is a relatively specific sign of invasive disease.

D. Magnetic Resonance Spectroscopic Imaging

In addition to high spatial resolution imaging by proton MRI, technology for spatially resolved spectroscopy of the prostate has been under development for some years. This usually involves a high-field magnet (at least 1.5 T) and an intrarectal coil. Proton spectroscopic data can be acquired from a three-dimensional array of voxels. These voxels are about two orders of magnitude larger than the voxels used for proton imaging, but can be superimposed on proton MRI maps to permit reasonably accurate spatial identification of the intraprostatic region supplying specific spectra.

Spectral analysis relies on the fact that normal prostate tissue and the tissue of benign prostatic hypertrophy secrete relatively large amounts of citrate; prostate adenocarcinoma elaborates much less citrate, but produces a relatively elevated amount of choline; the ratios between the spectral peaks for these molecules are used to distinguish voxels containing neoplasm from those that do not (123,124).

Currently, the potential uses for magnetic resonance spectroscopic imaging (MRSI) of the prostate might be original diagnosis, biopsy guidance, local staging, and evaluation of recurrent following local therapy.

With regard to diagnosis, several studies have shown that MRSI analysis of small groups of patients containing those without tumor and those with tumor can identify and localize tumors with reasonable, if less than perfect, sensitivity and specificity (125–128). But no sufficiently large or sufficiently well-controlled investigation has addressed whether MRSI is effective in screening for disease in a large sample reflecting either the population at large or those at increased risk because of an elevated PSA. And given that many prostate tumors are considerably smaller than the MRSI voxels, it is unlikely that sensitivity can ever be very high until considerable improvements in spatial resolution can be made.

Series have been published to investigate whether patients whose prostate biopsies have been negative, even though their elevated PSA levels suggest tumor, might be aided by using MRSI to guide further attempts at biopsy. The data show that biopsies using information from MRI and MRSI converts some of these patients from being false negative (for the original biopsy) to true positive for the MR-guided biopsies, but there are few data to show that adding MRSI information to the MRI information is of significant benefit in guiding these biopsies (129). Furthermore, the studies lack controls to investigate the possibility that the subsequent biopsies might have retrieved tumor tissue even without MR guidance. For patients who have had hormonal therapy (130) or who have had intraprostatic hemorrhage from a recent biopsy, localization of tumor by MRI can be difficult; MRSI may permit tumor identification in these circumstances (131), however, so if MRI-guided biopsy ever becomes wide-spread, MRSI may be of benefit.

There are also series that investigate whether MRSI might improve the accuracy of MRI for prostate staging (130,132). In one, the addition of MRSI data to MRI data enabled inexperienced readers to become as accurate as experienced readers were with MRI alone, but, for experienced readers, MRSI data did not improve accuracy. However, MRSI may help in assessing overall tumor volume, which is also a factor in staging. But whether this information actually changes treatment decisions for the better has yet to be investigated.

The feasibility of using MRSI to localize prostate cancer in aiding placement of radioactive seeds for brachytherapy and adjusting local doses for external beam therapy has been established (133,134). But whether this capacity actually improves outcomes, either in terms of disease control or complication reduction, is not yet known. In patients who have had local therapy to destroy prostate tumors—in particular, cryotherapy—MRSI is likely to be better in detecting local tumor recurrence than MRI (135,136). This has the potential for indicating salvage therapy in patients who do not have disseminated disease, but whether these management choices, aided by MRI, benefit patient outcome, also remains to be determined.

In summary, there seems to be little doubt that MRSI can with reasonable accuracy detect foci of intraprostatic tumor, at least when the tumor nodules are not small, and the technique holds promise for diagnosis, staging, prognosis, radiotherapy planning, and determining the need for salvage therapy. But series of sufficient size and sufficiently rigorous design to determine whether any of these functions will be of clinical benefit remain for the future (insufficient evidence).

E. Positron Emission Tomography

There has been considerable investigation of the role of 18-fluorodeoxyglucose positron emission tomography (FDG-PET) scanning in patients with prostate cancer (137–149). Although carbon-11 acetate (137,140,142,150–152) and carbon-11 choline (141,150–156) have been found to have certain advantages over FDG, FDG is most available and most frequently used.

There are no data supporting the use of PET scanning as a screen for detecting prostate cancer.

When used in patients with known prostate cancer in order to test its sensitivity, FDG-PET has yielded extremely disparate results, with reported sensitivities ranging from 19% to 83% (143,145,150). Sensitivity is probably higher among patients with higher histologic grades (145). No authors suggest that, among patients with palpable prostate nodules or elevated PSA values, FDG-PET can substitute for biopsy diagnosis of prostate cancer, or to identify a subset of patients with marginal findings who ought to undergo biopsy.

In patients undergoing initial staging of prostate cancer, FDG-PET has been assessed in a number of series (143,145,147,149). The sensitivity for disease in lymph nodes has been reported as ranging from 0% to 67%, and in bones from 57% to 75%. This performance does not support utilization of FDG-PET for routine clinical staging.

In evaluating patients who have undergone therapy and who are at risk for recurrence, FDG-PET has also been tested (137,139,140,144). Sensitivities for detecting recurrence have been reported from 9% to 75%, and are, not surprisingly, better in patients whose PSA levels and PSA velocities are higher (144). Sensitivity appears to be higher for nodal disease than skeletal disease (137); specificity, accuracy, PPV, and NPV have been found to be 100%, 83%, 100%, and 67% in one publication (139). Although some of these figures appear impressive, the reported NPV and the range of reported sensitivities do not constitute strong evidence for routine use of FDG-PET.

IV. How Accurate Is Bone Scan for Detecting Metastatic Prostate Cancer?

Summary of Evidence: Radionuclide bone scan should be performed to evaluate for possible skeletal metastases in subjects with a PSA value of 10 or more (strong evidence).

Supporting Evidence: During the evaluation of patients with recently diagnosed prostate cancer, assessment of metastatic disease is crucial. Prostate cancer frequently metastasizes to bones and pelvic nodes; either may occur first. For skeletal metastases, the standard imaging technique is a radionuclide bone scan. Although this is not a terribly expensive test, the number of patients with initial diagnoses of prostate cancer each year is very large; if it were possible to stratify these patients into those with significant or negligible risk of skeletal metastases so that many might not have to undergo bone scanning, savings would be considerable.

The simplest and must frequently cited parameter for assessing metastatic potential is PSA. A large number of investigations have found that when the PSA value is less than 10 ng/mL, the rate of positive bone scans is so low that the scan may be omitted (157–164). Others have suggested a higher threshold—less than 20 ng/mL (165–170). Given that the occasional poorly differentiated prostate cancer may produce very little PSA, and given the difficulty of establishing absolute biologic thresholds, it is not surprising that, on rare occasion, a patient with a very low PSA may still have a positive bone scan; at least some authors suggest that, no matter what the PSA, an initial scan should be obtained as a baseline.

Other characteristics of individual tumors are, not surprisingly, also related to the likelihood of metastatic disease; those that indicate likelihood of metastasis independent of PSA levels have been proposed to be used in conjunction with PSA in determining which patients should undergo bone scanning. Bone alkaline phosphate levels (171–173) have been found useful in this regard; indeed, at least one group found alkaline phosphate levels alone to be better determinants of a threshold than PSA (174). Gleason score and clinical stage have also been found to be independent risk factors for positive scans (175), although not by all investigators (176).

The false-negative rate for bone scans is not accurately known, although it is certainly true that in patients with high PSA levels there may be skeletal disease even in the face of a normal bone scan (163). The false-positive rate for bone scans is not well known either; in most cases, foci of increased activity due to fracture, Paget's disease, and degenerative spondylitis may be demonstrated to be false-positive indicators of metastatic disease by their characteristic pattern and by follow-up examinations with radiography and CT.

A. Special Case: Which Patients Should Undergo Imaging After Initial Treatment to Look for Metastatic Disease?

Follow-up imaging after initial treatment of prostate cancer should be instituted depending on the likelihood that it will aid in future therapeutic decisions. Metastatic disease is usually treated by maneuvers intended to reduce the effect of testosterone upon the tumors, including surgical orchiectomy and drugs that block the release or action of testosterone. Occasionally salvage therapy is tried—that is, prostatectomy after initial radiotherapy, or local radiotherapy after prostatectomy—if it is felt that disease has recurred locally after the initial treatment and that distant metastases are not likely. After initial treatment, serial PSA determinations are the usual surveillance mechanism to detect recurrent disease. When PSA levels begin to rise, there may still be a question of whether therapy should be initiated if the patient is asymptomatic and disease cannot be identified in any other way.

After primary local radiotherapy or prostatectomy, serial PSA determinations are usually used since it is felt that progressive elevation of PSA is more sensitive than any imaging technique and can detect recurrent disease at an earlier stage; most authorities suggest, therefore, that in the absence of PSA elevations, no imaging is necessary (177–183). There are a few publications that suggest that on rare occasion bone scans may detect recurrent disease prior to PSA (184); given that a small percentage of poorly differentiated tumor may not produce much PSA, this should not be entirely surprising. Other investigators feel that bone alkaline phosphate determinations may indicate recurrent disease and the need for imaging prior to PSA elevations (185).

Salvage therapy requires both proof that there is local recurrent tumor, and, to whatever degree possible, that there is no metastatic disease. Local tumor proof usually requires biopsy, which may be digitally guided if a nodule is palpable, but ultrasound has also been shown to demonstrate residual tumor (186,187), as has MRI (188) and even MR spectroscopy (189). Computed tomography is ineffective at this task (190). With regard to distant metastases, a clearly positive bone scan or CT is usually felt to be accurate. There are undoubtedly false positives, but little work is available to quantify this problem, and there are undoubtedly false-negative imaging examinations in patients with recurrent distant disease. In general, after primary local therapy, patients whose lowest posttherapy PSA is relatively high, and in whom subsequent rises in PSA happen quickly after therapy and proceed with a high velocity, are more likely to have distant recurrences, and vice versa.

Positron emission tomography scanning has been tried to search for recurrent disease; FDG-PET has found to be only moderately sensitive and may fail to demonstrate small bone metastases (191–194). Carbon-11 acetate may be more sensitive (195–197).

In patients who have metastatic disease, imaging may be useful. The number and intensity of metastases demonstrated by bone scan (198) mimics the amount of disease as indicated by tumor markers, and tumor burden as demonstrated by bone scans is of prognostic value (199,200). Tumor volume in nodes as measured by CT also may be used for prognosis (201); when evaluating patients for recurrent disease by CT, enlarged nodes almost always appear in the pelvis first, unless the patient has had a lymphadenectomy, in which case the first enlarged nodes may be found in the upper abdomen (202).

Take-Home Figure

Figure 7.1 is a flow chart for evaluating and treating patients suspected of having prostate cancer.

Imaging Case Studies

These cases highlight the advantages and limitations of imaging in patients with prostate cancer.

Case 1

A 65-year-old man's prostate biopsy is positive for adenocarcinoma. His Gleason score is 6 and his PSA is 7.1. A bone scan was performed despite the published data suggesting that he has a very low probability of having a true positive result for metastatic disease. Focal regions of increased

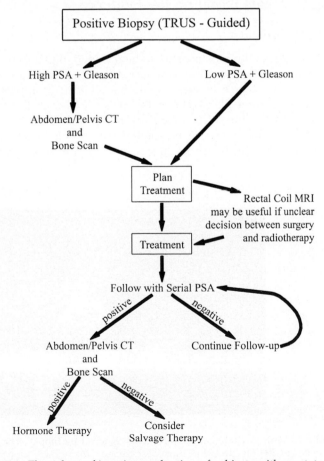

Figure 7.1. Flow chart of imaging evaluation of subjects with prostate cancer.

activity in sites that are common locations for metastatic prostate cancer were identified. Computed tomography revealed that the changes were all due to degenerative disease, however, corroborating the predictive value of the PSA and Gleason data, and illustrating the value of these numbers in analyzing images (Fig. 7.2).

Case 2

A 59-year-old man's prostate cancer was recently diagnosed by biopsy. Computed tomography and bone scan showed no evidence of metastases. His Gleason score is 9 and his PSA is 21, which suggest that he is likely to have disseminated disease, and would probably have recurrent disease after prostatectomy. He continued to request radical surgery, stating that he had heard that surgery was his only chance for cure. Magnetic resonance imaging revealed gross tumor invasion of the seminal vesicles (the low-intensity regions replacing the bright lumina of the seminal vesicles), which both increased the likelihood of disseminated disease to the level at which surgery was felt to be inappropriate, precluded effective treatment by brachytherapy, and provided guidance for designing conformal external-beam radiotherapy (Fig. 7.3).

Imaging Protocols Based on the Evidence

Transrectal Ultrasound

Diagnostic images of the prostate should be recorded in planes both sagittal and transverse to the apex-to-base axis of the gland. Images are obtained at 6 to 9 MHz. Transverse images should be obtained at approximately 5-mm intervals; for large glands it may be necessary to angle the probe left and right to image the two sides of the gland independently. With the probe imaging in the sagittal plane, the midsagittal view should be accompanied by views produced with the probe angled to each side. There is no stan-

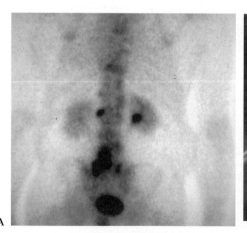
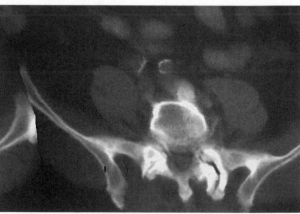

A   B

Figure 7.2. Case 1. A: A 65-year-old man with prostate cancer recently diagnosed by biopsy. The Gleason score is 6 and his PSA is 5. Active foci originally interpreted as metastases despite the unlikelihood given the Gleason and PSA. B: CT reveals abnormality to be degenerative spondylitis.

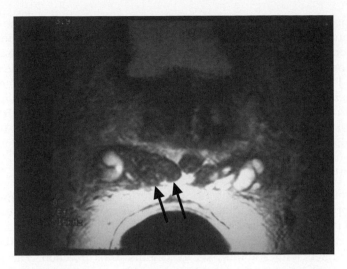

Figure 7.3. Case 2. A 59 year old man with recently diagnosed prostate cancer, Gleason score 9, and PSA 21. T2–weighted MRI reveals low-intensity tumor invading the seminal vesicle lumen, primarily on the right (arrows).

dard for the angle between successive views; obviously, the larger the gland the more images need to be obtained.

Although color Doppler and contrast-enhanced imaging have been described, they are not universally applied.

Computed Tomography

Evaluation of prostate cancer patients by CT involves a limited focus, which is to determine whether metastases are seen in lymph nodes or bones. Most patients have simultaneous skeletal scintigraphy, so that limiting the range of CT to the abdomen and pelvis—or even to the pelvis alone—is not likely to reduce sensitivity significantly.

Since node size is critical, a slice thickness that does not cause partial-volume averaging of structures as small as 1 cm in diameter is crucial; slices no thicker than 5 mm are ideal. Oral and intravenous contrast are ideal but not absolutely necessary. Inspection of the skeleton using bone windows is crucial.

Magnetic Resonance Imaging

Staging prostate cancer by MRI involves evaluation of the extent of any local extracapsular extent of tumor and detection of lymphatic disease that may have enlarged pelvic lymph nodes. The standard examination is limited to the prostate and periprostatic regions and pelvis; abdominal imaging is usually not routine.

Most imaging has been performed with 1.5-T magnets, with either a body coil or wraparound phased array pelvic coils. A series of T1-weighted spin-echo transverse images is performed, no thicker than 5 mm with the gap no greater than 1 mm. The TR should be several hundred milliseconds and the TE should be as short as the scanner permits.

Focused imaging of the prostate should be performed with an intrarectal coil, coupled with a body coil or wraparound pelvic coil. Imaging includes transverse T1-weighted spin-echo and T2-weighted fast spin-echo images of the prostate and seminal vesicles with T2-weighted sagittal and coronal series. Paramagnetic contrast agents are not routinely utilized. The reference axis for these images may be either the long axis of the entire body or the long axis of the prostate gland. The TR should be 4000 or 5000 ms, and effective TE from 90 to 110 ms. Slices should be no more than 4 mm thick, and slice gap should not exceed 1 mm.

Radionuclide Bone Scan

The protocol for scanning patients with prostate cancer is no different from that appropriate for scanning adults for other malignancies that metastasize to the skeleton; 20 mCi of technetium 99m (Tc-99m) ethylene hydroxydiphosphonate (HDP) or Tc-99m methylene diphosphonate (MDP) are administered with scanning $2\frac{1}{2}$ to 3 hours after injection. The patient should drink sufficient fluid that he can void immediately before scanning, since the isotope accumulates in the bladder and may obscure pelvic metastases.

If planar scanning is performed, both anterior and posterior views should be obtained. A parallel-hole collimator should be used. A scan speed of 10 to 15 cm/minute usually provides adequate recorded activity. If single photon emission computed tomography (SPECT) scanning is performed, a dual- or triple-head camera can be used; a 128×128 matrix with 30 seconds per frame and 360-degree acquisition should provide good images.

Positron Emission Tomography Scan

Although compounds currently under investigation may prove to be more effective than 18F-FDG, this isotope continues to be the most frequently employed one for oncologic imaging; 10 mCi is an appropriate dose. It is important that the patient's blood glucose level not be elevated. Patients should fast for 4 to 6 hours prior to the procedure so that blood glucose does not exceed 160 mg/dL; the level should be checked before administering the isotope intravenously. Sixty minutes should elapse before beginning the scan, during which time the patient must continue to fast. The patient should empty his bladder immediately before the scan begins.

Future Research

- Can any imaging technique—especially metabolism-dependent modalities like magnetic resonance spectroscopy (MRS) and PET—be used to determine which cases of prostate cancer safely may be managed by watchful waiting?
- Which clinical or serologic thresholds should be used to indicate imaging in detection and characterization of recurrent disease after initial therapy, and which modalities should be used?
- Can the initial research that suggests that superparamagnetic agents and lymph node imaging by MRI can detect tumor in normal-sized nodes be replicated?

References

1. Jemal A, Tiwari RC, Murray T, et al. CA Cancer J Clin 2004;54:8–29.
2. Ciatto S, Bonardi R, Lombardi C, et al. Tumori 2002;88(4):281–283.
3. Cupp MR, Oesterling JE. Mayo Clin Proc 1993;68(3):297–306.
4. Mandell MJ, Hopper KD, Jarowenko MV, et al. Crit Rev Diagn Imaging 1991;32(4):273–300.
5. Lee F, Littrup PJ, Torp-Pedersen ST, et al. Radiology 1988;168(2):389–394.
6. Lee F, Gray JM, McLeary RD, et al. Radiology 1986;158(1):91–95.
7. Lee F, Gray JM, Mc Leary RD, et al. Prostate 1985;7(2):117–129.
8. Ellis WJ, Chelner MP, Preston SD, et al. J Urol 1994;152(5 pt 1):1520–1525.
9. Shinohara K, Wheeler TM, Scardino PT, et al. J Urol 1989;142(1):76–82.
10. Ciatto S, Bonardi R, Lombardi C, et al. Int J Biol Markers 2001;16(3):179–182.
11. Rietergen JB, Kranse R, Kirkels WJ, et al. Br J Urol 1997;79(suppl 2):57–63.
12. Ciatto S, Bonardi R, Gervasi G, et al. Radiol Med 2002:103(3):219–224.
13. Flanigan RC, Catalona WJ, Richie JP, et al. J Urol 1994;152(5 pt a):1506–1509.
14. Chancellor MB, Van Appledorn CA. Urology 1993;41(6):590–593.
15. Carter HB, Hamper UM, Sheth S, et al. J Urol 1989;142(4):1008–1010.
16. Gustafsson O, Carlsson P, Norming U, et al. Prostate 1995;26(6):299–309.
17. Norming U, Gustafsson O, Nyman CR. Acta Oncol 1991;30(2):277–279.
18. Ciatto S, Bonardi R, Mazzotta A, et al. Tumori 1995;81(4):225–229.
19. Babaian RJ, Dinney CP, Ramirez EI, et al. Urology 1993;41(5):421–425.
20. Cooner WH, Mosley BR, Rutrherfor CL Jr. et al. J Urol 1990;143:1146.
21. Yamamoto T, Ito K, Ohi M, et al. Urology 2001;58(6):994–998.
22. Kuligowska E, Barish MA, Fenlon HM, et al. Radiology 2001;220(3)757–764.
23. Halpern EJ, Rosenberg M, Gomella LG. Radiology 2001;219(1):219–225.
24. Palken M, Cobb OE, Simons CE. J Urol 1991;145(1):86–90, discussion 90–92.
25. Benson MC, Whang IS, et al. J Urol 1992;147(3 pt 2):815–816.
26. Bazinet M, Meshref AW, et al. Comments. Urology 1994;44(1):150–151, 43(1):44–51, discussion 51–52.
27. Bretton PR, Evans WP, et al. Cancer 1994;74(11)11:2991–2995.
28. Kochanska-Dziurowic AA, Mielniczuk MR, et al. Comment. Br J Urol 1998; 82(6):933, 81(6):834–838.
29. Men S, Cakar B, et al. J Exp Clin Cancer Res 2001;20(4):473–480.
30. Catalona WJ, Richie JP, et al. J Urol 1994;152(6 pt 1):2046–2048; 152(6 pt 1): 2031–2036.
31. Zlotta AR, Djavan B, et al. Comment. J Urol 1997;157(4):1335–1336; 157(4): 1315–1321.
32. Horiguchi A, Nakashima J, et al. Prostate 2003;56(1):23–29.
33. Freedland SJ, Kane CJ, et al. J Urol 2003;169(3):969–973.
34. Turkeri L, Tarcan T, Biren T. Int J Urol 1996;3(6):459–461.
35. Leibowitz CB, Staub PG. Aust Radiol 1996;40(3):240–243.
36. Hammerer P, Huland H. J Urol 1994;151(1):99–102.
37. de la Taille A, Antiphon P, Salomon L, et al. Urology 2003;61(6):1181–1186.
38. Kojima M, Hayakawa T, Saito T, et al. Int J Urol 2001;8(6):301–307.
39. Ravery V, Goldblatt L, Royer B, et al. J Urol 2000;164(2):393–396.
40. Presti JC Jr, Chang JJ, Bhargava V, et al. J Urol 2000;163(1):163–167.
41. Babaian RJ, Toi A, Kamoi K, Troncoso P, et al. J Urol 2000;163(1):152–157.
42. Chen ME, Troncoso P, Johnston DA, et al. J Urol 1997;158(6):2168–2175.
43. Lippman HR, Ghiatas AA, Sarosdy MF. J Urol 1992;147(3 pt 2):827–829.
44. Park SJ, Miyake H, Hara I, et al. Int J Urol 2003;10(2):68–71.
45. Fleshner NE, O'Sullivan M, Premdass C, et al. Urology 1999;53(2):356–358.
46. Melchior SW, Brawer MK. J Clin Ultrasound 1996;24(8):463–471.
47. Franco OE, Arima K, Yanagawa M. Br J Urol Int 2000;85(9):1049–1052.
48. Frauscher F, Klauser A, Volgger H, et al. J Urol 2002;1767(4):1648–1652.
49. Abu-Yousef MM, Narayana AS. Radiology 1985;156(1):175–180.

50. Young MP, Jones DR, Griffiths GJ, et al. Eur Urol 1993;24(4):479–482.
51. Magnusson A, Fritjofsson A, Norlen BJ, Wicklund H. Scand J Urol Nephrol 1988;22(1):7–10.
52. Friedman AC, Seidmon EJ, Radecki RD, Lev-Toaff A, Caroline DF. Urology 1988;31(6):530–537.
53. Perrapato SD, Carothers GG, Maatman TJ, Soechtig CE. Urology 1989;33(2):103–105.
54. Ohori M, Egawa S, Shinohara K, Wheeler TM, Scardino PT. Br J Urol 1994;74(1):72–79.
55. Okihara K, Kamoi K, Lane RB, et al. J Clin Ultrasound 2002;30(3):123–131.
56. Deliveliotis CH, Varkarakis J, Trakas N, et al. Int Urol Nephrol 1999;31(1):83–87.
57. Liebross RH, Pollack A, Lankford SP, et al. Cancer, 1999;85(7):1577–1585.
58. Smith JA Jr, Scardino PT, Resnick MI, et al. J Urol 1997;157(3):902–906.
59. Colombo T, Schips L, Augustin H, et al. Minerva Urol Nefrol 1999;51(1):1–4.
60. Huch Boni RA, Boner JA, Debatin JF, et al. Clin Radiol 1995;50(9):593–600.
61. Rorvik J, Halvorsen OJ, Servoll E, Haukaas S. Br J Urol 1994;73(1);65–69.
62. Hamper UM, Sheth S, Walsch PC, Holtz PM, Epstein JI. AJR 1990;155(5):1015–1019.
63. Andriole GL, Coplen DE, Mikkelsen DJ, Catalona WJ. J Urol 1989;142(5):1259–1261.
64. Vijverberg PL, Giessen MC, Kurth KH, Dabhoiwala NF, de Reijke TM, van den Tweel JG. Eur J Surg Oncol 1992;18(5):449–455.
65. Wolf JS Jr, Shinohara K, Narayan P. Br J Urol 1992;70(5):534–541.
66. Presti JC Jr, Hricak H, Narayan PA, Shinohara K, White S, Carroll PR. AJR 1996;166(1):103–108.
67. Gerber GS, Goldberg R, Chodak GW. Urology 1992;40(4):311–316.
68. Ukimura O, Troncoso P, Ramirez EI, Babaian RJ. J Urol 1998;159(4):1251–1259.
69. Augustin H, Graefen M, Palisaar J, et al. J Clin Oncol 2003;21(15):2860–2868.
70. Sanders H, el-Galley R. World J Urol 1997;15(6):336–338.
71. Werner-Wasik M, Whittington R, Malkowicz SB, et al. Urology 1997;50(3):385–389.
72. Cornud F, Hamida K, Flam T, et al. AJR 2003;175(4):1161–1168.
73. Sauvain JL, Palascak P, Bourscheid D, et al. Eur Urol 2003;44(1):21–30.
74. Ismail M, Petersen RO, Alexander AA, Newschaffer C, Gomella LG. Urology 1997;50(6):906–912.
75. Garg S, Flortling B, Chadwick D, Robinson MC, Hamdy FC. J Urol 1999;162(4):1318–1321.
76. Giri PG, Walsh JW, Hazra TA, Texter JH, Koontz WW. Int J Radiat Oncol Biol Phys 1982;8(2):283–287.
77. Sawczuk IS, deVere White R, Gold RP, Olsson CA. Urology 1983;21(1):81–84.
78. Platt JF, Bree RL, Schwab RE. AJR 1987;149(2):315–318.
79. Friedman AC, Seidmon EJ, Radecki PD, Lev-Toaff A, Caroline DF. Urology 1988;31(6):530–537.
80. Engeler CE, Wasserman, NF, Zhang G. Urology 1992;40(4):346–350.
81. Borley N, Fabrin K, Sriprasad S, et al. Scand J Urol Nephrol, 2003;37(5):382–386.
82. Magnusson A, Fritjorfsson A, Norlen BJ, Wicklund H. Scand J Urol Nephrol 1988;22(1):7–10.
83. Tiguert R, Gheiler EL, Tefilli MV, et al. Urology 1999;53(2):367–371.
84. Burcombe RJ, Ostler PJ, Ayoub AW, Hoskin PJ. Clin Oncol 2000;12(1):32–35.
85. Lee N, Newhouse JH, Olsson CA, et al. Urology 1999;54(3):490–494.
86. Spencer JA, Chng WJ, Hudson E, Boon AP, Whelan P. Br J Radiol 1998;7(851):1130–1135.
87. Huncharek M, Muscat J. Abdom Imaging 1996;21(4):364–367.
88. Levran Z, Gonzalez JA, Diokno AC, Jafri SZ, Steinert BW. Br J Urol 1995;75(6):778–781.

89. Rifkin MD, Zerhouni EA, Gatsonis CA, et al. N Engl J Med 1990;323(10): 621–626.
90. Tempany CM, Rahmouni AD, Epstein JI, et al. Radiology 1991;181(1):107–112.
91. Schiebler ML, Yankaskas BC, Tempany C, et al. Invest Radiol 1992;27(8): 575–577.
92. Tempany CM, Zhou X, Zerhouni EA, et al. Radiology 1994;192(1):47–54.
93. Mukamel E, de Kernion JB, Hannah J, et al. J Urol (Paris) 1988;94(8):381–388.
94. Tuzel E, Sevinc M, Obuz F, et al. Urol Int 1998;61(4):227–231.
95. Friedman AC, Seidmon EJ, Radecki PD, et al. Urology 1988;31(6):530–537.
96. Rorvik J, Halvorsen OJ, Albrektsen G, et al. Clin Radiol 1999;54(3):164–169.
97. Jager GJ, Barentsz JO, de la Rosette JJ, et al. Radiologe 1994;34(3):129–133.
98. Cornud F, Belin X, Flam T, et al. Br J Urol 1996;77(6):843–850.
99. Bartolozzi C, Menchi I, Lencioni R, et al. Eur Radiol 1996;6(3):339–345.
100. Bates TS, Gillatt DA, Cavanagh PM, et al. Br J Urol 1997;79(6):927–932.
101. Sheu MH, Wang JH, Chen KK, et al. Chung Hua I Hsueh Tsa Chih 1998;61(5):243–252.
102. Rorvik J, Halvorsen OJ, Albrektsen G, et al. Eur Radiol 1999;9(1):29–34.
103. Ekici S, Ozen H, Agildere M, et al. Br J Urol Int 1999;83(7):796–800.
104. May F, Treumann T, Dettmar P, et al. Br J Urol Int 2001;87(1):66–69.
105. Borley N, Fabrin K, Sriprasad S, et al. Scand J Urol Nephrol 2003;37(5):382–386.
106. D'Amico A, Altschuler M, Whittington R, et al. Clin Perf Qual Health Care 1993;1(4):219–222.
107. D'Amico AV, Whittington R, Schnall M, et al. Cancer 1995;75(9):2368–2372.
108. Huch Boni RA, Boner JA, Debatin JF, et al. Clin Radiol 1995;50(9):593–600.
109. D'Amico AV, Whittington R, Malkowicz SB, et al. Urology 1997;49(3A suppl):23–30.
110. Getty DJ, Seltzer SE, Tempany CM, et al. Radiology 1997;204(2):471–479.
111. D'Amico AV, Whittington R, Malkowicz SB. Urology 2000;55(4):572–577.
112. Horiguchi A, Nakashima J, Horiguch Y, et al. Prostate 2003;56(1):23–29.
113. Seltzer SE, Getty DJ, Tempany CM, et al. Radiology 1997;202(1):219–226.
114. Huch Boni RA, Boner JA, Lutolf UM, et al. J Comput Assist Tomogr 1995; 19(2):232–237.
115. Brown G, Macvicar DA, Ayton V, et al. Clin Radiol 1995;50(9):601–606.
116. Padhani AR, Gapinski CJ, Macvicar DA, et al. Clin Radiol 2000;55(2):99–109.
117. Ogura K, Maekawa S, Okubo K, et al. Urology 2001;57(4):721–726.
118. Harisinghani MG, Barentsz J, Hahn PF, et al. N Engl J Med 2003;348(25): 2491–2499.
119. Cheng GC, Chen MH, Whittington R, et al. Int J Radiat Oncol Biol Phys 2003; 55(1):64–70.
120. D'Amico AV, Whittington R, Malkowicz B, et al. J Urol 2000;164(3 pt 1): 759–763.
121. Soulie M, Aziza R, Escourrou G, et al. Urology 2001;58(2):228–232.
122. Huncharek M, Muscat J. Cancer Invest 1995;13(1):31–35.
123. Kurhanewicz J, Vigneron DB, Nelson SJ, et al. Urology 1995;45(3):459–466.
124. Narayan P, Jajodia P, Kurhanewicz J, et al. J Urol 1991;146(1):66–74.
125. Hasumi M, Suzuki K, Taketomi A, et al. Anticancer Res 2003;23(5b):4223–4227.
126. Hasumi M, Suzuki K, Oya N, et al. Anticancer Res 2002;22(2B):1205–1208.
127. Garcia-Segura JM, Sanchez-Chapado M, Ibarburen C, et al. Magn Reson Imaging 1999;17(5):755–765.
128. Heerschap A, Jag GJ, van der Graaf M, et al. Anticancer Res 1997;17(3A): 1455–1460.
129. Yuen JS, Thng CH, Tan PH, et al. J Urol 2004;171(4):1482–1486.
130. Scheidler J, Srivastava A, Males RG. Radiology 2001;221(2):380–390.
131. Kaji Y, Kurhanewicz J, Hricak H, et al. Radiology 1998;206(3):785–790.
132. Yu KK, Scheidler J, Hricak H, et al. Radiology 1999;213(2):481–488.
133. Pouliot J, Kim Y, Lessard E, et al. Int J Radiat Oncol Biol Phys 2004;59(4): 1196–1207.

134. Zaider M, Zelefsky MJ, Lee EK, et al. Int J Radiat Oncol Biol Phys 2000; 47(4):1085–1096.
135. Parivar F, Hricak H, Shinohara K, et al. Urology 1996;48(4):594–599.
136. Kurhanewicz J, Vigneron DB, Hricak H, et al. Radiology 1996;200(2):489–496.
137. Fricke E, Machtens S, Hofmann M, et al. Eur J Nucl Med Mol Imaging 2003;30(4):607–611.
138. Sung J, Espiritu JI, Segall GM, et al. BJU Int 2003;92(1):24–27.
139. Chang CH, Wu HC, Tsai JJ, et al. Urol Int 2003;70(4):311–315.
140. Oyama N, Miller TR, Dehdashti F, et al. J Nucl Med 2003;44(4):549–555.
141. Picchio M, Messa C, Landoni C, et al. J Urol 2003;169(4):1337–1340.
142. de Jong IJ, Pruim J, Elsinga PH, et al. Eur Urol 2002;42(1):18–23.
143. Oyama N, Akino H, Kanamaru H, et al. J Nucl Med 2002;43(2):181–186.
144. Seltzer MA, Barbaric Z, Belldegrun A, et al. J Urol 1999;162(4):1322–1328.
145. Oyama N, Akino H, Zusuki Y, et al. Jpn J Clin Oncol 1999;29(12):623–629.
146. Sanz G, Robles JE, Gimenez M, et al. BJU Int 1999;84(9):1028–1031.
147. Heicappell R, Muller-Mattheis V, Reinhardt M, et al. Eur Urol 1999;36(6): 582–587.
148. Yeh SD, Imbriasco M, Larson SM, et al. Nucl Med Biol 1996;23(6):693–697.
149. Shreve PD, Grossman HB, Gross MD, et al. Radiology 1996;199(3):751–756.
150. Effert PJ, Bares R, Handt S, et al. J Urol 1996;155(3):994–998.
151. Kotzerke J, Volkmer BG, Glatting G, et al. Nuklearmedizin 2003;42(1):25–30.
152. Kato T, Tsukamoto E, Kuge Y, et al. Eur J Nucl Med Mol Imaging 2002; 29(11):1492–1495.
153. Kotzerke J, Volkmer BG, Neumaier B, et al. Eur J Nucl Med Mol Imaging 2002;29(10):1380–1384.
154. de Jong IJ, Pruim J, Elsinga PH, et al. Eur Urol 2003;44(1):32–38, discussion 38–39.
155. deJong IJ, Pruim J, Elsinga PH, et al. J Nucl Med 2003;44(3):331–335.
156. Kotzerke J, Prang J, Neumaier B, et al. Eur J Nucl Med 2000;27(9):1415–1419.
157. Lin K, Szabo Z, Chin BB, Civelek AC. Clin Nucl Med 1999;24(8):579–582.
158. Ataus S, Citci A, Alici B, et al. Int Urol Nephrol 1999;31(4):481–489.
159. Wolff JM, Bares R, Jung PK, Buell U, Jakse G. Urol Int 1996;56(3):169–173.
160. Gleave ME, Coupland D, Drachenberg D, et al. Urology 1996;47(5):708–712.
161. Huncharek M, Muscat J. Cancer Invest 1995;13(1):31–35.
162. Sassine AM, Schulman C. Eur Urol 1993;23(3):348–351.
163. Pantelides ML, Bowman SP, George NJ. Br J Urol 1992;70(3):299–303.
164. Woff JM, Zimny M, Borchers H, et al. Eur Urol 1998;33(4):376–381.
165. O'Sullivan JM, Norman AR, Cook GJ, Fisher C, Dearnaley DP. BJU Int 2003;92(7):685–689.
166. Rydh A, Tomic R, Tavelin B, Hietala SO, Damber JE. Scand J Urol Nephrol 1999;33(2):89–93.
167. Spencer JA, Chng WJ, Hudson E, Boon AP, Whelen P. Br J Radiol 1998; 71(851):1130–1135.
168. Stokkel MP, Zwinderman AH, Zwartendijk J, Pauwels EK, Van Eck-Smith BL. Int J Biol Markers 1998;13(2):70–76.
169. Kemp PM, Maguire GA, Bird NJ. Br J Urol 1997;79(4):611–614.
170. Levran Z, Gonzalez JA, Diokno AC, Jafri SZ, Steinert BW. Br J Urol 1995; 75(6):778–781.
171. Lorente JA, Valenzuela H, Morote J, Gelabert A. Eur J Nucl Med 1999; 26(6):625–632.
172. Morote J, Lorenta JA, Encabo G, Cancer 1996;78(11):2374–2378.
173. Lorente JA, Morote J, Raventos C, Encabo G, Valenzuela H. J Urol 1996; 155(4):1348–1351.
174. Wymenga LF, Boomsma JH, Groenier K, Piers DA, Mensink HJ. BJU Int 2001; 88(3):226–230.
175. Lee N, Fawaaz R, Olsson CA, et al. Int J Radiat Oncol Biol Phys 2000;48(5): 1443–1446.

176. Vijayakumar V, Vijayakumar S, Quadri, SF, Blend MJ. Am J Clin Oncol 1994; 17(5):432–436.
177. Colberg JW, Ornstein DK, et al. J Urol 1999;161(2):520–523.
178. Lorente JA, Morote J, Raventos C, et al. J Urol 1996;155(4):1348–1351.
179. Oommen R, Geethanjali FS, Gopalakrishnan G, et al. Br J Radiol 1994;67(797):469–471.
180. Mulders PF, Fernandez del Moral P, Theeuwes AG, et al. Eur Urol 1992; 21(1):2–5.
181. Corrie D, Timmons JH, Bauman JM, et al. Cancer 1988;61(12):2453–2454.
182. Huben RP, Schellhammer PF. J Urol 1982;128(3):510–522.
183. Yap BK, Choo R, Deboer G, et al. Cancer managed with watchful observation alone? Br J Urol Int 2003;91(7):613–617.
184. Kagan AR, Steckel RJ. Med Pediatr Oncol 1993;21(5):327–332.
185. Murphy GP, Troychak MJ, Cobb OE, et al. Prostate 1997;33(2):141–146.
186. Salomon CG, Flisak ME, Olson MC, et al. Radiology 1993;189(3):713–719.
187. Wasserman NF, Kapoor DA, Hildebrandt WC, et al. Radiology 1992;185(2): 367–372.
188. Silverman JM, Krebs TL. AJR 1997;168(2):379–385.
189. Parivar F, Hricak H, Shinohara K, et al. Urology 1996;48(4):594–599.
190. Older RA, Lippert MC, Gay SB, et al. Acad Radiol 1995;2(6):470–474.
191. Jadvar H, Pinski JK, Conti PS. Oncol Rep 2003;10(5):1485–1488.
192. Salminen E, Hogg A, Binns D, et al. Acta Oncol 2002;41(5):425–429.
193. Hofer C, Laubenbacher C, Block T, et al. Eur Urol 1999;36(1):31–35.
194. Shreve PD, Grossman HB, Gross MD, et al. Radiology 1996;199(3):751–756.
195. Fricke E, Machtens S, Hofmann M, et al. Eur J Nucl Med Mol Imag 2003; 30(4):607–611.
196. Oyama N, Miller TR, Dehdashti F, et al. J Nucl Med 2003;44(4):549–555.
197. Kotzerke J, Volkmer BG, Neumaier B, et al. Eur J Nucl Med Mol Imag 2002;29(10):1380–1384.
198. Koizumi K, Uchiyama G, Komatsu H. Ann Nucl Med 1994;8(4):225–230.
199. Sabbatini P, Larson SM, Kremer A, et al. J Clin Oncol 1999;17:948–957.
200. Soloway MS, Hardeman SW, Hichen D, et al. Cancer 1988;61:195–202.
201. Cheng L, Bergstralh EJ, Cheville JC, et al. Am J Surg Pathol 1998;22(12): 1491–1500.
202. Spencer JA, Golding SJ. Clin Radiol 1994;49(6):404–407.

8

Neuroimaging in Alzheimer Disease

Kejal Kantarci and Clifford R. Jack, Jr.

Key Points

- By differentiating potentially treatable causes, structural imaging with either computed tomography (CT) or magnetic resonance imaging (MRI) influences patient management during the initial evaluation of dementia (strong evidence).
- No evidence exists on the choice of either CT or MRI for the initial evaluation of dementia (insufficient evidence).
- Diagnostic accuracy of positron emission tomography (PET) and single photon emission computed tomography (SPECT) to distinguish patients with Alzheimer disease (AD) from normal is not higher than that for clinical evaluation (moderate evidence).
- Hippocampal atrophy on MRI-based volumetry and regional decrease in cerebral perfusion on SPECT correlates with the pathologic stage in AD (moderate evidence).

- Positron emission tomography, SPECT, and dynamic susceptibility contrast-enhanced MRI are not cost-effective for the diagnostic workup of AD with the assumed minimal effectiveness of the drug donepezil hydrochloride (moderate evidence).
- Use of PET in early dementia can increase the accuracy of clinical diagnosis without adding to the overall costs of the evaluation (moderate evidence).
- Longitudinal decrease in MRI-based hippocampal volumes, N-acetylaspartate (NAA) levels on ^{1}H magnetic resonance spectroscopy (MRS), glucose metabolism on PET, and cerebral blood flow on SPECT is associated with the rate of cognitive decline in patients with AD (moderate evidence).
- The validity of imaging techniques as surrogate markers for therapeutic efficacy in AD has not been tested in a positive disease-modifying drug trial (insufficient evidence).

Definition and Pathophysiology

Alzheimer disease (AD) is a progressive neurodegenerative dementia. The pathologic hallmarks of AD are accumulation of neurofibrillary tangles and senile plaques. The neurofibrillary pathology, which is associated with cognitive dysfunction, neuron and synapse loss, involves the limbic cortex early in the disease course, and extends to the neocortex as the disease progresses. In addition to the histopathologic changes, there is a gradual loss of cholinergic innervation in AD, which has been the basis for cholinesterase inhibitor therapy.

Epidemiology

Alzheimer disease is the most common cause of dementing illnesses. The prevalence of AD increases with age, and the disease is becoming a significant health problem as the aging population increases in size (1,2). In the United States, the prevalence of AD was 2.32 million in 1997, and it is projected that 8.64 million people will have the disease by 2047 (3,4).

Overall Cost to Society

The average lifetime cost per patient is estimated to be $174,000. The cost to U.S. society of AD has been estimated at $100 billion per year (5).

Goals

The goals of imaging are to (1) exclude a potentially reversible cause of dementia in subjects with possible AD, (2) identify subjects at risk for AD, (3) quantify the stage of disease to enable tracking of treatment response, and (4) identify subjects who may respond to therapy. Although no currently available treatments have been proven to stabilize or reverse the neurodegenerative process, a number of putative disease modifying agents are now in development with early clinical trials (6,7). The primary targets of such interventions are people who are at risk or who are at the mild to moderate stages of the disease. Imaging markers that can accurately discriminate individuals at risk, and are sensitive to disease onset and progression are needed for trials involving disease-modifying therapies.

Methodology

A literature search was conducted using Medline. The search included articles published from January 1966 through February 2004. The main search term was *Alzheimer* or *Alzheimer's disease*. Other terms combined with the main topic were *clinical diagnosis*, *clinical criteria*, *neuroimaging*, *MRI*, *MR spectroscopy*, *PET*, *SPECT*, and *cost-effectiveness*. The search yielded 3284 articles. Animal studies, non–English-language articles, and articles published before 1980 were excluded, and only articles relevant to our search questions were included for review.

I. How Accurate Are the Clinical Criteria for the Diagnosis of Alzheimer Disease?

Summary of Evidence: There is strong evidence that the *Diagnostic and Statistical Manual of Mental Disorders*, 3rd edition revised (DSM-IIIR) and the National Institute of Neurologic, Communicative Disorders, and Stroke–Alzheimer Disease and Related Disorders Association NINCDS-ADRDA criteria are reliable for the diagnosis of dementia and AD (strong evidence). There are, however, limitations to the data supporting clinical criteria for the diagnosis of AD. Diagnostic accuracy of clinical criteria may vary with the extent of the disease and the skills of the clinician. Clinical criteria for AD need to be validated by clinicians with different levels of expertise and at different clinical settings if such criteria will have widespread use to identify patients for therapeutic interventions (insufficient evidence).

Supporting Evidence: The clinical diagnosis of AD in a living person is labeled either possible or probable AD. Definite diagnosis of AD requires tissue examination, through biopsy or autopsy, of the brain. Histopathologic hallmarks of the disease are neurofibrillary tangles and senile plaques, which show marked heterogeneity in the pathologic progression of AD, and are also encountered to a lesser extent in elderly individuals with normal cognition (8–12). Thus the boundary between the histopathologic changes in elderly individuals considered to be cognitively normal and patients with AD is quantitative, not qualitative. The most recent recommendations for postmortem diagnosis of AD by the work group sponsored by the National Institute on Aging and the Reagan Research Institute of the Alzheimer's Association (13) defines AD as a clinicopathological entity, emphasizing the importance of clinical impression for pathologic diagnosis.

The diagnostic accuracy of clinical criteria is assessed by using the pathologic diagnosis as a standard. A shortcoming of this approach is that clinical and pathologic findings do not correlate perfectly. For example, some clinically demented patients do not meet the pathologic criteria for AD or any other dementing illness. Similarly, some patients who are clinically normal have extensive pathologic changes of AD. However, from a practical standpoint, by taking pathologic diagnosis as a gold standard, it is possible to assess the diagnostic accuracy of clinical or neuroimaging criteria for the diagnosis of AD. The two commonly used clinical criteria that were subject to assessment for the diagnosis of dementia and AD are the DSM-IIIR (14) and the NINCDS-ADRDA criteria (15).

When both the DSM-IIIR and NINCDS-ADRDA criteria are applied to the diagnosis, clinical-pathologic correlation ranges from 75% to 90% in studies involving a broad spectrum of patients (16–18) (strong evidence). The disagreement between clinical and pathologic diagnosis in 10% to 25% of the cases provides the motivation to develop neuroimaging markers that can accurately identify the effects of AD pathology even in the presymptomatic phase.

The sensitivity of the DSM-IIIR and NINCDS-ADRDA criteria for the diagnosis of AD ranges from 76% to 98% and the specificity from 61% to 84% (19–23), providing strong evidence that the accuracy of the two commonly used clinical criteria for identifying pathologically diagnosed AD is good, but show marked variability across academic centers. When community-based and clinic-based patients were evaluated by the same physicians, both the sensitivity and specificity of the clinical diagnosis were lower for the community- than for the clinic-based cohorts (92% and 79% for community vs. 98% and 84% for clinic) (19) (strong evidence).

Interrater agreement on the diagnosis of dementia and AD with the DSM-IIIR and NINCDS-ADRDA criteria has been good [κ = 0.54–0.81 for DSM-IIIR (24,25), and κ = 0.51–0.72 for NINCDS-ADRDA criteria (26,27) in population-based studies (strong evidence)].

II. Does Neuroimaging Increase the Diagnostic Accuracy of Alzheimer Disease in the Clinical Setting?

A. Structural Neuroimaging

Summary of Evidence: The traditional use of structural neuroimaging to differentiate potentially reversible or modifiable causes of dementia such as brain tumors, subdural hematoma, normal pressure hydrocephalus, and vascular dementia from AD is widely accepted (28). There is strong evidence that structural imaging influences patient management during the initial evaluation of dementia. There is moderate evidence that the diagnostic precision of structural neuroimaging is higher with volume measurements than visual evaluation, especially in mildly demented cases, but the figures are still comparable to clinical evaluation.

Supporting Evidence: Besides the potential causes of dementia mentioned above, structural neuroimaging can also identify anatomic changes that occur due to the pathologic involvement in AD (29). Neurofibrillary pathology, which correlates with neuron loss and cognitive decline in patients with AD, follows a hierarchical topologic progression course in the brain (10,30–32). It initially involves the anteromedial temporal lobe and limbic cortex. As the disease progresses it spreads over to the neo-cortex (30). The macroscopic result of this pathologic involvement is atrophy, which is related to the decrease in neuron density (33). For this reason, the search for anatomic imaging markers of AD has targeted the anteromedial temporal lobe, particularly the hippocampus and entorhinal cortex, which are involved earliest and most severely with the neurofibrillary pathology and atrophy in AD.

Visual evaluation or measurements of the anteromedial temporal lobe width with computed tomography (CT) detected 80% to 95% of the pathologically confirmed AD cases (23,35). However, the accuracy declined to 57% when only mild AD cases with low pretest probability were quota studied, and the clinical diagnosis with the NINCDS-ADRDA criteria was more accurate than CT measurements for identifying AD patients at pathologically early stages of the disease (strong evidence) (35).

One study with a pathologically confirmed cohort (34) revealed that structural neuroimaging can help to identify vascular dementia or vascular component of AD (mixed dementia) by increasing the sensitivity of the clinical evaluation from 6% to 59%, and management of the vascular component may in turn slow down cognitive decline (strong evidence).

1. Special Case: Volumetric Measurements

A reliable and reproducible method for quantifying medial temporal lobe atrophy is magnetic resonance imaging (MRI)-based volume measurements of the hippocampus and the entorhinal cortex (29,36). Antemortem hippocampal atrophy was not found to be specific for AD in a pathologically confirmed cohort; however, hippocampal volumes on MRI correlated well with the pathologic stage of the disease ($r = -0.63$; $p = 0.001$) (37). Structural neuroimaging changed the clinical diagnosis in 19% to 28% of the cases, and changed patient management in 15% (38) (strong evidence).

Visual evaluation of the anteromedial temporal lobe for atrophy on MRI to differentiate patients with AD from normal subjects had a sensitivity of 83% to 85% and a specificity of 96% to 98% in clinically confirmed cohorts (38,39). Although visual evaluation of the temporal lobe accurately distinguishes AD patients in experienced hands, evidence is lacking on the precision of visual evaluation at different clinical settings. Diagnostic accuracy of this technique for distinguishing AD patients from normal has been 79% to 94% in clinically confirmed cohorts (40,41), being comparable in mildly and moderately demented cases (42). Routine use of volumetry techniques for the diagnosis of AD may be time-consuming and cumbersome in a clinical setting. However, the intimate correlation between pathologic involvement and hippocampal volumes is encouraging for the use of hippocampal volumetry as an imaging marker for disease progression (moderate evidence).

By differentiating potentially treatable causes, structural imaging with either CT or MRI influences patient management during the initial evaluation of dementia (strong evidence). Evidence is lacking for the choice of either CT or MRI. Computed tomography may be appropriate when a brain tumor or subdural hematoma is suspected, and MRI may be the modality of choice for vascular dementia because of its superior sensitivity to vascular changes. The decision should be based on clinical impression at this time (insufficient evidence).

B. Functional Neuroimaging

Summary of Evidence: Single photon emission computed tomography (SPECT) and positron emission tomography (PET) are the two widely investigated functional neuroimaging techniques in AD. Measurements of regional glucose metabolism with PET, and regional perfusion measurements with SPECT indicate a metabolic decline and a decrease in blood flow in the temporal and parietal lobes of patients with AD relative to normal elderly. There is moderate evidence that the diagnostic accuracy of either SPECT or PET is not higher than the clinical criteria in AD. Nonetheless, both functional imaging techniques appear promising for differentiating other dementia syndromes (frontotemporal dementia and dementia with Lewy bodies) from AD due to differences in regional functional involvement.

Supporting Evidence: With visual evaluation of SPECT images for temporoparietal hypoperfusion, the sensitivity for distinguishing AD patients from normal differed from 42% to 79% at a specificity of 86% to 90%, being lower in patients with mild AD than in patients with severe AD in both clinically and pathologically confirmed cases (43–45), and not superior to the clinical diagnosis based on NINCDS-ADRDA criteria (46) (strong evidence). The regional decrease in cerebral perfusion with SPECT correlated with the neurofibrillary pathology staging of AD (47) (strong evidence); SPECT increased the accuracy of clinical evaluation for identifying AD pathology, but cases with other types of dementia were not included (48) (moderate evidence).

The sensitivity and specificity of the temporoparietal metabolic decline on PET for differentiating patients with pathologically confirmed AD from normal subjects was 63% and 82%, respectively, similar to the sensitivity (63%) but lower than the specificity (100%) of clinical diagnosis in the same cohort (49) (strong evidence). On the other hand, occipital hypometabolism on PET distinguished pathologically confirmed patients with dementia with Lewy bodies from AD patients with a comparable specificity (80%) and higher sensitivity (90%) than clinical evaluation (strong evidence) (50,51).

Visual evaluation of SPECT images for temporoparietal hypoperfusion distinguished clinically confirmed AD patients from those with frontotemporal dementia by correctly classifying 74% of AD patients with decreased blood flow in the parietal lobes and 81% of frontotemporal dementia patients with decreased blood flow in the frontal lobes (52) (moderate evidence).

Visual interpretation of PET images for temporoparietal glucose metabolism was reliable ($\kappa = 0.42$–0.61) (53), and PET was more useful than SPECT for differentiating clinically confirmed patients with AD from normal elderly (54). With automated data analysis methods, PET could distinguish clinically confirmed AD cases from normal with a sensitivity of 93% at 93% specificity (55) (moderate evidence).

C. Other Magnetic Resonance Techniques

Summary of Evidence: Due to the ease of integrating an extra pulse sequence into the standard structural MRI exam, and the advantage of obtaining metabolic or functional information different from that of the anatomic

MRI, other magnetic resonance (MR) techniques have also been investigated for the diagnosis of AD. The utility of these MR techniques remains to be confirmed with the standard of histopathology (moderate evidence).

Supporting Evidence: One of the most extensively studied MR techniques for the diagnosis of AD is ^{1}H MR spectroscopy (^{1}H MRS), which provides biochemical information from hydrogen proton–containing metabolites in the brain (Fig. 8.1). A decrease in the ratio of the neuronal metabolite *N*-acetylaspartate (NAA) to the metabolite myoinositol (MI) distinguished AD patients from normal with a sensitivity of 83% and specificity of 98% in a clinically confirmed cohort (56). A decrease in NAA levels on ^{1}H MRS of the frontal lobe also distinguished clinically diagnosed patients with frontotemporal dementia from patients with AD with an accuracy of 84% (57) (moderate evidence). Another functional imaging technique, dynamic susceptibility MRI, has been proposed as an alternative to SPECT for the quantitation of temporoparietal hypoperfusion in AD, and the sensitivity and specificity of this technique have been comparable to those of SPECT (58) (moderate evidence).

The diagnostic accuracy of other quantitative MRI techniques, such as diffusion weighted MRI (DWI) and magnetization transfer MRI to distin-

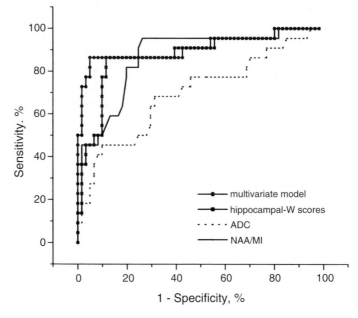

Figure 8.1. Receiver operating characteristic (ROC) plots of magnetic resonance (MR) measurements in distinguishing patients with a clinical diagnosis of Alzheimer disease (AD) from cognitively normal elderly. MRI-based hippocampal volumetry (W scores), hippocampal apparent diffusion coefficients (ADC) on diffusion weighted MRI, *N*-acetylaspartate/myoinositol (NAA/MI) on ^{1}H MR spectroscopy, and the multivariate model derived from these three MR measurements were plotted. While the multivariate model is slightly more accurate in distinguishing AD from normal, there is no significant difference between the hippocampal W scores and NAA/MI in distinguishing the two groups. The hippocampal ADC, on the other hand, is less accurate than hippocampal W scores and NAA/MI. [*Source:* Kantarci et al. (110), with permission from S. Karger AG, Basel.]

guish AD patients from normal elderly in clinically confirmed cohorts, was lower than that of clinical evaluation (59,60), and evidence is lacking on the diagnostic accuracy of either functional MRI or phosphorus (^{31}P) MRS in AD (insufficient evidence).

III. Can Neuroimaging Identify Individuals at Elevated Risk for Alzheimer Disease and Predict Its Future Development?

A. Prodromal Alzheimer Disease, or Mild Cognitive Impairment

Summary of Evidence: There is moderate evidence that quantitative MR techniques and PET are sensitive to the structural and functional changes in patients with amnestic mild cognitive impairment (MCI). Magnetic resonance–based evaluation of the hippocampal volumes is associated with the rate of future development of AD in individuals with MCI based on clinically confirmed cases, and PET can predict subsequent clinical behavior in cognitively normal elderly.

Supporting Evidence: Risk groups for AD are composed of individuals identified through either clinical examination or family history and genetic testing who have a greater probability of developing AD than members of the general population, and in whom the relevant exposures are absent. The rationale for identifying imaging criteria for those at elevated risk comes from recent advances in disease-modifying therapies. Individuals with elevated probability of developing AD are the primary targets of these treatment trials aimed at preventing or delaying the neurodegenerative process. Thus, biomarkers that can accurately distinguish individuals at risk and predict if and when they will develop AD are required in order to utilize these interventions before the neurodegenerative disease advances and irreversible damage occurs.

Aging is a risk factor for AD, and elderly individuals who develop AD pass through a transitional phase of a decline in memory function before meeting the clinical criteria for AD (61). This early symptomatic or prodromal phase has several clinical definitions some of which are MCI, age-associated memory impairment, clinical dementia rating score of 0.5, cognitive impairment, or minimal impairment. While the clinical criteria for each syndrome show similarities, they are subtly different. Longitudinal studies show that individuals with MCI, specifically amnestic MCI are at a higher risk of developing AD than normal elderly (62). Patients with MCI have the earliest features of AD pathology with neuron loss and atrophy in the anteromedial temporal lobe, specifically the entorhinal cortex, which is involved in memory processing (63). There is strong evidence that there is an association between pathologic involvement and cognitive impairment in the evolution of AD (8,10,11). Hence patients with MCI reside between normal aging and AD, both in the pathologic and in the cognitive continuum (Fig. 8-2) (strong evidence).

In concordance with the pathologic evolution of AD, MR-based volumetry identified smaller hippocampal and entorhinal cortex volumes in patients with MCI than in normal elderly (36,64) (Fig. 8-3). Among several regions in the temporal lobe, reduced hippocampal volumes on MRI and hippocampal glucose metabolism on PET were the best discriminator of

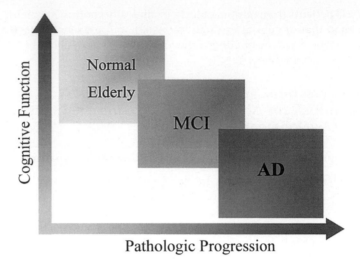

Pathologic Progression

Figure 8.2. In the cognitive continuum, people with mild cognitive impairment (MCI) reside at a transitional clinical state between cognitively normal elderly, and people with AD. People with MCI are also at an intermediate stage between asymptomatic elderly individuals with early pathologic involvement of AD to people with established AD.

patients with MCI from normal elderly (65). Hippocampal volumes were also comparable to entorhinal cortex volumes for distinguishing patients with MCI (36,65), elderly individuals with mild memory problems, and very mild AD (66,67) from normal (moderate evidence). Other quantitative MRI techniques, such as DWI and magnetization transfer MRI measurements, have also revealed that the diffusivity of water is increased and magnetization transfer ratios are decreased in the hippocampi of patients with MCI relative to normals, both of which indicate an increase in free

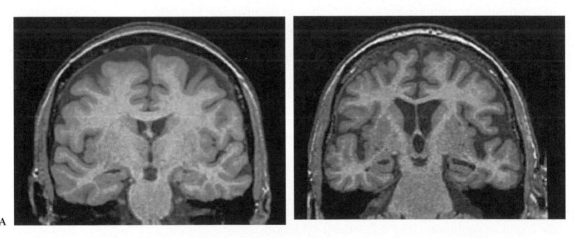

A   B

Figure 8.3. T1-weighted three-dimensional spoiled gradient echo images at the level of hippocampal heads in a 76-year-old cognitively normal subject (A), a 77-year-old patient with MCI (B), a 75-year-old patient with AD (C), and a 95-year-old cognitively normal subject (D). Patients with AD, MCI, and the 95-year-old cognitively normal subject have brain atrophy, which is marked in the hippocampi and the temporal lobes in the MCI and AD subject, compared to the younger normal subject. Atrophy is more severe in the AD subject than in the MCI subject. In this case, the age-adjusted regional and global volume measurements would be useful in differentiating atrophy due to normal aging from atrophy due to AD pathology.

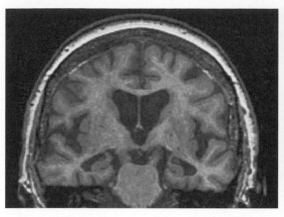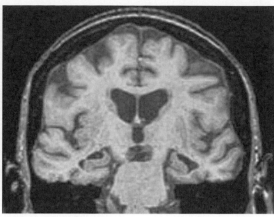

C

D

Figure 8.3. *Continued*

water, presumably due to hippocampal neuronal damage (59,68) (moderate evidence).

Because all patients with MCI do not develop AD at a similar rate, markers that can predict the rate of development of AD have important implications for assessing the effectiveness of therapies aimed at preventing or delaying development of AD in patients with MCI. Premorbid hippocampal and parahippocampal volumes (69), visual ranking of hippocampal atrophy (70,71), and measurements of entorhinal cortex volume (67) were associated with future development of AD in patients with mild memory difficulties and MCI. Positron emission tomography (72–74) and SPECT (75–77) have also been shown to predict subsequent development of MCI and AD in clinically determined normal elderly individuals, people with memory impairment, MCI, and questionable AD (moderate evidence).

Two ^{1}H MRS studies revealed that MI/creatine (Cr) levels are higher in both MCI and AD patients than in normal elderly. Furthermore, NAA/Cr levels were lower in AD, but not in MCI patients, than in normal elderly in the posterior cingulate gyri of clinically confirmed cases (78,79) (Fig. 8.4). Similar findings were encountered from neocortical regions in mild AD patients (80), which suggest that MI/Cr levels increase before a significant decrease in the neuronal metabolite NAA/Cr (moderate evidence).

The finding of an early increase in MI/Cr in MCI is encouraging because NAA/Cr is a marker for neuronal integrity. Thus an increase in MI/Cr levels in patients with MCI may predict future development of AD before substantial neuronal damage occurs. This hypothesis remains to be tested with longitudinal studies on these individuals (insufficient evidence).

No study has yet investigated the pathologic correlates of neuroimaging findings in patients with MCI (insufficient evidence).

B. Asymptomatic Apolipoprotein E ε4 Carriers

Summary of Evidence: The most recognized susceptibility gene in sporadic AD is Apolipoprotein E (ApoE) ε4 allele, which has been shown to influence age of onset (81) and amyloid plaque burden (82) in AD. Posterior cingulate gyrus hypometabolism, and the rate of decline in glucose metabolism on PET, is associated with ApoE genotype in people with normal cognition (moderate evidence).

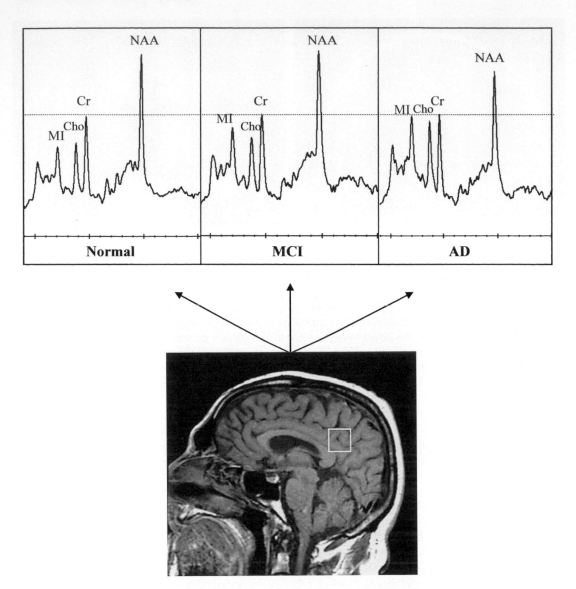

Figure 8.4. Examples of ^{1}H MR spectra obtained from the posterior cingulate volume of interest (VOI) with an echo time of 30 ms in an 81-year-old cognitively normal subject, a 77-year-old patient with MCI, and a 79-year-old patient with AD. The VOI is placed on a midsagittal T1-weighted localizing image, which includes right and left posterior cingulate gyri and inferior precunei. The ^{1}H MR spectra are scaled to the creatine (Cr) peak (dashed line). Cr peak is found to be stable in AD and is commonly used as an internal reference for quantitation of other metabolite peaks. Myoinositol (MI)/Cr ratio is higher in the patient with MCI than the normal subject. Choline (Cho)/Cr and MI/Cr ratio is higher, and N-acetylaspartate (NAA)/Cr ratio is lower in the patient with AD than in both the patient with MCI and the normal subject.

Supporting Evidence: While some studies showed that ApoE genotype does not have any influence on hippocampal volumes (83,84), others found an association between ApoE genotype and medial temporal lobe atrophy (85,86). The dissociation between hippocampal volumes and ApoE genotype may increase the accuracy of both markers for predicting development of AD in the elderly, when combined in prediction models. Posterior cingulate gyrus hypometabolism, and the rate of decline in glucose metabolism on PET on the other hand, is associated with ApoE genotype in people with normal cognition (87–89) (moderate evidence).

Evidence is lacking on the predictive value of PET for development of AD in carriers versus noncarriers of the ApoE ε4 allele, which requires further investigation with longitudinal studies. No studies were identified on the neuroimaging correlates of ApoE genotype in pathologically confirmed cohorts (insufficient evidence).

IV. Is Neuroimaging Cost-Effective for the Clinical Evaluation of Alzheimer Disease?

Summary of Evidence: Current treatment options for AD may reduce the social and economic costs of the disease by slowing the rate of cognitive decline, improving the quality of life, and delaying nursing home placement. Neuroimaging may contribute to identification of individuals with early AD who may benefit from such therapies. Use of PET in early dementia can increase the accuracy of clinical diagnosis without adding to the overall costs of the evaluation (moderate evidence). However, the cost-effectiveness analysis revealed that the addition of SPECT, dynamic susceptibility contrast-enhanced MRI, and PET to the diagnostic workup of AD was not cost-effective considering the currently available treatment options (moderate evidence).

Supporting Evidence: One study indicated that PET increases the diagnostic accuracy for early AD, reducing the rate of false-negative and false-positive diagnoses and avoiding unnecessary treatment costs and late interventions, without increasing the costs of evaluation and management of AD (90). On the other hand, the cost-effectiveness analysis of SPECT, dynamic susceptibility contrast-enhanced MRI (91), and PET (92,93) for the diagnosis of AD revealed that the addition of functional neuroimaging to the diagnostic workup of AD in an AD clinic is not cost-effective considering the assumed effectiveness of the drug donepezil hydrochloride (moderate evidence).

The cost-effectiveness of a diagnostic modality is directly related to the effectiveness of the therapy for the condition being diagnosed. Thus, cost-effectiveness studies on the diagnostic procedures in AD should be viewed in the context of minimal effectiveness of currently available treatment options. The outcome of cost-effectiveness analyses of diagnostic modalities in AD could change dramatically when more effective therapies become available. No study investigated the cost-effectiveness of neuroimaging in clinical decision making in pathologically confirmed cohorts (insufficient evidence).

V. Can Neuroimaging Measure Disease Progression and Therapeutic Efficacy in Alzheimer Disease?

Summary of Evidence: Recent advances in treatments aimed at inhibiting the pathologic process of AD created a need for biologic markers that can accurately measure the effectiveness of therapeutic interventions. Neuropsychologic measures of memory and cognitive function can monitor the symptomatic progression in patients with AD. Yet, monitoring biologic

progression is only possible with markers closely related to the neurodegenerative pathology. The usefulness of neuroimaging as a surrogate for
therapeutic efficacy in AD remains to be tested in trials with large cohorts
and positive therapeutic outcomes. Currently, there is insufficient evidence
that neuroimaging can be a surrogate for therapeutic efficacy in AD (insufficient evidence).

Supporting Evidence: Magnetic resonance (MR)-based hippocampal volumetry and regional perfusion on SPECT correlate with the stage of pathologic involvement in AD (37,47) (strong evidence). Serial measurements of
whole brain volumes using the boundary shift integral method on MRI
(94–96) and MR- based hippocampal volumetry (97,98) revealed that the
rate of atrophy is associated with cognitive decline in patients with AD
over time. Serial MR measures of the rate of atrophy in AD may be a valuable surrogate in drug trials. Serial brain to ventricular volume ratio measurements on MRI indicate that to detect a 20% excess rate of atrophy with
90% power in AD in 6 months, 135 subjects would be required in each
arm of a randomized placebo-controlled trial, and for 30% excess rate of
atrophy, 61 subjects would be required (99) (moderate evidence).

Magnetic resonance–based volume measurements of the whole brain
and the hippocampus are valid macroscopic measures of ongoing atrophy
in AD. Functional imaging techniques, on the other hand, provide markers
related to the neurodegenerative pathology at the microscopic level. Longitudinal decrease of the neuronal metabolite NAA on ^{1}H MRS (100,101),
regional glucose metabolism on PET (102), and cerebral blood flow on
SPECT (103,104) are associated with the cognitive decline in AD (moderate evidence).

Although it is possible to monitor AD pathology once it is established,
irreversible damage characterized by neuron and synapse loss in the
anteromedial temporal lobe starts earlier (8–12). The effectiveness of
disease-modifying treatments is expected to be greatest on those patients
who are at the very early stages of pathologic involvement but have not
yet met the current clinical criteria for AD. For these treatment trials, the
most crucial stage for monitoring pathologic progression is the prodromal
phase, such as MCI (62). The rate of hippocampal volume loss measured
with serial MRI exams in patients with MCI and normal elderly individuals correlates with cognitive decline, as these individuals progress in the
cognitive continuum from normal to MCI and to AD (105) (moderate evidence). Similarly, the decrease in whole brain volumes (106) and cerebral
metabolism on PET (107) is associated with cognitive decline in patients
under the genetic risk of developing AD, although the outcome of these
risk groups is not known at this time (moderate evidence).

Clinical rating scales and neuropsychological tests are regarded as the
gold standard for assessing disease progression and therapeutic efficacy in
AD. However, imaging markers may be more accurate in measuring pathologic progression. Estimated sample sizes required to power an effective
therapeutic trial (25% to 50% reduction in rate of deterioration over 1 year)
in MCI indicate that the required sample sizes are substantially smaller for
MRI volumetry than commonly used cognitive tests or clinical rating scales
at the early stages of disease progression (108). These data support the use
of MRI along with clinical and psychometric measures as surrogate markers
of disease progression in AD therapeutic trials (Moderate evidence).

Take-Home Tables

Table 8.1. Sensitivity and specificity of neuroimaging techniques in distinguishing Alzheimer disease (AD) from normal elderly

Source	No. of controls	No. of AD patients	Neuroimaging modality	Sensitivity (%)	Specificity (%)
Jack et al. (42)	126	94	MRI (hippocampal volumes)	CDR 0.5 : 78 CDR 1 : 84 CDR 2 : 87	80
O'Brien et al. (38)	40	77	MRI (visual evaluation)	83	80
Laasko et al. (41)	42	55	MRI (hippocampal volumes)	82–90	86–98
Wahlund et al. (39)	66	41	MRI (visual evaluation + MMSE scores)	95	96
Xu et al. (36)	30	30	MRI (hippocampal volumes)	83	80
Herholtz et al. (55)	110	395	PET (automated analysis)	93	93
Silverman et al. (109)*	97	18	PET (visual evaluation)	94	73
Claus et al. (43)	60	48	SPECT (visual evaluation)	42–79**	90
Shonk et al. (56)	65	32	¹H MRS (myoinositol/N-acetylaspartate)	83	98
Kantarci et al. (110)	61	22	¹H MRS (N-acetylaspartate/myoinositol)	82	80

CDR, clinical dementia rating scale; MMSE, mini–mental status examination; MRI, magnetic resonance imaging; MRS, magnetic resonance spectroscopy; PET, positron emission tomography; SPECT, single photon emission computed tomography.
* The diagnoses were pathologically confirmed.
** Mild to severe AD.

Table 8.2. Suggested diagnostic evaluation for suspected dementia or mild cognitive impairment (MCI)

Detailed clinical evaluation
Structural imaging with CT or MRI
PET and SPECT if the diagnosis is still uncertain

Suggested Protocols

Computed Tomography Imaging

- *CT without contrast:* Axial 5- to 10-mm images should be used to assess for cerebral hemorrhage, mass effect, normal pressure hydrocephalus or calcifications.
- *CT with contrast:* Axial 5- to 10-mm enhanced images should be used in patients with suspected neoplasm, infection, or other focal intracranial lesion. If indicated, CT angiography can be performed as part of the enhanced CT.

Magnetic Resonance Imaging

- A scout image is acquired to ensure symmetric positioning of the brain within the field of view.
- Sagittal T1-weighted spin-echo sequence (TR/TE = 500/20) is used for standard diagnostic purposes and measuring intracranial volume where applicable.
- Coronal three-dimensional volumetric acquisition is used with 124 partitions and 1.6-mm slice thickness (TR/TE/flip angle = 23/6/25).
- Axial double spin echo (TR/TE = 2200/ 30 and 80) or axial fast FLAIR (fluid-attenuated inversion recovery) sequences (TR/TE/TI = 16000/ 140/2600) are used for standard diagnostic purposes and assessment of cerebrovascular disease.
- In patients with suspected neoplasm, infection, or focal intracranial lesions, gadolinium-enhanced T1-weighted conventional spin-echo (TR/TE = 500/20) images should be acquired in at least two planes.

Fluorodeoxyglucose–Positron Emission Tomography and Single Photon Emission Computed Tomography Imaging

- Standard brain fluorodeoxyglucose (FDG)-PET and SPECT protocols can be used.
- The intravenously injection of the radiopharmaceutical should take place in a controlled environment with minimal sensory input (dimly lit room with minimal ambient noise).
- The dose of radiopharmaceuticals [FDG for PET, technetium-99m (Tc-99m) ECD (bicisate) or Tc-99m HMPAO (exametazime) for SPECT] may differ between scanners.

Future Research Areas

- Validating the clinical criteria for AD by clinicians with different levels of expertise and at different clinical settings.

- Determining the choice of either CT or MRI for the initial evaluation of dementia in large-scale clinical trials.
- Validating the usefulness of PET, SPECT, and MR techniques for the diagnosis of AD with autopsy confirmation in large-scale clinical trials.
- Determining the cost-effectiveness of neuroimaging techniques as effective treatments become available for AD.
- Determining the usefulness of neuroimaging as a surrogate for therapeutic efficacy in trials with positive therapeutic outcomes.

References

1. Kokmen E, Beard CM, O'Brien PC, et al. Neurology 1993;43:1887–1892.
2. Beard CM, Kokmen E, O'Brien PC, et al. Neurology 1995;45:75–79.
3. Advisory Panel on Alzheimer Disease and Related Dementias: Acute and Long-Term Care Services. NIH publication 96–4136. Washington, DC: U.S. Department of Health and Human Services, 1996.
4. Brookmeyer R, Gray S, Kawas C. Am J Public Health 1998;88(9):1337–1342.
5. 2001–2002 Alzheimer Disease Progress Report. National Institutes of Health publication No. 03–5333, July 2003, p. 2.
6. Knapp MJ, Knopman DS, Solomon PR, et al. JAMA 1994;271(13):985–991.
7. Rogers SL, Farlow MR, Doody RS, et al. Neurology 1998;50(1):136–145.
8. Price JL, Morris JC. Ann Neurol 1999;45:358–368.
9. Schmitt FA, Davis DG, Wekstein DR, Smith CD, et al. Neurology 2000;55:370–376.
10. Grober E, Dickson D, Sliwinski MJ, et al. Neurobiol Aging 1999;20(6):573–579.
11. Delacourte A, David JP, Sergeant N, et al. Neurology 1999;52:1158–1165.
12. Morris JC, Storandt M, McKeel DW Jr, et al. Neurology 1996;46:707–719.
13. The National Institute on Aging, and Reagan Institute Working Group on Diagnostic Criteria for the Neuropathological Assessment of Alzheimer Disease. Neurobiol Aging 1997;18(4):S1–S2.
14. American Psychiatric Association. Diagnostic and Statistical Manual of Mental Disorders, 3rd ed., revised. DSM-IIIR. Washington, DC: APA, 1987.
15. Mc Khann GM, Drachman D, Folstein M, et al. Neurology 1984;34:939–944.
16. Lim A, Tsuang D, Kukull W, et al. J Am Geriatr Soc 1999;47(5):564–569.
17. Victoroff J, Mack WJ, Lyness SA, et al. Am J Psychiatry 1995;152(10):1476–1484.
18. Galasko D, Hansen LA, Katzman R. Arch Neurol 1994;51(9):888–895.
19. Massoud F, Devi G, Stern Y, et al. Arch Neurol 1999;56(11):1368–1373.
20. Blacker D, Albert MS, Bassett SS, et al. Arch Neurol 1994;51(12):1198–1204.
21. Kukull WA, Larson EB, Reifler BV, et al. Neurology 1990;40(9):1364–1369.
22. Massoud F, Devi G, Moroney JT. J Am Geriatr Soc 2000;48:1204–1210.
23. Jobst KA, Barnetson LP, Shepstone BJ. Int Psychogeriatr 1998;10(3):271–302.
24. Fratiglioni L, Grut M, Forsell Y, et al. Arch Neurol 1992;49(9):927–932.
25. Graham JE, Rockwood K, Beattie BL, et al. Neuroepidemiology 1996;15(5):246–256.
26. Blacker D, Albert MS, Bassett SS, et al. Arch Neurol 1994;51(12):1198–204 1994.
27. Baldereschi M, Amato MP, Nencini P, et al. Neurology 1994;44(2):239–242.
28. Knopman DS, DeKosky ST, Cummings JL, et al. Neurology 2001;56:1143–1153.
29. Jack CR Jr, Petersen RC, O'Brien PC, et al. Neurology 1992;42:183 188.
30. Braak H, Braak E. Acta Neuropathol (Berl) 1991;82:239–259.
31. Gomez-Isla T, Hollister R, West H, et al. Ann Neurol 1997;41:17–24.
32. Arriagata PV, Growdon JH, Hedley-Whyte ET, et al. Neurology 1992;42:631–639.
33. Bobinski M, de Leon MJ, Wegiel J, et al. Neuroscience 2000;95(3):721–725.
34. Chui H, Qian Z. Neurology 1997;49(4):925–935.
35. Nagy Z, Hindley NJ, Braak H. Dementia Geriatr Cogn Disord 1999;10(2):109–114.

36. Xu Y, Jack CR Jr, O'Brien PC, et al. Neurology 2000;54:1760–1767.
37. Jack CR Jr, Dickson DW, Parisi JE, et al. Neurology 2002;58:750–757.
38. O'Brien JT, Desmond P, Ames D, Schweitzer I, Chiu E, Tress B. Psychol Med 1997;27(6):1267–1275.
39. Wahlund LO, Julin P, Johansson SE, et al. J Neurol Neurosurg Psychiatry 2000; 69(5):630–635.
40. Juottonen K, Laasko MP, Insausti R, et al. Neurobiol Aging 1998;19(1):15–22.
41. Laasko MP, Soininen H, Partanen K, et al. Neurobiol Aging 1998;19(1):23–3.
42. Jack CR, Petersen RC, Xu Y, et al. Neurology 1997;49:786–794.
43. Claus JJ, van Harskamp F, Breteler MM. Neurology 1994;44(3 pt 1):454–461.
44. Van Gool WA, Walstra GJ, Teunisse S, et al. J Neurol 1995;242(2):401–405.
45. Bonte FJ, Weiner MF, Bigio EH, et al. Radiology 1997;202(3):793–797.
46. Mattman A, Feldman H, Forster B, et al. Can J Neurol Sci 1997;24(1):22–28.
47. Bradley KM, O'Sullivan VT, Soper ND, et al. Brain 2002;125(8):1772–1781.
48. Jagust W, Thisted R, Devous MD, et al. Neurology 2001;56:950–956.
49. Hoffman JM, Welsh-Bohmer KA, Hanson MW, et al. J Nucl Med 2000;41(11): 1920–1928.
50. Minoshima S, Foster NL, Sima AA, et al. Ann Neurol 2001;50(3):358–365.
51. McKeith IG, Ballard CG, Perry RH, et al. Neurology 2000;54:1050–1058.
52. Pickut BA, Saerens J, Marien P, et al. J Nucl Med 1997;38(6):929–934.
53. Hoffman JM, Hanson MW, Welsh KA, et al. Invest Radiol 1996;31(6):316–322.
54. Messa C, Perani D, Lucignani G, et al. J Nucl Med 1994;35(2):210–216.
55. Herholz K, Salmon E, Perani D, et al. Neuroimage 2002;17:302–316.
56. Shonk TK, Moats RA, Gifford PG, et al. Radiology 1995;195:65–72.
57. Ernst T, Chang L, Melchor R, et al. Radiology 1997;203:829–836.
58. Harris GJ, Lewis RF, Satlin A, et al. AJNR 1998;19(9):1727–1732.
59. Kantarci K, Jack CR, Xu YC, et al. Radiology 2001;219:101–107.
60. Hanyu H, Asano T, Iwamoto T, et al. AJNR 2000;21:1235–1242.
61. Petersen RC, Smith GE, Ivnik RJ, et al. Neurology 1994;44:867–872.
62. Petersen RC, Smith GE, Waring SC, et al. Arch Neurol 1999;56:303–308.
63. Kordower JH, Chu Y, Stebbins GT, et al. Ann Neurol 2001;49:202–213.
64. Du AT, Schuff N, Amend D, et al. J Neurol Neurosurg Psychiatry 2001;71(4): 431–432.
65. De Santi S, de Leon MJ, Rusinek H, et al. Neurobiol Aging 2001;22(4):529–539.
66. Dickerson BC, Goncharova I, Sullivan MP, et al. Neurobiol Aging 2001; 22(5):747–754.
67. Killany RJ, Gomez-Isla T, Moss M, et al. Ann Neurol 2000;47:430–439.
68. Kabani NJ, Sled JG, Shuper A, et al. Magn Reson Med 2002;47:143–148.
69. Jack CR, Petersen RC, Xu Y, et al. Neurology 1999;52:1397–1403.
70. Visser PJ, Scheltens P, Verhey FR, et al. J Neurol 1999;246(6):477–485.
71. de Leon MJ, Golomb J, George AE, et al. AJNR 1993;14:897–906.
72. de Leon MJ, Convit A, Wolf AT, et al. Proc Natl Acad Sci 2001;286:2120–2127.
73. Chetelat G, Desgranges B, de la Sayette V, Viader F, Eustache F, Baron JC. Neurology 2003;60:1374–1377.
74. Drzezga A, Lautenschlager N, Siebner H, et al. Eur J Nucl Med Mol Imaging 2003;30(8):1104–1113.
75. Huang C, Wahlund LO, Svensson L, Winblad B, Julin P. BMC Neurology 2002; 2(1):9.
76. Tanaka M, Fukuyama H, Yamauchi H, et al. J Neuroimaging 2002;12(2): 112–118.
77. Johnson KA, Jones K, Holman BL, et al. Neurology 1998;50:1563–1571.
78. Kantarci K, Jack CR, Xu YC, et al. Neurology 2000;55(2):210–217.
79. Catani M, Cherubini A, Howard R. Neuroreport 2001;12(11):2315–2317.
80. Huang W, Alexander GE, Chang L, et al. Neurology 2001;57:626–632.
81. Tsai MS, Tangalos E, Petersen R, et al. Am J Human Genet 1994;54:643–649.
82. Gomez-Isla T, West HL, Rebeck GW, et al. Ann Neurol 1996;39:62–70.
83. Jack CR, Petersen RC, Xu Y, et al. Ann Neurol 1998;43:303–310.

84. Barber R, Gholkar A, Scheltens P, et al. Arch Neurol 1999;56(8):961–965.
85. Geroldi C, Pihlajamaki M, Laasko MP, et al. Neurology 1999;53:1825–1832.
86. Lehtovirta M, Soininen H, Laasko MP, et al. J Neurol Neurosurg Psychiatry 1996;60:644–649.
87. Small GW, Mazziotta JC, Collins MT, et al. JAMA 1995;273:942–947.
88. Reiman EM, Caselli RJ, Yun LS, et al. N Engl J Med 1996;334:752–758.
89. Small GW, Ercoli LM, Silverman DH, et al. Proc Natl Acad Sci 2000; 97(11):6037–6042.
90. Silverman DH, Gambhir SS, Huang HW. J Nucl Med 2002;43(2):253–266.
91. McMahon PM, Araki SS, Neumann PJ, et al. Radiology 2000;217:58–68.
92. McMahon PM, Araki SS, Sandberg EA, Neumann PJ, Gazelle GS. Radiology 2003;228:515–522.
93. Kulasingam SL, Samsa GP, Zarin DA, et al. Value Health 2003;6(5):542–550.
94. Freeborough PA, Fox NC. IEEE Trans Med Imaging 1997;15:623–629.
95. Fox NC, Cousens S, Scahill R, et al. Arch Neurol 2000;57(3):339–344.
96. Fox NC, Warrington EK, Rossor MN. Lancet 1999;353:2125.
97. Jack CR, Petersen RC, Xu Y, et al. Neurology 1998;51:993–999.
98. Laasko MP, Lehtovirta M, Partanen K, et al. Biol Psychiatry 2000;47(6):557–561.
99. Bradley KM, Bydder GM, Budge MM, et al. Br J Radiol 2002;75(894):506–513.
100. Adalsteinsson E, Sullivan EV, Kleinhans N, et al. Lancet 2000;355:1696–1697.
101. Jessen F, Block W, Träber F, et al. Neurology 2001;57(5):930–932.
102. Smith GS, de Leon MJ, George AE, et al. Arch Neurol 1992;49:1142–1150.
103. Brown DR, Hunter R, Wyper DJ, et al. J Psychiatr Res 1996;30(2):109–126.
104. Shih WJ, Ashford WJ, Coupal JJ, et al. Clin Nucl Med 1999;24(10):773–777.
105. Jack CR, Petersen RC, Xu Y, et al. Neurology 2000;55:484–489.
106. Fox NC, Crum WF, Scahill RI, et al. Lancet 2001;358:201–205.
107. Reiman EM, Caselli RJ, Chen K, et al. Proc Natl Acad Sci 2001;98:3334–3339.
108. Jack CR, Shiung MM, Gunter JL, et al. Neurology 2004;62:591–600.
109. Silverman DHS, Small GW, Chang CY, et al. JAMA 2001;286(17):2120–2127.
110. Kantarci K, Xu YC, Shiung MM, et al. Dementia Geriatr Cogn Disord 2002;14(4):198–207.

9

Neuroimaging in Acute Ischemic Stroke

Katie D. Vo, Weili Lin, and Jin-Moo Lee

Key Points

- Noncontrast computed tomography (CT) is currently accepted as the gold standard for the detection of intracranial hemorrhage, though rigorous data is lacking (limited evidence). Magnetic resonance imaging (MRI) is equivalent to CT in the detection of intracranial hemorrhage (strong evidence), but its role in the evaluation of thrombolytic candidates has not been studied.
- Noncontrast CT of the head should be performed in all patients who are candidates for thrombolytic therapy to exclude intracerebral hemorrhage (strong evidence).
- Magnetic resonance (MR) (diffusion-weighted imaging) is superior to CT for detection of cerebral ischemia within the first 24 hours of symptom onset (moderate evidence); however, some argue that iden-

tification of ischemia merely confirms a clinical diagnosis and does not necessarily influence acute clinical decision making, or outcome.

- Advanced functional imaging such as MR perfusion, MR spectroscopy, CT perfusion, xenon CT, single photon emission computed tomography (SPECT), and positron emission tomography (PET) show promise in improving patient selection and individualizing therapeutic time windows (limited evidence), but the data are inadequate for routine use in the current management of stroke patients.

Definition and Pathophysiology

This chapter focuses on imaging within the first few hours of stroke onset, where issues relating to the decision to administer thrombolytics are of paramount importance. *Stroke* is a clinical term that describes an acute neurologic deficit due to a sudden disruption of blood supply to the brain. Stroke is caused by either an occlusion of an artery (ischemic stroke or cerebral ischemia/infarction) or rupture of an artery leading to bleeding into or around the brain (hemorrhagic stroke or intracranial hemorrhage). The vast majority of strokes are ischemic (88%), whereas 9% are intracerebral hemorrhages and 3% are subarachnoid hemorrhages (1). Ischemic stroke can be divided into several subtypes based on etiology: small-vessel strokes (40%), large-vessel atherothrombotic strokes (20%), cardioembolic strokes (20%), and strokes from unknown etiologies (20%) (2). Risk factors for stroke include age, male gender, race (African American), previous history of stroke, diabetes, hypertension, heart disease, smoking, and alcohol. Treatment of ischemic stroke can be divided into acute therapies, consisting of thrombolysis with tissue plasminogen activator (tPA) and management of secondary complications (edema, herniation, hemorrhage); and preventative therapies, aimed at reducing the risk of recurrent stroke.

Epidemiology

It is estimated that approximately 731,000 new or recurrent strokes occur annually, and that a new stroke occurs every 45 seconds in United States (1,3). This number is expected to increase as the population ages. The third leading cause of mortality after heart disease and cancer, stroke results in approximately 160,000 deaths per year, leaving 4.6 million stroke survivors in the United States. Fifteen to 30% of stroke survivors are permanently disabled or require institutional care, making it the leading cause of severe long-term disability and the leading diagnosis from hospital to long-term care (1,4,5).

Overall Cost to Society

The estimated direct and indirect costs of stroke are $53.6 billion in 2004, with 62% of the cost related directly to medical expenditures (1). Acute inpatient hospital costs account for 70% of the first-year post-stroke cost;

the contribution of diagnostic tests during the initial hospitalization accounts for 19% of total hospital costs (6). These diagnostic tests included MR or CT (91% of patients), echocardiogram (81%), noninvasive carotid artery evaluation (48%), angiography (20%), and electroencephalography (6%).

Goals

The primary goal of neuroimaging in patients presenting with acute neurologic deficits is to differentiate between ischemic and hemorrhagic stroke, and to exclude other diagnoses that may mimic stroke. Other emerging goals in acute stroke patients are to determine if brain tissue is viable and thereby amenable to interventional therapies, and to determine the localization of vascular occlusion.

Methodology

A comprehensive Medline search (United States National Library of Medicine database) for original articles published between 1966 and July 2004 using the Ovid and Pubmed search engines was performed using a combination of the following key terms: *ischemic stroke, hemorrhage, diagnostic imaging, CT, MR, PET, SPECT, angiography, gadolinium, circle of Willis, carotid artery, brain, technology assessment, evidence-based medicine,* and *cost.* The search was limited to English-language articles and human studies. The abstracts were reviewed and selected based on well-designed methodology, clinical trials, outcomes, and diagnostic accuracy. Additional relevant articles were selected from the references of reviewed articles and published guidelines.

I. What Is the Imaging Modality of Choice for the Detection of Intracranial Hemorrhage?

Summary of Evidence: Computed tomography (CT) is widely accepted as the gold standard for imaging intracerebral hemorrhage; however, it has not been rigorously examined in prospective studies, and thus the precise sensitivity and specificity is unknown (limited evidence). For the evaluation of thrombolytic candidates (exclusion of intracerebral hemorrhage), however, CT is clearly the modality of choice based on strong evidence (level I) from randomized controlled trials (7,8). By many measures MR is at least as sensitive as CT in the detection of intracerebral hemorrhage, and it is suspected to be more sensitive during the subacute and chronic phases. A recent study indicates that the sensitivity and accuracy of MR in detecting intraparenchymal hemorrhage is equivalent to CT even in the hyperacute setting (within 6 hours of ictus) (strong evidence) (9).

Supporting Evidence

A. Computed Tomography

It is essential that an imaging study reliably distinguish intracerebral hemorrhage from ischemic stroke because of the divergent management of these two conditions. This is especially critical for patients who present within 3 hours of symptom onset under consideration for thrombolytic therapy. Noncontrast CT is currently the modality of choice for detection of acute intracerebral hemorrhage. Acute hemorrhage appears hyperdense for several days due to the high protein concentration of hemoglobin and retraction of clot, but becomes progressively isodense and then hypodense over a period of weeks to months from breakdown and clearing of the hematoma by macrophages. Rarely acute hemorrhage can be isodense in severely anemic patients with a hematocrit of less than 20% or $10\,g/dL$ (10,11). Although it has been well accepted that CT can identify intra-parenchymal hemorrhage with very high sensitivity, surprisingly few studies have been conducted to support this (12,13). In 1974, shortly after the introduction of the EMI scanner, Paxton and Ambrose (14) diagnosed 66 patients with intracerebral hemorrhages with this novel modality; the study was observational, lacking autopsy confirmation, and thus accuracy was not determined (insufficient evidence). Subsequently, in an autopsy series of 79 patients, EMI did not detect four out of 17 patients with hem-orrhages—all were brainstem hemorrhages (limited evidence) (15). There is little doubt that the sensitivity of current third-generation CT scanners for the detection of intracerebral hemorrhage is far superior to the first-generation scanners; however, it is of interest that the precise sensitivity and specificity of this well-accepted modality is unknown, and the level of evidence supporting its use is limited (level III).

Four studies evaluating third-generation CT scanners in patients with nontraumatic subarachnoid hemorrhage identified by CT or cerebrospinal fluid (CSF) have been reported (16–19). The overall sensitivity of CT was 91% to 92%, but was dependent on the time interval between symptom onset and scan time. Sensitivity was 100% (80/80) for patients imaged within 12 hours, 93% (134/144) within 24 hours, and 84% (31/37) after 24 hours (level III) (18,19). These numbers were confirmed by two other studies that demonstrated a sensitivity of 98% (117/119) for scans obtained within 12 hours, 95% (1313/1378) within 24 hours, 91% (1247/1378) between 24 and 48 hours, and 74% after 48 hours (1017/1378) (moderate evidence) (16,17). These studies relied on a diagnosis made by CT, or by blood detected in CSF in the absence of CT findings. No studies with autopsy confirmation have been reported.

Therefore, although CT is commonly regarded as the modality of choice for imaging intracranial hemorrhage, the precise sensitivity and specificity is unknown and is dependent on time after onset, concentration of hemo-globin, and size and location of the hemorrhage (limited evidence).

B. Magnetic Resonance Imaging

Like CT, the appearance and detectability of hemorrhage on magnetic res-onance imaging (MRI) depends on the age of blood and the location of the hemorrhage (intraparenchymal or subarachnoid). In addition, the strength of the magnetic field, and type of MR sequence influences its sensitivity (20). As the hematoma ages, oxyhemoglobin in blood breaks down sequen-tially into several paramagnetic products: first deoxyhemoglobin, then methemoglobin, and finally hemosiderin. Iron in hemoglobin is shielded from surrounding water molecules when oxygen is bound, resulting in a molecule (oxyhemoglobin) with diamagnetic properties. As a result, the MR signal is similar to that of normal brain parenchyma, making it diffi-cult to detect on any MR sequence, including susceptibility weighted sequences (echo-planar imaging [EPI] T2* or gradient echo). In contrast, iron exposed to surrounding water molecules in the form of deoxyhemoglobin creates signal loss, making it easy to identify on susceptibility-weighted and T2-weighted (T2W) sequences (21,22). Thus the earliest detection of hemorrhage depends on the conversion of oxyhemoglobin to deoxyhemoglobin, which was believed to occur after the first 12 to 24 hours (20,23). However, this early assumption has been questioned with reports of intraparenchymal hemorrhage detected by MRI within 6 hours, and as early as 23 minutes from symptom onset (24–26). One of the studies prospectively demonstrated that MRI detected all nine patients with CT-confirmed intracerebral hemorrhage (ICH), suggesting the potential of MRI for the hyperacute evaluation of stroke (limited evidence) (24–26). More recently, a blinded study comparing MRI (diffusion-, T2-, and T2*-weighted images) to CT for the evaluation of ICH within 6 hours of onset demonstrated that ICH was diagnosed with 100% sensitivity and 100% accuracy by expert readers using MRI; CT-detected ICH was used as the gold standard (strong evidence) (9).

Data regarding the detection of acute subarachnoid and intraventricular hemorrhage using MRI is limited. While it is possible that the conversion of blood to deoxyhemoglobin occurs much earlier than expected in hypoxic tissue, this transition may not occur until much later in the oxygen-rich environment of the CSF (20,27). Thus the susceptibility-weighted sequence may not be sensitive enough to detect subarachnoid blood in the hyperacute stage. This problem is further compounded by severe susceptibility artifacts at the skull base, limiting detection in this area. The use of the fluid-attenuated inversion recovery (FLAIR) sequence has been advocated to overcome this problem. Increased protein content in bloody CSF appears hyperintense on FLAIR and can be readily detected. Three case-control series using FLAIR in patients with CT-documented subarachnoid or intraventricular hemorrhage demonstrated a sensitivity of 92% to 100% and specificity of 100% compared to CT and was superior to CT during the subacute to chronic stages (limited evidence) (28–30). Hyperintense signal in the CSF on FLAIR can be seen in areas associated with prominent CSF pulsation artifacts (i.e., third and fourth ventricles and basal cisterns) and in other conditions that elevate protein in the CSF such as meningitis or after gadolinium administration (level III) (31–33); however, these conditions are not usually confused with clinical presentations suggestive of subarachnoid hemorrhage.

At later time points in hematoma evolution (subacute to chronic phase) when the clot demonstrates nonspecific isodense to hypodense appearance on CT, MRI has been shown to have a higher sensitivity and specificity than CT (limited evidence) (28,34,35). The heightened sensitivity of MRI susceptibility-weighted sequences to microbleeds that are not otherwise detected on CT makes interpretation of hyperacute scans difficult, especially when faced with decisions regarding thrombolysis (Fig. 9.1). Patient outcome regarding the use of thrombolytic treatment in this subgroup of patients with microbleeds is not known; however, in one series of 41 patients who had MRI prior to intraarterial tPA, one of five patients with microbleeds on MRI developed major symptomatic hemorrhage compared to three of 36 without (36), raising the possibility that the presence of microbleeds may predict the subsequent development of symptomatic hemorrhage following tPA treatment. As this finding was not statistically significant, a larger study is required for confirmation.

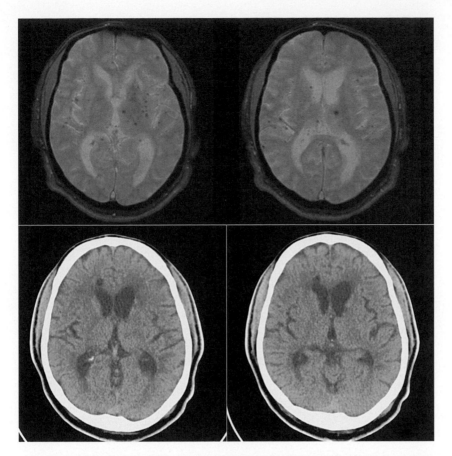

Figure 9.1. Microhemorrhages. Top row: Two sequential magnetic resonance (MR) images of T2* sequence show innumerable small low signal lesions scattered throughout both cerebral hemispheres compatible with microhemorrhages. Bottom row: Noncontrast axial computed tomography (CT) at the same anatomic levels does not show the microhemorrhages.

II. What Are the Imaging Modalities of Choice for the Identification of Brain Ischemia and the Exclusion of Stroke Mimics?

Summary of Evidence: Based on moderate evidence (level II), MRI (diffusion-weighted imaging) is superior to CT for positive identification of ischemic stroke within the first 24 hours of symptom onset, allowing exclusion of stroke mimics. However, some argue that despite its superiority, positive identification merely confirms a clinical diagnosis and does not necessarily influence acute clinical decision making or outcome.

Supporting Evidence

A. Computed Tomography

Computed tomography images are frequently normal during the acute phase of ischemia and therefore the diagnosis of ischemic stroke is contingent upon the exclusion of stroke mimics, which include postictal state, systemic infection, brain tumor, toxic-metabolic conditions, positional vertigo, cardiac disease, syncope, trauma, subdural hematoma, herpes encephalitis, dementia, demyelinating disease, cervical spine fracture, conversion disorder, hypertensive encephalopathy, myasthenia gravis, and Parkinson disease (37). Based purely on history and physical examination alone without confirmation by CT, stroke mimics can account for 13% to 19% of cases initially diagnosed with stroke (37,38). Sensitivity of diagnosis improves when noncontrast CT is used but still 5% of cases are misdiagnosed as stroke, with ultimate diagnoses including paresthesias or numbness of unknown cause, seizure, complicated migraine, peripheral neuropathy, cranial neuropathy, psychogenic paralysis, and others (39).

An alternative approach to excluding stroke mimics, which may account for the presenting neurologic deficit, is to directly visualize ischemic changes in the hyperacute scan. Increased scrutiny of hyperacute CT scans, especially following the early thrombolytic trials, suggests that some patients with large areas of ischemia may demonstrate subtle early signs of infarction, even if imaged within 3 hours after symptom onset. These early CT signs include parenchymal hypodensity, loss of the insular ribbon (40), obscuration of the lentiform nucleus (41), loss of gray–white matter differentiation, blurring of the margins of the basal ganglia, subtle effacement of the cortical sulci, and local mass effect (Fig. 9.2). It was previously believed that these signs of infarction were not present on CT until 24 hours after stroke onset; however, early changes were found in 31% of CTs performed within 3 hours of ischemic stroke (moderate evidence) (42). In addi-

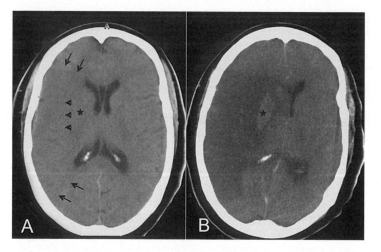

Figure 9.2. Early CT signs of infarction. A: Noncontrast axial CT performed at 2 hours after stroke onset shows a large low-attenuated area involving the entire right middle cerebral artery distribution (bounded by arrows) with associated effacement of the sulci and sylvian fissure. There is obscuration the right lentiform nucleus (*) and loss of the insular ribbon (arrowhead). B: Follow-up noncontrast axial image 4 days later confirms the infarction in the same vascular distribution. There is hemorrhagic conversion (*) in the basal ganglia with mass effect and subfalcine herniation.

tion, early CT signs were found in 81% of patients with CTs performed within 5 hours of middle cerebral artery (MCA) stroke onset (demonstrated angiographically) (moderate evidence) (43). Early CT signs, however, can be very subtle and difficult to detect even among very experienced readers (moderate evidence) (44–46). Moreover, the presence of these early ischemic changes in only 31% of hyperacute strokes precludes its reliability as a positive sign of ischemia.

Early CT signs of infarction, especially involving more than 33% of the MCA distribution, have been reported to be associated with severe stroke, increased risk of hemorrhagic transformation (46–49), and poor outcome (50). Because of these associations, several trials involving thrombolytic therapy including the European Cooperative Acute Stroke Study (ECASS) excluded patients with early CT signs in an attempt to avoid treatment of patients at risk for hemorrhagic transformation (8,46,51,52). Although ECASS failed to demonstrate efficacy of intravenous tPA administered within 6 hours of stroke onset, a marginal treatment benefit was observed in the target population (post-hoc analysis), excluding patients with early CT signs that were inappropriately enrolled in the trial (46). The National Institute of Neurological Disorders and Stroke (NINDS) t-PA stroke trial (7), which did demonstrate efficacy, did not exclude patients with early CT signs, and retrospective analysis of the data showed that early CT signs were associated with stroke severity but not with increased risk of adverse outcome after t-PA treatment (42). Thus, based on current data, early CT signs should not be used to exclude patients who are otherwise eligible for thrombolytic treatment within 3 hours of stroke onset (strong and moderate evidence) (7,42).

B. Magnetic Resonance Imaging

Unlike CT and conventional MR, new functional MR techniques such as diffusion-weighted imaging (DWI) allow detection of the earliest physiologic changes of cerebral ischemia. Diffusion-weighted imaging, a sequence sensitive to the random brownian motion of water, is capable of demonstrating changes within minutes of ischemia in rodent stroke models (53–55). Moreover, the sequence is sensitive, detecting lesions as small as 4mm in diameter (56). Although the in vivo mechanism of signal alteration observed in DWI after acute ischemia is unclear, it is believed that ischemia-induced energy depletion increases the influx of water from the extracellular to the intracellular space, thereby restricting water motion, resulting in a bright signal on DW images (57,58). Diffusion-weighted imaging has become widely employed for clinical applications due to improvements in gradient capability, and it is now possible to acquire DW images free from artifacts with an echo planar approach. Because DW images are affected by T1 and T2 contrast, stroke lesions becomes progressively brighter due to concurrent increases in brain water content, leading to the added contribution of hyperintense T2W signal known as "T2 shine-through." To differentiate between true restricted diffusion and T2 shine-through, bright lesions on DWI should always be confirmed with apparent diffusion coefficient (ADC) maps, which exclusively measure diffusion. For stroke lesions in adults, although there is wide individual variability, ADC signal remains decreased for 4 days, pseudo-normalizes at 5 to 10 days, and increases thereafter (56). This temporal evolution of DWI signal allows one to determine the age of a stroke.

The high sensitivity and specificity of DWI for the detection of ischemia make it an ideal sequence for positive identification of hyperacute stroke, thereby excluding stroke mimics. Two studies evaluating DWI for the detection of ischemia within 6 hours of stroke onset reported an 88% to 100% sensitivity and 95% to 100% specificity with a positive predictive value (PPV) of 98.5% and negative predictive value (NPV) of 69.5%, using final clinical diagnosis as the gold standard (moderate and limited evidence) (59,60). In another study, 50 patients were randomized to DWI or CT within 6 hours of stroke onset, and subsequently received the other imaging modality with a mean delay of 30 minutes. Sensitivity and specificity of infarct detection among blinded expert readers was significantly better when based on DWI (91% and 95%, respectively) compared to CT (61% and 65%) (moderate evidence) (61). The presence of restricted diffusion is highly correlated with ischemia, but its absence does not rule out ischemia: false negatives have been reported in transient ischemic attacks and small subcortical infarctions (moderate evidence) (60,62–64). False-positive DWI signals have been reported in brain abscesses (65), herpes encephalitis (66,67), Creutzfeldt-Jacob disease (68), highly cellular tumors such as lymphoma or meningioma (69), epidermoid cysts (70), seizures (71), and hypoglycemia (72) (limited evidence). However, the clinical history and the appearance of these lesions on conventional MR should allow for exclusion of these stroke mimics. Within the first 8 hours of onset, the stroke lesion should be seen only on DWI, and its presence on conventional MR sequences suggests an older stroke or a nonstroke lesion. The DWI images, therefore, should not be interpreted alone but in conjunction with conventional MR sequences and within the proper clinical context.

Acute DWI lesion volume has been correlated with long-term clinical outcome, using various assessment scales including the National Institutes of Health Stroke Scale (NIHSS), the Canadian Neurologic Scale, the Barthel Index, and the Rankin Scale (moderate evidence) (73–77). This correlation was stronger for strokes involving the cortex and weaker for subcortical strokes (73,74), which is likely explained by a discordance between infarct size and severity of neurologic deficit for small subcortical strokes.

In addition to DWI, MR perfusion-weighted imaging (PWI) approaches have been employed to depict brain regions of hypoperfusion. They involve the repeated and rapid acquisition of images prior to and following the injection of contrast agent using a two-dimensional (2D) gradient echo or spin echo EPI sequence (78,79). Signal changes induced by the first passage of contrast in the brain can be used to obtain estimates of a variety of hemodynamic parameters, including cerebral blood flow (CBF), cerebral blood volume (CBV), and mean transit time (MTT, the mean time for the bolus of contrast agent to pass through each pixel) (79–81). These parameters are often reported as relative values since accurate measurement of the input function cannot be determined. However, absolute quantification of CBF has also been reported (82). Thus, hypoperfused brain tissue resulting from ischemia demonstrates signal changes in perfusion-weighted images, and may provide information regarding regional hemodynamic status during acute ischemia (insufficient evidence).

III. What Imaging Modality Should Be Used for the Determination of Tissue Viability—the Ischemic Penumbra?

Summary of Evidence: Determination of tissue viability using functional imaging has tremendous potential to individualize therapy and extend the therapeutic time window for some. Several imaging modalities, including MRI, CT, PET, and SPECT, have been examined in this role. Operational hurdles may limit the use of some of these modalities in the acute setting of stroke (e.g., PET and SPECT), while others such as MRI show promise (limited evidence). Rigorous testing in large randomized controlled trials that can clearly demonstrate that reestablishment of perfusion to regions "at risk" prevents progression to infarction is needed prior to their use in routine clinical decision making.

Supporting Evidence

A. Magnetic Resonance Imaging

The combination of DWI and PWI techniques holds promise in identifying brain tissue at risk for infarction. It has been postulated that brain tissue dies over a period of minutes to hours following arterial occlusion. Initially, a core of tissue dies within minutes, but there is surrounding brain tissue that is dysfunctional but viable, comprising the ischemic penumbra. If blood flow is not restored in a timely manner, the brain tissue at risk dies, completing the infarct (83). The temporal profile of signal changes seen on DWI and PWI follows a pattern that is strikingly similar to the theoretical construct of the penumbra described above. On MR images obtained within hours of stroke onset, the DWI lesion is often smaller than the area of perfusion defect (on PWI), and smaller than the final infarct (defined by T2W images obtained weeks later). If the arterial occlusion persists, the DWI lesion grows until it eventually matches the initial perfusion defect, which is often similar in size and location to the final infarct (chronic T2W lesion) (Fig. 9.3) (limited evidence) (84,85). The area of normal DWI signal but abnormal PWI signal is known as the diffusion-perfusion mismatch and has been postulated to represent the ischemic penumbra. Diffusion-perfusion mismatch has been reported to be present in 49% of stroke patients during the hyperacute period (0 to 6 hours) (limited evidence) (86). Growth of the DWI lesion over time has been documented in a randomized trial testing the efficacy of the neuroprotective agent citicoline. Mean lesion volume in the placebo group increased by 180% from the initial DWI scan (obtained within 24 hours of stroke onset) to the final T2W scan obtained 12 weeks later. Interestingly, lesion volume grew by only 34% in the citicoline-treated group, suggesting a treatment effect (moderate evidence) (87). However, efficacy of the agent was not definitively demonstrated using clinical outcome measures (88). The ultimate test of the hypothesis that mismatch represents "penumbra," will come from studies that correlate initial mismatch with salvaged tissue after effective treatment. One small prospective series of 10 patients demonstrated that patients with successful recanalization after intraarterial thrombolysis showed larger areas of mismatch that were salvaged compared to patients that were not successfully recanalized (limited evidence) (89).

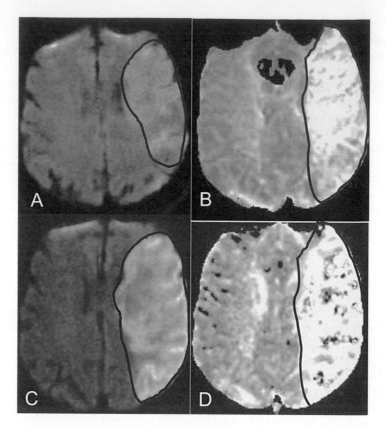

Figure 9.3. Evolution of the right middle cerebral distribution infarction on magnetic resonance imaging (MRI). A,B: MRI at 3 hours after stroke onset shows an area of restricted diffusion on diffusion-weighted imaging (DWI) (A) with a larger area of perfusion defect on perfusion-weighted imaging (PWI) (B). The area of normal DWI but abnormal PWI represents an area of diffusion-perfusion mismatch. C,D: Follow-up MRI at 3 days postictus shows interval enlargement of the DWI lesion (C) to the same size as the initial perfusion deficit (B). There is now a matched diffusion-perfusion (C,D).

The promise of diffusion-perfusion mismatch is that it will provide an image of ischemic brain tissue that is salvageable, and thereby individualize therapeutic time windows for acute treatments. The growth of the lesion to the final infarct volume may not occur until hours or even days later in some individuals (limited evidence) (84,85), suggesting that tissue may be salvaged beyond the 3-hour window in some. One of the assumptions underlying the hypothesis that diffusion-perfusion mismatch represents salvageable tissue is that the acute DWI lesion represents irreversibly injured tissue. However, it has been known for some time that DWI lesions are reversible after transient ischemia in animal stroke models (90,91), and reversible lesions in humans have been reported following a transient ischemic attack (TIA) (92) or after reperfusion (93). These data suggest that at least some brain tissue within the DWI lesion may represent reversibly injured tissue.

Additional new experimental MR techniques such as proton MR spectroscopy (MRS) and T2 Blood Oxygen Level Dependent (BOLD) and 2D multiecho gradient echo/spin echo have also been explored for the identification of salvageable tissue (94,95). Magnetic resonance spectroscopy is an MR technique that measures the metabolic and biochemical changes within the brain tissues. The two metabolites that are commonly measured following ischemia are lactate and N-acetylaspartate (NAA). Lactate signal is not detected in normal brain but is elevated within minutes of ischemia in animal models, remaining elevated for days to weeks (96). The lactate signal can normalize with immediate reperfusion (97). N-acetylaspartate, found exclusively in neurons, decreases more gradually over a period of hours after stroke onset in animal stroke models (98). It has been suggested that an elevation in lactate with a normal or mild reduction in NAA during the acute period of ischemia may represent the ischemic penumbra (94), though this has not been examined in a large population of stroke patients. The cerebral metabolic rate of oxygen consumption ($CMRO_2$) has been measured in acute stroke patients using MRI, and a threshold value has been proposed to define irreversibly injured brain tissue (level III) (82). Though preliminary, these results appear to be in agreement with data obtained using PET (see below) (99,100). Measurement of $CMRO_2$ has theoretical advantages over other measures (e.g., CBF, CBV), as the threshold value for irreversible injury is not likely to be time-dependent (101). Clearly research into the identification of viable ischemic brain tissue is at a preliminary stage. However, such techniques may be important for future acute stroke management. These new imaging approaches will require extensive validation and assessment in well-designed clinical trials.

B. Computed Tomography

In addition to anatomic information, CT is capable of providing some physiologic information, accomplished with either intravenous injection of nonionic contrast or inhalation of xenon gas. Like PWI, perfusion parameters can be obtained by tracking a bolus of contrast or inhaled xenon gas in blood vessels and brain parenchyma with sequential CT imaging. Using spiral CT technology, the study can be completed in 6 minutes.

Stable xenon (Xe) has been employed as a means to obtain quantitative estimates of CBF in vivo. Xenon, an inert gas with an atomic number similar to iodine, can attenuate x-rays like contrast material. However, unlike CT contrast, the gas is freely diffusable and can cross the blood–brain barrier. Sequential imaging permits the tracking of progressive accumulation and washout of the gas in brain tissue, reflected by changes in Hounsfield units over time, and quantitative CBF and CBV maps can be calculated (102). The quantitative CBF value from xenon-enhanced CT has been shown to be highly accurate compared with radioactive microsphere and iodoantipyrine techniques under different physiologic conditions and wide range of CBF rates in baboons (correlation coefficient $r = 0.67$ to 0.92, $p < .01$ and $<.001$) (103,104). The major advantage of the xenon CT is that it allows absolute quantification of the CBF, which may help to define a threshold value from reversible to irreversible cerebral injury. Low CBF (<15 mL/100 g/min) correlated with early CT signs of infarction, proximal M1 occlusion, severe edema, and life-threatening herniation. Very low CBF values (<7 mL/100 g/min) predicted irreversibly injured tissue (105,106). In addition, xenon CT has been shown to be effective in obtaining cerebral vascular reserve (CVR) in patients with occlusive disease (107). Poor CVR has been shown to be a risk factor for stroke in patients with high-grade carotid stenosis or occlusion (108). However, to ensure a sufficient signal-to-noise ratio for Xe-CT perfusion, a high concentration of Xe is needed, which itself may cause respiratory depression, cerebral vasodilation, and thus confound the measurements of CBF (109).

In addition to inhalation xenon gas, bolus nonionic contrast can also be used to generate a CT perfusion map. Rapid repeated serial images of the brain are acquired during the first-pass passage of intravenous contrast to generate relative CBF, CBV, and MTT. The CT perfusion maps obtained within 6 hours of stroke onset in patients with MCA occlusion had significantly higher sensitivity for the detection of stroke lesion volume compared to noncontrast CT, and the perfusion volume correlated with clinical outcome (limited evidence) (105,110). Cerebral blood flow maps generated by CT perfusion in 70 acute stroke patients predicted the extent of cerebral infarction with a sensitivity of 93% and a specificity of 98% (limited evidence) (111). A major limitation to this technique is that only relative CBF map can be obtained, thus precluding exact determination of the transition from ischemia to infarction.

C. Positron Emission Tomography (PET)

Positron emission tomography imaging has provided fundamental information on the pathophysiology of human cerebral ischemia. Quantitative measurements of cerebral perfusion and metabolic parameters can be obtained, namely CBF, CBV, MTT, oxygen extraction fraction (OEF), and $CMRO_2$, using multiple tracers and serial arterial blood samplings. Based on the values of these hemodynamic parameters, four distinct successive pathophysiologic phases of ischemic stroke have been identified: autoregulation, oligemia, ischemia, and irreversible injury (112). Oligemia (low CBF, elevated OEF with normal $CMRO_2$) and ischemia (low CBF, elevated OEF but decreased $CMRO_2$) are sometimes termed misery perfusion, and have been postulated to represent the ischemic penumbra (113). During misery perfusion, a decline in $CMRO_2$ heralds the beginning of a transition from reversible to irreversible injury. Irreversible injury is reflected in tissue with $CMRO_2$ below 1.4 mL/100 g/min (99,100). In three serial observational studies of acute ischemic stroke, elevation of OEF in the setting of low CBF has been suggested to be the marker of tissue viability in ischemic tissue (level II) (114–116). The CBF in ischemic tissue with elevated OEF is between 7 and 17 mL/100 g/min. Elevated OEF has been observed to persist up to 48 hours after stroke onset (115). Progression to irreversible injury is reflected in decreased OEF (114,115). Furthermore, in a prospective blinded longitudinal cohort study of 81 patients with carotid occlusion, elevated OEF was found to be an independent predictor for subsequent stroke and potentially defining a subgroup of patients who may benefit from revascularization (moderate evidence) (117). However, confirmation of tissue viability in the region of elevated OEF is best accomplished by large randomized controlled trials that can clearly demonstrate that reestablishment of perfusion to this region prevents progression to infarction. Such studies have not been done and are difficult to implement since PET is limited to major medical centers and requires considerable expertise and time. Moreover, the requirement for intraarterial line placement precludes its use for evaluating thrombolytic candidates. Despite these hurdles one study assessed PET after thrombolysis in 12 ischemic stroke patients within 3 hours of symptoms onset (118). Due to the above-mentioned hurdles, only relative CBF was obtained prior to and following intravenous thrombolysis (118). In all patients, early reperfusion of severely ischemic tissue ($<12\,mL/110\,g/min$ in gray matter) predicted better clinical outcome and limited infarction.

D. Single Photon Emission Computed Tomography (SPECT)

The most commonly used radiopharmaceutical agent for SPECT perfusion study is technetium-99m pertechnetate hexamethyl-propylene amine oxime (99m Tc-HMPAO). This lipophilic substance readily crosses the blood–brain barrier and interacts with intracellular glutathione, which prevents it from diffusing back. However, due to technical problems including incomplete first-pass extraction from blood, incomplete binding to glutathione leading to back diffusion, and metabolism within the brain, absolute quantification of the CBF cannot be determined. However, SPECT technology is much more accessible than PET and is more readily available. In a multicenter prospective trial with 99mTc-bicisate (99mTc-ECD, an agent with better brain-to-background contrast) of 128 patients with ischemic stroke and 42 controls, SPECT had a sensitivity of 86% and specificity of 98% for localization of stroke compared with final clinical, diagnostic, and laboratory studies (119). The sensitivity decreased to 58% for lacunar stroke (119). Perfusion studies with HMPAO-SPECT in early ischemic stroke demonstrated that patients with severe hypoperfusion on admission had poor outcome at 1 month (120). Furthermore, reperfusion of ischemic tissue with 65% to 85% reduction of regional CBF (rCBF) compared to the contralateral hemisphere decreased the final infarct volume but had no affect on regions with reduction greater than 85% (121).

IV. What Is the Role of Noninvasive Intracranial Vascular Imaging?

Summary of Evidence: With the development of different delivery approaches for thrombolysis in acute ischemic stroke, there is a new demand for noninvasive vascular imaging modalities. While some data are available comparing magnetic resonance angiography (MRA) and computed tomography angiography (CTA) to digital substraction angiography (DSA) (moderate and limited evidence), strong evidence in support of the use of such approaches for available therapies is lacking. Prospective studies examining clinical outcome after the use of screening vascular imaging approaches to triage therapy are needed.

Supporting Evidence

A. Computed Tomography Angiography

One advantage of CTA is that it can be performed immediately following the prerequisite noncontrast CT for all stroke patients. Using spiral CT, the entire examination can be completed in 5 minutes with 100 cc of nonionic intravenous contrast, with an additional 10 minutes required for image reconstruction. The sensitivity and specificity of CTA for trunk occlusions of the circle of Willis are 83% to 100% and 99% to 100%, respectively, compared to DSA in several case series (limited evidence) (122–126). Few studies have examined the sensitivity of CTA for distal occlusions. In one study the reliability in assessing MCA branch occlusion was significantly lower (123).

B. Magnetic Resonance Angiography

In addition to tissue evaluation, MR is capable of noninvasively assessing the intracranial vascular status of stroke patients using MRA. One of the most commonly used MRA techniques is the 2D or 3D time-of-flight technique. Stationary background tissue is suppressed while fresh flowing intravascular blood has bright signal. The source images are postprocessed using a maximal intensity projection (MIP) to display a 3D image of the blood vessel. However, the sensitivity and specificity of MRA are somewhat limited when compared to DSA. In a prospective nonconsecutive study of 50 patients, MRA had a sensitivity of 100% and a specificity of 95% for occlusion and 89% sensitivity and specificity for stenosis of the intracranial vessels compared to DSA (limited evidence) (127). In another study of 131 patients with 32 intracranial steno-occlusive lesions, MRA had a sensitivity of 85% and specificity of 96% for internal carotid artery (ICA) pathology, and for MCA lesions, 88% sensitivity and 97% specificity (moderate evidence) (128). A recent comparison of MRA and DSA in 24 children presenting with cerebral infarction demonstrated that all lesions detected on DSA were present on MRA; however, distal vascular lesions and the degree of stenosis were more accurately detected with DSA (moderate evidence) (129). In another study, DSA and MRA were compared to surgical and histologic findings of specimens removed during endarterectomy; MRA was 89% and DSA was 93% in agreement with histologic specimens in determining the degree of stenosis, and plaque morphology was in agreement in 91% of cases for MRA and 94% for DSA (130).

These findings are not surprising given the known technical limitations associated with MRA. First, the ability of MRA to accurately depict the vessel lumen is limited due to the fact that complete or partial signal voids in regions of high or turbulent flow normally occur (spin dephasing), leading to an overestimation of the extent of stenosis. Second, the inability to acquire high-resolution images due to limited signal-to-noise ratios and loss of contrast between blood and brain parenchyma for slow-flowing spins (spin saturation) makes it difficult for MRA to depict distal and small vessels. Therefore, while MRA is able to provide images of the cerebral vasculature noninvasively, cautious interpretation of lumen definition is warranted. Although contrast-enhanced MRA of the extracranial arteries appears to be better at defining the degree of stenosis than the time-of-flight MRA technique (131,132), assessment of the intracranial vessels with contrast is limited due to venous contamination. However, while it may be possible to overcome this limitation with new technical development including ultrafast imaging techniques and better timing of the arrival of contrast, data regarding its accuracy has not yet been defined (133). Whether MRA can provide screening for future thrombolytic/interventional approaches remains to be seen.

V. What Is the Role of Acute Neuroimaging in Pediatric Stroke?

Summary of Evidence: Due to the low incidence of stroke in the pediatric population, few studies are available regarding risk factors, recurrence, and outcome. Moreover, the efficacy of acute therapies has not been examined in this population, limiting the utility of acute neuroimaging in pediatric stroke for early therapeutic decision making.

Supporting Evidence: In contrast to stroke in the adult population, pediatric stroke is an uncommon disorder with a very different pathophysiology. The overall incidence of ischemic stroke is 2 to 13 per 100,000 children, with the highest rate occurring in the perinatal period (26.4 per 100,000 infants less than 30 days old) (134). The incidence of ischemic stroke has increased over the past two decades, probably due to better population-based studies (the Canadian Pediatric Stroke Registry), more sensitive imaging techniques (fetal MR, DWI), and an increased survival of immature neonates due to improved treatment modalities (extracorporeal membrane oxygenation). The etiologies of ischemic stroke in children are due to nonatherosclerotic causes such as congenital heart disease, sickle cell anemia, coagulation disorders, arterial dissection, varicella zoster infection, inherited metabolic disorders, and moyamoya, and is found to be idiopathic in one third of the cases (134,135).

To date, there are no randomized clinical trials for the treatment of acute ischemic stroke in the pediatric population. Indeed, there is only one published randomized controlled trial for stroke prevention [the Stroke Prevention Trial (STOP) in Sickle Cell Anemia], which showed that blood transfusions greatly reduced the risk of stroke in children with sickle cell anemia who have peak mean blood flow velocities greater than 200 cm per second measured by transcranial Doppler ultrasonography in the ICA or proximal MCA (strong evidence) (136). Though there is no Food and Drug Administration (FDA)-approved treatment for children with acute ischemic stroke, several case reports have documented the use of intravenous tPA in this setting (insufficient evidence) (137–139).

The lack of proven therapeutic interventions for acute pediatric stroke limits the utility of acute neuroimaging for early therapeutic decision making. However, the diagnosis and differentiation of stroke subtypes may still be important for preventative measures. This is true especially in neonates and infants, where neurologic deficits may be subtle and difficult to ascertain. In this regard, MRI (with T1W, T2W, FLAIR, as well as DWI) may be superior to CT in the early identification of ischemic lesions and exclusion of stroke mimics (extrapolated from adult data).

Take-Home Table

Table 9.1 summarizes sensitivity, specificity and strength of evidence of neuroimaging in acute intraporenchymal hemorrhage, acute subarachnoid hemorrhage, and acute ischemic infarction.

Table 9.1. Diagnostic performance for patients presenting with acute neurological deficits

	Sensitivity	Specificity	Reference	Evidence
Acute intraparenchymal hemorrhage (<6 hours)				
CT	100%*	100%*		*
MRI	100%	100%	61	Strong
Acute subarachnoid hemorrhage (<12 hours)				
CT	98–100%		16,17	Moderate
MRI (FLAIR)	92–100%	100%	28–30	Limited
Acute ischemic infarction (<6 hours)				
CT	61%	65%	9	Moderate
MRI	91%	95%	9	Moderate

* Although the exact sensitivity or specificity of CT for detecting intraparenchymal hemorrhage is unknown (limited evidence), it serves as the gold standard for detection in comparison to other modalities.

Acute Imaging Protocols Based on the Evidence

Head CT: indicated for all patients presenting with acute focal deficits
    Noncontrast examination
    Sequential or spiral CT with 5-mm slice thickness from the skull base to
        the vertex
Head MR: indicated if stroke is in doubt
    Axial DWI (EPI) with ADC map, GRE, or ep T2*, FLAIR, T1W
    Optional sequences (insufficient evidence for routine clinical practice):
        MRA of the circle of Willis (3D TOF technique)
        PWI (EPI FLASH, 12 slices per measurement for 40 measurements,
            with 10- to 15-sec injection delay, injection rate of 5 cc/sec with
            single or double bolus of gadolinium, followed by a 20-cc saline
            flush)
        Axial T1W postcontrast

Areas of Future Research

- Use of neuroimaging to select patients for acute therapies:
  - Imaging the ischemic penumbra to extend the empirically determined therapeutic windows for certain individuals
  - Predict individuals at high risk for hemorrhagic conversion
  - As more therapies are made available, neuroimaging has the potential to help determine which modality might be most efficacious (e.g., imaging large vessel occlusions for use of intraarterial thrombolysis or clot retrieval).
- Use of neuroimaging to predict outcome:
  - Useful for prognostic purposes, or for discharge planning
  - Useful as a surrogate measure of outcome in clinical trials

References

1. American Heart Association. 2004 Heart Disease and Stroke Statistics Update. Dallas: AHA, 2004.
2. Bogousslavsky J, Van Melle G, Regli F. Stroke 1988;19(9):1083–1092.
3. Broderick J, et al. Stroke 1998;29(2):415–421.
4. MMWR 2001;50(7).
5. Sacco RL, et al. Am J Epidemiol 1998;147(3):259–268.
6. Diringer MN, et al. Stroke 1999;30(4):724–728.
7. NINDS. N Engl J Med 1995;333(24):1581–1587.
8. Furlan A, et al. JAMA 1999;282(21):2003–2011.
9. Fiebach JB, et al. Stroke 2004;35(2):502–506.
10. New PF, Aronow S. Radiology 1976;121(3 pt 1):635–640.
11. Smith WP Jr, Batnitzky S, Rengachary SS. AJR 1981;136(3):543–546.
12. Culebras A, et al. Stroke 1997;28(7):1480–1497.
13. Beauchamp NJ Jr, et al. Radiology 1999;212(2):307–324.
14. Paxton R, Ambrose J. Br J Radiol 1974;47(561):530–565.
15. Jacobs L, Kinkel WR, Heffner RR Jr. Neurology 1976;26(12):1111–1118.
16. Adams HP Jr, et al. Neurology 1983;33(8):981–988.
17. van der Wee N, et al. J Neurol Neurosurg Psychiatry 1995;58(3):357–359.
18. Sames TA, et al. Acad Emerg Med 1996;3(1):16–20.
19. Sidman R, Connolly E, Lemke T. Acad Emerg Med 1996;3(9):827–831.
20. Bradley WG Jr. Radiology 1993;189(1):15–26.
21. Gomori JM, et al. Radiology 1985;157(1):87–93.
22. Edelman RR, et al. AJNR 1986;7(5):751–756.
23. Thulborn K, Atlas SW. Intracranial hemorrhage. In: Atlas SW, ed. Magnetic resonance imaging of the brain and spine. 1991:175–222. New York: Raven Press, 1991.
24. Schellinger PD, et al. Stroke 1999;30(4):765–768.
25. Patel MR, Edelman RR, Warach S. Stroke 1996;27(12):2321–2324.
26. Linfante I, et al. Stroke 1999;30(11):2263–2267.
27. Bradley WG Jr, Schmidt PG. Radiology 1985;156(1):99–103.
28. Noguchi K, et al. Radiology 1997;203(1):257–262.
29. Noguchi K, et al. Radiology 1995;196(3):773–777.
30. Bakshi R, et al. AJNR 1999;20(4):629–636.
31. Bakshi R, et al. AJNR 2000;21(3):503–508.
32. Dechambre SD, et al. Neuroradiology 2000;42(8):608–611.
33. Melhem ER, Jara H, Eustace S. AJR 1997;169(3):859–862.
34. Ogawa T, et al. AJR 1995;165(5):1257–1262.
35. Hesselink JR, et al. Acta Radiol Suppl 1986;369:46–48.
36. Kidwell CS, et al. Stroke 2002;33(1):95–98.
37. Libman RB, et al. Arch Neurol 1995;52(11):1119–1122.
38. Norris JW, Hachinski VC. Lancet 1982;1(8267):328–331.
39. Kothari RU, et al. Stroke 1995;26(12):2238–2241.
40. Truwit CL, et al. Radiology 1990;176(3):801–806.
41. Tomura N, et al. Radiology 1988;168(2):463–467.
42. Patel SC, et al. JAMA 2001;286(22):2830–2838.
43. von Kummer R, et al. AJNR 1994;15(1):9–15; discussion 16–18.
44. Schriger DL, et al. JAMA 1998;279(16):1293–1297.
45. Grotta JC, et al. Stroke 1999;30(8):1528–1533.
46. Hacke W, et al. JAMA 1995;274(13):1017–1025.
47. Toni D, et al. Neurology 1996;46(2):341–345.
48. Larrue V, et al. Stroke 1997;28(5):957–960.
49. Larrue V, et al. Stroke 2001;32(2):438–441.
50. von Kummer R, et al. Radiology 1997;205(2):327–333.
51. Hacke W, et al. Lancet 1998;352(9136):1245–1251.
52. Clark WM, et al. JAMA 1999;282(21):2019–2026.

53. Kucharczyk J, et al. Magn Reson Med 1991;19(2):311–315.
54. Reith W, et al. Neurology 1995;45(1):172–177.
55. Mintorovitch J, et al. Magn Reson Med 1991;18(1):39–50.
56. Warach S, et al. Ann Neurol 1995;37(2):231–241.
57. Moseley ME, et al. Magn Reson Med 1990;14(2):330–346.
58. Hoehn-Berlage M, et al. J Cereb Blood Flow Metab 1995;15(6):1002–1011.
59. Gonzalez RG, et al. Radiology 1999;210(1):155–162.
60. Lovblad KO, et al. AJNR 1998;19(6):1061–1066.
61. Fiebach JB, et al. Stroke 2002;33(9):2206–2210.
62. Marks MP, et al. Radiology 1996;199(2):403–408.
63. Kidwell CS, et al. Stroke 1999;30(6):1174–1180.
64. Ay H, et al. Neurology 1999;52(9):1784–1792.
65. Ebisu T, et al. Magn Reson Imaging 1996;14(9):1113–1116.
66. Ohta K, et al. J Neurol 1999;246(8):736–738.
67. Sener RN. Comput Med Imaging Graph 2001;25(5):391–397.
68. Bahn MM, et al. Arch Neurol 1997;54(11):1411–1415.
69. Gauvain KM, et al. AJR 2001;177(2):449–454.
70. Chen S, et al. AJNR 2001;22(6):1089–1096.
71. Chu K, et al. Arch Neurol 2001;58(6):993–998.
72. Hasegawa Y, et al. Stroke 1996;27(9):1648–1655; discussion 1655–1656.
73. Lovblad KO, et al. Ann Neurol 1997;42(2):164–170.
74. Schwamm LH, et al. Stroke 1998;29(11):2268–2276.
75. Barber PA, et al. Neurology 1998;51(2):418–426.
76. Tong DC, et al. Neurology 1998;50(4):864–870.
77. van Everdingen KJ, et al. Stroke 1998;29(9):1783–1790.
78. Villringer A, et al. Magn Reson Med 1988;6(2):164–174.
79. Rosen BR, et al. Magn Reson Med 1991;19(2):285–292.
80. Rosen BR, et al. Magn Reson Med 1990;14(2):249–265.
81. Ostergaard L, et al. Magn Reson Med 1996;36(5):726–736.
82. Lin W, et al. J Magn Reson Imaging 2001;14(6):659–667.
83. Astrup J, Siesjo BK, Symon L. Stroke 1981;12(6):723–725.
84. Baird AE, et al. Ann Neurol 1997;41(5):581–589.
85. Beaulieu C, et al. Ann Neurol 1999;46(4):568–578.
86. Perkins CJ, et al. Stroke 2001;32(12):2774–2781.
87. Warach S, et al. Ann Neurol 2000;48(5):713–722.
88. Clark WM, et al. Neurology 2001;57(9):1595–1602.
89. Uno M, et al. Neurosurgery 2002;50(1):28–34; discussion 34–35.
90. Minematsu K, et al. Stroke 1992;23(9):1304–1310; discussion 1310–1311.
91. Hasegawa Y, et al. Neurology 1994;44(8):1484–1490.
92. Kidwell CS, et al. Ann Neurol 2000;47(4):462–469.
93. Fiehler J, et al. Stroke 2002;33(1):79–86.
94. Barker PB, et al. Radiology 1994;192(3):723–732.
95. Grohn OH, Kauppinen RA. NMR Biomed 2001;14(7–8):432–440.
96. Decanniere C, et al. Magn Reson Med 1995;34(3):343–352.
97. Bizzi A, et al. Magn Reson Imaging 1996;14(6):581–592.
98. Sager TN, Laursen H, Hansen AJ. J Cereb Blood Flow Metab 1995;15(4): 639–646.
99. Powers WJ, et al. J Cereb Blood Flow Metab 1985;5(4):600–608.
100. Touzani O, et al. Brain Res 1997;767(1):17–25.
101. Baron JC. Cerebrovasc Dis 1999;9(4):193–201.
102. Gur D, et al. Science 1982;215(4537):1267–1268.
103. Wolfson SK Jr, et al. Stroke 1990;21(5):751–757.
104. DeWitt DS, et al. Stroke 1989;20(12):1716–1723.
105. Firlik AD, et al. Stroke 1997;28(11):2208–2213.
106. Firlik AD, et al. J Neurosurg 1998;89(2):243–249.
107. Pindzola RR, et al. Stroke 2001;32(8):1811–1817.
108. Webster MW, et al. J Vasc Surg 1995;21(2):338–344; discussion 344–345.

109. Plougmann J, et al. J Neurosurg 1994;81(6):822–828.
110. Lev MH, et al. Stroke 2001;32(9):2021–2028.
111. Mayer TE, et al. AJNR 2000;21(8):1441–1449.
112. Baron JC, et al. J Cereb Blood Flow Metab 1989;9(6):723–742.
113. Baron JC, et al. Stroke 1981;12(4):454–459.
114. Wise RJ, et al. Brain 1983;106(pt 1):197–222.
115. Heiss WD, et al. J Cereb Blood Flow Metab 1992;12(2):193–203.
116. Furlan M, et al. Ann Neurol 1996;40(2):216–226.
117. Grubb RL Jr, et al. JAMA 1998;280(12):1055–1060.
118. Heiss WD, et al. J Cereb Blood Flow Metab 1998;18(12):1298–1307.
119. Brass LM, et al. J Cereb Blood Flow Metab 1994;149(suppl 1):S91–98.
120. Giubilei F, et al. Stroke 1990;21(6):895–900.
121. Sasaki O, et al. AJNR 1996;17(9):1661–1668.
122. Katz DA, et al. Radiology 1995;195(2):445–449.
123. Knauth M, et al. AJNR 1997;18(6):1001–1010.
124. Shrier DA, et al. AJNR 1997;18(6):1011–1020.
125. Wildermuth S, et al. Stroke 1998;29(5):935–938.
126. Verro P, et al. Stroke 2002;33(1):276–278.
127. Stock KW, et al. Radiology 1995;195(2):451–456.
128. Korogi Y, et al. Radiology 1994;193(1):187–193.
129. Husson B, et al. Stroke 2002;33(5):1280–1285.
130. Liberopoulos K, et al. Int Angiol 1996;15(2):131–137.
131. Cloft HJ, et al. Magn Reson Imaging 1996;14(6):593–600.
132. Willig DS, et al. Radiology 1998;208(2):447–451.
133. Okumura A, et al. Neurol Res 2001;23(7):767–771.
134. Lynch JK, et al. Pediatrics 2002;109(1):116–123.
135. Kirkham FJ, et al. J Child Neurol 2000;15(5):299–307.
136. Adams RJ, et al. N Engl J Med 1998;339(1):5–11.
137. Gruber A, et al. Neurology 2000;54(8):1684–1686.
138. Carlson MD, et al. Neurology 2001;57(1):157–158.
139. Thirumalai SS, Shubin RA. J Child Neurol 2000;15(8):558.

10

Adults and Children with Headache: Evidence-Based Role of Neuroimaging

L. Santiago Medina, Amisha Shah, and Elza Vasconcellos

Key Points

- In adults, benign headache disorders usually start before the age of 65 years. Therefore, in patients older than 65 years, secondary causes should be suspected.
- Although most headaches in children are benign in nature, a small percentage is caused by serious diseases, such as brain neoplasm.
- Computed tomography (CT) imaging remains the initial test of choice for (1) new-onset headache in adults and (2) headache suggestive of subarachnoid hemorrhage (limited evidence).
- Neuroimaging is recommended in adults with nonacute headache and unexplained abnormal neurologic examination (moderate evidence).

- Computed tomography angiography and magnetic resonance (MR) angiography have sensitivities greater than 85% for aneurysms greater than 5 mm. The sensitivity of these two examinations drops significantly for aneurysms less than 5 mm (moderate evidence).
- In adults with headache and known primary neoplasm suspected of having brain metastatic disease, MR imaging with contrast is the neuroimaging study of choice (moderate evidence).
- Neuroimaging is recommended in children with headache and an abnormal neurologic examination or seizures (moderate evidence).
- Sensitivity and specificity of MR imaging is greater than CT for intracranial lesions. For intracranial surgical space-occupying lesions, however, there is no difference in diagnostic performance between MR imaging and a CT (limited evidence).

Definition and Pathophysiology

Headaches can be divided into primary and secondary (Table 10.1). Primary causes include migraine, cluster, and tension-type headache disorders, and secondary etiologies include neoplasms, arteriovenous malformations, aneurysm, infection and hydrocephalus. Diagnosis of primary headache disorders is based on clinical criteria as set forth by the International headache Society (1). Neuroimaging should aid in the diagnosis of secondary headache disorders.

Table 10.1. Common causes of primary and secondary headache

Primary headaches
  Migraine
  Cluster
  Tension-type
Secondary headaches
  Intracranial space occupying lesions
    Neoplasm
    Arteriovenous malformation
    Abscess
    Hematoma
  Cerebrovascular disease
    Intracranial aneurysms
    Occlusive vascular disease
  Infection
    Sinusitis
    Meningitis
    Encephalitis
  Inflammation
    Vasculitis
    Acute disseminated encephalomyelitis
  Increased intracranial pressure
    Hydrocephalus
    Pseudotumor cerebri

Epidemiology

Adults

Headache is a very common symptom among adults, accounting for 18 million (4%) of the total outpatient visits in the United States each year (2). In any given year, more than 70% of the U.S. population has a headache (3). An estimated 23.6 million people in the U.S. have migraine headaches (4,5).

In the elderly population, 15% of patients 65 years or older, versus 1% to 2% of patients younger than 65 years, presented with secondary headache disorders such as neoplasms, strokes, and temporal arteritis (4,6). Brain metastases are the most common intracranial tumors, far outnumbering primary brain neoplasms (7). Approximately 58% of primary brain neoplasms in adults are malignant (7). Common primary malignant neoplasms include astrocytomas and glioblastomas (7). Benign brain tumors account for 38% of primary brain neoplasms (7). Despite being benign, they may have aggressive characteristics causing significant morbidity and mortality (7). Meningioma is the most common type (7).

Children

In approximately 50% of patients with migraines, the headache disorder starts before the age of 20 years (4). In the U.S., adolescent boys and girls have a headache prevalence of 56% and 74%, and a migraine prevalence of 3.8% and 6.6%, respectively (2). A small percentage of headaches in children are secondary in nature.

A primary concern in children with headache is the possibility of a brain tumor (8,9). Although brain tumors constitute the largest group of solid neoplasms in children and are second only to leukemia in overall frequency of childhood cancers, the annual incidence is low at 3 in 100,000 (9). Primary brain neoplasms are far more prevalent in children than they are in adults (10). They account for almost 20% of all cancers in children but only 1% of cancers in adults (4). Central nervous system (CNS) tumors are the second cause of cancer-related deaths in patients younger than 15 years (11).

Overall Cost to Society

The prevalence of migraine is highest in the peak productive years of life between the ages of 25 and 55 years (12,13). The direct and indirect annual cost of migraine has been estimated at more than $5.6 billion (14).

Goals of Neuroimaging

- Diagnose the secondary causes of headache (Table 10.1) so that appropriate treatment can be instituted.
- Exclude secondary etiologies of headache in patients with atypical primary headache disorders.
- Decrease the risk of brain herniation prior to lumbar puncture by excluding intracranial space occupying lesions.

Table 10.2. Suggested guidelines for neuroimaging in adult patients with new-onset headache

First or worst headache
Increased frequency and increased severity of headache
New-onset headache after age 50
New-onset headache with history of cancer or immunodeficiency
Headache with fever, neck stiffness, and meningeal signs
Headache with abnormal neurologic examination

Methodology

A Medline search was conducted using Ovid (Wolters Kluwer, New York, New York) and PubMed (National Library of Medicine, Bethesda, Maryland). A systematic literature review was performed from 1966 through August 2003. Keywords included (1) *headache*, (2) *cephalgia*, (3) *diagnostic imaging*, (4) *clinical examination*, (5) *practice guidelines*, and (6) *surgery*.

I. Which Adults with New-Onset Headache Should Undergo Neuroimaging?

Summary of Evidence: The most common causes of secondary headache in adults are brain neoplasms, aneurysms, arteriovenous malformations, intracranial infections, and sinus disease. Several history and physical examination findings may increase the yield of the diagnostic study discovering an intracranial space-occupying lesion in adults. Table 10.2 shows the scenarios that should warrant further diagnostic testing (limited evidence) (3,4,15). The factors outlined in Table 10.2 increase the pretest probability of finding a secondary headache disorder.

II. What Neuroimaging Approach Is Most Appropriate in Adults with New-Onset Headache?

Summary of Evidence: The data reviewed demonstrate that 11% to 21% of patients presenting with new-onset headache have serious intracranial pathology (moderate and limited evidence) (4,16,17). Computed tomography (CT) examination has been the standard of care for the initial evaluation of new-onset headache because CT is faster, more readily available, less costly than magnetic resonance imaging (MRI), and less invasive than lumber puncture (4). In addition, CT has a higher sensitivity than MRI for subarachnoid hemorrhage (SAH) (18,19). Unless further data become available that demonstrate higher sensitivity of MRI, CT is recommended in the assessment of all patients who present with new-onset headache (limited evidence) (4). Lumbar puncture is recommended in those patients in which the CT scan is nondiagnostic and the clinical evaluation reveals abnormal neurologic findings, or in those patients in whom SAH is strongly suspected (limited evidence) (4). Figure 10.1 is a suggested decision tree to evaluate adult patients with new-onset headache.

Supporting Evidence for Clinical Guidelines and Neuroimaging in New-Onset Headache: Duarte and colleagues (16) studied 100 consecutive patients over

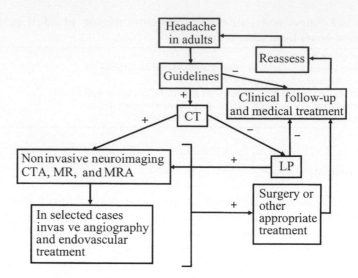

Figure 10.1. Decision tree for use in adults with new-onset headache. For those patients who meet any of the guidelines in Table 10.2, computed tomography (CT) is suggested. For patients who do not meet these criteria or those with negative diagnostic workup, clinical observation with periodic reassessment is recommended. If CT is positive, further workup with CT angiography or magnetic resonance imaging (MRI) plus MR angiography is recommended. In selected case, conventional angiography and endovascular treatment may be warranted. If CT is negative, lumbar puncture is advised. In patients with suspected metastatic brain disease, contrast-enhanced MRI is recommended. In patients with suspected intracranial aneurysm, further assessment with CT angiography or MR angiography is warranted. CTA, CT angiography; LP, lumbar puncture; MRA, MR angiography. [*Source:* Medina et al. (29), with permission from Elsevier.]

a 1-year period (moderate evidence). Inclusion criteria included patients admitted to the neurology unit with recent onset of headache. Recent onset of headache was defined by the authors as persistent headache of less than 1 year's duration. All the patients studied had an unenhanced and enhanced CT. Lumbar puncture, MRI, and MR angiogram were performed in selected cases. Tumors were identified in 21% of the patients, which comprised 16% of the patients with a negative neurologic examination.

A smaller-scale prospective study examined the association of acute headache and SAH (limited evidence) (20). All patients were examined using state-of-the art CT. Patients had a mean headache duration of approximately 72 hours (20). Of the 27 patients studied, 20 had a negative CT and four were diagnosed with SAH. Among the remaining three patients, one had a frontal meningioma, another had a hematoma associated with SAH, and the other had diffuse meningeal enhancement caused by bacterial meningitis. Lumbar puncture was performed in 19 of the patients with negative CT, yielding five additional cases of SAH. Hence, CT did not demonstrate SAH in five of nine patients.

A retrospective study of 1111 patients with acute headache who had CT evaluation found 120 (10.8%) abnormalities, including hemorrhage, infarct, and neoplasm (limited evidence) (17). All imaging studies were done at two teaching institutions over a 3-year period. There were statistical differences in the percentage of intracranial lesions based on the setting in which the CT was ordered. The inpatient rate (21.2%) was twice that of emergency patients (11.7%) and three times more than outpatients (6.9%; $p < .005$). Of 155 CT studies performed for headache as the sole presenting symptom (14.0%), nine (5.8%) patients had acute intracranial abnormalities. One study in the outpatient setting that studied 726 patients with new headaches found no serious intracranial disease (limited evidence) (6). The difference in prevalence of disease among emergency patients, inpatients, and outpatients is probably related to patient selection bias.

III. What Is the Role of Neuroimaging in Adults with Migraine or Chronic Headache?

Summary of Evidence: Most of the available literature (moderate and limited evidence) suggests that there is no need for neuroimaging in patients with migraine and normal neurologic examination. Neuroimaging is indicated in patients with nonacute headache and unexplained abnormal neurologic examination, or in patients with atypical features or headache that does not fulfill the definition of migraine.

Supporting Evidence: Evidence-based guidelines on the use of diagnostic imaging in patients presenting with migraine have been developed by a multispecialty group called the U.S. Headache Consortium (21). Data were examined from 28 studies (moderate and limited evidence), six not blinded prospective and 22 retrospective studies. The specific recommendations from the U.S. Headache Consortium were (1) neuroimaging should be considered in patients with nonacute headache and unexplained abnormal findings on the neurologic examination, (2) neuroimaging is not usually warranted in patients with migraine and normal findings on neurologic examination, and (3) a lower threshold for CT or MRI may be applicable in patients with atypical features or with headache that do not fulfill the definition of migraine.

The study by Joseph and colleagues (22) (limited evidence) in 48 headache patients found five patients with neoplasms and one with an arteriovenous malformation. Of these patients, five had physical signs and one had headache on exertion. Weingarten and colleagues (23) (limited evidence) extrapolated data from 100,800 adult patients enrolled in a health maintenance organization and estimated that, in patients with chronic headache and a normal neurologic examination, the chance of finding abnormalities on CT requiring neurosurgical intervention were as low as 0.01% (1 in 10,000).

In 1994, the American Academy of Neurology provided a summary statement on the use of neuroimaging in patients with headache and a normal neurologic examination based on a review of the literature (moderate and limited evidence) (24). It concluded that routine imaging "in adult patients with recurrent headaches that have been defined as migraine—including those with visual aura—with no recent change in pattern, no history of seizures, and no other focal neurologic signs of symptoms . . . is not warranted (4)". This statement was based on a 1994 literature review by Frishberg (25) of 17 articles published between 1974 and 1991 that were limited to studies with more than 17 subjects per study (moderate evidence). All patients had normal neurologic examinations. Of 897 CT or MRI studies performed in patients with migraine, only three tumors and one arteriovenous malformation were noted, resulting in a yield of 0.4% (4 in 1000). The summary statement mentions, however, that "patients with atypical headache patterns, a history of seizure, or focal neurological signs or symptoms, CT or MRI may be indicated" (4,24).

IV. What Is the Role of Imaging in Patients with Headache and Subarachnoid Hemorrhage Suspected of Having an Intracranial Aneurysm?

Summary of Evidence: In North America, 80% to 90% of nontraumatic SAH is caused by the rupture of nontraumatic cerebral aneurysms (26). Computed tomography angiography and MR angiography have sensitivities greater than 85% for aneurysms greater than 5 mm. The sensitivity of these two examinations drops significantly for aneurysms less than 5 mm.

Supporting Evidence: White et al. (27) searched the literature from 1988 through 1998 to find studies with 10 or more subjects in which the conventional angiography results were compared with noninvasive imaging. They included 38 studies that scored more than 50% on evaluation criteria by using intrinsically weighted standardized assessment to determine suitability for inclusion (moderate evidence). The rates of aneurysm accuracy for CT angiography and MR angiography were 89% and 90%, respectively. The study showed greater sensitivity for aneurysms larger than 3 mm than for aneurysms 3 mm or smaller for CT angiography (96% verses 61%) and for MR angiography (94% versus 38%).

White et al. (28) also performed a prospective blinded study in 142 patients who underwent intraarterial digital subtraction angiography to detect aneurysms (moderate evidence). Results were compared with CT angiography and MR angiography. The accuracy rates per patient for the best observer were 87% and 85% for CT angiography and MR angiography, respectively. The accuracy rates for brain aneurysm for the best observer were 73% and 67% for CT angiography and MR angiography, respectively. The sensitivity for the detection of aneurysms 5 mm or larger was 94% for CT angiography and 86% for MR angiography. For aneurysms smaller than 5 mm, sensitivities for CT angiography and MR angiography were 57% and 35%, respectively.

V. What Is the Recommended Neuroimaging Examination in Adults with Headache and Known Primary Neoplasm Suspected of Having Brain Metastases?

Summary of Evidence: In patients older than 40 years, with known primary neoplasm, brain metastasis is a common cause of headache (29). Most studies described in the literature suggest that contrast-enhanced MRI is superior to contrast-enhanced CT in the detection of brain metastatic disease, especially if the lesions are less than 2 cm (moderate evidence). In patients with suspected metastases to the central nervous system, enhanced brain MRI is recommended.

Supporting Evidence: Davis and colleagues (30) (moderate evidence) studied imaging studies in 23 patients that compared contrast-enhanced

MRI with double dose-contrast enhanced CT. Contrast-enhanced MRI demonstrated more than 67 definite or typical brain metastases. The double dose-delayed CT revealed only 37 metastatic lesions. The authors concluded that MRI with enhancement is superior to double dose-contrast enhanced CT scan for detecting brain metastasis, anatomic localization, and number of lesions.

Golfieri and colleagues (31) reported similar findings (moderate evidence). They studied 44 patients with small cell carcinoma to detect cerebral metastases. All patients were studied with contrast-enhanced CT scan and gadolinium-enhanced MRI. Of all patients, 43% had cerebral metastases. Both contrast-enhanced CT and gadolinium-enhanced MRI detected lesions greater than 2 cm. For lesions less than 2 cm, 9% were detected only by gadolinium-enhanced T1-weighted images. The authors concluded that gadolinium-enhanced T1-weighted images remain the most accurate technique in the assessment of cerebral metastases.

Sze and colleagues (32) performed prospective and retrospective studies in 75 patients (moderate evidence). In 49 patients, MRI and contrast-enhanced CT were equivalent. In 26 patients, however, results were discordant, with neither CT nor MRI being consistently superior; MRI demonstrated more metastases in nine of these 26 patients, but contrast-enhanced CT better depicted lesions in eight of 26 patients.

VI. When Is Neuroimaging Appropriate in Children with Headache?

Summary of Evidence: Table 10.3 summarizes the neuroimaging guidelines in children with headaches. Theses guidelines reinforce the primary importance of careful acquisition of the medical history and performance of a thorough examination, including a detailed neurologic examination (33). Among children at risk for brain lesions based on these criteria, neuroimaging with either MRI or CT is valuable in combination with close clinical follow-up (Fig. 10.2).

Supporting Evidence: In 2002 the American Academy of Neurology and Child Neurology Society published evidence-based neuroimaging recommendations for children (34). Six studies (one prospective and five retrospective) met inclusion criteria (moderate evidence). Data on 605 of 1275 children with recurrent headache who underwent neuroimaging found only 14 (2.3%) with nervous system lesions that required surgical treatment. All 14 children had definite abnormalities on neurologic examination. The recommendations from this study were as follows: (1)

Table 10.3. Suggested guidelines for neuroimaging in pediatric patients with headache

Persistent headaches of less than 1 month's duration
Headache associated with abnormal neurologic examination
Headache associated with seizures
Headache with new onset of severe episodes or change in the type of headache
Persistent headache without family history of migraine
Family or medical history of disorders that may predispose one to CNS lesions, and clinical or laboratory findings that suggest CNS involvement

Neuroimaging should be considered in children with an abnormal neurologic examination or other physical findings that suggest CNS disease. Variables that predicted the presence of a space-occupying lesion included (a) headache of less than 1 month's duration, (b) absence of family history of migraine, (c) gait abnormalities, and (d) occurrence of seizures. (2) Neuroimaging is not indicated in children with recurrent headaches and a normal neurologic examination. (3) Neuroimaging should be considered in children with recent onset of severe headache, change in the type of headache, or if there are associated features suggestive of neurologic dysfunction.

Medina and colleagues (33) performed a 4-year retrospective study of 315 children with no known underlying CNS disease who underwent brain imaging for a chief complaint of headache (moderate evidence). All patients underwent brain MRI. Sixty-nine patients also underwent brain CT. Clinical data were correlated with findings from MRI and CT, and the final diagnosis, by means of logistic regression. Thirteen (4%) of patients had surgical space-occupying lesions—nine malignant neoplasms, three hemorrhagic vascular malformations, and one arachnoid cyst. Medina and colleagues identified seven independent multivariate predictors of a surgical lesion, the strongest of which were sleep-related headache [odds ratio 5.4, 95% confidence interval (CI): 1.7–17.5] and no family history of migraine (odds ratio 15.4, 95% CI: 5.8–41.0). Other predictors included vomiting, absence of visual symptoms, headache of less than 6 months' duration, confusion, and abnormal neurologic examination findings. A positive correlation between the number of predictors and the risk of surgical lesion was noted ($p < .0001$). No difference between MRI and CT was noted in detection of surgical space-occupying lesions, and there were no false-positive or false-negative surgical lesions detected with either modality on clinical follow-up.

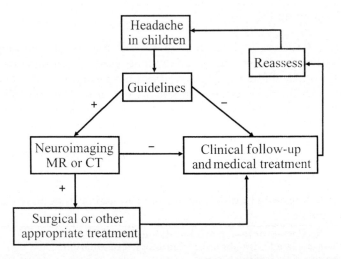

Figure 10.2. Decision tree for use in children with headache. Neuroimaging is suggested for patients who meet any of the guidelines in Table 10.3. For patients who do not meet these criteria or those with negative findings from imaging studies, clinical observation with periodic reassessment is recommended. [*Source:* Medina et al. (33), with permission from the Radiological Society of North America.]

Table 10.4. Diagnostic performance of imaging

Variable	Baseline (%)	Range (%)	Reference
Diagnostic tests			
MR imaging			
Sensitivity	92	82–100	33, 39, 40
Specificity	99	81–100	33, 40
CT			
Sensitivity	81	65–100	33, 39, 40
Specificity	92	72–100	33, 39, 40

VII. What Is the Sensitivity and Specificity of Computed Tomography and Magnetic Resonance Imaging?

Summary of Evidence: The sensitivity and specificity of MRI are greater than those of CT for intracranial lesions. For surgical intracranial space-occupying lesions, however, there is no difference between MRI and CT in diagnostic performance.

Supporting Evidence: The sensitivity and specificity of CT and MRI for intracranial lesions are shown in Table 10.4. Medina and colleagues (33) (moderate evidence) showed that the overall sensitivity and specificity with MRI (92% and 99%, respectively) were higher than with CT (81% and 92%, respectively). Comparison of patients who underwent MRI and CT revealed no statistical significant disagreement between the tests for surgical space-occupying lesions (McNemar test, $p = 0.75$). The U.S. Headache Consortium evidence-based guidelines from systematic review of the literature concluded that MRI may be more sensitive than CT in identifying clinically insignificant abnormalities, but MRI may be no more sensitive than CT in identifying clinically significant pathology (21).

VIII. What Is the Cost-Effectiveness of Neuroimaging in Patients with Headache?

Summary of Evidence: No well-designed cost-effectiveness analysis (CEA) in adults could be found in the literature, but CEA in children with headache suggests that MRI maximizes the quality-adjusted life years (QALY) gained at a reasonable cost-effectiveness ratio in patients at high risk of having a brain tumor. Conversely, the strategy of no imaging with close clinical follow-up is cost saving in low-risk children. Although the CT-MRI strategy maximizes QALY gained in the intermediate-risk patients, its additional cost per QALY gained is high. In children with headache, appropriate selection of patients and diagnostic imaging strategy may maximize quality-adjusted life expectancy and decrease costs of medical workup.

Supporting Evidence: Medina and colleagues (35) reported a CEA in children with headaches. This study assessed the clinical and economic consequences of three diagnostic strategies in the evaluation of children with headache suspected of having a brain tumor: MRI, CT followed by MRI for positive results (CT-MRI), and no neuroimaging with close clinical follow-up. A decision-analysis Markov model and CEA were performed incorporating the risk group pretest or prior probability, MRI and CT sensitivity and specificity, tumor survival, progression rates, and cost per strategy. Outcomes were based on QALY gained and incremental cost per QALY gained.

The results were as follows: For low-risk children with chronic non-migraine headaches of more than 6 months' duration as the sole symptom [pretests probability of brain tumor, 0.01% (1 in 10,000)], close clinical observation without neuroimaging was less costly and more effective than the two neuroimaging strategies. For the intermediate-risk children with migraine headache and normal neurologic examination [pretest probability of brain tumor, 0.4% (4 in 1000)], CT-MRI was the most effective strategy but cost more than $1 million per QALY gained compared with no neuroimaging. For high-risk children with headache of less than 6 months' duration and other clinical predictors of a brain tumor, such as an abnormal neurologic examination (pretest probability of brain tumor, 4%), the most effective strategy was MRI, with a cost-effectiveness ratio of 113,800 per QALY gained compared with no imaging.

The cost-effectiveness ratio in the high-risk children with headache is in the comparable range of annual mammography for women aged 55 to 64 years at $110,000 per life-year saved (36), of colonoscopy for colorectal cancer screening for persons older than 40 years at $90,000 per life-year saved (37,38), and of annual cervical cancer screening for women beginning at age 20 years at $220,000 per life-year saved (36,38).

Imaging Case Studies

Case 1: Colloid Cyst

The patient presented with headache and vomiting (Fig. 10.3).

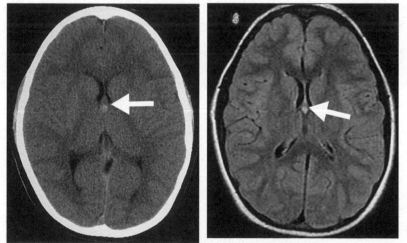

Figure 10.3. A: Unenhanced CT shows a small focal lesion with increased density at the level of the foramen of Monro (arrow). B: Axial FLAIR sequence shows increased T2-weighted signal in the lesion (arrow). No hydrocephalus noted. Neuroimaging findings consistent with colloid cyst.

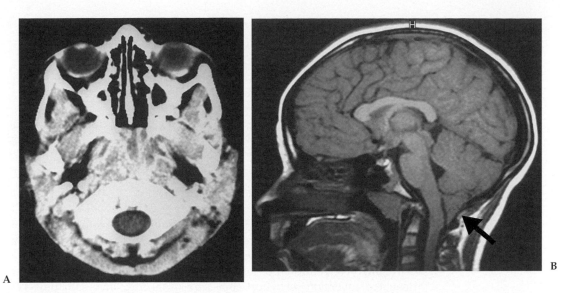

Figure 10.4. A: Unenhanced CT at craniocervical junction was interpreted as unremarkable. B: Sagittal MRI T1-weighted image shows pointed cerebellar tonsils extending more than 5mm below the foramen magnum (arrow) consistent with Chiari I. No cervical cord hydrosyrinx noted.

Case 2: Chiari I

The patient presented with persistent headaches (Fig. 10.4).

Case 3: Brainstem Infiltrative Glial Neoplasm

The patient presented with ataxia and headaches (Fig. 10.5).

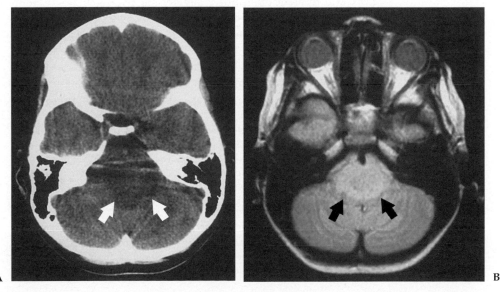

Figure 10.5. A: Unenhanced CT through posterior fossa is limited by beam hardening artifact. A hypodense lesion is seen in the pons (arrows). B: Axial proton density MR image better depicts the anatomy and extent of the lesion without artifact effects (arrows).

Suggested Protocols

CT Imaging

CT without contrast: axial 5- to 10-mm nonspiral images should be used to assess for subarachnoid hemorrhage, tumor hemorrhage, or calcifications.

CT with contrast: axial 5- to 10-mm nonspiral enhanced images should be used in patients with suspected neoplasm, infection, or other focal intracranial lesion. If indicated, CT angiography can be performed as part of the enhanced CT.

MR Imaging

Basic brain MR protocol sequences include sagittal T1-weighted conventional spin-echo (repetition time, 600 ms; echo time 11 ms [600/11]), axial proton density-weighted conventional or fast spin echo (2000/15), axial T2-weighted conventional or fast spin-echo (3200/85), axial FLAIR (fluid-attenuated inversion recovery) spin-echo (8800/152, inversion time [TI] 2200 ms), and coronal T2-weighted fast spin-echo (3200/85) images (33). In patient with suspected neoplasm, infection or focal intracranial lesions gadolinium enhanced T1-weighted conventional spin-echo (600/11) images should be acquired in at least two planes (16,20).

Future Research

- Large-scale prospective studies to validate risk factors and prediction rules of significant intracranial lesions in children and adults with headache.
- Large diagnostic performance studies comparing the sensitivity, specificity and receiver operating characteristic (ROC) curves of neuroimaging in adults and children with headache.
- Cost-effectiveness analysis of neuroimaging in adults with headaches.

References

1. Headache Classification Committee of the International Headache Society. Cephalalgia 1988;8(suppl):1–96.
2. Linet MS, Stewart WF, Celentano DD, et al. JAMA 1989;261:2211–2216.
3. Silberstein SD. Headache 1992;32:396–407.
4. Field AG, Wang E. Emerg Clin North Am 1999;17:127–152
5. Stewart WF, Lipton RB, Celentano DD, et al. JAMA 1992;267:64–69.
6. Hale WE, May FE, Marks RG, et al. Headache 1987;27:272–276.
7. Hutter A, Schwetye K, Bierhals A, McKinstry RC. Clin North Am 2003; 13:237–250.
8. Honig PJ, Charney EB. Am J Dis Child 1982;136:121–124.
9. The Childhood Brain Tumor Consortium. J Neurooncol 1991;10:31–46.
10. Rorke L, Schut L. Introductory survey of pediatric brain tumors. In: McLaurin RL, ed. Pediatric Neurosurgery, 2nd ed. Philadelphia: WB Saunders, 1989: 335–337.
11. Silverberg E, Lubera J. Cancer 1986;36:9–23.
12. Pryse-Phillips W, Findlay H, Tugwell P, et al. Can J Neurol Sci 1992;19:333–339.
13. Lipton RB, Stewart WF. Neurology 1993;43:S6–S10

14. de Lissovoy G, Lazarus SS. Neurology 1994;44(suppl):S56–62.
15. Evans RW. Med Clin North Am 2001;85:865–885.
16. Duarte J, Sempere AP, Delgado JA, et al. Acta Neurol Scand 1996;94:67–70.
17. Kahn CEJ, Sanders GD, Lyons EA, et al. Can Assoc Radiol J 1993;44:189–193.
18. Prager JM, Mikulis DJ. Med Clin North Am 1991;75:525–544.
19. Edelman RR, Warach S. N Engl J Med 1993;328:708–715.
20. Lledo A, Calandre L, Martinez-Menendez B, et al. Headache 1994;34:172–174.
21. Scott Morey S. Am Fam Physician 2000;62:1699–1701.
22. Joseph R, Cook GE, Steiner TJ, et al. Practitioner 1985;229:477–481.
23. Weingarten S, Kleinman M, Elperin L, et al. Arch Intern Med 1992; 152:2457–2462.
24. Quality Standards Subcommittee of the American Academy of Neurology. Neurology 1994;44:1353–1354.
25. Frishberg BM. Neurology 1994;44:1191–1197.
26. Gentry LR, Gordersky JC, Thopson BH. MR imaging. Radiology 1989;171: 177–187.
27. White PM, Wardlaw JM, Easton V. Radiology 2000;217:361–370.
28. White PM, Teasdale EM, Wardlaw JM, et al. Radiology 2001;219:739–749.
29. Medina LS, D'Souza B, Vasconcellos E. Neuroimag Clin North Am 2003; 13:225–235.
30. Davis PA, Hudgins PA, Peterman SB, et al. AJNR 1991;12:293–300.
31. Golfieri R, Cherryman GR, Oliff JF, et al. Radiol Med (Torino) 1991;82:27–34.
32. Sze G, Shin J, Krol G, et al. Radiology 1988;168:187–194.
33. Medina LS, Pinter JD, Zurakowski D, et al. Radiology 1997;202:819–824.
34. Lewis D, Ashwal S, Dahl G, et al. Neurology 2002;51:490–498.
35. Medina LS, Kuntz KM, Pomeroy SL. Pediatrics 2001;108:255–263.
36. Tengs T, Adams M, Pliskin J, et al. Risk Analysis 1995;15:369–390.
37. England W, Halls J, Hunt V. Med Decis Making 1989;9:3–13.
38. Eddy DM. Gynecol Oncol 1981;12(2 pt 2):S168–187.
39. Haughton VM, Rimm AA, Sobocinski KA, et al. Radiology 1986;160:751–755.
40. Orrison WJ, Stimac GK, Stevens EA, et al. Work in progress. Radiology 1991;181:121–127.

11

Neuroimaging of Seizures

Byron Bernal and Nolan Altman

Issues	
	I. Is neuroimaging appropriate in patients with febrile seizures?
	II. What neuroimaging examinations do patients with acute nonfebrile symptomatic seizures need?
	III. What is the role of neuroimaging in patients with first unprovoked seizures?
	IV. What is the most appropriate study in the workup of patients with temporal lobe epilepsy of remote origin?
	V. When should functional imaging be performed in seizure patients and what is the study of choice?

Key Points

- The main goal of neuroimaging in seizures is to rule out focal lesions that could threaten the patient's life (i.e., neoplasm or other intracranial space-occupying lesion).
- The most important role of neuroimaging in epilepsy is to identify the structural substrate of the epileptogenic focus.
- Neuroimaging is not recommended for a simple febrile seizure (limited evidence).
- Computed tomography scan is the best imaging study in the evaluation of patients with acute nonfebrile symptomatic seizures because it detects important abnormalities, such as acute intracranial hemorrhage, that may require immediate medical or surgical treatment (limited evidence).
- Magnetic resonance imaging (MRI) is the neuroimaging study of choice in the workup of first unprovoked seizures (moderate evidence).
- Focal neurologic deficit is an important predictor of an abnormality in the neuroimaging examination (moderate evidence).
- Magnetic resonance (MR) evaluation should be performed in non-acute symptomatic seizure patients with confusion and postictal deficits (moderate evidence).

- Magnetic resonance should be performed in children with unexpected cognitive or motor delays or children under 1 year of age, with remote symptomatic seizures (moderate evidence).
- Patients with focal seizures, abnormal EEG, or generalized epilepsy should be imaged (moderate evidence).
- Magnetic resonance imaging is the imaging modality of choice in temporal lobe epilepsy (moderate evidence).
- Ictal single photon emission computed tomography (SPECT) is the best neuroimaging examination to localize seizure activity (moderate evidence).

Definitions

A seizure is a symptom; epilepsy is a disease. Seizures occur as the result of an electrical discharge in the brain. Epilepsy is a disease characterized by more than one seizure. The International League Against Epilepsy (1) has proposed a classification of the epileptic syndromes, epilepsies, and related seizure disorders. Five main parameters are considered: age, etiology (symptomatic, cryptogenic, or idiopathic), electroclinical features (generalized vs. partial), prognosis (benign vs. malignant), and response to treatment (responsive vs. refractory epilepsy).

Numerous categories are produced from the combination of these factors, which creates confusion in the classification of seizures and epilepsies not only for the general physician but also for specialists. Based on clinical findings, seizures are usually divided into symptomatic and nonsymptomatic seizures. The term *symptomatic* indicates that the seizure is a symptom with an underlying cause. This may be systemic (e.g., hyponatremia, hypocalcemia) or localized (e.g., tumor, cortical dysplasia, abscess). Seizures are categorized as acute symptomatic or remote symptomatic, depending on how long the underlying cause predated the seizure. *Acute symptomatic seizures* occur as the result of a proximate precipitant, such as fever, electrolyte imbalance, drug intoxication, alcohol withdrawal, brain trauma, central nervous system (CNS) infection, or aggressive neoplasm. In *remote symptomatic seizures* the lesion is preexistent and the seizure is the main or only symptom (e.g., cortical dysplasia, ganglioglioma, hippocampal sclerosis, scar, or gliosis). Nonsymptomatic seizures include cryptogenic and idiopathic seizures. In *cryptogenic seizures* (or epilepsy), no cause can be found, even though one is clinically suspected by focal electroencephalography (EEG) or lateralized neurologic examination. In *idiopathic generalized epilepsy* there are no focal clinical signs or clear macrostructural cause for the epilepsy. In these cases a genetic factor is presumed to be present. The term *unprovoked seizures* is used for seizures in patients without history or abnormal neurologic examination. They may turn out to be cryptogenic, idiopathic, or remote symptomatic after the appropriate workup. Partial seizures have a focal origin demonstrated by clinical semiology or EEG. Partial seizures are divided into simple and complex, the latter affecting the patient's awareness.

Epidemiology

The prevalence of epilepsy in industrialized countries is between 5 and 10 cases per 1000 persons (2); hence, epilepsy affects between 1.5 to 3.0 million in the United States. Higher prevalence of epilepsy has been reported in developing countries (3), with a few exceptions. The incidence of epilepsy is age dependent. It peaks at the extremes of life, ranging from 100 to 140 per 100,000 in neonates and infants, and about 140 cases per 100,000 persons in the elderly; 50% of cases occur under the age of 1 year or over 60 years of age (2). The incidence is lowest in early adulthood (25 per 100,000), followed by an increase during late adulthood (4). A different age-specific distribution is seen in developing countries, with a second peak in early adulthood (5,6).

Specific Epidemiologic Data

Febrile seizures affect children between 6 months and 6 years of age. The cumulative incidence of febrile seizures is 2% in children (7). The two most important predictors for first episode of febrile seizures are age less than 1 year and family history of febrile seizures (8). The overall incidence of febrile seizures recurrence is 35% (9). The recurrence of seizures after a focal febrile seizure lasting more than 15 minutes (complex febrile seizure) is two- to fourfold compared to an initial simple febrile seizure (10).

Acute afebrile symptomatic seizures affect 31 of 100,000 people per year and accounts for 40% of all new-onset afebrile seizures. The incidence is highest in the neonatal period (100 per 100,000 inhabitants), with a second peak in patients older than 75 years (123 per 100,000).

The probability of recurrent seizures after an initial *unprovoked seizure* is 36% by 1 year of age, and increases yearly up to 56% by 5 years (11). The presence of neurodevelopmental abnormalities increases the probability of future unprovoked seizures (12). The recurrence of all types of seizures ranges between 24% and 67% (13). Of all patients with recurrent seizures, up to 20%, may have a intractable epilepsy (14).

Overall Cost to Society

Murray et al. (15) analyzed the cost of neuroimaging in the U.S. health care system in 1994 for adult refractory epilepsy. Computed tomography (CT) was used in 60% of new and in 5% of existing cases of epilepsy, whereas magnetic resonance imaging (MRI) was requested in 90% of new and 12% of existing cases (15). Cost was determined by multiplying the CT or MRI incidence rate of usage by the incidence of new-onset seizures and by the cost of the exam. The cost for an MRI of the brain in the U.S. is between $1200 and $2000 (16). Therefore, the CT and MRI workup expenses of new-onset seizures in the U.S. is between $28,000 and $84,000 per 100,000 inhabitants per year.

A French cohort study on medical costs of epilepsy in 1942 patients (17) reported that neuroimaging studies accounted for 8% of the total health care costs for these patients.

Bronen et al. (18) have reported the economic impact of replacing CT with MRI for refractory epilepsy, based on the assumption that the higher sensitivity of MRI in lesion detection would result in reducing the costs of interoperative electrocorticography otherwise needed to localize the site of the epileptogenic focus. They found that in 29 of 117 patients the replacement of CT by MRI eliminated the need for surgical placement of intracranial electrodes with potential savings of $1,450,000 in 29 patients.

Goals

The main goal of the neuroimaging in seizures and epilepsy is to rule out focal lesions that could threaten the patient's life. Neuroimaging also allows the identification of the structural substrate of the epileptogenic focus. Neuroimaging may increase or decrease the pretest probability of having a particular etiology or confirm a clinical diagnosis.

Methodology

For each of the procedures MRI, CT, single photon emission computed tomography (SPECT), positron emission tomography (PET), magnetic resonance spectroscopy (MRS), and functional MRI (fMRI), a systematic review of the literature from January 1, 1982, to January 31, 2004, for abstracts in English and for human subjects only, was performed utilizing PubMed (National Library of Medicine, Bethesda, Maryland) with the following terms: *epilepsy, seizure, evidence-based review,* and *neuroimaging evidence.* Titles and abstracts were reviewed to determine the appropriateness of content. Articles were excluded if they studied fewer than 30 patients, lacked pathologic verification, had no standard of reference, or had no significant influence on clinical decision making. Articles about MRI using less than 1.5 T were also excluded. The specificity, sensitivity, likelihood ratios, probability, predictors, and techniques were summarized for each procedure.

Seizures were divided into two main categories—new-onset seizures and established epilepsy—with particular emphasis on partial types. Adult and childhood epilepsy were addressed as well as febrile and temporal lobe epilepsy due to their clinical and radiologic importance.

Each of the selected articles was reviewed, abstracted and classified by two reviewers. Of a total of 606 abstracts, 131 articles met inclusion criteria and the full text was reviewed in detail.

I. Is Neuroimaging Appropriate in Patients with Febrile Seizures?

Summary of Evidence: Neuroimaging is not recommended for a simple febrile seizure (limited evidence).

Supporting Evidence: No level I or II (strong or moderate evidence) articles were found. In a level III article (limited evidence), Offringa et al. (19) reported an evidence-based medicine study for the management of febrile seizures and the role of neuroimaging in regard to detection of meningitis. The overall prevalence of meningitis detected by CT/MRI scans was

1.2% of 2100 cases of seizures associated with fever. This manuscript, as well as the study by the American Academy of Pediatricians (20) (limited evidence) suggests that CT and MRI are not recommended for a simple febrile seizure.

II. What Neuroimaging Examinations Do Patients with Acute Nonfebrile Symptomatic Seizures Need?

Acute nonfebrile symptomatic seizures occur in nonfebrile patients having neurologic findings pointing to an underlying abnormality. It excludes meningitis, encephalitis, abscess, and empyema.

Summary of Evidence: Computed tomography scan is the best imaging study in the evaluation of patients with acute symptomatology, as it is sensitive for finding abnormalities such as acute intracranial hemorrhage, which may require immediate medical or surgical treatment. It is also fast and readily available (limited evidence).

Supporting Evidence: No articles meeting the criteria for level I or II (strong or moderate evidence) were found. Several level III (limited evidence) studies were found as discussed. Eisner and colleagues (21) reported a study with 163 patients, who presented to the emergency room with first seizure (Table 11.1). All patients older than 6 years of age who had recent head trauma, focal neurologic deficit, or focal seizure activity underwent head CT. Of 19 patients, five (26%) had CT abnormalities, including one subdural hematoma, resulting in a change of medical care. Earnest and colleagues (22) found CT abnormalities in 6.2% of 259 patients with alcohol withdrawal seizures. In 3.9% medical management was changed because of the CT result. Reinus and colleagues (23) retrospectively evaluated the medical records of 115 consecutive patients who had seizures after acute trauma and underwent a noncontrast cranial CT. An abnormal neurologic examination predicted 95% (19 of 20) of the positive CT scans $p < .00004$.

Henneman et al. (24) conducted a retrospective study on 333 patients with new-onset seizures, not associated with acute head trauma, hypo-

Table 11.1. Neuroimaging in acute symptomatic seizures (CT/MRI)

Author	No. of patients	CT/MRI	% of positive	Comments
Eisner et al., 1986 (21)	163	19	25	Positive results in 3% of the total of patients
Earnest et al., 1988 (22)	259	259	6.2	Only patients with seizures after alcohol withdrawal were included; 3.9% of patients resulted in significant treatment changes
Reinus et al., 1993 (23)	115	?	36	Post–acute head trauma (60 patients had previous seizure disorder)
Henneman et al., 1994 (24)	333	325	41	Seizures no associated with head trauma

glycemia from diabetic therapy, or alcohol or recreational drug use. Of the 325 patients studied with CT scans, 134 (41%) had clinically significant results.

Bradford and Kyriakedes (25) reported an evidence-based review (limited evidence) of diagnostic tests in this population. The authors report a diagnostic yield of 87% for CT. Predictors of abnormal CT scans in patients with new onset of seizures had the following risk factors: head trauma, abnormal neurologic findings, focal or multiple seizures (within a 24-hour period), previous CNS disorders, and history of malignancy. The article concludes that there are supportive data to perform CT scanning in the evaluation of all first-time acute seizures of unknown etiology.

III. What Is the Role of Neuroimaging in Patients with First Unprovoked Seizures?

Summary of Evidence: Magnetic resonance imaging is the neuroimaging study of choice in the workup of first unprovoked seizures (moderate evidence). Neuroimaging is positive in 3% to 38% of cases. The probability is higher in patients with partial seizures and focal neurological deficit (Fig. 11.1). Neuroimaging is advised in children under 1 year of age and in those with significant unexplained cognitive or motor impairment, or prolonged postictal deficit. Significant neuroimaging findings impacting medical care are found in up to 50% of adults and in 12% of children.

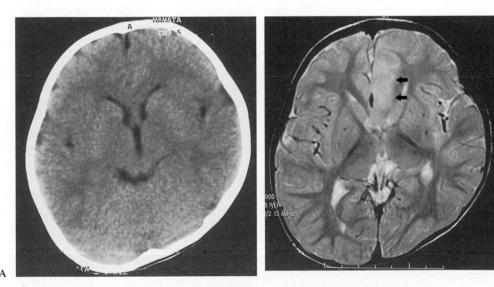

Figure 11.1. Computed tomography (CT) vs. magnetic resonance imaging (MRI) sensitivity in nonacute symptomatic seizure. This figure illustrates the higher sensitivity of MRI in the detection of cortical dysplasia. The transverse CT (A) is compared to the MRI (B) in a child with intractable epilepsy and postural plagiocephaly. The region of cortical dysplasia in the left parasagittal frontal lobe is clearly seen only on the MRI exam by the loss of gray–white matter interface and the increased T2-weighted signal intensity.

Table 11.2. Neuroimaging in first unprovoked seizure

Author	Patients	CT/MRI	% of positives	Comments
Shinnar et al., 2001 (26)	218	186/59	34/22	1.8% significant findings
King et al., 1998 (27)	300	263/14	17/8	
Hirtz et al., 2000 (28)	(EBM review)		18–34	In children: significant findings in less than 7%
Maytal et al., 2000 (29)	66	66/20	21	None with significant findings
Hopkins et al., 1988 (30)	408	408/0	?	3% tumors
Schoenenberger and Heim, 1994 (31)	119	119/0	34	17% with significant findings
Garvey et al., 1998 (32)	50	50/0	17	12% with significant findings

Supporting Evidence: No level I (strong evidence) studies were available (Table 11.2). One level II study (moderate evidence) was found describing a cohort study in which neuroimaging studies were performed in 218 of 411 children (26); CT was performed in 159 and MRI in 59 cases. The cohort was followed for a mean of 10 years and none of the patients had evidence of neoplasm (accepted as the reference standard); 21% of the 218 exams were abnormal. The most frequent diagnoses were encephalomalacia (16 cases) and cerebral dysgenesis (11 cases). Six children had gray-matter migration disorders, which were seen only on MRI. In this study, a higher number of MRIs (34%) than CT studies (22%) were abnormal. In four cases (1.8%) the results altered both the diagnosis and the acute management of the patient. Children in this study who had a neurologic deficit (56% vs. 12%, $p < .001$), or abnormal EEG and partial seizures ($p < .05$) were more likely to have abnormal imaging.

A level III (limited evidence) case series study of 300 adults and children with an unexplained first seizure was reported by King et al. (27) in 1998; 92% of these patients had neuroimaging. A total of 263 patients had MRI and 14 had only CT. Epileptogenic lesions were found in 38 patients (13%). Of these, 17 had neoplasms that changed the patient's medical care. Magnetic resonance imaging detected abnormalities in 17% of patients. Computed tomography was performed in 28 of the 38 cases, with lesions on MRI being concordant with MRI in only 12 cases. Computed tomography missed a cavernous angioma and eight tumors. Magnetic resonance imaging was done in 50 patients with generalized epilepsy and only one had a neoplasm causing partial epilepsy.

In pediatric studies, neuroimaging diagnostic performance was similar to that in the adult literature according to an evidence-based study by Hirtz et al. (28) (limited evidence). However, the overall effect of neuroimaging on medical management was less in children than in adults (28).

The role of CT in evaluating children with new-onset unprovoked seizure was analyzed in a retrospective (limited evidence) study by Maytal et al. (29). Of 66 patients, 21.2% had abnormal CT results. The seizure etiology was clinically determined to be cryptogenic in 33 patients. Two of these children (6%) had abnormal nonspecific CT findings that did not require intervention. No abnormal CT results were seen in 13 cases with complex febrile seizures.

In a level III (limited evidence) study of 408 adults, CT scanning found tumors in 3% of patients. These patients were more likely to have recurrent seizures (30). Other studies have shown a higher percentage of positive imaging results in this population. A total of 119 adult patients with new-onset seizure underwent CT of the brain. Focal structural brain lesions were found in 40 patients (34%; 95% confidence interval, 25% to 42%). In 50% of the patients, the imaging findings prompt an important change in therapeutic management. The major predictor for finding a focal lesion on CT was the presence of a focal neurologic deficit (sensitivity of 50%, specificity of 89%) (31). Another study evaluated 50 patients referred for CT from a group of 107 children with first unprovoked seizure. A total of 19 children had brain abnormalities on CT. Of these, six patients had significant changes in medical workup or treatment (32).

The Quality Standards Subcommittee of the America Academy of Neurology, the Child Neurology Society, and the American Epilepsy Society have published a special report on practice guidelines in the evaluation of first nonfebrile seizures in children (unprovoked seizure) based on evidence-based medicine (EBM) (28) (limited evidence). The selection criteria included some small sample studies that lack stringent EBM criteria. This review article included studies in adults and in children. Analysis of the results found a range of 0% to 7% of children had lesions on CT that changed management of epilepsy (i.e., tumors, hydrocephalus, arachnoid or porencephalic cysts, and cysticercosis). Focal lesions on CT were more common in adults (18–34%).

Overall, MRI found more lesions than CT but did not always change medical management (i.e., atrophy, mesial temporal sclerosis, and brain dysgenesis). This report concluded that there is insufficient evidence to support the recommendation for routine neuroimaging after the first unprovoked seizure. Neuroimaging, however, may be indicated in cases of focal seizures associated with positive neurologic clinical findings. If a neuroimaging study is required, MR is the preferred modality. Emergency imaging with CT or MR should be performed in cases of long-lasting postictal focal deficit, or in those patients who remain confused several hours after the seizure. Nonurgent imaging studies with MRI should be considered in children less than 1 year of age, significant and unexplained cognitive or motor impairment, a partial seizure, EEG findings not consistent with benign partial epilepsy of childhood, and primary generalized epilepsy.

IV. What Is the Most Appropriate Study in the Workup of Patients with Temporal Lobe Epilepsy of Remote Origin?

Summary of Evidence: Magnetic resonance imaging is the imaging modality of choice in temporal lobe epilepsy (moderate evidence). The seizure focus may be lateralized by MR volumetric techniques. Magnetic reso-

Table 11.3. Neuroimaging in temporal lobe epilepsy (TLE) and other partial seizures

Author	Patients	CT/MRI	% of positives	Comments
Harvey et al., 1997 (33)	63	48/58	23/36.5	Study done with two magnets: 0.3 T and 1.5 T; etiologies: 13 HS, 8 tumors, 1 cortical dysplasia, 1 arachnoidal cyst, 1 hamartoma
Kramer et al., 1998 (34)	143	117/42	(35)	Study in children and adolescents: 8 diffuse atrophy, 8 porencephalic cyst, 6 tumors, 6 neurocutaneous syndrome, 6 dysgenesis; neither an abnormality in the neurologic exam nor the type of seizure were predictors for finding a tumor
Lee et al., 1998 (36)	274	0/186	97	Patients with intractable TLE; 65% had HS, 32 had abnormalities in the rest of the temporal lobe; 42 tumors in pediatric patients
Berg et al., 2000 (35)	359	(312)	(13.8)	All pediatric patients; in 3 normal-CT cases the MRI was abnormal; the strongest predictor of abnormal imaging was abnormal motor examination
Sinclair et al., 2001 (37)	42	39/42	31/64	Patients with intractable partial epilepsy; postoperative findings: 13 tumors, 8 HS, 5 dual pathology, 4 cortical dysplasia, 4 tuberous sclerosis, 1 porencephalic cyst
Spencer, 1994 (38)	809	?	43–55	370 patients with temporal lobe abnormalities; the lowest % for extratemporal lobe epilepsy

Note: The reported data in parenthesis are not divided due to lack of further information.

nance sensitivity reaches 97% for hippocampal sclerosis using FLAIR (fluid-attenuated inversion recovery) imaging. Loss of digitations of the hippocampal head has a sensitivity of 92% for hippocampal sclerosis. Quantitative measurement of hippocampal size has a higher sensitivity than qualitative inspection with 76% versus 71%, respectively.

Supporting Evidence: No level I (strong evidence) studies are available (Table 11.3). There is one prospective cohort level II study (moderate evidence) of neuroimaging in temporal lobe epilepsy of childhood (33). Sixty-three children with new-onset temporal lobe epilepsy were included; MRI was performed in 58 (92%) and CT in 48 (76%). The MRI was abnormal in 23 children (36.5%) and included unilateral hippocampal sclerosis (HS) in 12, bilateral HS in one, temporal lobe tumor in eight, arachnoid cyst in one, and cortical dysplasia in one. Computed tomography was positive in 23% of cases, which included all tumors, but failed to detect cases of HS. Computed tomography demonstrated calcifications in the posterior area of the hippocampus in one case that was not detected on MR. This lesion was shown to be a small hamartoma pathologically. The authors proposed three groups to classify partial seizures based on the relationship among neuroimaging findings, prior history, and age:

Group I: Developmental temporal lobe epilepsy (10 patients). Seizures begin in mid- to late childhood (mean age 8.2 years) and neurobehavioral problems are infrequent. This epilepsy is associated with tumors and malformations that are usually long-standing and nonprogressive cortical lesions such as gangliogliomas, dysembryoplastic neuroepithelial tumors, and pilocytic xanthochromic astrocytomas.

Group II: Temporal lobe epilepsy with hippocampal sclerosis (18 patients), included children with significant prior clinical history of neurologic insult, including complicated febrile seizures, hypoxic-ischemic encephalopathy, and meningitis.

Group III: Cryptogenic temporal lobe epilepsy (34 patients) in whom no etiology could be determined.

A level III study (limited evidence) by Kramer et al. (34) studied the predictive value of abnormal neurologic findings on the neuroimaging of 143 children with partial seizures. Fifty patients had neuroimaging abnormalities and 36 had abnormal clinical findings. The neurologic exam findings of hemiparesis, mental retardation, and neurocutaneous stigmata were risk factors in predicting abnormal neuroimaging findings. However, the abnormality detected on neurologic examination or the type of seizure was not a predictive parameter in determining tumor resectability as shown by neuroimaging.

A level III study (limited evidence) by Berg and coworkers (35) reported the neuroimaging findings in a group of 613 children with newly diagnosed temporal lobe epilepsy. A total of 359 patients had partial seizures. Of this group, 312 (86.9%) underwent imaging; 283 had MRI alone or with CT. Relevant abnormalities were found in 43 (13.8% of those imaged). The strongest predictor of abnormal imaging was an abnormal motor examination (odds ratio: 18.9; 95% confidence interval, 9.9% to 36.3%; $p < .0001$).

The MR findings in 186 of 274 consecutive patients who underwent temporal lobectomy for intractable epilepsy were retrospectively reviewed (moderate evidence) (Table 11.4) (36). This was a blinded study with

Table 11.4. MRI sensitivity and specificity in temporal lobe epilepsy

Item	Sensitivity (%)	Specificity (%)	Reference
Hippocampal lesion	93	83	Lee et al., 1998 (36)
Nonhippocampal temporal lobe lesion	97	97	Lee et al., 1998
Global sensitivity for tumor detection	83	97	Lee et al., 1998
High T2 signal for hippocampal sclerosis	93	74	Lee et al., 1998
High FLAIR signal for hippocampal sclerosis	97	?	Jack et al., 1996 (43)

pathology as the reference standard. Magnetic resonance imaging detected 121 hippocampal/amygdala abnormalities (sensitivity and specificity of 93% and 83%, respectively) and 60 other abnormalities in the remainder of the temporal lobe (sensitivity and specificity of 97% and 97%, respectively). Increased signal of the hippocampus on T2-weighted images had a sensitivity of 93% and specificity of 74% in predicting mesial temporal sclerosis (Fig. 11.2). Forty-two temporal tumors were detected with a sensitivity and specificity of 83 and 97%, respectively.

The sensitivity of CT and MRI in temporal lobe pathology was recently reported by Sinclair et al. (37) (limited evidence). Forty-two pediatric patients were studied. All patients underwent temporal lobectomy for intractable epilepsy, hence providing histopathology as the reference standard. Magnetic resonance imaging found abnormalities in 27 cases (64%) and CT scan in 12 of 39 cases (31%). Magnetic resonance imaging was clearly more sensitive than CT in the detection of pathology.

The MRI sensitivity in demonstrating the epileptogenic zone determined by EEG (a weak standard reference) was investigated in a level III study (limited evidence). The weakness of the reference standard is in part compensated by the number of cases. Pooled data of 809 patients, of whom 370 had temporal lobe abnormalities, were analyzed (38). The sensitivity of MR was 55% for temporal epileptogenic zones and 43% for extratemporal regions as determined by EEG.

Moore et al. (39) addressed the incidence of hippocampal sclerosis in normal subjects in a level III article (limited evidence). They studied 207 patients referred for hearing loss with high-resolution MR and found two cases of unsuspected HS. Retrospective chart review revealed that both

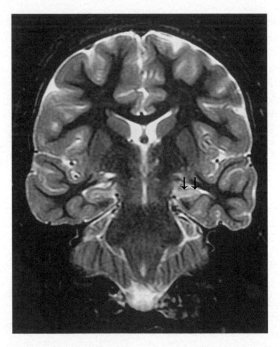

Figure 11.2. T2-inversion recovery MRI. The image corresponds to a patient with intractable epilepsy and EEG findings of left temporal origin. Coronal image at the level of the temporal lobes demonstrates left hippocampal sclerosis characterized by reduction in size, and increased signal intensity (arrows), compared to the normal right hippocampus.

Table 11.5. MRI sensitivity and specificity for hippocampal sclerosis

Author	Patients	Sensitivity	Specificity	Comments
Spencer, 1994 (38)	153	71	?	Review
Moore et al., 1999 (39)	207	100	100	Study conducted in "normal volunteers"; 2 had HS and prior history of seizures in detail chart review
Jack et al., 1990 (40)	41	76	100	Quantitative volumetric measurement of the hippocampus
Oppenheim, 1998 (42)	63	92	100	Based on loss of digitations in hippocampal head
Jack et al., 1996 (43)	36	97	?	FLAIR sequence was compared to SE (91% sensitivity)

patients had seizures. One of them had seizure onset 18 months prior to the MR study that was believed to be associated with hemorrhage from an arteriovenous malformation ipsilateral to the HS.

The most important neuroimaging findings in HS are small size (atrophy) and intense T2 signal of the hippocampus (Table 11.5). These signs have been quantified in a level III retrospective study (limited evidence) of 41 MRI of patients who underwent temporal lobectomy (40). The authors compared measurements of the left and right hippocampal formations and found them to have 76% sensitivity and 100% specificity for correct seizure lateralization.

Watson et al. (41) performed a comparison among different types of epilepsy with volumetric measuring of the hippocampus in 110 patients with chronic epilepsy of whom 81 had partial seizures (limited evidence) and 17 had pathologically proven HS. All 17 patients with HS had reduced absolute hippocampal volumes, greater than 2 standard deviations (SD) below the mean of the control group. The degree of reduced hippocampal size correlates well with the severity of the HS. Hippocampal volumes were within normal range in all patients with generalized epilepsy, and in extratemporal and extrahippocampal temporal lesions.

Oppenheim et al. (42) proposed that the loss of digitations of the hippocampal head on MRI be considered a major criterion of hippocampal sclerosis along with signal abnormality and reduced volume. In a level III case-series study (limited evidence) of 193 patients with intractable epilepsy evaluated retrospectively for atrophy, 63 patients were diagnosed as having mesial temporal sclerosis based on T2 signal changes and loss of digitations of the hippocampal head; 24 of these patients underwent surgery and HS was confirmed in all of them. A control group of 60 patients with frontal seizures and normal MRI was also studied. The digitations of the hippocampal head were evaluated in the two groups. Digitations were not visible in 51 and poorly visible in eight of the 63 patients with mesial temporal sclerosis. Of 24 hippocampi in which HS was confirmed histologically, 22 had no MRI-visible digitations. In the control group digitations were sharply visible in 55 and poorly visible in five. The sensitivity and specificity of complete loss of hippocampal head digitations in HS was 92 and 100%, respectively.

Jack et al. (43) in a level II study (moderate evidence) compared the accuracy of FLAIR sequence with that of conventional dual spin-echo (SE) sequence in the identification of increased signal of HS. The study was blinded and controlled with a reference standard criterion of the histopathologic examination. A total of 36 patients were included. The sensitivity was 97% for FLAIR versus 91% for SE in the diagnosis of HS.

The MRI findings as predictors of outcome of temporal lobectomy were assessed in a cohort (moderate evidence) study of 135 patients (44). Sixty months after surgery, 69% of patients with neuroimaging lesions, 50% with HS, and 21% with normal MRIs had no postoperative seizures. Outcome was worse in those with normal MRI examinations.

V. When Should Functional Imaging Be Performed in Seizure Patients and What Is the Study of Choice?

Summary of Evidence: Functional neuroimaging can provide additional data in seizure patients (Table 11.6). The sensitivity of SPECT for localizing epileptogenic focus increases from interictal (44%) to ictal examinations (97%) (moderate evidence). The sensitivity is lower in cases of extratemporal partial epilepsy in which only the ictal exam is reliable (sensitivity of 92%). Subtraction techniques of the interictal from the ictal study may be helpful; however, the ictal study remains the preferred examination. Positron emission tomography (PET) is more sensitive than interictal SPECT in localizing temporal and extratemporal epilepsy but far less sensitive than ictal SPECT for the localization of epileptogenic foci. More research is needed on MR spectroscopy as a tool to lateralize the epilepsy

Table 11.6. Functional neuroimaging in epileptic focus detection

Author	Procedure	No. of patients	Ictal Sen/Spec	Postictal Sen/Spec	Interictal Sen/Spec	Comments
Spencer, 1994 (38)	PET	312	—	—	84/86* 33/95**	
Spencer, 1994 (38)	SPECT	80	90/73* 81/93**	90/73*	66/68* 60/93**	Compared to EEG False localization was found in 10–25%
Newton et al., 1995 (46)	SPECT	177	97/* 92/*	71/* 46/**	48/* —	
Devous et al., 1998 (45)	SPECT	624	97/*	75/*	44/*	Compared to EEG and/ or surgical outcome

Sen, sensitivity; Spec, specificity.
* In temporal lobe epilepsy.
** In extratemporal lobe epilepsy.

Table 11.7. Functional MRI in language lateralization for epilepsy surgery

Author	Paradigm	No. of patients	Reference standard	Sensitivity (%)	Comments
Woermann et al., 2003 (49)	Word generation	100	Bilateral IAT	91	Cases with localization-related epilepsy; discordant categorization between fMR and IAT includes absence of IAT lateralization in 2 cases
Gaillard et al., 2002 (50)	Reading and naming	30	Bilateral IAT	93	All cases temporal lobe epilepsy; no disagreement with reference standard

IAT, intracarotid amobarbital test.

focus. Functional MRI can help to lateralize language in the workup of patients for epilepsy surgery (limited evidence). Functional MRI has a sensitivity greater than 91% for language lateralization, when the intracarotid Amytal test (Wada test) is used as the reference standard (Table 11.7). fMRI influences the seizure team's diagnostic and therapeutic decision making (moderate evidence).

Supporting Evidence: No level I studies (strong evidence) were found. In the level II meta-analysis study (moderate evidence) reported by Spencer (38), ictal SPECT was performed in 108 patients. Eighty epileptogenic foci were localized by SPECT in the temporal lobe. In temporal lobe epilepsy the diagnostic sensitivity for ictal or postictal SPECT is 90% and the specificity of 73%. In extratemporal lobe epilepsy ictal SPECT sensitivity decreases to 81% and specificity increases to 93% when using EEG criteria as the standard of reference. False localization was found in 5% of cases. Interictal SPECT sensitivity and specificity were found to be significantly lower, at 66% and 68%, respectively, for temporal lobe, and at 60% and 93%, respectively, for extratemporal regions when compared to EEG. False localization was found in 10% to 25%. A later level II study (moderate evidence) by Devous et al. (45) presented a second meta-analysis of SPECT brain imaging in partial epilepsy (temporal and extratemporal). The pooled data were gathered from 624 interictal, 101 postictal, and 136 ictal cases. The vast majority of patients were adults. The reference standard was EEG or surgical outcome (162 cases). The results from this study showed that the sensitivity of technetium-99m labeled hexamethyl-propylene amine oxime (HMPAO) SPECT in localizing a temporal lobe epileptic focus increases from 44% in interictal studies to 75% in postictal studies and reaches 97% in ictal studies. False positives, when compared to surgical outcome, were 4.4% for interictal and 0% for postictal and ictal studies.

A level III study (limited evidence) by Newton et al. (46) of 177 patients with partial epilepsy showed similar results. In 119 patients with known unilateral temporal lobe epilepsy, correct localization by ictal SPECT was demonstrated in 97% of cases. Postictal SPECT was correct in 71% of cases and interictal SPECT in 48% of cases. In extratemporal epilepsy, the yield of ictal SPECT studies was 92% and that of postictal SPECT studies was 46%. The interictal SPECT was of little value in extratemporal epilepsy.

Lewis et al. (47) reported a small level III case series (limited evidence) of 38 patients with seizures not associated with HS using subtraction techniques of interictal SPECT from ictal SPECT. In 58% of the studies the subtraction images "contributed additional information" but were confusing in 9%.

In a level III study (limited evidence) of 312 patients pooled by Spencer (38), PET was compared to EEG for localization. A total of 205 patients had reduced temporal lobe metabolism of which 98% were concordant with EEG findings. Thirty-two patients had hypometabolism in an extratemporal location, which was concordant with EEG in 56% of cases. The abnormalities in 75 patients were not localized by PET, 36 of whom had temporal lobe EEG abnormalities. The diagnostic sensitivity for fluorodeoxyglucose (FDG)-PET was 84% (specificity of 86%) for temporal, and 33% (specificity of 95%) for extratemporal epilepsy, respectively.

A level III study (limited evidence) of single-voxel proton MR spectroscopy (MRS) was performed to lateralize seizures; MRS was compared with MRI and PET in a case series of 33 HS patients (48). Ratios <0.8 for N-acetylaspartate (NAA)/choline (Cho), and 1.0 for NAA/creatine (Cr) were regarded as abnormal. The sensitivity of MRS and PET in lesion lateralization was 85% for both, using MRI as the reference standard. False lateralization rates for MRS and PET were 3% and 6%, respectively. The concordance between MRS and PET was 73%. These results did not influence medical decisions making.

Functional MRI is a new technique based on the ability to detect small amounts of paramagnetic susceptibility produced by blood-oxygen level changes linked to brain cortical activity. Although fMRI is still under investigation and is without Food and Drug Administration (FDA) approval, it has shown promise as an examination that might replace the more invasive and expensive Wada intracarotid amobarbital exam in the lateralization and location of language in patients who are candidates for epilepsy surgery.

Most fMRI papers are based on small samples. One level III case-series paper (limited evidence) (49) describes procedures and results of language dominance lateralization in 100 patients with partial epilepsy performing a covert word generation task. The reference standard was a bilateral Wada intracarotid amobarbital test (IAT) performed in all cases. The results impacted clinical decision making. There was 91% concordance between both tests. Divergent results between the tasks included two cases in which the IAT showed absence of lateralization. Discordance was much higher in cases of left-sided extratemporal epilepsy (25%). In another level III case-series paper (limited evidence), Gaillard et al. (50) described the findings of language lateralization in a group of 30 patients with temporal lobe epilepsy. They used IAT in 21 cases as the reference standard. Eighteen cases had temporal resection and further follow-up. There were no divergent results (i.e., methods pointing to the opposite side). One case showed bilateral fMRI activation and lateralized IAT. Two cases had bilateral IAT and left lateralized fMRI.

The Miami Children's Hospital Group, in a prospective study (moderate evidence), enrolled prospectively 60 subjects to determine the role of fMRI in the diagnostic evaluation and surgical treatment of patients with seizure disorders. In 35 (58.3%) of the 60 patients, the seizure team thought that fMRI results altered patient and family counseling. In 38 (63.3%) of the 60 patients, fMRI avoided further studies including Wada test. In 31 (51.7%) and 25 (41.7%) of the 60 patients, fMRI altered intraoperative mapping plans and surgical approach plans, respectively. In five (8.3%) patients, a two-stage surgery with extraoperative direct electrical stimulation mapping was averted and resection could be accomplished in a one-stage surgery. In four (6.7%) patients, the extent of surgical resection was altered because eloquent areas were identified close to the seizure focus. The authors concluded that fMRI influences the seizure team's diagnostic and therapeutic decision making (51).

A recent study compared the costs of fMRI and IAT (Wada test) in the workup of language lateralization in patients who where candidates for epilepsy surgery (52). Two age-matched groups were studied prospectively. Twenty-one patients had fMRI and 18 IAT. Total direct costs of the Wada test ($1130.01 ± $138.40) and of fMRI ($301.82 ± $10.65) were significantly different (p < .001). The cost of the Wada test was 3.7 times higher than that of fMRI.

Take Home Figure

Figure 11.3 provides a decision-making algorithon for children and adults with seizure disorders.

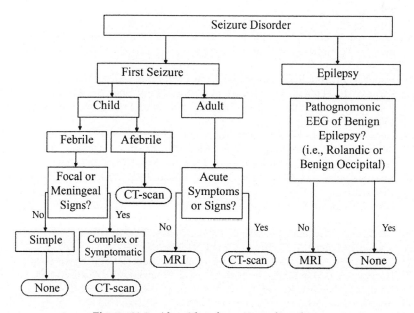

Figure 11.3. Algorithm for seizure disorders.

Future Research

- To define better the different seizure risk groups so neuroimaging can be tailored appropriately.
- To determine the advantages, limitations, indications, and pitfalls of new imaging studies such as functional MRI and MR spectroscopy.
- To determine the impact that imaging has in the outcome of patients with seizure disorders.
- To perform formal cost-effectiveness analysis of the role of imaging in patients with seizure disorders.

References

1. Commission on Classification and Terminology of the International League Against Epilepsy. Epilepsia 1989;34:592–596.
2. Bell GS, Sander JW. Seizure 2001;10:306–316.
3. Senanayake N, Roman GC. Bull WHO 1993;71:247–225.
4. Hauser WA, Annegers JF, Kurland LT. Epilepsia 1993;34:453–468.
5. Lavados J, Germain L, Morales A, et al. Acta Neurol Scand 1992;85:249–256.
6. Rwiza HT, Kilonzo GP, Haule J, et al. Epilepsia 1992;33:1051–1056.
7. Hauser WA, Annegers JF, Rocca WA. Mayo Clin Proc 1996;71:576–586.
8. Berg AT, Shinnar S, Hauser WA, et al. J Pediatr 1990;116:329–337.
9. Knudsen FU. Arch Dis Child 1985;60:1045–1049.
10. Offringa M, Bossuyt PMM, Lubsen J, et al. J Pediatr 1994;124:574–584.
11. Annegers JF, Shirts SB, Hauser WA, et al. Epilepsia 1986;27:43–50.
12. Berg AT, Shinnar S. Neurology 1996;47:562–568.
13. Berg AT, Shinnar S. Neurology 1991;41:965–972.
14. Shorvon SD. Epilepsia 1996;37(suppl 2):S1–S3.
15. Murray MI, Halpern MT, Leppik IE. Epilepsy Res 1996;23:139–148.
16. Ho SS, Kuzniecky RI. J Neuroimaging 1997;7:236–241.
17. De Zelicourt M, Buteau L, Fagnani F, et al. Seizure 2000;9:88–95.
18. Bronen RA, Fulbright RK, Spencer SS, et al. Magn Reson Imaging 1997;15:857–862.
19. Offringa M, Moyer VA. West J Med 2001;175:254–259.
20. American Academy of Pediatrics Provisional Committee on Quality Improvement, Subcommittee on Febrile Seizures. Pediatrics 1996;97:769–772; discussion 773–775.
21. Eisner RF, Turnbull TL, Howes DS, et al. Ann Emerg Med 1986;15:33–39.
22. Earnest MP, Feldman H, Marx JA, et al. Neurology 1988;38:1561–1565.
23. Reinus WR, Wippold FJ 2nd, Erickson KK. Ann Emerg Med 1993;22:1298–1303.
24. Henneman PL, DeRoos F, Lewis RJ. Ann Emerg Med 1994;24:1108–1114.
25. Bradford JC, Kyriakedes CG. Emerg Med Clin North Am 1999;17:203–220.
26. Shinnar S, O'Dell C, Mitnick R, et al. Epilepsy Res 2001;43:261–269.
27. King MA, Newton MR, Jackson GD, et al. Lancet 1998;352:1007–1011; comments 1855–1857.
28. Hirtz D, Ashwal S, Berg A, et al. Neurology 2000;55:616–623.
29. Maytal J, Krauss JM, Novak G, et al. Epilepsia 2000;41:950–954.
30. Hopkins A, Garman A, Clarke C. Lancet 1988;1:721–726.
31. Schoenenberger RA, Heim SM. BMJ 1994;309:986–989.
32. Garvey MA, Gaillard WD, Rusin JA, et al. J Pediatr 1998;133:664–669.
33. Harvey AS, Berkovic SF, Wrennall JA, et al. Neurology 1997;49:960–968.
34. Kramer U, Nevo Y, Reider-Groswasser I, et al. Seizure 1998;7:115–118.
35. Berg A, Testa FM, Levy SR, et al. Pediatrics 2000;106:527–532.
36. Lee DH, Gao F-Q, Rogers JM, et al. AJNR 1998;19:19–27.

37. Sinclair DB, Wheatley M, Aronyk K, et al. Pediatr Neurosurg 2001;35:239–246.
38. Spencer SS. Epilepsia 1994;35(suppl):S72–S89.
39. Moore KR, Swallow CE, Tsuruda JS. AJNR 1999;20:1609–1612.
40. Jack CR Jr, Sharbrough FW, Twomey CK, et al. Radiology 1990;175:423–429.
41. Watson C, Cendes F, Fuerst D, et al. Arch Neurol 1997;54:67–73.
42. Oppenheim C, Dormont D, Biondi A, et al. AJNR 1998;19:457–463.
43. Jack Jr. CR, Rydberg CH, Krecke KN, et al. Radiology 1996;1996:367–373.
44. Berkovic SF, McIntosh AM, Kalnins RM, et al. Neurology 1995;45:1358–1363.
45. Devous Sr. MD, Thisted RA, Morgan GF, et al. J Nucl Med 1998;39:285–293.
46. Newton MR, Berkovic SF, Austin MC, et al. J Neurol Neurosurg Psychiatry 1995;59:26–30.
47. Lewis PJ, Siegel A, Siegel AM, et al. J Nucl Med 2000;41:1619–1626.
48. Park S-W, Chang K-H, Kim H-D, et al. AJNR Am J Neuroradiol 2001;22:625–631.
49. Woermann FG, Jokeit H, Luerding R, et al. Neurology 2003;61:699–701.
50. Gaillard WD, Balsamo L, Xu B, et al. Neurology 2002;59:256–265.
51. Medina LS, Bernal B, Dunoyer C, et al. Radiology 2005;236:247–253.
52. Medina LS, Aguirre E, Bernal B, Altman NR. Radiology 2004;230:49–54.

12

Imaging Evaluation of Sinusitis: Impact on Health Outcome

Yoshimi Anzai and William E. Neighbor, Jr.

Key Points

- Acute bacterial sinusitis is overdiagnosed clinically and antibiotics are overprescribed, leading to antibiotics resistant infections. We need to differentiate patients with acute bacterial sinusitis who may benefit from antibiotic treatment from those with an uncomplicated upper respiratory viral infection (strong evidence).
- Although a computed tomography (CT) scan is frequently performed to assist in the diagnosis of sinusitis, no adequate data exist on the

sensitivity and specificity of sinus CT for diagnosis of acute bacterial sinusitis (limited evidence).
- The diagnosis of chronic sinusitis is based on clinical grounds. No gold standard exists to confirm clinical diagnosis. Computed tomography findings for chronic sinusitis often do not correlate with patients' clinical symptoms (limited evidence).
- Computed tomography influences surgeons' decision regarding which patients will undergo sinus surgery, in addition to providing anatomic information to guide endoscopic sinus surgery (limited evidence).

Definitions and Pathophysiology

The term *sinusitis* technically refers to inflammation of the mucosa of the paranasal sinuses. The paranasal sinuses are lined by mucosa and connect to the nasal cavity. Normal mucous secretions contain antibodies and, together with the ciliary function, work to clear bacteria from the sinuses. Thus, maintaining the mucociliary flow and an intact local mucosal surface are key host defenses against infection (1). Sinusitis is often accompanied by inflammation of the nasal cavity; thus, some prefer the term *rhinosinusitis* rather than sinusitis.

Sinusitis is classified as acute, subacute, or chronic, based on the duration of the illness. Acute sinusitis refers to sinusitis symptoms lasting fewer than 4 weeks, and chronic sinusitis refers to sinusitis lasting more than 12 weeks. Subacute sinusitis falls in between these two. The etiologies of sinusitis include infection (bacterial, viral, and fungal), allergy, noxious chemical exposures, and systemic disease such as metabolic, genetic, or endocrine abnormalities. Bacterial infection commonly follows viral sinusitis. Among bacterial infections, *Streptococcus pneumoniae* and *Haemophilus influenzae* are the most common organisms. Anaerobic bacteria account for 10% of cases and are usually of dental origin. For viral sinusitis, rhinoviruses, influenza, and parainfluenza viruses also invade the sinuses and potentially lead to secondary bacterial infection (2).

Epidemiology

Sinusitis is a highly prevalent disease, affecting 33 million Americans (3). The prevalence of sinusitis has increased in the last decade according to the National Ambulatory Medical Care Survey (from 0.2% of diagnoses at office visits in 1990 to 0.4% in 1995). Fourteen percent of Americans claim to have had a previous diagnosis of sinusitis (4). The Centers for Disease Control and Prevention (CDC) reported that chronic sinusitis is the most common chronic condition for people younger than 45 years and, after hypertension, the second most common for people between 45 and 65 years. The prevalence of sinusitis among children is even higher than adults, and may be as high as 32% in young children (5–7). Men and women are equally affected. Sinusitis is more common in the Midwest and the southern regions of the United States than at the coasts.

Table 12.1. Risk factors for sinusitis

Asthma
Allergy (peripheral eosinophilia)
Aspirin sensitivity
Cystic fibrosis
Kartagener syndrome
Wegener granulomatosis
Sarcoidosis
Cocaine abuse
Smoking
Polyp
Immunocompromised patients
   Cancer
   Organ transplant
   AIDS

The prevalence of acute bacterial sinusitis (ABS) among patients presenting with sinusitis symptoms is not well known since an unequivocal diagnosis of ABS requires sinus puncture and a culture of the aspirate showing more than 10^4 colony-forming units (CFUs) per milliliter in sinus aspirate (8). Sinus puncture is not performed in routine clinical practice because it is invasive and costly. The literature suggests that up to 38% of patients presenting with symptoms of sinusitis in an adult general medicine clinic may have ABS (9).

Certain groups of patients are more susceptible to sinus infection than others. The risk factors for sinusitis are summarized in Table 12.1. Asthma and allergy are the two most common associations with sinusitis (10,11). Samter's triad refers to sensitivity to acetylsalicylic acid, asthma, and sinonasal polyposis. Patients with Samter's triad usually respond less well to surgical treatment (12). Other risk factors include impaired mucociliary function such as cystic fibrosis (13) or Kartagener syndrome (immobile cilia syndrome). Wegener granulomatosis is a systemic vasculitis, commonly involves the paranasal sinuses, and often results in chronic sinusitis. Bone erosion of the nasal septum or turbinate has also been reported in Wegener granulomatosis (14). Another granulomatous disease involving the paranasal sinuses is sarcoidosis (15). Nasal cocaine use also contributes to the development of severe chronic sinusitis as well as osteocartilaginous necrosis and perforation of the nasal septum (16,17).

Immunocompromised patients in general have a higher risk of developing sinus infection. These include patients with organ transplant, underlying malignancy, autoimmune disease treated with steroids, as well as HIV. Recently an increasing number of patients with HIV present with medically refractory sinusitis (18) and may present with pseudomonas sinusitis. Another study indicated that sinusitis in HIV patients involved the posterior sinuses, such as the sphenoid and posterior ethmoid sinuses (19).

Overall Cost to Society

Sinusitis has a significant economic impact on health care organizations. In 1992, Americans spent $200 million on prescription medications and more than $2 billion for over-the counter medications to treat sinusitis (20). The Medical Expenditure Panel Survey (MEPS) by Agency Research and Quality (AHRQ) reported 11 million doctor visits and 1.3 million outpatients visit due to sinusitis in 1999 (21). Approximately 200,000 sinus surgeries are performed each year. The study using data from Agency for Health Care Policy and Research (AHCPR's) 1987 National Medical Expenditure Survey (inflated to 1996 dollars) estimated overall health care expenditures attributable to sinusitis were $5.8 billion, of which 31% ($1.8 billion) was for children 12 years or younger. They concluded that sinusitis needs to be recognized as a serious, debilitating, costly disease that warrants precise diagnosis and effective specific therapy (9). This estimate of costs does not include time lost from work by patients. According to the MEDSAT group, between 1990 and 1992 approximately 73 million restricted activity days were reported by patients with sinusitis, which is a 50% increase over the corresponding total tabulated between 1986 and 1988 (22). Indirect costs due to lost days from work or decreased productivity are enormous. Gliklich and Metson (23), using the SF-36 questionnaire, evaluated the health impact of chronic sinusitis on 158 patients, and reported that chronic sinusitis placed a significantly greater health burden on bodily pain and social functioning than do congestive heart failure, angina, or back pain (23).

Goals

The overall goal for the diagnosis of acute sinusitis is to differentiate patients with acute bacterial sinusitis who may benefit from antibiotic treatment from those with uncomplicated upper respiratory tract viral infection. There is insufficient evidence regarding the validity of sinus CT for the diagnosis of acute bacterial sinusitis.

The goal of sinus CT for chronic sinusitis is to provide objective information to support the clinical diagnosis, to provide detailed anatomy for surgical planning, and to predict which patients most benefit from endoscopic sinus surgery.

Methodology

A Medline search was performed using PubMed (National Library of Medicine, Bethesda, Maryland) for original research publications discussing the diagnostic performance and effectiveness of imaging strategies in the evaluation of sinusitis. Clinical predictors of acute and chronic sinusitis were also included in the literature search, which covered the years 1966 to 2003. The search strategy employed different combinations of the following three terms: (1) *sinusitis*, (2) *CT scan* OR *imaging*, and (3) *infection*. Additional articles were identified by reviewing the reference lists of relevant papers. This review was limited to human studies and the English-language literature. The author performed an initial review of the titles and abstracts of the identified articles followed by review of the full text in articles that were relevant.

I. Acute Sinusitis: How Can We Identify Patients with Acute Sinusitis Who Will Benefit from Antibiotic Treatment?

Summary of Evidence: How to determine which sinusitis patients should receive antibiotic treatment and how to distinguish those patients from ones with uncomplicated upper respiratory tract infection are questions that have been studied in detail in the clinical literature. The majority of the literature supports using clinical guidelines to select patients with acute bacterial sinusitis and recommends the first-line antibiotic treatment (amoxicillin) for patients with severe symptoms and illness longer than 7 days. Imaging studies are not routinely recommended for initial diagnosis of acute sinusitis (limited evidence). Evidence of imaging accuracy for diagnosis of acute sinusitis is very limited (Table 12.2).

Supporting Evidence: Most cases of acute sinusitis diagnosed in ambulatory care are caused by uncomplicated viral upper respiratory tract infections. Bacterial and viral sinusitis are difficult to differentiate on clinical grounds. The clinical literature suggests that the diagnosis of acute bacterial sinusitis should be reserved for patients with sinusitis symptoms lasting 7 days or more who have maxillary pain or tenderness in the face or teeth (especially when unilateral) and purulent nasal secretions (24,25).

A meta-analysis study evaluated by the Canadian Sinusitis Symposium in 1996 revealed that diagnosis should be made based on clinical history and physical examination (26). Five clinical findings comprising three symptoms—maxillary toothache, poor response to decongestants, and a history of colored nasal discharge—and two signs—purulent nasal secretion and abnormal transillumination result—are the best predictors of acute bacterial sinusitis (moderate evidence). These five criteria are called William's criteria. On the other hand, Gonzales et al. (25) reported that purulent nasal secretions alone predict neither bacterial infection nor benefit from antibiotic treatment. Transillumination is a useful technique in the hands of experienced personnel, but only negative findings are useful (limited evidence). Radiography is not warranted when the likelihood of acute sinusitis is high or low but is useful when the diagnosis is in doubt (limited evidence). First-line therapy should be a 10-day course of amoxicillin (strong evidence) and a decongestant (limited evidence). Patients allergic to amoxicillin and those not responding to first-line therapy should be switched to a second-line agent such as macrolide or cephalosporin.

Sinus puncture and culture of the aspirate, although a standard reference, is invasive and costly, and thus not a practical or feasible diagnostic method to identify patients who benefit from antibiotic treatment. Moreover, sinus puncture is technically feasible only for maxillary sinusitis, not for the remainder of the paranasal sinuses.

Nasal swab and culture from the middle meatus is also reported but the correlation with nasal swab with sinus puncture remains weak. Endoscopic-guided swab culture is more accurate to sample secretion from a sinus of interest. However, this is usually performed by otolaryngologists, resulting in higher cost, and thus is not feasible for routine use.

II. Acute Sinusitis: How Accurate Are Imaging Studies for the Diagnosis of Acute Bacterial Sinusitis?

Summary of Evidence: There is no single report from the U.S. concerning testing sensitivity or specificity of CT compared with a sinus puncture and culture of aspirate, which is the gold standard of acute bacterial sinusitis. Only one report measured positive predictive value (PPV) compared with

Table 12.2. Diagnostic performance of clinical examination, radiography, computed tomography, and ultrasound for acute sinusitis

Authors	Study design	Gold standard	Modality	Diagnostic performance	Comments	Reference
Varonen	Meta-analysis	Sinus puncture	Radiography Clinical exam US	ROC curve: 0.82 ROC curve: 0.75 Less accurate	11 articles, 1144 patients included Maxillary sinusitis only	32
Engles	Meta-analysis	Sinus puncture	Radiography Clinical exam* US	Sensitivity: 73% Specificity: 80% ROC curve: 0.83 ROC: 0.74 Variable results	Supported from AHRQ 13 articles Exam incorporated with risk factors	31
Low	Prospective	Radiography	Clinical exam	5 independent factors If more than 4, prob of dz: 81% If more than 3, prob of dz: 63%	247 adult male patients	26
Lindbaek	Prospective	Sinus puncture	CT	90% PPV	Using fluid level and opacification No NPV data	30
Lindbaek	Prospective	CT	Clinical exam**	Sensitivity: 66% Specificity: 81%	**Combination of three or more clinical signs Double sickening, purulent secretion, high ESR	34
Shapiro	Clinical trial	Radiography	US Clinical exam***	Sensitivity: 44–58% Specificity: 55–61% positive correlation	75pt with acute sinus symptoms Maxillary sinusitis only ***Copius and purulent rhinorrhea ($p < .001$)	28
Chen	Clinical series	CT	Radiography Maxillary Others	Sensitivity: 81% Specificity: 73% Sensitivity: 41–52% Specificity: 85–93%	Radiography correlated well with CT only for maxillary sinus disease	33

CT, computed tomography; ESR, erythrocyte sedimentation rate; PPV, positive predictive value; US, ultrasound.

the gold standard of sinus aspiration. Sinus radiography has been reported to have moderate sensitivity. Sinus CT is reported to be more sensitive than sinus radiography, but little is known about its specificity (insufficient evidence).

Supporting Evidence

A. Imaging Modalities for Sinusitis

The diagnostic imaging study for sinusitis is primarily sinus CT. Sinus radiography is rarely performed. There are two main types of sinus CT currently performed in most institutions: limited (or screening) and full (complete) sinus CT. The limited sinus CT was developed to replace sinus radiography (27). Direct coronal images with 3- to 5-mm thickness of the sinuses are obtained every 10 mm from the frontal to the sphenoid sinuses for a limited sinus CT. The limited sinus CT, however, is a quick, more definitive test that is easy to perform and interpret compared with sinus radiography. The limited sinus CT is often referred to as a screening sinus CT to rule out sinusitis, although it is not truly a screening test since the patients have sinusitis symptoms. Full sinus CT is performed using 2.5-mm contiguous coronal images through the sinuses. This study is primarily ordered by otolaryngologists to evaluate detailed anatomy of the ostiomeatal complex. No intravenous contrast is necessary for sinus CT, unless complications of sinusitis are suspected, such as orbital abscess, epidural or brain abscess, or cavernous sinus thrombosis.

Despite wide clinical application of magnetic resonance imaging (MRI), it has not been used routinely as a diagnostic imaging study for sinusitis patients. Ultrasound has been occasionally used for evaluation of the maxillary sinus disease, but the sensitivity of ultrasound is reported to be poor (28). Since the paranasal sinuses are surrounded by bone and contain air, ultrasound has limited value for evaluation of the sinuses.

B. Imaging Criteria for Acute Bacterial Sinusitis

The imaging hallmarks of ABS are the presence of air-fluid level (particularly unilateral) and severe opacification of a sinus (Fig. 12.1). A mild mucosal thickening (less than 4 mm) without fluid level is a nonspecific CT finding that is frequently seen in asymptomatic subjects who undergo head CT or orbital CT for other medical complaints, as well as in patients with a common cold (upper respiratory viral infection) (29), allergy, or asthma (Fig. 12.2). There is no microbiologic proof that those patients with only mucosal thickening do not have ABS, since sinus puncture is not justified for patients without fluid level in the sinus. A double-blinded, placebo controlled, randomized control study of antibiotic therapy for patients with sinusitis symptoms and only mucosal thickening on CT revealed no clinical improvements in patients with antibiotic compared with placebo group, suggesting that those patients with only mucosal thickening do not benefit from antibiotic treatment (30).

It is important for radiologists not to overdiagnose acute sinusitis for patients with mucosal thickening only, since such a CT report contributes to overuse of antibiotic treatment for patients presenting with sinusitis symptoms. The term *sinusitis* means to some primary care physicians acute bacterial infection of the sinus.

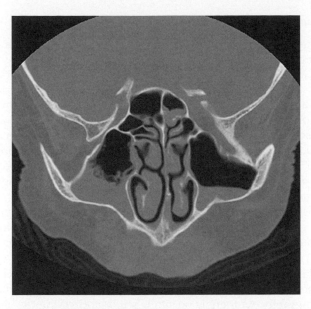

Figure 12.1. A coronal computed tomography image shows presence of air-fluid level in both maxillary sinuses, with bubbly thick mucus secretion in the right maxillary sinus, suspicious for acute sinusitis.

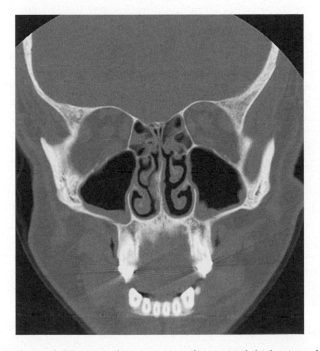

Figure 12.2. Coronal CT image shows nonspecific mucosal thickening of maxillary sinuses bilaterally. The finding is commonly seen in asymptomatic subjects, and patients with allergy, asthma, common cold, or chronic sinusitis.

C. Accuracy of Imaging Studies for Acute Bacterial Sinusitis

A meta-analysis of diagnostic tests for acute sinusitis by Engels et al. (31) report that compared with puncture/aspiration, radiography offers a moderate ability to diagnose acute bacterial sinusitis (summary receiver operator curve area, 0.83). Using sinus opacity or fluid as the criterion for sinusitis, radiography had a sensitivity of 73% and a specificity of 80%. The authors conclude that radiography and clinical evaluation appear to provide useful information for the diagnosis of sinusitis. Varonen et al. (32) also report that clinical examination is a rather unreliable method for diagnosing ABS, even in the hands of experienced specialists, and recommend using radiography or ultrasound to improve the accuracy of diagnosis (32) (limited evidence).

The most comprehensive evidence-based report on the diagnosis and treatment of acute bacterial sinusitis was published by the Agency for Health Care Research and Quality (AHCRQ) authored by Lau et al. (9). According to their report, sinus radiography has a moderate sensitivity (76%) and specificity (79%). They conclude that limited evidence suggests that diagnoses based on clinical criteria may be as accurate as those using sinus radiography. As there is no single study addressing the accuracy of sinus CT for diagnoses of acute bacterial sinusitis compared with sinus puncture, there are no statements in the AHRQ report regarding the diagnostic value of CT.

Despite the lack of evidence, CT scan is occasionally used as a proxy for the gold standard. When comparing sinus radiography and CT, there are a number of reports that sinus radiography has limited sensitivity and specificity. Chen et al. (33) compared the diagnostic performance of sinus radiography and CT in 53 asthmatic children and concluded that sinus radiography has a sensitivity of 81% for maxillary sinus disease, and 41% to 52% for the other sinuses using CT as a standard reference.

It is reasonable to assume that sinus CT is more sensitive for detection of ABS than sinus radiography. The question is the specificity of sinus CT, which depends on the diagnostic criteria used to determine whether the CT is considered positive for ABS. An explicit statement of diagnostic criteria is lacking in many studies with the report only stating that the sinus CT was normal or abnormal. Thus, CT scan has been criticized for the over-diagnosis of ABS.

A study from Netherlands by Lindbaek et al. (34) reported that, compared with sinus puncture and culture of the secretion, sinus CT has a 90% PPV for acute bacterial sinusitis using the presence of an air-fluid level or total opacification of the sinus as diagnostic criteria. Since patients with negative sinus CT did not undergo sinus puncture, no data regarding negative predictive values (NPVs) were available in their study. Also, predictive values highly depend on the prevalence of disease in a study population.

D. Special Case: Pediatric Acute Sinusitis

Imaging diagnosis of acute sinusitis in children is challenging. The paranasal sinuses are in the process of development, and mucosal thickening or fluid collection is physiologically seen in such developing sinuses. Once sinuses are well developed and pneumatized, then diagnosis with sinus CT or radiography is similar to what is observed in an adult population.

A clinical practice guideline regarding the diagnosis, evaluation, and treatment of children with acute bacterial sinusitis recommends that the diagnosis of acute bacterial sinusitis be based on clinical criteria in children 6 years or younger who present with upper respiratory symptoms that are either persistent or severe (35). Although controversial, imaging studies may be necessary to confirm a diagnosis of acute bacterial sinusitis in children older than 6 years. Computed tomography scans of the paranasal sinuses should be reserved for children who present with complications of ABS or who have very persistent or recurrent infections and are not responsive to medical management (moderate evidence).

There are only five controlled randomized trials and eight case series on antibiotic therapy for ABS in children. A placebo-controlled randomized trial by Garbutt et al. (36) found no significant difference in the clinical improvement of children treated with antibiotics compared with those given a placebo. However, children with complications or suspected complications of ABS should be treated promptly and aggressively with antibiotics and, when appropriate, drainage.

E. Special Case: Cost-Effectiveness Analysis in Acute Sinusitis

A few studies have rigorously addressed the cost-effectiveness of diagnosis and treatment for acute sinusitis. Balk et al. (37) reported on strategies for diagnosing and treating suspected acute bacterial sinusitis. They created a Markov model to examine four strategies for acute sinusitis: (1) no antibiotic treatment, (2) empirical antibiotic treatment, (3) clinical criteria-guided treatment, and (4) radiography-guided treatment. The model simulated a 14-day course of illness and included sinusitis prevalence and symptom severity. They concluded that the use of clinical criteria-guided treatment was cost-effective in most cases. The empirical use of antibiotics was cost-effective with higher prevalence. Sinus radiography-guided treatment was never cost-effective for initial treatment.

A meta-analysis by the AHRQ also reported that treatment of uncomplicated sinusitis with amoxicillin or folate inhibitors based on clinical criteria is the most cost-effective strategy (38). Fagnan (39) also stated that sinus radiography and CT generally were not cost-effective in making an initial diagnosis. Most of the literature suggests that sinus radiography is not recommended for the diagnosis of routine cases. The role of sinus radiograph is limited based on the literature, which is in part due to the limited sensitivity or specificity but also to the added cost for diagnosis of this highly prevalent disease. A practice guide based on consensus of Canadian and American experts in infectious diseases, microbiology, otolaryngology, and family medicine states that radiography is not warranted when the likelihood of acute sinusitis is high or low but is useful when the diagnosis is in doubt (limited evidence) (26).

The limitations of these cost-effectiveness analyses (CEAs) include the unrealistic assumption that patients receive the first-line antibiotic, amoxicillin, which is inexpensive. Increasing numbers of physicians, however, prescribe more expensive broad-spectrum antibiotics, in part due to prevalent amoxicillin-resistant infections in the community. Moreover, the model used in the CEA by Balk et al. (37) did not account for downstream societal cost of increasing antibiotic resistant infection. If a diagnosis of acute sinusitis is made by a definitive test, such as CT, it may potentially reduce necessity of antibiotic treatment.

III. Chronic Sinusitis: How Can We Diagnose Chronic Sinusitis?

Summary of Evidence: A diagnosis of chronic sinusitis is usually based on clinical history and physical examination. It is not a pathologic diagnosis, and thus patients' symptoms drive medical care. Sinus CT may show mucosal thickening in various degrees, from minimal mucosal thickening to severe opacification of the paranasal sinuses. Mucosal thickening on CT is nonspecific and could be subtle, since many patients have been treated with antibiotics or antiinflammatory medication prior to CT. Occasionally, bone thickening or sclerosis of the affected sinus is seen, suggestive of chronic periosteal inflammation.

Supporting Evidence

A. Clinical Diagnosis of Chronic Sinusitis

The diagnosis of chronic sinusitis is on clinical grounds. Sinusitis symptoms lasting more than 12 weeks are considered to be chronic sinusitis. No gold standard exists to confirm a diagnosis. Chronic sinusitis symptoms are relatively nonspecific and subtle compared with those of acute sinusitis, including fatigue, cough, postnasal drip, sleep deprivation, and headache. Other conditions may mimic chronic sinusitis, such as migraine, depression, gastroesophageal reflux disease, degenerative disease of temporomandibular joint, head and neck malignancies, or skull base lesions. Thus, when a patient presents with symptoms of chronic sinusitis, the physician needs to know if it is really a sinus-related disease or some other conditions, mimicking chronic sinusitis.

B. Diagnostic Accuracy of Imaging Studies

Since there is no gold standard for the diagnosis of chronic sinusitis, no accuracy data of imaging studies for chronic sinusitis are available. However, several studies have reported correlation of two imaging modalities (CT and plain films) or imaging study with a patient's clinical symptoms (Table 12.3). In a prospective study of 113 patients with chronic sinusitis who underwent plain sinus radiography, Gonzalez Morales et al. (40) found that 60% had abnormalities on plain films. The remaining 40% with normal plain films underwent sinus CT, which showed abnormality in the ethmoid sinuses in all patients. Garcia et al. (41) reported that in 91 pediatric patients with chronic sinusitis, plain films missed significant disease in the frontal, sphenoid, and ethmoid sinuses. A significant difference in diagnostic performance between limited sinus CT and full sinus CT was not found. A prospective study comparing sinus CT and sinus plain radiography read by two radiologists and two emergency physicians showed that sinus CT had higher sensitivity and higher interobserver agreement ($\kappa = 0.74$–0.79) compared with plain radiography ($\kappa = 0.30$–0.39)

Table 12.3. Correlation of clinical symptoms and diagnostic imaging study for chronic sinusitis

Authors	Study design	Patient population	Modality	Results	Reference
Stewart	Clinical trial	254 pts 2 academic centers	CT vs. symptoms	Severity of CT did not correlate with severity of symptoms	44
Arango	Prospective	53 pts in a tertiary care	CT vs. symptoms	CT positive patients had worse symptoms score Extent of disease on CT did not correlate with symptoms score	47
Bhattacharyya	Prospective	221 pts	CT vs. symptoms	CT did not correlate with patients' clinical symptoms Patients with facial pain had lower CT scores than those without	46
Gonzalez	Prospective	113 pts	CT vs. radiography	60% of patients had abnormality on radiography 40% of pts with negative radiograph had ethmoid disease on CT Radiograph had sensitivity of 60% (CT: reference of standard)	40
Garcia	Clinical series	91 pediatric pts	CT vs. radiography	Radiography had sensitivity of 75% for maxillary, 54% for ethmoid, 20% for frontal, and 0% for sphenoid sinusitis (CT is reference of standard)	41
Burke	Clinical series	30 ER pts	CT vs. radiography	Higher sensitivity of sinus CT using CT as reference of standard	42
Lee	Clinical series	33 pediatric pts	CT vs. radiography	Sensitivity and specificity for maxillary sinus: 74% and 76% Sensitivity and specificity for ethmoid sinus: 41% and 44% CT as reference of standard	43

(42). Another study by Lee et al. (43) also confirmed better diagnostic performance of sinus CT compared with plain films in 33 pediatric patients with chronic sinusitis. In that report, sensitivity and specificity of sinus plain films were 74% and 76% for maxillary sinus disease, and 41% and 44% for ethmoid sinus disease, respectively.

There is conflicting evidence whether CT scan correlates with patients' clinical symptoms (44–46). Patients with severe clinical symptoms may not have substantial mucosal thickening on CT. Arango and Kountakis (47) reported, on the other hand, that higher clinical symptom scores were seen in patients with severe abnormality on CT, compared with patients with normal or minimum findings on CT, and that the differences between these two groups were statistically significant. The fact that patient symptom scores did not correlate with the extent of the disease on CT may not necessarily indicate poor accuracy of sinus CT. When sinus CT is normal for a patient with a clinical diagnosis of chronic sinusitis, it is uncertain whether sinus CT underestimates disease or the patient warrants other diagnoses.

C. Imaging Findings of Chronic Sinusitis

Sinus CT may show mucosal thickening in various degrees, from minimal mucosal thickening to severe opacification of the paranasal sinuses. Frequently, for various reasons, sinus CT shows no or only minimal mucosal abnormality. Those patients with persistent chronic sinusitis symptoms have taken antiinflammatory medication as well as nasal spray; thus the degree of mucosal inflammation is usually subtle. Some ear, nose, and throat (ENT) surgeons schedule CT scan 4 to 6 weeks after antibiotic treatment, in order to see fine bone detail, which is often obscured by mucosal disease. Alternatively, those patients may have some other disease mimicking chronic sinusitis. At the other extreme, sinus CT may show severe opacification of all paranasal sinuses. Occasionally, bone thickening or sclerosis of the affected sinus is seen, suggestive of chronic periosteal inflammation. Polypoid soft tissue masses seen within the nasal cavity along with complete sinus opacification is suggestive of sinonasal polyposis (Fig. 12.3), which is often associated with allergy or asthma.

Chronic sinusitis is occasionally caused by fungi, such as aspergillosis or mucormycosis. There are three distinct categories of sinus fungal infection, allergic fungal sinusitis, invasive fungal sinusitis, and fungal ball (also called sinus mycetoma). Allergic fungal sinusitis patients are usually young and immunocompetent. Males are more frequently affected than females. Chronic inspissated secretion may appear in a high attenuation central region separated from the sinus wall on noncontrast CT (Fig. 12.4) (48). The lesion involves multiple sinuses and is often bilateral. Bone destruction and expansion is frequent, mimicking tumor. Treatment is usually surgical debridement and antifungal medication. Invasive fungal sinusitis is seen in immunocompromised or diabetic patients. Acute invasive fungal sinusitis presents with a rapid clinical deterioration and has very poor prognosis. Imaging studies often show infiltrative soft tissue abnormalities with gross bone destruction. Mucormycosis is one of the most common organisms in this entity. Fungal ball is a chronic fungal infection within the sinus, resulting in a well-defined expansile soft tissue mass with mottled foci of calcification.

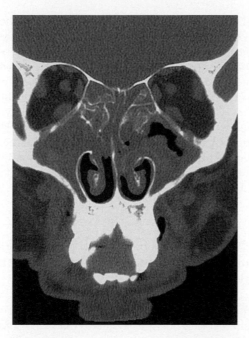

Figure 12.3. A coronal CT image shows severe opacification of all paranasal sinuses with soft tissue fullness within the nasal cavity, suspicious for sinonasal polyposis. Notice thick mucosal thickening of maxillary sinuses bilaterally. Sclerotic changes are also seen in the ethmoid septi, suggestive of chronic inflammation.

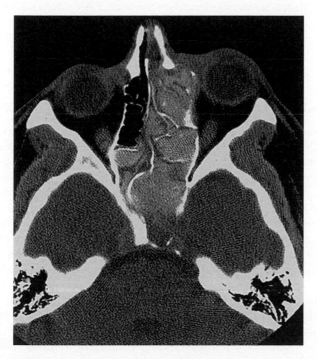

Figure 12.4. Allergic fungal sinusitis. A noncontrast axial CT image shows high attenuation soft tissue fullness within the ethmoid and sphenoid sinuses bilaterally with expansile bone erosion along the left laminae papyracea.

Although MRI is not a primary imaging study for the evaluation of sinusitis, signal characteristics of sinus secretions were evaluated in chronic sinusitis patients. Som et al. (49) reported MR signal intensity changes as a function of protein concentration of sinus secretions. Normal sinus secretions consist predominantly of water; thus it appears as low T1 and high T2 signal intensities. As the sinus secretions become more viscous, the T1 signal intensity increases and the T2 signal intensity slowly decreases. Furthermore, as sinus secretions become more desiccated and sludge-like, they appear as low intensity in both T1 and T2 signals (50), and may become signal void. Fungal sinusitis is also associated with signal void on MRI as paramagnetic substance deposition such as manganese is fairly commonly seen with fungal infection.

IV. Chronic Sinusitis: What Is the Role of Imaging in Chronic Sinusitis? Does Imaging Change Treatment Decision Making?

Summary of Evidence: The roles of sinus CT for chronic sinusitis patients are to support clinical diagnosis, to evaluate the extent of disease, and to provide detailed anatomy to assist treatment planning. The literature suggests that sinus CT findings do not always correlate with patients' clinical symptoms. Whether patients with a normal CT but with persistent clinical symptoms should undergo surgery remains controversial. There is not enough evidence that sinus CT predicts clinical outcomes or that sinus CT affects treatment decisions. Evidence for the CEA of diagnosis and treatment of chronic sinusitis is lacking (insufficient evidence).

Supporting Evidence

A. The Role of Sinus Computed Tomography for Chronic Sinusitis

Despite a lack of evidence and problems related to the diagnosis of chronic sinusitis by CT, it remains the imaging study of choice for patients with chronic sinusitis. One of the roles of sinus CT is to determine whether a patient is truly suffering from chronic sinusitis, as symptoms related to chronic sinusitis are often vague and nonspecific (i.e., headache or facial pain). Completely normal sinus CT performed when a patient is having symptoms without prior medical treatment should suggest other diagnoses. Sinus CT is also indicated for patients who do not respond to medical management and to evaluate any obstructive lesions such as a polyp, inverting papilloma, or sinonasal cancer or anatomic abnormalities impairing mucociliary drainage of the sinus (insufficient evidence).

Once diagnosis of chronic sinusitis is supported clinically and radiographically, an imaging evaluation for chronic sinusitis patients should include the extent of the disease. The distribution of sinus involvement may indicate a mucosal abnormality at the ostiomeatal complex. One should also look for potential complications associated with sinusitis, such as orbital cellulitis/abscess, mucocele or pyocele, epidural or brain abscess using a soft tissue window.

B. The Role of Sinus Computed Tomography Before and After Endoscopic Sinus Surgery

Chronic sinusitis develops from persistent or recurrent sinus inflammation, resulting in impaired ciliary function of the mucosa. Functional endoscopic sinus surgery (FESS) has been developed to repair mucociliary drainage of the sinus (51,52). Once surgery is indicated, CT is essential for providing detailed sinus anatomy as well as the status of ostiomeatal complex prior to FESS (insufficient evidence). Careful attention to key anatomic structures of the ostiomeatal complex is needed. These include ethmoid infundibulum, uncinate process, perpendicular plate and basal lamella of the middle turbinate, ethmoid bulla, nasofrontal duct, sphenoethmoid recess, and fovea ethmoidalis. Although certain anatomic variations such as concha bullosa, paradoxical middle turbinate, and nasal septum deviation can narrow the ostiomeatal complex (53,54), whether or not these anatomical variations cause increased risk of developing chronic sinusitis is not known.

Functional endoscopic sinus surgery has been reported, primarily in the surgical literature, to provide improved clinical outcomes for patients with chronic sinusitis (51,55,56). However, a study evaluating the methodologic quality of FESS investigations reports that most outcome studies of endoscopic sinus surgery lack a control group (57); thus the efficacy of FESS has not been well established. Moreover, a substantial portion of patients who had endoscopic sinus surgery have recurrent symptoms and seek further medical care. Those patients may receive a second or third surgery and undergo additional CT scan prior to the additional surgery.

Common CT findings following FESS include uncinectomy, partial middle turbinectomy, and bulla ethmoidectomy. The extensive middle and inferior turbinectomies are no longer recommended since it may cause dryness or crusting of the nasal cavity, as well as turbulent air flow within the nasal cavity, resulting in perception of difficulty in breathing through the nose. One needs to look for a residual uncinate process for a patient with persistent symptoms after sinus surgery.

C. Computed Tomography Prediction of Clinical Outcome for Chronic Sinusitis

The value of sinus CT for predicting the clinical outcome of patients with chronic sinusitis is highly controversial (limited evidence). Stewart et al. (58) reported that the severity of sinus CT findings was a strong predictor of improved clinical outcome in 57 patients. Patients with severe pretreatment CT abnormality showed significantly larger improvement and lower absolute levels of symptoms after treatment. Kennedy (52), on the other hand, reported a strong correlation between the extent of disease on CT and a poor surgical outcome in 120 patients with chronic sinusitis. Wang et al. (59) also reported that in 230 consecutive patients the extent of disease on sinus CT predicts clinical outcome of endoscopic sinus surgery for chronic sinusitis in that the extent of disease was a consistent predictor ($p < 0.05$) for bleeding, complication occurrence, medical resource utilization, subjective sinus-specific health status, and physicians' objective evaluation of surgical outcomes. Another study of endoscopic sinus surgery indicated that advanced staging of CT and a previous history of sinus surgery correlated with poor clinical outcome (60). Mantoni et al. (61), on the other hand, reported that severity of sinus CT abnormality after FESS does not correlate well with a clinical relief of patients' symptoms.

D. Does Sinus Computed Tomography Affect Treatment Decision Making in Chronic Sinusitis?

Chronic sinusitis is managed either medically or surgically. Because sinus CT has uncertain diagnostic accuracy and poor correlation with patients' clinical symptoms for chronic sinusitis, some otolaryngologists advocate that a treatment decision should be based solely on clinical grounds (44,46). Surgery is indicated when the maximum medical treatment fails to resolve the patient's symptoms. However, there is no consensus as to what represents the maximum medical treatment. Moreover, the basis of treatment decisions, medical versus surgical, for patients with chronic sinusitis is not universally established. Whether or not a patient should be treated surgically, despite normal sinus CT, remains controversial (62). It is an open question whether treatment decisions are purely based on physical examination and clinical history alone, or if sinus CT alters the treatment decisions by ENT surgeons (limited evidence).

We prospectively administered questionnaires to a surgeon specializing in endoscopic sinus surgery each time he saw a patient for suspected sinusitis (63). After obtaining a clinical history and physical examination, we first asked his treatment decision without a sinus CT, and then again after reviewing the sinus CT. The abstracted clinical information of 27 patients was presented to two other otolaryngologists, and the same questionnaires were administered before and after reviewing the sinus CT. Sinus CT altered dichotomous treatment decisions (surgical versus nonsurgical) by the surgeon in one third of patients (9/27) and there was a tendency to offer the surgical treatment after reviewing the sinus CT more than before. The agreement among surgeons with clinical history and physical examination alone was poor but was much improved after reviewing sinus CT. The results of this study indicate that sinus CT provides pivotal objective information that affects treatment decisions and improves the agreement of treatment plans among surgeons (limited evidence).

E. Special Case: Cost-Effectiveness Analysis in Chronic Sinusitis

There has been no CEA for chronic sinusitis from the U.S. or Europe. Only one recent study from Taiwan assessed cost utility analysis of endoscopic sinus surgery. It measured the cumulative cost of treating chronic sinusitis with FESS based on severity of disease. Utility assessment was performed with the six-item Chronic Sinusitis Survey. The study revealed an average cost-utility ratio of $70,221 and a high cost-utility ratio of $103,872 (after conversion to U.S. dollars at 1999 rates) for treatment of more severe sinusitis cases due to the high cost and the limited utility gain (64). Some patients were admitted for surgery with an average length of stay of 2.4 days (standard deviation 1.2). The cost structure in their study showed that 66% of the total cost was the operation fee. Endoscopic sinus surgery is primarily performed on an outpatient basis in the U.S. Evidence is lacking in this field, and future research is needed (insufficient evidence).

Health care costs for patients with chronic sinusitis were investigated in health maintenance organizations (HMOs) in the state of Washington. This study found that adult patients with chronic sinusitis have more nonurgent outpatient visits and fill more prescriptions than adult patients without a history of chronic sinusitis, not including endoscopic sinus surgery. The

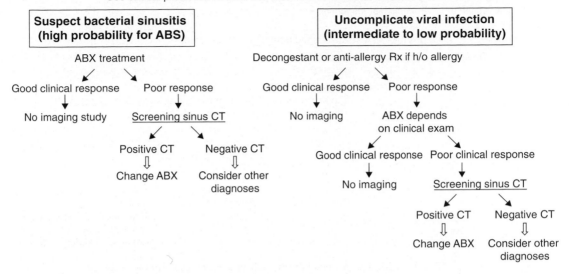

Figure 12.5. Decision tree for imaging evaluation and management of acute bacterial sinusitis (ABS). ABX, antibiotics; h/o, history of.

marginal total cost was $206 and the overall direct cost in the U.S. in 1994 was estimated to have been $4.3 billion (65).

Take-Home Figures

Decision trees for imaging evaluation and management of acute and chronic sinusitis are shown in Figures 12.5 and 12.6.

Suggested Imaging Protocol

1. Noncontrast screening sinus CT
   5-mm-thick coronal images every 10 mm
   140 KVP, 200 MA
   Indications: sinusitis symptoms not responding to medical treatment
   Diagnosis of sinusitis is in doubt, rule out sinusitis
   Recent sinusitis, need to evaluate response to treatment
2. Noncontrast fine-cut maxillofacial CT
   2.5 mm thick helical
   140 KVP, 200 MA
   Indications: patients with chronic or recurrent sinusitis symptoms, need
      to evaluate anatomical abnormality
   Patients with chronic sinusitis failed to respond to the maximal medical
      treatment; considering endoscopic sinus surgery
3. Axial fine-cut maxillofacial CT with coronal and sagittal reformat
   0.625- to 1.25-mm helical scanning with coronal and sagittal reformat
   140 KVP, 175 MA

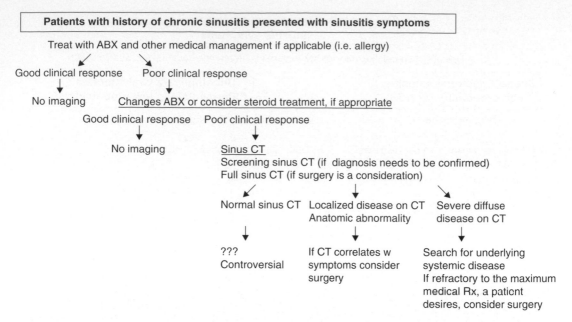

Figure 12.6. Decision tree for evaluation and management of chronic sinusitis.

Indications: patients require imaging-guided monitoring for endoscopic sinus surgery for skull base lesions or complex sinus surgery

Future Research

- Randomized controlled trial of antibiotic for patients with mucosal thickening only on CT in order to determine if this group of patients benefits from antibiotic treatment for acute sinusitis.
- Cost-effectiveness analysis based on more realistic model assumptions regarding types and durations of antibiotic treatment for acute sinusitis.
- Randomized controlled trial of endoscopic sinus surgery compared with sham surgery in order to determine the efficacy of FESS for patients with chronic sinusitis.
- Prospective outcome assessment for chronic sinusitis patients treated medically or surgically in order to determine if CT findings predict treatment response.

Summary

Acute sinusitis
- Despite inaccurate clinical diagnosis of acute or chronic sinusitis, the initial treatment decision is based on clinical diagnosis.
- For patients present with acute sinusitis symptoms, if clinical suspicion for acute bacterial sinusitis is high, patients should be treated with antibiotics.
- If clinical suspicion for acute bacterial sinusitis is intermediate or low, decongestant and conservative management is appropriate. Imaging study is indicated when patients failed to respond to the initial treatment.

Chronis sinusitis
- For patients with clinical diagnosis of chronic sinusitis, imaging study is indicated when patients failed to respond to medical management, in order to determine if symptoms are related to sinusitis, or to evaluate strutural abnormalities.
- Sinus CT provides objective information as to how diffuse or localized disease is, and if symptoms are related to sinusitis, assisting treatment decisions for patients with chronic sinusitis.

References

1. Gwaltney JM Jr, Jones JG, Kennedy DW. Ann Otol Rhinol Laryngol Suppl 1995; 167:22–30.
2. Gwaltney JM Jr, Sydnor A Jr, Sande MA. Ann Otol Rhinol Laryngol Suppl 1981; 90:68–71.
3. Collins J. National Center for Health Statistics Advanced Data 1988;1155: 1981–1916.
4. Willett LR, Carson JL, Williams JW Jr. J Gen Intern Med 1994;9:38–45.
5. Ioannidis JP, Lau J. Pediatrics 2001;108:51–58.
6. Clement PA, Bluestone CD, Gordts F, et al. Int J Pediatr Otorhinolaryngol 1999; 49:S95–100.
7. Garbutt JM, Gellman EF, Littenberg B. Qual Life Res 1999;8:225–233.
8. Turner BW, Cail WS, Hendley JO, et al. J Allergy Clin Immunol 1992;90:474–478.
9. Lau J, DZ, Engles E, et al. Diagnosis and Treatment of Acute Bacterial Rhinos-inusitis. Rockville, MD: Agency for Health Care Policy and Research, 1999.
10. Newman LJ, Platts-Mills TA, Phillips CD, Hazen KC, Gross CW. JAMA 1994; 271:363–367.
11. Senior BA, Kennedy DW, Tanabodee J, Kroger H, Hassab M, Lanza DC. Oto-laryngol Head Neck Surg 1999;121:66–68.
12. Amar YG, Frenkiel S, Sobol SE. J Otolaryngol 2000;29:7–12.
13. April MM, Zinreich SJ, Baroody FM, Naclerio RM. Laryngoscope 1993;103: 985–990.
14. Yang C, Talbot JM, Hwang PH. Am J Rhinol 2001;15:121–125.
15. Anderhuber W, Walch C, Braun H. Laryngorhinootologie 1997;76:315–317.
16. Lancaster J, Belloso A, Wilson CA, McCormick M. J Laryngol Otol 2000;114:630–633.
17. Schweitzer VG. Laryngoscope 1986;96:206–210.
18. Del Borgo C, Del Forno A, Ottaviani F, Fantoni M. J Chemother 1997;9:83–88.
19. Godofsky EW, Zinreich J, Armstrong M, Leslie JM, Weikel CS. Am J Med 1992; 93:163–170.
20. Collins JG. Vital Health Stat 1997;10:1–89.
21. National Center for Health Statistics: Sinusitis. NCHS, Hyattsville, MD, 2002.
22. Kaliner MA, Osguthorpe JD, Fireman P, et al. Otolaryngol Head Neck Surg 1997; 116:S1–20.
23. Gliklich RE, Metson R. Otolaryngol Head Neck Surg 1995;113:104–109.
24. Hickner JM, Bartlett JG, Besser RE, Gonzales R, Hoffman JR, Sande MA. Ann Emerg Med 2001;37:703–710.
25. Gonzales R, Bartlett JG, Besser RE, et al. Ann Emerg Med 2001;37:690–697.
26. Low DE, Desrosiers M, McSherry J, et al. Can Med Assoc J 1997;156:S1–14.
27. Hudgins PA, Mukundan S. AJNR 1997;18:1850–1854.
28. Shapiro GG, Furukawa CT, Pierson WE, Gilbertson E, Bierman CW. J Allergy Clin Immunol 1986;77:59–64.
29. Gwaltney JM Jr, Phillips CD, Miller RD, Riker DK. N Engl J Med 1994;330:25–30.
30. Lindbaek M, Hjortdahl P, Johnsen UL. BMJ 1996;313:325–329.
31. Engels EA, Terrin N, Barza M, Lau J. J Clin Epidemiol 2000;53:852–862.

32. Varonen H, Makela M, Savolainen S, Laara E, Hilden J. J Clin Epidemiol 2000; 53:940–948.
33. Chen LC, Huang JL, Wang CR, Yeh KW, Lin SJ. Asian Pac J Allergy Immunol 1999;17:69–76.
34. Lindbaek M, Hjortdahl P, Johnsen UL. Fam Med 1996;28:183–188.
35. American Academy of Pediatrics. Pediatrics 2001;108:798–808.
36. Garbutt JM, Goldstein M, Gellman E, Shannon W, Littenberg B. Pediatrics 2001; 107:619–625.
37. Balk EM, Zucker DR, Engels EA, Wong JB, Williams JW Jr, Lau J. J Gen Intern Med 2001;16:701–711.
38. Benninger MS, Sedory Holzer SE, Lau J. Otolaryngol Head Neck Surg 2000; 122:1–7.
39. Fagnan LJ. Am Fam Physician 1998;58:1795–1802, 1805–1796.
40. Gonzalez Morales JE, Leal de Hernandez L, Gonzalez Spencer D. Usefulness of simple paranasal sinus radiographs and axial computed tomography in the diagnosis of chronic sinusitis (in Spanish). Rev Alerg Mex 1998;45:17–21.
41. Garcia DP, Corbett ML, Eberly SM, et al. J Allergy Clin Immunol 1994;94: 523–530.
42. Burke TF, Guertler AT, Timmons JH. Acad Emerg Med 1994;1:235–239.
43. Lee HS, Majima Y, Sakakura Y, Inagaki M, Sugiyama Y, Nakamoto S. Nippon Jibiinkoka Gakkai Kaiho 1991;94:1250–1256.
44. Stewart MG, Sicard MW, Piccirillo JF, Diaz-Marchan PJ. Am J Rhinol 1999; 13:161–167.
45. Piccirillo JF, Merritt MG Jr, Richards ML. Otolaryngol Head Neck Surg 2002; 126:41–47.
46. Bhattacharyya T, Piccirillo J, Wippold FJ. Arch Otolaryngol Head Neck Surg 1997;123:1189–1192.
47. Arango P, Kountakis SE. Laryngoscope 2001;111:1779–1782.
48. Mukherji SK, Figueroa RE, Ginsberg LE, et al. Radiology 1998;207:417–422.
49. Som P, Dillon W, Fullerton G, et al. Radiology 1989;172:515–520.
50. Som PM, Brandwein M. In: Som PM, Curtin HD, eds. Head and Neck Imaging, 3rd ed. St. Louis: Mosby, 1996;125–315.
51. Kennedy DW, Senior BA. Otolaryngol Clin North Am 1997;30:313–330.
52. Kennedy DW. Laryngoscope 1992;102:1–18.
53. Calhoun KH, Waggenspack GA, Simpson CB, Hokanson JA, Bailey BJ. Otolaryngol Head Neck Surg 1991;104:480–483.
54. Yousem DM, Kennedy DW, Rosenberg S. J Otolaryngol 1991;20:419–424.
55. Senior BA, Kennedy DW, Tanabodee J, Kroger H, Hassab M, Lanza D. Laryngoscope 1998;108:151–157.
56. Metson R, Gliklich RE. Arch Otolaryngol Head Neck Surg 1998;124:1090–1096.
57. Lieu JE, Piccirillo JF. Arch Otolaryngol Head Neck Surg 2003;129:1230–1235.
58. Stewart MG, Donovan DT, Parke RB, Bautista MH. Otolaryngol Head Neck Surg 2000;123:81–84.
59. Wang PC, Chu CC, Liang SC, Tai CJ. Otolaryngol Head Neck Surg 2002; 126:154–159.
60. Marks SC, Shamsa F. Am J Rhinol 1997;11:187–191.
61. Mantoni M, Larsen P, Hansen H, Tos M, Berner B, Orntoft S. Eur Radiol 1996;6:920–924.
62. Kennedy DW. JAMA 2000;283:2143–2150.
63. Anzai Y, Weymuller EA, Yueh B, Maronian N, Jarvik JG. The impact of sinus computed tomography on treatment decisions for chronic sinusitis. Arch Otolaryngol Head Neck Surg 2004;130(4):423–428.
64. Wang PC, Chu CC, Liang SC, Tai CJ. Otolaryngol Head Neck Surg 2004; 130:31–38.
65. Murphy MP, Fishman P, Short SO, Sullivan SD, Yueh B, Weymuller EA Jr. Otolaryngol Head Neck Surg 2002;127:367–376.

13

Neuroimaging for Traumatic Brain Injury

Karen A. Tong, Udo Oyoyo, Barbara A. Holshouser, and Stephen Ashwal

Issues

Key Points

- Head injury is not a homogeneous phenomenon and has a complex clinical course. There are different mechanisms, varying severity, diversity of injuries, secondary injuries, and effects of age or underlying disease.
- Classifications of injury and outcomes are inconsistent. Differences in diagnostic procedures and practice patterns prevent direct comparison of population-based studies.

233

- There are a variety of imaging methods that measure different aspects of injury, but there is not one all-encompassing imaging method.
- Plain films have limited use for evaluating traumatic brain injury (moderate evidence).
- Computed tomography (CT) is an important part of the initial evaluation and currently is the imaging modality of choice for screening of life-threatening lesions requiring surgical intervention. It is probably more useful for predicting short-term/crude (survival versus mortality) outcomes (moderate evidence).
- Magnetic resonance imaging (MRI) is more sensitive than CT and is useful for secondary evaluation. It is more useful for predicting long-term outcome, although utility remains controversial (moderate evidence). Functional MRI holds promise for predicting neuropsychological outcomes (limited evidence).
- Accurate prognostic information is important for determining management, but there are different needs for different populations. In severe traumatic brain injury, information is important for acute patient management, long-term rehabilitation, and family counseling. In mild or moderate traumatic brain injury, patients with subtle impairments may benefit from counseling and education.

Definition and Pathophysiology

Head trauma is difficult to study because it is a heterogeneous entity that encompasses many different types of injuries that may occur together (Table 13.1). Definitions of age groups, injuries and outcomes are also variable. Classification of injury severity is usually defined by the Glasgow Coma Scale (GCS) score, a scale ranging from 3 to 15, which is often grouped into mild, moderate, or severe categories. There is inconsistency in the timing of measurement, with some investigators using initial or field GCS while others use postresuscitation GCS. Grouping of GCS scores also vary. There is no universal definition of mild or minor head injury (1), as some use GCS scores of 13 to 15 (2,3), while others use 14 to 15 (1) and others use only 15. Variable definitions result in inconsistencies in imaging recommendations. Moderate traumatic brain injury (TBI) is defined by a GCS of 9 to 12. Severe TBI is defined by a GCS of 3 to 8.

Classification and measures of outcome are even more variable. The most commonly used outcome measure is the Glasgow Outcome Scale (GOS) (4). It is an overall measure based on degree of independence and ability to participate in normal activities, with five categories: 5, good recovery; 4, moderate disability; 3, severe disability; 2, vegetative state (VS); and 1, death. The GOS is often dichotomized, although grouping is variable. Recently modified, the extended GOS (5) has eight categories: 8, good recovery; 7, good recovery with minor physical or mental deficits; 6, moderate disability, able to return to work with some adjustments; 5, works at a lower level of performance; 4, severe disability, dependent on others for some activities; 3, completely dependent on others; 2, VS; and 1, death. Less common outcome scales include: the Differential Outcome Scale (DOS) (6), the Rappaport Disability Rating Scale (DRS) (7), the Dis-

Table 13.1. Types of head injury (excluding penetrating/missile injuries and nonaccidental trauma)

Primary injuries
- Peripheral, nonintracranial
  - Scalp or soft tissue injury
  - Facial or calvarial fractures
- Extraaxial
  - Extradural or epidural hemorrhage
  - Subdural hemorrhage
  - Traumatic subdural effusion or "hygroma"
  - Subarachnoid hemorrhage
  - Intraventricular hemorrhage
- Parenchymal
  - Contusion
    - Hemorrhagic
    - Nonhemorrhagic
    - Both
  - Shearing injury or "diffuse axonal injury"
    - Hemorrhagic
    - Nonhemorrhagic
    - Both
- Vascular
  - Arterial dissection/laceration/occlusion
  - Dural venous sinus laceration/occlusion
  - Carotid-cavernous fistula

Secondary injuries
- Cerebral edema
- Focal infarction
- Diffuse hypoxic-ischemic injury
- Hydrocephalus
- Infection

ability Score (DS) (8), the FIM instrument (9), the Supervision Rating Scale (SRS) (10), and the Functional Status Examination (FSE) (11,12).

The timing of outcome measurement also varies. Some investigators measure outcomes at discharge and at 3, 6, or 12 months (or more) after injury. This may be problematic because outcomes often improve with time. However, there is moderate to strong evidence that 6 months is an appropriate time point to measure outcomes for clinical trials (13). Neuropsychological assessment is the most sensitive measure of outcome, although this is difficult to perform in severely injured patients, resulting in selection bias. There is a wide variety of psychometric scales for various components of cognitive function such as intellect, orientation, attention, language, speech, information processing, motor reaction time, memory, learning, visuoconstructive ability, verbal fluency, mental flexibility, executive control, and personality. Currently, research has not been able to demonstrate strong relationships between neuroimaging in the acute period and long-term neuropsychological impairment (14,15).

Epidemiology in the United States

There is difficulty in determining the prevalence of TBI because many less severely injured patients are not hospitalized, and cases with multiple injuries may not be included. Estimates are often based on existing disabilities. Approximately 1.74 million/year suffer mild TBI that results in a physician visit or temporary disability of at least 1 day (16) and more than 1 million visits per year to emergency departments are for TBI-related injuries (17). There are more than 230,000 TBI-related hospitalizations/year (17), perhaps up to 500,000/year (18), which account for 12% of all hospital admissions (18). Traumatic brain injury is responsible for nearly 40% of all deaths from acute injuries (16). Between 1989 and 1998, there were approximately 53,000 TBI-related deaths/year, for a rate of 20.6/100,000 population (17). The major causes of TBI-related deaths are firearms (40%), motor vehicle accidents (MVAs) (34%), and falls (10%) (17). The risk of TBI peaks between the ages of 15 and 30 (16), with the highest TBI-related death rates occurring in American Indian/Alaska natives, males, and persons over the age of 75 (17).

Overall Cost to Society

From 1989 to 1998 there has been an overall decline in TBI-related deaths, probably due to multiple factors including improvements in medical care, use of evidence-based guidelines, and injury-prevention efforts (17). An estimated 5.3 million U.S. residents live with permanent TBI-related disabilities (17). Direct costs are estimated at $4 billion/year (16). In 1995, total direct and indirect costs of TBI were estimated at $56 billion/year (17). There are few data on the costs of TBI related solely to imaging. There has been one small study (limited evidence) that determined that 60% of patients were found to have additional lesions on MRI, but because none of these additional findings changed management, MRI resulted in a non–value-added benefit incremental increase of $1891 per patient and a $3152 incremental increase in charges to detect each patient with a lesion not identified on CT (19).

Goals of Neuroimaging

- To detect the presence of injuries that may require immediate surgical or procedural intervention.
- To detect the presence of injuries that may benefit from early medical therapy.
- To determine the prognosis of patients to tailor rehabilitative therapy or help with family counseling.

Methodology

A search of the Medline/PubMed electronic database (National Library of Medicine, Bethesda, Maryland) was performed using the following keywords: (1) *head injury, head trauma, brain injury, brain trauma, traumatic brain injury*, or *TBI*; and (2) *CT, computed tomography, computerized tomography, MR, magnetic resonance, spectroscopy, diffusion, diffusion tensor, functional magnetic, functional MR*, *T2*, *FLAIR, GRE, gradient-echo*. No time limits were applied for the searches, which were repeated several times up to April 16, 2004. Searches were limited to the English-language literature, abstracts, and human subjects. A search of the National Guideline Clearinghouse at www.guideline.gov was also performed using the following key words: (1) *head injury, head trauma*, and *brain injury*; and (2) *parameter* and *guideline.*

I. Which Patients with Head Injury Should Undergo Imaging in the Acute Setting?

Summary of Evidence: The need for acute imaging is generally based on the severity of injury. It is agreed that severe TBI (based on GCS score) indicates the need for urgent CT imaging to determine the presence of lesions that may require surgical intervention (strong evidence). There is greater variability concerning recommendations for imaging of patients with mild or moderate TBI, although there are several recent guidelines (strong evidence) summarized in take-home Tables 13.2 and 13.3.

Supporting Evidence: There are several clinical prediction rules (strong evidence) for evaluating mild/minor head injury in adults, based on prospective studies. The Canadian Head CT Rule (2001) (20) was developed from prospective analysis of 3121 patients with GCS scores of 13 to 15. A CT scan was recommended if a patient had any of the following: GCS score <15 after 2 hours; suspected open or depressed skull fracture; any sign of basal skull fracture; episode(s) of vomiting; age greater than 65 (associated with high risk for neurosurgical intervention); amnesia for the period occurring 30 minutes or more before impact; or an injury due to a dangerous mechanism, such as being struck by or ejected from a motor vehicle (associated with a medium risk for brain injury on CT). Another guideline by Haydel and colleagues (21) was developed after prospective analysis of 520 patients in the first phase and 909 patients in the second phase. After recur-

Table 13.2. Suggested guidelines for acute neuroimaging in adult patient with mild TBI (Glasgow Coma Scale score 13 to 15)

If GCS 13–15, CT recommended if patient has any one of the following:
- **High risk**
  - GCS remains <15 at 2 hours after injury
  - Suspected open or depressed skull fracture
  - Any clinical sign of basal skull fracture
  - Two or more episodes of vomiting
  - Aged 65 years or older
- **Medium risk**
  - Possible loss of consciousness
  - Amnesia for period before impact, of at least 30-minute time span
  - Dangerous mechanism (pedestrian versus motor vehicle, ejected from motor vehicle, fall from greater than 3 feet or five stairs)
  - Any transient neurologic deficit
  - Headache, vomiting

If GCS of 15, patient can be discharged without CT scan if:
- **Low risk**
  - GCS remains 15
  - No loss of consciousness or amnesia
  - No neurologic/cognitive abnormalities
  - No headache, vomiting

CT, computed tomography, TBI, traumatic brain injury, GCS, Glasgow coma scale.
Source: Modified from the Canadian Head CT Rule (20), EAST guidelines (2), and the Neurotraumatology Committee of the World Federation of Neurosurgical Societies (1).

Table 13.3. Suggested guidelines for acute neuroimaging in adult patient with severe TBI (GCS 3–8)

- CT scan patient with severe TBI as soon as possible to determine if require surgical intervention
- If initial scan is normal, but patient has neurologic deterioration, repeat CT scan or consider MRI as soon as possible
- If initial scan is abnormal, but patient status is unchanged, repeat CT scan within 24 to 36 hours to determine possible progressive hemorrhage or edema requiring surgical intervention, particularly if initial scan showed:
  ○ Any intracranial hemorrhage
  ○ Any evidence of diffuse brain injury
- If initial scan is abnormal, repeat CT scan or consider MRI as soon as possible if GCS worsens
- Consider MRI within first few days if:
  ○ Suspect secondary injury such as focal infarction, diffuse hypoxic-ischemic injury or infection

TBI, traumatic brain injury; CT, computed tomography; MRI, magnetic resonance imaging; GCS, Glasgow coma scale.

sive partitioning of variables in the first phase, seven variables were tested in the second phase: headache, vomiting, age over 60 years, drug or alcohol intoxication, short-term memory deficits, physical evidence of trauma above the clavicles, and seizure. All patients with positive CT scans had at least one variable, resulting in 100% sensitivity (21). An older guideline (1995), prospectively analyzed 51 clinical variables in 540 patients in the first phase and 10 remaining variables in 273 patients in the second phase. The resulting sensitivity and negative predictive value were 96% and 94%, respectively (22).

A guideline, "Practice Management Guidelines for the Management of Mild Traumatic Brain Injury," developed by the Eastern Association for the Surgery of Trauma (EAST) Practice Management Guidelines Work Group (2001) (2), was based on level II evidence from several studies (three retrospective and one uncontrolled prospective). They reported that 3% to 17% of patients with mild injuries had significant CT findings, although they noted that there was no uniform agreement as to what constitutes a positive CT scan in different studies. They also reported that a patient with a normal head CT had a 0% to 3% probability of neurologic deterioration. Therefore, if a patient had a GCS of 15 and no neurologic/cognitive abnormalities, it was recommended that the patient be discharged. A CT scan was recommended for all patients with transient neurologic deficits.

One guideline for severe TBI, "Management and Prognosis of Severe Traumatic Brain Injury" (2000), was developed by the American Association of Neurological Surgeons (AANS), and approved by the American Society of Neuroradiology, the American Academy of Neurology, the American College of Surgeons, the American College of Emergency Physicians, the Society for Critical Care Medicine, and the American Academy of Physical Medicine and Rehabilitation (23,24). An extensive review of the CT literature supported the need for CT in the acute period. Computed tomography was reported to be abnormal in 90% of patients with severe head injury. Computed tomography is included as a necessary step in the algorithm of initial management.

II. What Is the Sensitivity and Specificity of Imaging for Injury Requiring Immediate Treatment/Surgery?

Summary of Evidence: Computed tomography is the mainstay of imaging in the acute period. The majority of evidence relates to the use of CT for detecting injuries that may require immediate treatment or surgery. Speed, availability, and lesser expense of CT studies remain important factors for using this modality in the acute setting. Sensitivity of detection also increases with repeat scans in the acute period (strong evidence).

Supporting Evidence: The incidence of injury-related abnormalities on CT is related to the severity of injury. After minor head injury, the incidence is approximately 6% (25) and increases up to 15% in the elderly population (26); those with GCS 13 or 14 have higher frequency of abnormalities than those with GCS 15 (27). The incidence of CT abnormalities in moderate head injury (with GCS of 9 to 13) has been reported to be 61% (28). The sensitivity of CT for detecting abnormalities after severe TBI (GCS below 9) varies from 68% to 94%, while normal scans range from approximately 7% to 12% (29). Several studies have shown that the timing of CT studies also affects the sensitivity. Oertel and colleagues (30) (strong evidence) prospectively studied 142 patients with moderate or severe injury who had undergone more than one CT scan within the first 24 hours, and found that the initial CT scan did not detect the full extent of hemorrhagic injuries in almost 50% of patients, particularly if scanned within the first 2 hours. The likelihood of progressive hemorrhagic injury that potentially required surgical intervention was greatest for parenchymal hemorrhagic contusions (51%), followed by epidural hematoma (EDH) (22%), subarachnoid hemorrhage (SAH) (17%), and subdural hemorrhage (SDH) (11%). Servadei and colleagues (31) (strong evidence) prospectively studied 897 patients with more than one CT scan, and found that 16% of patients with diffuse brain injury demonstrated significant evolution of injury. This was more frequent in those with midline shift, often evolving to mass lesions. Similar results have been seen in retrospective studies (32). Therefore, it is useful to perform repeat CT scans in the acute period, particularly after moderate and severe injury, although the timing has not been clearly determined.

III. What Is the Sensitivity and Specificity of Imaging for All Brain Injuries?

Summary of Evidence: The sensitivity and specificity of MRI for brain injury is generally superior to CT, although most studies have been retrospective and very few head-to-head comparisons have been performed in the recent decade. Computed tomography is clearly superior to MRI for the detection of fractures, but MRI outperforms CT in detection of most other lesions (limited to moderate evidence), particularly diffuse axonal injury (DAI). However, MRI is expensive and not widely available, which also hinders research. Because different sequences vary in the ability to detect certain lesions, it is often difficult to compare results. Although MRI facilitates more detailed analysis of injuries, including metabolic and physiologic measures, further evidence-based research is needed.

Supporting Evidence: Magnetic resonance imaging has higher sensitivity than CT, though most comparison studies were performed in the late 1980s and early 1990s (with older generation or lower field scanners). Orrison and colleagues (33) (moderate evidence) retrospectively studied 107 patients with MRI and CT within 48 hours and showed that MRI had an overall sensitivity of 97% compared to 63% for CT, even when a low-field MRI scanner was used, with better sensitivity for contusion, shearing injury, and subdural and epidural hematoma. Ogawa and colleagues (34) (moderate evidence) detected more lesions with conventional MRI than with CT, with the exception of subdural and subarachnoid hemorrhages, in a prospective study of 155 patients, although they were studied at variable time points. Other studies (moderate evidence), showed better detection of nonhemorrhagic contusions and shearing injuries (35) and of brainstem lesions (36).

Some lesions, such as DAI, are clearly better detected with MRI, and have been reported in up to 30% of patients with mild head injury with normal CT (37) (limited evidence). However, sensitivity depends on the sequence, field strength, and type of lesion. Gradient echo (GRE) sequences are best for detecting hemorrhagic DAI, although the proportion of hemorrhagic versus nonhemorrhagic DAI is not truly known. An early report (limited evidence) suggested that fewer than 20% of DAI lesions were visibly hemorrhagic (38), but this is likely to be erroneously low, due to poor sensitivity of the imaging methods available at that time. We have recently studied a new susceptibility-weighted imaging (SWI) sequence (at 1.5 T) that is a modified GRE sequence, and have shown significantly better detection of small hemorrhagic shearing lesions compared to conventional GRE (39) (limited evidence). Scheid and colleagues (moderate evidence) (40) prospectively studied 66 patients using high-field (3.0 T) MRI and found that T2*-weighted GRE sequences detected significantly more lesions than conventional T1- or T2-weighted sequences. The fluid-attenuated inversion recovery (FLAIR) sequence is useful for detecting SAH, SDH, contusions, nonhemorrhagic DAI, and perisulcal lesions, but there are few studies comparing the sensitivity of FLAIR to other sequences. One study (limited to moderate evidence) found that FLAIR sequences were significantly more sensitive than spin echo (SE) sequences ($p < .01$) in detection of all lesions studied within 1 to 36 days (0.5 T), particularly in those who had DAI-type lesions (41).

Diffusion weighted imaging (DWI) has also recently been shown to improve the detection of nonhemorrhagic shearing lesions, although there are only a few small studies describing sensitivity. A small study (insufficient evidence) of patients scanned within 48 hours found that DWI identified an additional 16% of shearing lesions that were not seen on conventional MRI. The majority of DWI-positive lesions (65%) had decreased diffusion (42). Another descriptive study (limited evidence) characterized several different types and patterns of DWI lesions, although there was no comparison with other MRI sequences or analysis of diffusion changes over time (43). A recent study (limited evidence) found a strong correlation between apparent diffusion coefficient (ADC) histograms and GCS score (44). There are even fewer data on the sensitivity of diffusion tensor imaging (DTI). A few small studies (insufficient or limited evidence) have shown decreased anisotropy in brain parenchyma of TBI patients (45–47).

Although CT and MRI are often limited to observing structural abnormalities associated with TBI, magnetic resonance spectroscopy (MRS) can detect subtle cellular abnormalities that may more accurately estimate the extent of brain injury, particularly DAI. However, the sensitivity and specificity of MRS are not easily addressed, as only a small number of studies have been published. Several small studies have been performed using single voxel spectroscopy (SVS), although measured at variable time points. These have reported (insufficient evidence) decreased N-acetylaspartate (NAA) in the frontoparietal white matter (WM) (48,49), gray matter (GM) (50), or normal-appearing brain (51). Others have shown that NAA-derived ratios were decreased in areas particularly vulnerable to DAI (moderate evidence), such as the splenium of the corpus callosum (52,53). There has been insufficient evidence regarding the sensitivity of multivoxel magnetic resonance spectroscopic imaging (MRSI), although decreases in NAA have been detected in areas of visible T2 abnormality as well as normal-appearing regions compared to controls (54). There has been one small study using phosphorous MRS (insufficient evidence), which found alkaline pH, increased free intracellular magnesium, increased phosphocreatine to inorganic phosphate ratio (PCr/Pi), and reduced inorganic phosphate to adenosine triphosphate ratio (Pi/ATP) (55) in brains of severely injured patients. Further research regarding the sensitivity of MRS in TBI is warranted.

Several imaging methods permit in vivo assessment of regional metabolism or blood flow, which may be impaired after brain injury. These methods include CT, MRI, and nuclear medicine imaging techniques. The latter have been the most studied, although evidence remains limited. Most studies consist of small sample sizes, and have been performed in the subacute period. Single photon emission computed tomography (SPECT) can measure regional cerebral blood flow (CBF) and assess localized perfusion deficits that may correlate with cognitive deficits even in the absence of structural abnormalities. However, SPECT has low spatial and temporal resolution, does not permit imaging of transient cognitive events, and interpretation is often highly subjective. The SPECT studies generally show patchy perfusion deficits, often in areas with no visible injury on CT. One of the largest studies, although retrospective, was performed by Abdel-Dayem and colleagues (56) (moderate evidence), who reviewed SPECT findings in 228 subjects with mild or moderate TBI. They found focal areas of hypoperfusion in 77% of patients. However, there was no comparison to CT or MRI. Stamatakis and colleagues (57) (moderate evidence) studied 61 patients with SPECT and MRI, within 2 to 18 days after injury, and found that SPECT detected more extensive abnormality than MRI in acute and follow-up studies. A small study (limited evidence) of patients with persistent postconcussion syndrome after mild TBI found that SPECT showed abnormalities in 53% of patients, whereas MRI and CT showed abnormalities in only 9% and 4.6%, respectively (58)

Positron emission tomography (PET) can measure regional glucose and oxygen utilization, CBF at rest, and CBF changes related to performances of different tasks. Spatial and temporal resolution is also limited, although better than with SPECT. However, PET is not widely available. A few PET studies have reported various areas of decreased glucose utilization, even without visible injury. Bergsneider and colleagues (59) (limited to moderate evidence) prospectively studied 56 patients with mild to severe TBI, evaluated with 18F-fluorodeoxyglucose (FDG)-PET within 2 to 39 days of injury; 14 patients had subsequent follow-up studies. The authors state in this and previous reports that TBI patients demonstrate a triphasic pattern of glucose metabolism changes that consist of early hyperglycolysis, followed by metabolic depression, and subsequent metabolic recovery (after several weeks). There are few small studies evaluating sensitivity of xenon CT and even fewer describing the sensitivity of functional MRI (fMRI) or MR perfusion.

IV. Can Imaging Help Predict Outcome After Traumatic Brain Injury (TBI)?

Summary of Evidence: The study of outcome prediction after TBI is complex. Predictor variables may not be as accurate if measured too early, but may be less useful if measured too late. Evaluation of prognostic variables has ranged from studying individual measures to comprehensive multimodal evaluations. Many clinical predictors have been studied including age, gender, GCS, pupillary reactivity, intracranial pressure (ICP), coagulopathy, hypothermia, hypoxia, hypotension, hyperglycemia, and electrolyte imbalance, in addition to imaging findings. Thatcher and colleagues (60) (moderate evidence) studied 162 patients and showed that combined measures are more reliable and accurate than any single measure. There have been relatively few comprehensive studies of long-term prognostic indices compared to acute prognostic indices (e.g., death versus survival).

Analysis of CT predictors of outcome have yielded variable results in the literature. Abnormalities found on CT have been analyzed individually, collectively (in various combinations), or combined with clinical prognostic variables. Various studies have shown improvement in outcome prediction after severe TBI when adding CT information to clinical variables (moderate evidence). Computed tomography has been studied more extensively than other imaging modalities, although it is likely that MRI and other imaging methods will have greater value for predicting long-term outcome. Unfortunately, available evidence is sparse.

Supporting Evidence: Early research on CT predictors was performed with older technology that was less sensitive to the presence of injuries. Some studies analyzed the first scans while others analyzed the worst scans. Many studies used a crude categorization system, with limited information regarding the degree of abnormalities. Others have attempted to assess outcome prediction using more detailed classification schemes. Accordingly, there has been variability in the reported predictors and success at prediction.

A. Imaging Classification Schemes

Although there are a variety of classification schemes, very few have been used to predict clinical outcomes. The most widely studied classification scheme is based on CT findings in the Trauma Coma Databank (TCDB), developed by Marshall and colleagues (61), based on the status of cisterns, midline shift, and mass lesions. Categories include (a) diffuse injury I (normal): no visible intracranial pathology; (b) diffuse injury II (small lesions): cisterns are present, midline shift <5 mm, no lesions greater than 25 cc; (c) diffuse injury III (swelling): cisterns are compressed, midline shift <5 mm, no lesions greater than 25 cc; (d) diffuse injury IV (shift): midline shift of >5 mm, no lesions greater than 25 cc; (e) any surgically evacuated lesion; and (f) any nonevacuated mass lesion greater than 25 cc. The TCDB classification was developed in severely injured patients (GCS <8) and initially compared to discharge outcomes, although it has more recently been validated using 3- and 6-month GOS (62). It is reasonably good at predicting mortality, but it may not be as applicable to mild/moderately injured patients and has been criticized as poorly predictive of functional recovery (63). The TCDB classification has been variously modified, often to include the type, number (31,64), or location of lesions (65). In the AANS guideline (24), an extensive review of the previous CT literature (strong evidence) showed that the TCDB CT classification scheme strongly correlated with outcome.

B. Normal Scans

Extensive review (strong evidence) shows that normal CT scans in severe TBI patients are predictive of favorable outcome (61% to 78.5% positive predictive value) (29). In a recent study (moderate evidence) normal CT scans in moderate/severe TBI patients were associated with better neuropsychological performance at 6 months (66).

C. Brain Swelling

Brain swelling is a subjective finding and more difficult to evaluate as an outcome predictor. Partly compressed ventricles and cisterns are not as reliably measured as obliterated ventricles and cisterns (67). Marshall and colleagues (61) (strong evidence) studied the TCDB classification in 746 patients and reported that brain swelling on CT (categorized by diffuse injury III) was predictive of mortality, and that survivors showed a trend of worse GOS associated with increasing grade of diffuse injury. Compressed basal cisterns have been associated with a threefold risk of raised ICP, and a two- to threefold increase in mortality (24). However, brain swelling on CT does not appear to correlate with neuropsychological outcomes (14) (moderate evidence).

D. Midline Shift

Midline shift is felt to be less important than other CT parameters for predicting mortality or GOS score (24). However, some investigators have shown that midline shift may be predictive of worse outcomes based on rehabilitation measures such as greater need for assistance with ambulation, activities of daily living (ADLs), and supervision at rehabilitation discharge (68).

E. Hemorrhage

The presence of hemorrhage has different prognostic significance depending on the extent and location of blood. Traumatic subarachnoid hemorrhage is a significant independent prognostic indicator (24,69) (strong evidence), associated with a twofold increase in mortality, and a 70% positive predictive value for unfavorable outcome (24). Mortality is higher and outcome is worse with acute subdural hematoma compared to extradural hematoma (24). Hematoma volume correlates with outcome, and has 78% to 79% positive predictive value for unfavorable outcome (24). Another study (moderate evidence) found that patients with combined SDH and ICH on CT had poor outcome even after surgery compared to those with EDH or ICH alone (70). A small study (limited evidence) also found that intraventricular hemorrhage (IVH) in all four ventricles was significantly associated with poor outcome (71).

F. Number/Size/Depth of Lesions

Some investigators have attempted to evaluate the predictive ability of number, size, depth, or location of lesions. Van der Naalt and colleagues (6) (moderate evidence) studied 67 patients with mild/moderate TBI and found outcome (1 year extended GOS or DOS) was related to number, size, and depth of lesions on CT. Kido and colleagues (72) (moderate evidence) found GOS was correlated with the size of intracranial lesions (independent of compartment or brain region) on CT. A small MRI study (limited evidence) suggested that size, depth, and multiplicity of lesions correlated with neurobehavioral outcome (73).

Location of lesions is partly related to mechanism of injury and is associated with different outcomes. The most available evidence is related to brainstem injuries. Firsching and colleagues (65) (moderate evidence) studied 102 patients in coma with MRI in the first 8 days and found that mortality was 100% with lesions in the bilateral pons. Kampfl and colleagues (74) (moderate evidence) studied 80 patients and also showed that lesion location could predict recovery from posttraumatic VS by 12 months, whereas clinical variables such as initial GCS, age, and pupillary abnormalities were poor predictors. Logistic regression showed that corpus callosum and dorsolateral brainstem injuries were predictive of nonrecovery. This information is helpful in that almost half of the patients with initial VS may recover within 1 year (74). The association between extent or location of injuries and neuropsychological recovery has been less well studied, with only a few studies (limited evidence) that suggest that location of injury may be associated with specific neuropsychological impairments (73,75).

G. Diffuse Axonal Injury

It has been repeatedly demonstrated that CT and MRI findings are poor predictors of functional outcome of TBI patients, probably because DAI is frequently not detected (7). Because CT clearly underestimates DAI, this can lead to inaccurate prediction of outcome. The CT studies, many of which were performed with older generation CT scanners, predominantly report that DAI is associated with mortality (limited evidence) (76) or poor outcome (moderate evidence) (77,78). It has since been shown that patients with mild or moderate injuries can also have DAI (37) that is better detected with newer generation CT scanners or MRI, and can therefore have better outcomes than previously realized. Severe DAI can transform young productive individuals into dependent patients requiring institutionalized care, while milder DAI can result in neuropsychiatric problems, cognitive deficits including memory loss, concentration difficulties, decreased attention span, intellectual decline, headaches, and seizures (79).

The improved ability to detect DAI on CT even in milder injuries has also allowed comparison with neuropsychological outcome. Wallesch and colleagues (80) (moderate evidence) studied 60 patients with mild or moderate injuries who underwent neuropsychological assessment 18 to 45 weeks later. Patients with DAI identified on CT had relatively transient deficits of psychomotor speed, verbal short-term memory, and frontal lobe cognitive functions, whereas patients with frontal contusions had persistent behavior alterations.

The MRI studies also suggest an association between TBI severity and depth of axonal injury as well as outcomes. However, most MRI studies evaluating prognosis after DAI have consisted of small sample sizes. Small studies (limited or moderate evidence) have demonstrated that patients in VS are more likely to have DAI lesions in the corpus callosum and dorsolateral brainstem (81), compared with patients with mild TBI who were more likely to have lesions in the subcortical white matter without involvement of the corpus callosum or brainstem (77). The presence of hemorrhage in DAI lesions may also affect prognosis, although results depend on the MRI sequence. One study of VS (moderate evidence) found more nonhemorrhagic DAI lesions than hemorrhagic lesions, although only T1- and T2-weighted sequences were used (81). In contrast, another study (limited evidence) showed that hemorrhage in DAI lesions (detected by GRE) was associated with poor outcomes (6-month GOS), and that isolated nonhemorrhagic DAI lesions were not associated with poor outcome (82). There is also disagreement over whether the degree of hemorrhage correlates with outcomes, although this may be partly due to differences in outcome measures. One study (moderate evidence) found that the number of lesions (hypointense or hyperintense) detected by T2*-weighted GRE images correlated with duration of coma and 3-month GOS (83). However, another study (moderate evidence) (MRI sequence not specified) found no correlation between hemorrhagic lesion volume and neuropsychological outcome measures obtained more than 6 months after injury (84). A recent prospective study (moderate evidence) of 66 patients imaged with T2*-weighted GRE at 3.0 T, found no correlation between the total amount of microhemorrhages and patient outcomes measured by GOS. However, these patients were imaged in the chronic phase (40).

Magnetic resonance spectroscopy is able to detect abnormalities in structurally normal brain that are believed to reflect DAI, and has shown promise in predicting outcome, although there are only a few studies consisting of small sample sizes. Investigators have compared MRS findings from noncontused brain with various measures of clinical neurologic outcome such as GOS or DRS scores and found a general trend of reduced NAA corresponding to poor outcome (limited evidence) (50,52,53,85). However, results are difficult to compare since varied anatomic areas were studied and results were often acquired over a wide range of times after injury. It is uncertain whether the timing of MRS measurement affects outcome prediction. Subacute MRS studies have suggested that decreased NAA correlates with poor outcomes.

There have been few acute MRS studies evaluating outcome prediction. In a prospective MRS study (86) of 42 severely injured adults (limited to moderate evidence), we measured quantitative metabolite changes as soon as possible (mean of 7 days) after injury, in normal-appearing GM and WM. In contrast to other studies, we found no correlation between NAA-derived metabolites and outcomes at 6 to 12 months, possibly because our MRS studies were performed earlier. However, we found that gluta-mine/glutamate (Glx) and Cho were significantly elevated in occipital GM and parietal WM in patients with poor 6- to 12-month outcomes and that these two variables predicted outcome at 6 to 12 months with 89% accu-racy. A combination of Glx and Cho ratios with the motor component of the GCS score provided the highest predictive accuracy (97%). It may be that elevated Glx and Cho are more sensitive indicators of injury and pre-dictors of poor outcome when spectroscopy is obtained early after injury. This may be a reflection of early excitotoxic injury (i.e., elevated Glx) and of injury associated with membrane disruption secondary to diffuse axonal injury (i.e., increased Cho). An example of spectra from parietal and occipital GM in a TBI patient with poor outcome is shown in case study 2, below.

There have been no published results comparing data from MRSI to clin-ical outcomes. Our preliminary data (limited to moderate evidence) in 42 patients with severe TBI, taken with MRSI through the corpus callosum and surrounding GM and WM, showed significant decreases in NAA/Cre and increases in Cho/Cre ratios in areas of visibly injured and normal-appearing brain. Averaged ratios from all regions were able to differentiate between patients with mild, moderate, and severe/vegetative neurologic outcomes as measured with the GOS at 6 months compared with control values. The results suggest that decreased NAA-derived ratios and increased Cho/Cre ratios, detected by MRSI, are associated with worse outcomes.

There are other MRI techniques that can detect abnormalities in visibly normal brain, although there is little evidence regarding their role in outcome prediction. Small studies using magnetization transfer methods (limited evidence) have suggested that the magnetization transfer ratio (MTR) in normal or abnormal white matter (87) or the splenium (88) may be associated with outcomes. Diffusion weighted imaging has only recently been studied in the setting of TBI, and the relationship between ADC and clinical outcome has not been adequately investigated. Diffusion tensor imaging is an even more recent development. One study (limited evidence) compared 15 patients and 30 control subjects and found corre-lations between cerebral fractional anisotropy score in trauma (C-FAST) and short-term predictors such as death, length of hospital stay, or inten-sive care unit stay (45).

H. Combinations of Imaging Abnormalities and Progressive Brain Injury

Some studies have shown that combinations of imaging abnormalities are predictive of outcome, although not necessarily in agreement. Fearnside and colleagues (89) (strong evidence) prospectively studied 315 patients and found three CT findings—cerebral edema, intraventricular blood, and midline shift—to be highly predictive of mortality. Three other CT find-ings—subarachnoid hemorrhage, intracerebral hematoma, and intracere-bral contusion—were highly predictive of poor outcome in survivors (89). In contrast, Lannoo and colleagues (90) (moderate evidence) retrospec-tively reviewed 115 patients and found that subarachnoid, intracerebral, and subdural hemorrhage were predictive of mortality but not significantly related to morbidity. Wardlaw and colleagues (63) (moderate evidence) retrospectively reviewed 414 patients and developed a simple rating system of "overall appearance" of CT findings. They reported that massive injuries and SAH could predict poor prognosis (1-year GOS). Stein and colleagues (32) (moderate evidence) also showed, in a retrospective study of 337 patients, that delayed brain injury (44.5% of their population) was a significant independent predictor of outcome.

I. Abnormalities of Perfusion or Activation

The relationship between perfusion studies and outcome has still not been clearly demonstrated. The most extensive evidence has been with SPECT. However results vary, possibly related to the severity of injury or timing of studies. The largest study with patient outcomes was performed by Jacobs and colleagues (91) (moderate to strong evidence) who prospectively studied 136 patients with mild injury, within 4 weeks of injury. They found that SPECT had a high sensitivity and negative predictive value. A normal scan reliably excluded clinical sequelae of mild injury. A small study (limited evidence) of patients with severe TBI and diffuse brain injury showed that total CBF values initially increased above normal in the first 1 to 3 days and then decreased below normal in the subacute period of 14 to 42 days. The early CBF increase has been postulated to reflect vasodilatation due to high tissue CO_2 and lactic acidosis. The authors found that the initial elevation and subsequent drop in blood flow was more marked in the poor-outcome group (92). However, another small study (limited evidence) of patients with a spectrum of injury, studied within 3 weeks of brain injury, found that focal zones of hyperemia in normal-appearing brain was associated with slightly better outcomes than in patients without hyperemia (93). The SPECT findings have also been compared with neuropsychological outcomes, although studies have consisted of small sample sizes and have found varying results (58,94).

Several limited studies show poor correlation between PET findings and neuropsychological outcomes. Bergsneider and colleagues (59) (limited to moderate evidence) prospectively studied 56 patients with mild to severe TBI who underwent FDG-PET imaging within 2 to 39 days of injury; 14 patients had subsequent follow-up studies. These patients recovered metabolically, with similar patterns of changes in glucose metabolism, suggesting that FDG-PET cannot estimate degree of functional recovery. Several smaller studies have found inconsistent results. Although xenon CT has been studied in the past, there is insufficient evidence regarding correlation with outcome.

Magnetic resonance perfusion can also provide a measure of tissue perfusion similar to results found using PET or SPECT methods of CBF determination. However, there have been few data in the literature regarding its use in predicting outcome after TBI. To date there is one small study (insufficient evidence) that showed that patients who had reduced regional cerebral blood volume in areas of contusions had poorer outcome. A subset of these patients who had reduced regional cerebral blood volume in normal-appearing white matter had significantly poorer outcomes (95). Functional MRI (fMRI) can provide noninvasive, serial mapping of brain activation, such as with memory tasks. This form of imaging can potentially assess the neurophysiologic basis of cognitive impairment, with better spatial and temporal resolution than SPECT or PET. However, it is susceptible to motion artifact and requires extremely cooperative subjects, and therefore is more successful in mildly injured than moderately or severely injured patients. There have only been a few small studies (insufficient evidence) attempting to correlate fMRI with outcomes (96,97).

J. Measures of Atrophy

Quantification of the atrophy of various brain structures/regions (such as the corpus callosum, hippocampus, and ventricles) has also been studied with respect to predicting outcome, but it is time-consuming and often requires experienced raters and specialized software. Blatter and colleagues (98) (moderate evidence) studied 123 patients with moderate to severe TBI compared to 198 healthy volunteers using MRI volumetric analysis of total brain volume, total ventricular volume, and subarachnoid cerebrospinal fluid (CSF) volume. The TBI patients, particularly if studied later, had the greatest decrease in brain volume, suggesting that progressive brain atrophy in TBI patients occurs at a rate greater than with normal aging. However, because atrophy takes time to develop, it cannot be used acutely as an early predictor of outcome. Blatter and colleagues also showed that correlations with cognitive outcomes did not become significant until after 70 days. One study of late CT scans (moderate evidence) of Vietnam War veterans with penetrating or closed head injuries found that total brain volume loss and enlargement of the third ventricle were significantly related to cognitive abnormalities and return to work (99). Another study (moderate evidence) showed that frontotemporal atrophy on late MRI was predictive of 1-year outcome (measured by extended GOS or DOS) (6). In an MRI study (moderate evidence) of late MRI findings and neuropsychological outcome, hippocampal atrophy was correlated with verbal memory function, whereas temporal horn enlargement was correlated with intellectual outcome (100).

K. Combinations of Clinical and Imaging Findings

Numerous studies have attempted to analyze combinations of clinical and imaging findings to determine the best approach to predicting outcome. The diversity of TBI makes this a difficult but worthy task. There is agreement that there is no one single variable that can predict outcome after TBI. In fact, there is often disagreement between studies regarding the predictive value of certain clinical variables, including GCS. Ideally, a combined clinical and imaging approach to outcome prediction would likely be most accurate. Ratanalert and colleagues (101) (moderate evidence) studied 300 patients and reported that logistic regression showed that age, status of basal cisterns on initial CT, GCS at 24 hours, and electrolyte derangement strongly correlated with 6-month GOS score. Ono and colleagues (64) (moderate evidence) retrospectively studied 272 patients who were first divided into CT categories according to the TCDB classification and found that within certain groups additional variables such as age and GCS score were helpful predictors of outcome. Schaan and colleagues (102) (moderate evidence) studied the utility of creating a single score based on a weighted scale of clinical variables and CT findings including pupillary reaction, hemiparesis, brainstem signs, contusion, SDH, EDH, and cerebral edema. In their retrospective study of 554 patients, they divided the range of scores into three severity groups and found that there were significant differences in mortality and GOS scores between groups, suggesting that this approach had predictive value.

V. Is the Approach to Imaging Children with Traumatic Brain Injury Different from that for Adults?

Summary of Evidence: Pediatric TBI patients are known to have different biophysical features, risks, mechanisms, and outcomes after injury. There are also differences between infants and older children, although this remains controversial. Categorization of pediatric age groups is variable, and measures of injury or outcomes are inconsistent. The GCS and GOS have been used for pediatric studies, sometimes with modifications (103–105), or with variable dichotomization (103,106). For infants and toddlers, some investigators have used the Children's Coma Scale (CCS) (107). There are several pediatric adaptations of the GOS, such as the King's Outcome Scale for Childhood Head Injury (KOSCHI) (108), the Pediatric Cerebral Performance Category (PCPC), and the Pediatric Overall Performance Category (POPC) (109). Management guidelines are controversial. There are few pediatric studies regarding the use of imaging and outcome predictions. Guidelines in children are summarized in take-home Table 13.4.

Supporting Evidence: Within the pediatric population, age may be a confounding variable or effect modifier. Levin and colleagues (110) (moderate evidence) studied 103 children at one of the original four centers participating in the TCDB and found heterogeneity in 6-month outcomes based on age. The worst outcomes were found in newborns to 4-year-olds, and the best outcomes were found in 5- to 10-year-olds, while adolescents had intermediate outcomes. The authors suggested that studies involving severe TBI in children should analyze age-defined subgroups rather than pooling a wide range of pediatric ages.

There are few management guidelines in children, and they primarily pertain to mild head injury. A review of 108 articles published between 1966 and 1993 determined that outcome studies were inconclusive as to the

---

Table 13.4. Suggested guidelines for acute neuroimaging in pediatric patient with mild TBI (GCS 13–15) and no suspicion of nonaccidental trauma or comorbid injuries

- **CT scan if:**
  - History of loss of consciousness
  - Disoriented
  - Any neurologic dysfunction
  - Possible depressed or basal skull fracture

- **Observe or discharge if:**
  - No loss of consciousness
  - Oriented, neurologically intact

TBI, traumatic brain injury; CT, computed tomography.
Source: Modified from AAP guidelines (116) and the Cincinnati Children's Hospital (117).

impact of minor head trauma on long-term cognitive function in children, and that the literature on mild head trauma in children did not provide a sufficient basis for evidence-based recommendations for most of the key issues in clinical management (111). Shortly afterward, two guidelines for imaging of minor pediatric TBI (excluding nonaccidental trauma) were published. Management guidelines for minor closed head injury in children were developed by the American Academy of Pediatrics and the American Academy of Family Physicians in 1999 (112). Patients are categorized by whether or not they had brief loss of consciousness (LOC). After the literature review, the authors concluded that skull radiographs have low sensitivity and specificity for intracranial injury, and therefore low predictive value. They found no published studies that showed different outcomes between CT scanning early after minor head injury versus observation alone. They also reported no appreciable difference between CT and MRI in detecting clinically significant acute injury/bleeding requiring neurosurgical intervention. Their proposed algorithm recommends observation only if there was no LOC, and allowed a choice of observation versus CT if there was brief LOC. Because CT is more quickly and easily performed and less expensive than MRI, CT was recommended over MRI for the acute evaluation of children with minor head injury. An evidence-based clinical practice guideline for management of children with mild traumatic head injury was developed by Cincinnati Children's Hospital Medical Center in 2000 (113), although a summary of evidence was not detailed.

There are fewer studies on the utility of imaging in predicting outcome in pediatric TBI compared to that in adults. Many studies have consisted of relatively small sample sizes and used varying outcome, possibly accounting for conflicting reports regarding outcomes related to TBI in children. There have been several studies evaluating CT in predicting outcome in children with variable results. Suresh and colleagues (106) (moderate evidence) studied 340 children and compared CT findings to discharge GOS outcomes. They found that poor outcome (VS or death) occurred in 16% of their patients. In addition there was a range of outcomes that were worse with (in descending order) fractures, EDH, contusion, diffuse head injury, and acute SDH. Hirsch and colleagues (114) (moderate evidence) studied 248 children after severe TBI and compared initial CT findings to the level of consciousness (measured by a modified GCS score) at 1 year after injury. They found that children with normal CT or isolated SDH or EDH were least impaired, while children with diffuse edema had the most impairment. Those with parenchymal hemorrhage, ventricular hemorrhage, or focal edema had intermediate outcomes. A study of 82 children (moderate evidence) found that unfavorable prognosis (using a three-category Lidcombe impairment scale) was more likely to occur after shearing injury or intracerebral/subdural hematomas, whereas a better outcome was more likely in patients with epidural hematoma (115). Another study of 74 children (moderate evidence) found that the presence of traumatic subarachnoid hemorrhage on CT was an independent predictor of discharge outcome ($p < 0.001$) but did not find that DAI or diffuse swelling was associated with outcome. After stepwise logistic regression analysis, CT findings did not have prognostic significance compared to other variables such as GCS and the oculocephalic reflex (104). Another study (moderate evidence) compared 59 children and 59 adults and found that a CT finding of absent ventricles/cisterns was associated with a slightly lower frequency of poor outcome (6-month GOS) in children, suggesting that diffuse swelling may be more benign in children than in adults unless there was a severe primary injury or a secondary hypotensive insult (67).

There have been some studies evaluating MRI for outcome prediction in children with TBI. Prasad and colleagues (103) (moderate evidence) prospectively studied 60 children with acute CT and MRI. Hierarchical multiple regression indicated that the number of lesions, as well as certain clinical variables such as GCS (modified for children) and duration of coma, were predictive of outcomes up to 1 year (modified GOS). Several investigators have studied the correlation between depth of lesion and outcomes, with varying results. Levin and colleagues (116) (moderate evidence) studied 169 children prospectively as well as 82 patients retrospectively with MRI at variable time points, and showed a correlation between depth of brain lesions and functional outcome. Grados and colleagues (117) (moderate evidence) studied 106 children with a spoiled gradient echo (SPGR) (T1-weighted) MRI sequence obtained 3 months after TBI, and classified lesions into a depth-of-lesion model. Depth and number of lesions predicted outcome, but correlation was better with discharge outcomes than 1-year outcomes. Blackman and colleagues (118) (moderate evidence) studied 92 children in the rehabilitation setting (using variable imaging modalities) and used a depth-of-lesion classification (based on the Grados model) to study neuropsychological outcomes. They found that this classification had limited usefulness. Although patients with deeper lesions tended to have longer stays in rehabilitation, they were able to catch up after sufficient time had elapsed. In a recent study of hemorrhagic DAI lesions (moderate evidence), we found that the degree and location of hemorrhagic lesions correlated with GCS, duration of coma, and outcomes at 6 to 12 months after injury (119). Levin and colleagues (120) (moderate evidence) showed that in children, as in adults, corpus callosum area (measured on subacute MRI) correlated with functional outcome. They also found that the size of the corpus callosum decreased after severe TBI in contrast with mild/moderately injured children who showed growth of the corpus callosum on follow-up studies.

There are few MRS studies on pediatric outcomes after TBI. Ashwal and colleagues (121) (moderate evidence) demonstrated significant decreases in NAA-derived ratios and elevation of Cho/Cre measured in occipital GM within 13 days of neurologic insult. These metabolite changes correlated with poor neurologic outcome at 6 to 12 months after injury ($n = 52$) as measured with the PCPC. In a subgroup of these patients ($n = 24$) neuropsychological evaluations were performed at 3 to 5 years after neurologic insult. It was found that these metabolite changes strongly correlated with below-average functioning in multiple areas including full-scale IQ, memory, and sensorimotor and attention/executive functioning (122). Unlike adult studies, we have found that other metabolite abnormalities are associated with poor outcome, including presence of lactate (121) and elevated myoinositol (moderate evidence) (123). Our pediatric studies differed from our adult studies in that Glx, although elevated in pediatric TBI patients (moderate evidence), was not significantly different between outcome groups (124). There is little evidence regarding the predictive ability of other imaging methods such as DWI, DTI, or perfusion studies in children with TBI. Further investigation in all areas of pediatric head injury are warranted.

Take-Home Data

Table 13.1 lists the possible types of head injuries, excluding penetrating or missile injuries, or nonaccidental trauma. Table 13.2 lists suggested guidelines for acute CT imaging in adults with mild TBI, modified from the Canadian Head CT Rule (20), EAST guidelines (2), and the Neuro-traumatology Committee of the World Federation of Neurosurgical Societies (1). Table 13.3 lists suggested guidelines for acute neuroimaging in adult patients with severe TBI. Table 13.4 lists suggested guidelines for acute CT imaging in pediatric patients with mild TBI, modified from AAP guidelines (112), and the Cincinnati Children's Hospital (113).

Table 13.5 summarizes the principles, use, advantages and limitations of imaging in TBI.

Imaging Case Studies

The cases presented below highlight the advantages and limitations of the different neuroimaging modalities.

- Case study 1: Example of MR imaging for TBI: This case study illustrates imaging findings of DAI in a 10-year-old boy struck by a car (Fig. 13.1).
- Study 2: Example of MR spectroscopy. This case study illustrates the metabolite changes in single-voxel short echo time proton spectra (TE = 20 msec) from a 28-year-old man admitted to hospital with severe TBI (GCS of 4) following a motor vehicle accident, compared to a normal 27-year-old control subject (Fig. 13.2).

Table 13.5. Current imaging methods of traumatic brain injury (TBI)

Modality	Principle and advantages/limitations	Use in TBI	Potential correlation with outcome
CT	Based on x-rays, measures tissue density; rapid, inexpensive, widespread	Detects hemorrhage and surgical lesions	Short-term outcome—mortality versus survival
Xenon CT perfusion	Inhalation of stable xenon gas, which acts as a freely diffusible tracer; requires additional equipment and software that is available only in a few centers	Detects disturbances in CBF due to injury, edema, or infarction	Long-term outcome—global or neuropsychological
MRI	Uses radiofrequency (RF) pulses in magnetic field to distinguish tissues, employs many different techniques; currently has highest spatial resolution; complex and expensive	Detection of various injuries, sensitivity varies with different techniques	Long-term outcome—global or neuropsychological
MRI-FLAIR	Suppresses cerebrospinal fluid (CSF) signal	Detection of edematous lesions, particularly near ventricles and cortex, as well as extraaxial blood	Long-term outcome—global or neuropsychological
MRI-T2* GRE	Accentuates blooming effect, such as blood products	Detection of small parenchymal hemorrhages	Long-term outcome—global or neuropsychological

Table 13.5. *Continued*

Modality	Principle and advantages/limitations	Use in TBI	Potential correlation with outcome
MRI-DWI	Distinguishes water mobility in tissue	Detection of recent tissue infarction or traumatic cell death	Long-term outcome—global or neuropsychological
MRI-DTI	Based on DWI, maps degree and direction of major fiber bundles; requires special software	Detects impaired connectivity of white matter tracts, even in normal-appearing tissue	Long-term outcome—global or neuropsychological
MRI-MT	Suppression of "background" brain tissue containing protein-bound H_2O, enhances contrast between water and lipid-containing tissue	May detect microscopic neuronal dysfunction, even in normal-appearing tissue	Long-term outcome—global or neuropsychological
MRI-MRS	Analyzes chemical composition of brain tissue; requires special software	Metabolite patterns indicate neuronal dysfunction or axonal injury, even in normal-appearing tissue	Long-term outcome—global or neuropsychological
MR volumetry	Measure volumes of various brain structures or regions; time-consuming, requires special software	Detects atrophy of injured tissue, can quantitate progression over time	Long-term outcome—global or neuropsychological
fMRI	Measures small changes in blood flow related to brain activation; requires cooperative patient	Detects impairment or redistribution of areas of brain activation	Long-term outcome—neuropsychological
MR perfusion (global, non-fMRI)	Measures tissue perfusion using contrast or noncontrast methods; better temporal resolution than PET, SPECT; not as well studied	Detects disturbances in CBF due to injury, edema, or infarction	Long-term outcome—global or neuropsychological
SPECT	Photon emitting radioisotopes used to measure CBF	Detects disturbances in CBF due to injury, edema, or infarction	Long-term outcome—global or neuropsychological
PET	Positron-emitting radioisotopes act as freely diffusible tracers, used to measure CBF, metabolic rate (glucose metabolism or oxygen consumption), or response to cognitive tasks; available only in a few centers	Detects disturbances in CBF due to injury, edema, or infarction	Long-term outcome—global or neuropsychological

CT, computed tomography; MRI, magnetic resonance imaging; FLAIR, fluid-attenuated inversion recovery; GRE, gradient recalled echo; DWI, diffusion weighted imaging; DTI, diffusion tensor imaging; MT, magnetization transfer; MRS, magnetic resonance spectroscopy; fMRI, functional magnetic resonance imaging; SPECT, single photon emission computed tomography; PET, positron emission tomography; CBF, cerebral blood flow.

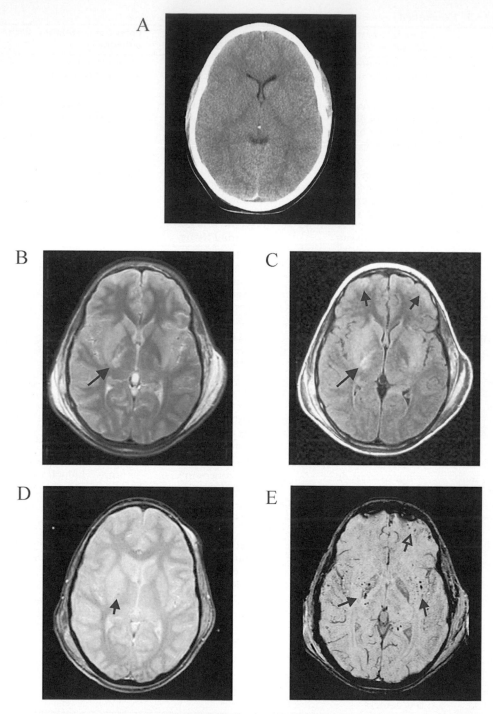

Figure 13.1. Magnetic resonance imaging findings of diffuse axonal injury (DAI) in a 10–year-old boy who was struck by a car. He had an initial Glasgow Coma Scale (GCS) score of 3, was in a coma for 11 days, and had elevated intracranial pressure (ICP). A: The admission CT scan was normal. B: An MRI was obtained 2 days after injury. Subtle hyperintense signal is seen in the right basal ganglia and posterior limb of the internal capsule (arrow), on the T2–weighted images. C: The fluid-attenuated inversion recovery (FLAIR) sequence accentuates the edema in those areas (long arrow), as well as along the periphery of the frontal lobes (short arrows). D: The standard T2*-GRE sequence shows a subtle punctuate hypointense focus in the right internal capsule (arrow). E: The susceptibility-weighted imaging (SWI) technique (a modified T2*-GRE sequence) shows multiple tiny hemorrhagic foci within the bilateral basal ganglia and capsular white matter (closed arrows) as well as within the left frontal contusion (open arrow).

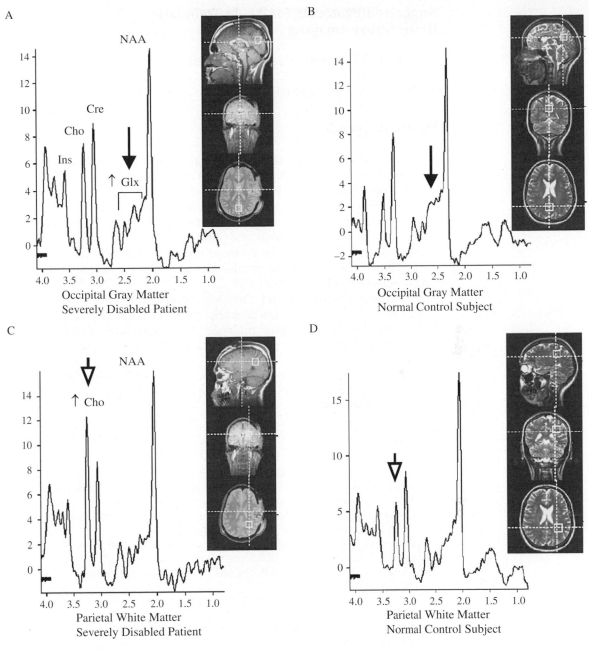

Figure 13.2. A 28-year-old man was admitted to the hospital with severe TBI (GCS of 4) following a motor vehicle accident. A: Single voxel short-echo magnetic resonance spectroscopy (MRS) image taken from the occipital gray matter shows increased glutamate/glutamine (Glx, arrows) compared to the control spectrum (B) in a normal 28-year-old man. C: Image taken from parieto-occipital white matter shows increased choline (Cho, arrowheads) compared to the control spectrum (D). Evaluation at 6 months after the injury revealed severe disabilities (GOS of 3) in this patient.

Suggested Protocols for Acute Traumatic Brain Injury Imaging

- CT: standard and bone algorithms, viewed with brain, intermediate, and bone windows.
- MRI: T1-weighted, T2-weighted, FLAIR, T2*-weighted GRE, DWI.

Future Research

- Clinical trials have been disappointing in TBI research, perhaps due to different mechanisms of injury included in the trials, but also probably due to nonuniformity in classification of injuries and outcomes. There is a need for a consistent, widely accepted classification of information to facilitate comparisons of different groups of patients and institutions. The vast amount of clinical and imaging data can yield elaborate approaches, but this must be balanced with practicality in clinical situation. The system should be simple, relevant, reliable, and acceptable to clinicians in routine practice (125).
- More research is needed, and ultimately a multimodal prognostic index for a wide range of disability probably needs to be developed.
- The link between imaging findings, neurobehavioral deficits, and outcome requires further research, particularly in patients with a mild TBI.
- Larger, prospective studies are needed to evaluate the sensitivity, specificity, predictive accuracy, and cost-effectiveness of various neuroimaging methods in TBI.

References

1. Servadei F, Teasdale G, Merry G, on behalf of the Neurotraumatology Committee of the World Federation of Neurosurgical Societies. J Neurotrauma 2001;18:657–664.
2. Cushman JG, Agarwal N, Fabian TC, et al.; EAST Practice Management Guidelines Work Group. J Trauma 2001;51:1016–1026.
3. Iverson GL, Lovell MR, Smith S, Franzen MD. Brain Inj 2000;14:1057–1061.
4. Jennett B, Bond M. Lancet 1975;1:480–484.
5. Jennett B, Snoek J, Bond MR, Brooks N. J Neurol Neurosurg Psychiatry 1981;44:285–293.
6. van der Naalt J, van Zomeren AH, Sluiter WJ, Minderhoud JM. J Neurol Neurosurg Psychiatry 1999;66:207–213.
7. Rappaport M, Hall KM, Hopkins K, Belleza BS, Cope DN. Arch Phys Med Rehabil 1982;63:118–123.
8. Schwab K, Grafman J, Salazar AM, Kraft J. Neurology 1993;43:95–103.
9. Guide for the Uniform Data Set for Medical Rehabilitation (including the FIM™ instrument), version 5.1. Buffalo, NY: State University of New York, 1997.
10. Boake C. Arch Phys Med Rehabil 1996;77:765–772.
11. Dikmen S, Machamer J, Miller B, Doctor J, Temkin N. J Neurotrauma 2001;18:127–140.
12. Temkin NR, Machamer JE, Dikmen SS. J Neurotrauma 2003;20:229–241.
13. Choi SC, Barnes TY, Bullock R, Germanson TA, Marmarou A, Young HF. J Neurosurg 1994;81:169–173.
14. Levin HS, Gary HEJ, Eisenberg HM, et al. J Neurosurg 1990;73:699–709.

15. Wilson JTL, Wiedmann KD, Hadley DM, et al. J Neurol Neurosurg Psychiatry 1988;51:391–39.
16. Torner JC, Choi S, Barnes TY. Epidemiology of head injuries. In: Marion D, ed. Traumatic Brain Injury. New York: Thieme, 1998:9–25.
17. Adekoya N, Thurman DJ, White DD, Webb KW. MMWR Surveill Summ 2002;51:1–14.
18. Meythaler JM, Peduzzi JD, Eleftheriou E, Novack TA. Arch Phys Med Rehabil 2001;82:1461–1471.
19. Fiser SM, Johnson SB, Fortune JB. Am Surg 1998;64:1088–1093.
20. Stiell IG, Wells FA, Vandemheen K, et al. Lancet 2001;357:1391–1396.
21. Haydel MJ, Preston CA, Mills TJ, Luber S, Blaudeau E, DeBlieux PMC. N Engl J Med 2000;343:100–105.
22. Madden C, Witzkc DB, Sanders AB, Valente J, Fritz M. Acad Emerg Med 1995;2:248–253.
23. Brain Trauma Foundation, American Association of Neurological Surgeons. Part I: Guidelines for the Management of Severe Traumatic Brain Injury. New York: Brain Trauma Foundation, 2000.
24. Brain Trauma Foundation, American Association of Neurological Surgeons. Part II: Early Indicators of Prognosis in Severe Traumatic Brain Injury. New York: Brain Trauma Foundation, 2000.
25. Eng J, Chanmugam A. Neuroimaging Clin North Am 2003;13:273–282.
26. Mack LR, Chan SB, Silva JC, Hogan TM. J Emerg Med 2003;24:157–162.
27. McAllister TW, Sparling MB, Flashman LA, Saykin AJ. J Clin Exp Neuropsychol 2001;23:775–791.
28. Fearnside M, McDougall P. Aust N Z J Surg 1998;68:58–64.
29. The Brain Trauma Foundation, American Association of Neurological Surgeons, Joint Section on Neurotrauma and Critical Care. J Neurotrauma 2000;17:597–627.
30. Oertel M, Kelly DF, McArthur D, et al. J Neurosurg 2002;96:109–116.
31. Servadei F, Murray GD, Penny K, et al. Neurosurgery 2000;46:70–75.
32. Stein SC, Spettell C, Young G, Ross SE. Neurosurgery 1993;32:25–30.
33. Orrison WW, Gentry LR, Stimac GK, Tarrell RM, Espinosa MC, Cobb LC. Am J Neuroradiol 1994;15:351–356.
34. Ogawa T, Sekino H, Uzura M, et al. Acta Neurochir 1992;suppl:8–10.
35. Hadley DM, Teasdale GM, Jenkins A, et al. Clin Radiol 1988;39:131–139.
36. Gentry LR, Godersky JC, Thompson B, Dunn VD. AJR 1988;150:673–682.
37. Mittl RL Jr, Grossman RI, Hiehle JF, et al. Am J Neuroradiol 1994;15:1583–1589.
38. Gentry LR, Godersky JC, Thompson B. AJR 1988;150:663–672.
39. Tong K, Ashwal S, Holshouser B, et al. Radiology 2003;227:332–339.
40. Scheid R, Preul C, Gruber O, Wiggins C, von Cramon DY. Am J Neuroradiol 2003;24:1049–1056.
41. Ashikaga R, Araki Y, Ishida O. Neuroradiology 1997;39:239–242.
42. Huisman TAGM, Sorensen AG, Hergan K, Gonzalez RG, Schaefer PW. J Comput Assist Tomogr 2003;27:5–11.
43. Hergan K, Schaefer PW, Sorensen AG, Gonzalez RG, Huisman TAGM. Eur Radiol 2002;12:2536–2541.
44. Shanmuganathan K, Gullapalli RP, Mirvis SE, Roys S, Murthy P. AJNR 2004;25:539–544.
45. Ptak T, Sheridan RL, Rhea JT, et al. AJR 2003;181:1401–1407.
46. Arfenakis K, Haughton VM, Carew JD, et al. AJNR 2002;23:794–802.
47. Jones DK, Dardis R, Ervine M, et al. Neurosurgery 2000;47:306–314.
48. Choe BY, Suh TS, Choi KH, Shinn KS, Park CK, Kang JK. Invest Radiol 1995;30:502–506.
49. Ricci R, Barbarella G, Musi P, Boldrini P, Trevisan C, Basaglia N. Neuroradiology 1997;39:313–319.
50. Ross BD, Ernst T, Kreis R, et al. J Magn Reson Imaging 1998;8:829–840.

51. Garnett MR, Blamire AM, Rajagopalan B, et al. Brain 2000;123:1403–1409.
52. Cecil KM, Lenkinski RE, Meaney DF, McIntosh TK, Smith DH. J Neurochem 1998;70:2038–2044.
53. Sinson G, Bagley LJ, Cecil KM, et al. Am J Neuroradiol 2001;22:143–151.
54. Wild JM, Macmillan CS, Wardlaw JM, et al. MAGMA 1999; 8:109–115.
55. Garnett MR, Corkill RG, Blamire AM, et al. J Neurotrauma 2001;18:231–240.
56. Abdel-Dayem HM, Abu-Judeh H, Kumar M, et al. Clin Nucl Med 1998;23:309–317.
57. Stamatakis EA, Wilson JT, Hadley DM, Wyper DJ. J Nucl Med 2002;43:476–483.
58. Kant R, Smith-Seemiller L, Isaac G, Duffy J. Brain Inj 1997;11:115–124.
59. Bergsneider M, Hovda DA, McArthur DL, et al. J Head Trauma Rehabil 2001;16:135–148.
60. Thatcher RW, Cantor DS, McAlaster R, Geisler F, Krause P. Ann N Y Acad Sci 1991;620:82–101.
61. Marshall LF, Marshall SB, Klauber MR, et al. J Neurotrauma 1992;9(suppl 1):287–292.
62. Vos PE, van Voskuilen AC, Beems T, Krabbe PF, Vogels OJ. J Neurotrauma 2001;18:649–655.
63. Wardlaw JM, Easton VJ, Statham P. J Neurol Neurosurg Psychiatry 2002;72:188–192.
64. Ono J, Yamaura A, Kubota M, Okimura Y, Isobe K. J Clin Neurosci 2001;8:120–123.
65. Firsching R, Woischneck D, Klein S, Reissberg S, Dohring W, Peters B. Acta Neurochir 2001;143:263–271.
66. Mataro M, Poca MA, Sahuquillo J, et al. J Neurotrauma 2001;18:869–879.
67. Lang DA, Teasdale GM, Macpherson P, Lawrence A. J Neurosurg 1994;80:675–680.
68. Englander J, Cifu DX, Wright JM, Black K. Arch Phys Med Rehabil 2003;84:214–220.
69. Servadei F, Murray GD, Teasdale GM, et al. Neurosurgery 2002;50:261–267.
70. Caroli M, Locatelli M, Campanella R, Balbi S, Martinelli F, Arienta C. Surg Neurol 2001;56:82–88.
71. LeRoux PD, Haglund MM, Newell DW, Grady MS, Winn HR. Neurosurgery 1992;31:678–684.
72. Kido DK, Cox C, Hamill RW, Rothenberg BM, Woolf PD. Radiology 1992;182:777–781.
73. Godersky JC, Gentry LR, Tranel D, Dyste GN, Danks KR. Acta Neurochirurgica 1990;(suppl 51):311–314.
74. Kampfl A, Schmutzhard E, Franz G, et al. Lancet 1998;351:1763–1767.
75. Wilson JTL, Hadley DM, Wiedmann KD, Teasdale GM. J Neurol Neurosurg Psychiatry 1995;59:328–331.
76. Tomei G, Sganzerla E, Spagnoli D, et al. J Neurosurg Sci 1991;35:61–75.
77. Cordobes F, Lobato RD, Rivas JJ, et al. Acta Neurochir 1986;81:27–35.
78. Wang HD, Duan GS, Zhang J, Zhou DB. Chin Med J 1998;111:59–62.
79. Parizel PM, Ozsarlak O, Van Goethem JW, et al. Eur Radiol 1998;8:960–965.
80. Wallesch C-W, Curio N, Kutz S, Jost S, Bartels C, Synowitz H. Brain Inj 2001;15:401–412.
81. Kampfl A, Franz G, Aichner F, et al. J Neurosurg 1998;88:809–816.
82. Paterakis K, KarantanasH, Komnos A, Volikas Z. J Trauma 2000;49:1071–1075.
83. Yanagawa Y, Tsushima Y, Tokumaru A, et al. J Trauma 2000;49:272–277.
84. Kurth SM, Bigler ED, Blatter DD. Brain Inj 1994;8:489–500.
85. Garnett MR, Blamire AM, Corkill RG, et al. Brain 2000;123:2046–2054.
86. Shutter L, Tong KA, Holshouser BA. J Neurotrauma 2004;21(12):1693–1705.
87. Bagley LJ, McGowan JC, Grossman RI, et al. J MRI 2000;11:1–8.
88. McGowan JC, Yang JH, Plotkin RC, et al. Am J Neuroradiol 2000;21:875–880.
89. Fearnside MR, Cook RJ, McDougall P, McNeil RJ. Br J Neurosurg 1993;7:267–279.

90. Lannoo E, Van Rietvelde F, Colardyn F, et al. J Neurotrauma 2000;17:403–414.
91. Jacobs A, Put E, Ingels M, Put T, Bossuyt A. J Nucl Med 1996;37:1605–1609.
92. Shiina G, Onuma T, Kameyama M, et al. AJNR 1998;19:297–302.
93. Sakas DE, Bullock MR, Patterson J, Hadley D, Wyper DJ, Teasdale GM. J Neurosurg 1995;83:277–284.
94. Kesler SR, Adams HF, Bigler ED. Brain Inj 2000;14:851–857.
95. Garnett MR, Blamire AM, Corkill RG, et al. J Neurotrauma 2001;18:585–593.
96. Christodoulou C, DeLuca J, Ricker JH, et al. Neurology 2003;60:1793–1798.
97. McAllister TW, Saykin AJ, Flashman LA, et al. Neurology 1999;53:1300–1308.
98. Blatter DD, Bigler ED, Gale SD, et al. Am J Neuroradiol 1997;18:1–10.
99. Groswasser Z, Reider-Groswasser II, Schwab K, et al. Brain Inj 2002;16:681–690.
100. Bigler ED, Blatter DD, Anderson CV, et al. Am J Neuroradiol 1997;18:11–23.
101. Ratanalert S, Chompikul J, Hirunpat S, Pheunpathom N. Br J Neurosurg 2002;16:487–493.
102. Schaan M, Jaksche H, Boszczyk B. J Trauma 2002;52:667–674.
103. Prasad MR, Ewing-Cobbs L, Swank PR, Kramer L. Pediatr Neurosurg 2002;36:64–74.
104. Pillai S, Praharaj SS, Mohanty A, Sastry Kolluri VR. Pediatr Neurosurg 2001;34:98–103.
105. Sganzerla EP, Tomei G, Guerra P, et al. Child's Nerv Syst 1989;5:168–171.
106. Suresh HS, Praharaj SS, Indira Devi B, Shukla D, Sastry Kolluri VR. Neurol India 2003;51:16–18.
107. Raimondi AJ, Hirschauer J. Head injury in the infant and toddler. Childs Brain 1984;11:12–35.
108. Crouchman M, Rossiter L, Colaco T, Forsyth R. Arch Dis Child 2001;84:120–124.
109. Fiser DH. J Pediatr 1992;121:69–74.
110. Levin HS, Aldrich EF, Saydjari C, et al. Neurosurgery 1992;31:435–443.
111. Homer CJ, Kleinman L. Pediatrics 1999;104:e78.
112. Committee on Quality Improvement, American Academy of Pediatrics. Commission on Clinical Policies and Research, American Academy of Family Physicians. Pediatrics 1999;104:1407–1415.
113. Cincinnati Children's Hospital Medical Center. Evidence Based Clinical Practice Guideline for Management of Children with Mild Traumatic Head Injury. Cincinnati: Cincinnati Children's Hospital Medical Center, 2000.
114. Hirsch W, Schobess A, Eichler G, Zumkeller W, Teichler H, Schluter A. Paediatr Anaesth 2002;12:337–344.
115. Tomberg T, Rink U, Pikkoja E, Tikk A. Acta Neurochir 1996;138:543–548.
116. Levin HS, Mendelsohn D, Lilly MA, et al. Neurosurgery 1997;40:432–440.
117. Grados MA, Slomine BS, Gerring JP, Vasa R, Bryan N, Denckla MB. J Neurol Neurosurg Psychiatry 2001;70:350–358.
118. Blackman JA, Rice SA, Matsumoto JA, et al. J Head Trauma Rehabil 2003;18:493–503.
119. Tong K, Ashwal S, Holshouser BA, et al. Ann Neurol 2004;56:36–50.
120. Levin HS, Benavidez DA, Verger-Maestre K, et al. Neurology 2000;54:647–653.
121. Ashwal S, Holshouser BA, Shu SK, et al. Pediatr Neurol 2000;23:114–125.
122. Brenner T, Freier MC, Holshouser BA, Burley T, Ashwal S. Pediatr Neurol 2003;28:104–114.
123. Ashwal S, Holshouser BA, Tong K, et al. Pediatr Res 2004;56:630–638.
124. Ashwal S, Holshouser BA, Tong K, et al. J Neurotrauma 2004;21:1539–1552.
125. Teasdale G, Teasdale E, Hadley D. J Neurotrauma 1992;9(suppl 1):249–257.

14

Imaging of Acute Hematogenous Osteomyelitis and Septic Arthritis in Children and Adults

John Y. Kim and Diego Jaramillo

Issues

I. What are the clinical findings that raise the suspicion for acute hematogenous osteomyelitis and septic arthritis to direct further imaging?

II. What is the diagnostic performance of the different imaging studies in acute hematogenous osteomyelitis and septic arthritis?

III. What is the natural history of osteomyelitis and septic arthritis, and what are the roles of medical therapy versus surgical treatment?

IV. Is there a role for repeat imaging in the management?

V. What is the diagnostic performance of imaging of osteomyelitis and septic arthritis in the adult?

VI. What are the roles of the different imaging modalities in the evaluation of acute osteomyelitis and septic orthritis?

Key Points

- The clinical presentation of acute osteomyelitis and septic arthritis can be nonspecific and sometimes confusing (moderate evidence).
- When signs and symptoms cannot be localized, bone scintigraphy is preferred over magnetic resonance imaging (MRI) (moderate evidence).
- When signs and symptoms can be localized, MRI is preferred (moderate to limited evidence).
- Ultrasound is the preferred imaging modality for evaluating joint effusions of the hip (moderate evidence).
- Magnetic resonance imaging is highly sensitive for the detection of osteomyelitis and its complications (abscess), but incurs added cost (moderate evidence).
- No data were found in the medical literature that evaluate the cost-effectiveness of the different imaging modalities in the evaluation of hematogenous osteomyelitis and septic joint (limited evidence).
- Overall, MRI is the imaging modality of choice to evaluate for osteomyelitis and septic arthritis in the adult population, including the diabetic patient and intravenous drug users. The ability to localize

symptoms and the inherent high spatial resolution allows exact anatomic detail that may be helpful for surgical planning (limited to moderate evidence).

Definition and Pathophysiology

Osteomyelitis is an infection of bone and bone marrow. Routes of infection include hematogenous spread, spread by contiguity, and direct infection by a penetrating wound (1). Hematogenous spread is the most common route in children, usually seeding the metaphyses of long bones due to sluggish blood flow patterns in this region (2,3). It arises in the setting of bacteremia. In children, the capillaries in the metaphyses are the terminal branches of the nutrient artery. The capillaries form loops that end in large venous sinusoids where there is decreased blood flow. The inflammatory response to infection leads to increased intraosseous pressure and stasis of blood flow, causing thrombosis and eventual bone necrosis (4). In children less than 18 months of age, transphyseal vessels allow metaphyseal infections to cross the physis and infect the epiphyses and joints. The most common bones affected by acute hematogenous osteomyelitis (AHO) are the tibia and femur (3); the most common organism is *Staphylococcus aureus*.

Acute septic arthritis is a bacterial infection of a joint. Most cases arise from hematogenous spread or contiguous spread from adjacent osteomyelitis in the metaphysis or epiphysis (5–7). The most common organism is *S. aureus* (3). The prognosis worsens with increasing delay of treatment due to lytic enzymes that destroy the articular and epiphyseal cartilage. In addition, increased pressure within the joint capsule reduces blood flow to the epiphyses. This can lead to long-term disability resulting from growth disturbances, dislocations, and malalignment (8,9).

There is evidence that acute osteomyelitis and septic arthritis are a spectrum of the same disease process (moderate evidence) (10). This hypothesis argues for a similar clinical approach and treatment for these two diseases.

The pattern of hematogenous spread of osteomyelitis and septic arthritis in the adult is different from the pediatric population. The unique vascular supply in the metaphysis normally seen in children is no longer present in adults, and most hematogenous infections arise in the diaphyseal marrow space, similar in pattern to hematogenous metastatic disease to the bone (11). Contiguous spread of infection from adjacent soft tissues is more prevalent in the adults than in children, although hematogenous spread is still more common (12). Contiguous infections can occur in trauma patients with open fractures, in bedridden patients with decubitus ulcers, and in patients with a diabetic foot. Localizing symptoms are more prevalent in the adult population as opposed to the pediatric population, allowing for more dedicated anatomic imaging with MRI, rather than a survey with radionuclide bone scanning.

Epidemiology

The annual incidence of osteomyelitis in children under 13 years of age is 1/5000 (13). With boys slightly more often affected than girls, fast-growing long bones such as the tibia and femur are the most affected regions.

Approximately 25% of cases affect the flat bones including the pelvis. Although a single bone is usually affected, polyostotic involvement has been reported in up to 6.8% of cases in infants and in 22% of neonates (4,14,15). The most common organisms are *S. aureus*, followed by β-hemolytic *Streptococcus*, Streptococcus pneumoniae, Escherichia coli, and *Pseudomonas aeruginosa* (3,16). Clinical presentation can be confusing, and many laboratory findings such as elevated sedimentation rate may be sensitive but not specific. Serial blood cultures are only positive in 32% to 60% of cases (1,17,18). Infections in infants and neonates are usually clinically silent, and toddlers may present with limping, pseudoparalysis, or pain on passive movement (19).

Half of the cases of septic arthritis occur in children less than 3 years of age (20). Approximately 53% are isolated cases of septic arthritis and 47% are cases of septic arthritis associated with osteomyelitis (21). Conversely, 30% of patients with osteomyelitis have adjacent septic arthritis (22). Boys are slightly more affected than girls (1.2:1), and the hip is the most affected joint (23). The most common symptoms are pain, fever, refusal to bear weight, and joint swelling. Most cases involve a single joint, although up to 15% of cases can affect multiple joints. Mortality rates of up to 7% have been reported (21). Similar organisms to those in osteomyelitis are found in septic arthritis, including *S. aureus* and *S. pneumoniae* (21,24). The most common sequelae of septic arthritis include joint instability, joint function limitation, and limb shortening (25).

Overall Cost to Society

No data were found in the medical literature on the overall cost to society from the diagnosis, treatment, and complications of acute hematogenous osteomyelitis or septic arthritis. Although there are several cost-effectiveness analyses evaluating the type, extent, and route of antibiotic administration in the treatment of osteomyelitis and septic arthritis, no cost-effectiveness data were found in the literature specifically incorporating imaging strategies in the management of acute hematogenous osteomyelitis or septic arthritis.

Goals

In acute hematogenous osteomyelitis and septic arthritis, the goal is early diagnosis and treatment to prevent the long-term sequelae of these diseases, which include growth disturbances, joint instability, chronic infection, malalignment, and limb deformity. The standard treatments include intravenous antibiotics and/or surgical debridement. Septic arthritis usually requires surgical therapy in order to decompress the intraarticular pressure. Surgical debridement may be necessary for osteomyelitis if frank pus can be aspirated from the bone, if there is necrotic bone present, or if there is failure to respond to antibiotic therapy (15,26).

Methodology

The authors performed a Medline search using PubMed (National Library of Medicine, Bethesda, Maryland) for data relevant to the diagnostic performance and accuracy of both clinical and radiographic examination of patients with acute hematogenous osteomyelitis and septic arthritis. The diagnostic performance of the clinical examination (history and physical exam) and surgical outcome was based on a systematic literature review performed for the years 1966 to 2004. The clinical examination search strategy used the following terms: (1) *acute hematogenous osteomyelitis*, (2) *septic arthritis*, (3) *pediatric*, (4) *children*, (5) *clinical examination*, (6) *epidemiology* or *physical examination* or *surgery*, and (7) *treatment* or *surgery*. The review of the diagnostic imaging literature was done for the same years. The search strategy used the following key words: (1) *acute hematogenous osteomyelitis*, (2) *septic arthritis*, (3) *magnetic resonance imaging* or *MRI*, (4) *bone scan*, (5) *ultrasound*, and (6) *imaging*, as well as combinations of these search strings. We excluded animal studies and non–English-language articles.

I. What are the Clinical Findings that Raise the Suspicion for Acute Hematogenous Osteomyelitis and Septic Arthritis to Direct Further Imaging?

Summary of Evidence: The clinical presentation of acute hematogenous osteomyelitis and septic arthritis can be confusing and nonspecific in the pediatric population. No single clinical finding in isolation leads to the diagnosis of osteomyelitis or septic arthritis. Repeat high-resolution imaging may be required to determine the need for surgical debridement, including extension into soft tissues or complications that are not amenable to systemic antibiotic therapy (limited evidence).

Supporting Evidence: Standard laboratory tests such as elevated sedimentation rate can be nonspecific or even normal (19) (limited evidence). Serial blood cultures are reported to be positive in 32% to 60% of cases (1,17,18) (moderate and limited evidence). Occasionally, direct aspiration of bone material may be needed for diagnosis. These aspirations can yield positive cultures in 87% of cases (27) (limited evidence).

The clinical presentation in the pediatric age group can be nonspecific. Infection in the neonate and infant is usually clinically silent. Toddlers can present with limping, pseudoparalysis, or pain on passive movement (4,28) (moderate to limited evidence).

Due to similarities in pathogenesis, there is also overlap in the clinical presentation of septic arthritis and osteomyelitis. Irritability, limping, or refusal to bear weight, along with elevated sedimentation rate or leukocytosis, are the most common presentations (15,23,24,29,30) (moderate to limited evidence). Kocher et al. (30) proposed probabilities for the presence of septic arthritis in the hip in order to guide further imaging and joint aspiration based on four clinical variables. These four predictors were leukocytosis greater than 12,000/mL, fever, inability to bear weight, and erythrocyte sedimentation rate (ESR) >40 mm/hr. If none of these predictors were present, there was a 0.2% chance of septic arthritis. The predicted probability of septic arthritis with one predictor was 3%, 40% with two predictors, 93.1% with three predictors, and 99.6% with four predictors. This constellation of clinical findings was most suggestive of osteomyelitis or septic arthritis and warranted further evaluation with imaging (moderate to limited evidence).

II. What Is the Diagnostic Performance of the Different Imaging Studies in Acute Hematogenous Osteomyelitis and Septic Arthritis?

Summary of Evidence: Although plain radiographs are neither sensitive nor specific, their low cost, ready availability, and ability to exclude other diseases that can produce similar symptoms (fractures, tumors) argue for their continued use as the initial evaluation (moderate to limited evidence) (31–35).

Several studies have shown that MRI and radionuclide bone scintigraphy have high sensitivity for detection of osteomyelitis (moderate evidence). Their relative merits have not been established. Bone scintigraphy has the advantage of whole-body imaging when symptoms cannot be localized, but has decreased specificity. This is especially true in the presence of superimposed disease processes such as a joint under pressure, or underlying bone diseases such as sickle cell or Gaucher's disease (moderate to limited evidence) (36–43).

Magnetic resonance imaging has the advantage of higher specificity and higher resolution to evaluate for soft tissue extension or complications, but has limited coverage of the body. This can be a disadvantage if symptoms cannot be localized or if there is polyostotic involvement (moderate to limited evidence).

Ultrasound is highly sensitive for the detection of a joint effusion, but not specific for the presence of infection. Based on the clinical predictors proposed by Kocher et al. (30), a decision to aspirate an effusion can be reliably made to exclude septic arthritis (moderate evidence) (44).

Supporting Evidence: Initial radiographs can detect deep soft tissue swelling and loss of soft tissue planes as early as 48 hours after onset of symptoms, but bone destruction is usually not detectable until 7 to 10 days after onset of symptoms (45). At least 30% of bone destruction is required before osteomyelitis becomes radiographically apparent (2). The sensitivity and specificity of plain radiographs are 43% to 75% and 75% to 83%, respectively (limited evidence) (32,46,47). If bone destruction is detected, however, no further imaging may be necessary. In addition, radiographs can detect other pathologies such as fractures and tumors that can clinically mimic osteomyelitis (moderate to limited evidence) (31–35,48).

The overall sensitivity and specificity for radionuclide bone scanning are 73% to 100% and 73% to 79% (moderate evidence) (36,41,49–53). In the neonate, however, the sensitivity of radionuclide bone scanning is decreased, ranging from 53% to 87% (54,55). Advantages of bone scintigraphy include the ability to image the entire body, delayed imaging with a single administration of tracer, and less sedation requirements. The ability to image the entire skeleton is ideal if symptoms cannot be localized or if there is polyostotic disease (limited to weak evidence) (33,51,52,56).

The sensitivity and specificity for MRI are 82% to 100% and 75% to 96% (moderate evidence) (33,57–64). Magnetic resonance imaging has the advantage of both high sensitivity and specificity. It can also display high-resolution images and evaluate for complications such as abscesses, joint effusions, and soft tissue extension that would require surgical intervention (63,65,66). The disadvantages include slighter higher cost relative to bone scintigraphy; prolonged imaging times, which may require sedation; and limited coverage.

Ultrasound is highly sensitive for the evaluation of joint effusions and can detect as little as 5 to 10cc of fluid within a joint (67). However, no ultrasound characteristics, including complexity of the fluid, the quantity of fluid, or adjacent hyperemia on color Doppler imaging, have been shown to be definitive in distinguishing septic arthritis from other non-infectious causes of joint effusions (68–71). Despite this limitation, the absence of fluid by ultrasound can be very helpful as septic arthritis is very unlikely in this setting (33,71,72). As outlined above, Kocher et al. (30) have provided clinical guidelines to direct joint aspiration. These include fever, the presence of elevated white count, an elevated sedimentation rate, and inability to bear weight (moderate evidence).

III. What Is the Natural History of Osteomyelitis and Septic Arthritis, and What Are the Roles of Medical Therapy Versus Surgical Treatment?

Summary of Evidence: Most uncomplicated cases of osteomyelitis require hospitalization and the institution of systemic intravenous antibiotic therapy. If there is a delay of more than 4 days prior to institution of therapy, there is increased poor outcomes and long-term sequelae (moderate evidence). Approximately 5% to 10% of cases require surgical intervention after initial antibiotic therapy, and up to 20% to 50% of all cases eventually require some form of surgery, including reconstruction and repeat debridements.

Approximately 5% to 10% of all cases have long-term sequelae such as growth disturbance, loss of function, malalignment, and deformity. Approximately 6% of cases develop chronic osteomyelitis (73).

Supporting Evidence: Most cases of acute osteomyelitis and septic arthritis are treated with antibiotics. If frank pus is aspirated from a joint, surgical debridement is required immediately. Patients are admitted for initiation of systemic antibiotic therapy. Average length of stay ranges from 3 to 7 days (16,24,74). Average course of systemic antibiotic therapy is approximately 11 to 14 days with an additional 4 weeks of outpatient oral antibiotic therapy (5,7,16,75). Many of the clinical signs and symptoms improve within 48 hours of initiation of systemic antibiotics, which is a reassuring sign. If there is no clinical improvement, further evaluation including imaging may be required to exclude complications not amenable to antibiotics alone, such as abscess collections, necrotic tissue, or extension into soft tissues.

Approximately 20% to 50% of all cases eventually require surgical intervention (28). Up to 10% of patients eventually have long-term sequelae, including growth disturbance, loss of function, malalignment, and deformity (8,9,16,23,28). Up to 6% of patients eventually have chronic osteomyelitis. There is evidence that a delay in initiation of therapy (>4 days after onset of symptoms), certain infecting organisms (methicillin-resistant *S. aureus*), and age of the patient (<6 months of age) are predictors of bad outcomes (moderate evidence) (3,7,16,73).

IV. Is There a Role for Repeat Imaging in the Management?

Summary of Evidence: Most patients respond clinically to systemic antibiotics within 48 hours. If there is no clinical response to therapy, repeat imaging should be performed to exclude complications that would require surgical intervention such as abscess collections, extensive soft tissue extension, or necrotic tissue. The performance characteristics of MRI are ideal in this setting (moderate to limited evidence).

Supporting Evidence: Approximately 95% to 98% of patients respond clinically to antibiotic therapy alone (76). Children usually respond quickly to antibiotics, on average within 48 hours. However, approximately 5% to 10% of patients eventually require surgical intervention (77,78). These patients require high-resolution imaging to evaluate for surgical disease. The literature supports the use of MRI for evaluation of necrosis, abscess collections, and soft tissue extension (63–65,79) (moderate evidence to limited evidence). This information can be helpful for the surgeon in planning the surgical approach and method of debridement. There are also some data in the literature suggesting that MRI should be the repeat imaging modality of choice if the site of infection is localized to the spine or pelvis. There is a higher incidence of abscess formation in these deep infections, which would require earlier surgical evaluation and treatment (33,57,63,80).

V. What Is the Diagnostic Performance of Imaging of Osteomyelitis and Septic Arthritis in the Adult?

Summary of Evidence: Overall, MRI appears to be the imaging modality of choice to evaluate for osteomyelitis and septic arthritis in the adult population, including the diabetic patient and intravenous drug users. The ability to localize symptoms and inherent high spatial resolution allows exact anatomic detail that may be helpful for surgical planning (limited to moderate evidence).

Supporting Evidence: Osteomyelitis in the diabetic foot represents a diagnostic challenge both clinically and by imaging. The diabetic foot is prone to infection and suboptimal healing due to the decreased blood supply from diabetic vasculopathy, decreased immune response, and repetitive trauma and abnormal mechanics from diabetic neuropathy (81). Because of these abnormalities, there are baseline abnormal imaging findings of the bones and joints without superimposed infection.

Radiographically, the diabetic foot has many features mimicking infection, including destruction, debris, and subluxation. The diabetic foot can also have abnormal findings without osteomyelitis on three-phase radionuclide bone scan (82). There is some evidence of using both bone scan with methylene diphosphanate (MDP) as well as a white blood cell scan to map out specific areas of infection (82–85) (limited to moderate evidence). Although it has excellent sensitivity and specificity (92 and 97% respectively), the technique is cumbersome and laborious (83). Its lower resolution relative to MRI also limits the imaging of anatomic detail for surgical planning (86,87).

Magnetic resonance imaging has both high sensitivity and specificity for evaluating osteomyelitis in the diabetic foot (88–91). Sensitivity ranges from 88% to 92% and specificity ranges from 82% to 100% (85,90,92) (moderate evidence). However, the diagnosis is frequently not made based on specific imaging characteristics, but by the location of the abnormality. The neuropathic foot inherently contains signal abnormalities similar to osteomyelitis. Imaging diagnosis is made by identifying signal abnormalities in the bone contiguous and in direct contact with adjacent skin ulcers and known pressure points in the diabetic foot (87).

Hematogenous osteomyelitis and septic arthritis also occurs in intravenous drug users. Many of these infections arise initially in the soft tissues, such as the psoas muscle, with subsequent involvement into the spine or sacroiliac (SI) joint (93,94). Septic arthritis with osteomyelitis is slightly more common in this population than osteomyelitis alone (95). The plain film is neither sensitive nor specific in commonly involved locations, such as the spine and SI joint. Computed tomography (CT) scan with intravenous contrast material has been shown to be very accurate in the identification of the soft tissue infections and abscesses, but not as accurate in the evaluation of the spinal osteomyelitis/discitis or sacroiliitis (96,97) (limited to moderate evidence). Magnetic resonance imaging is superior in evaluating these structures due to its higher contrast, signal-to-noise ratio, and multiplanar imaging.

Ultrasound can still detect joint effusions, but can be technically more difficult due to the larger amount of soft tissue in adults compared to the pediatric population (98,99). Magnetic resonance imaging is highly sensitive for the evaluation of septic arthritis (97,100,101). Hyperemia and synovitis can also be elucidated with the use of intravenous gadolinium, increasing the accuracy of septic arthritis (102).

VI. What Are the Roles of the Difference Imaging Modalities in the Evaluation of Acute Osteomyelitis and Septic Arthritis?

The decision tree in Figure 14.1 outlines the role of each imaging modality in the evaluation of suspected osteomyelitis. Table 14.1 summarizes the diagnostic performance of the imaging studies for osteomyelitis in children and adults. The plain radiograph is the initial imaging evaluation due to its relative low cost, rapid acquisition, and ready availability. If there is frank evidence of osteomyelitis on the radiograph, immediate antibiotic therapy can be instituted and further imaging may not be necessary, as up to 80% of patients are successfully treated with antibiotics alone.

If the radiograph is negative for osteomyelitis, and there are no localizing symptoms clinically, radionuclide bone scintigraphy is the next imaging modality, based on its ability to provide whole-body imaging.

If there are localized symptoms, MRI would be a better choice due to higher resolution, more specificity, and ability to immediately evaluate complications.

Repeat imaging with MRI should be considered in all patients who do not improve clinically after 48 hours of systemic antibiotic therapy, and to direct management of those who require surgical therapy. In addition, if immediate surgical therapy is planned, such as in cases of infections involving the spine or pelvis, earlier imaging with MRI may be of use.

If symptoms are referable to the hip, an ultrasound should be performed to rapidly evaluate for the presence of an effusion, and also to provide imaging-guided joint aspiration.

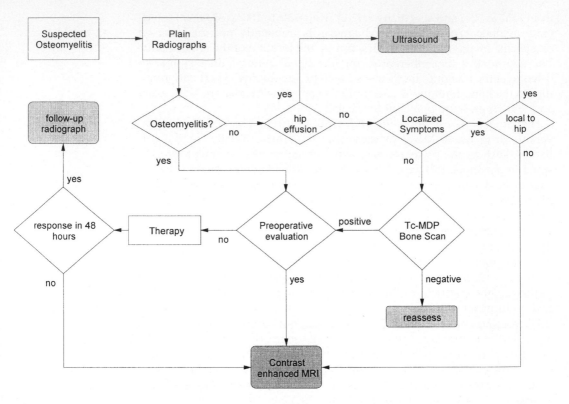

Figure 14.1. Algorithm for imaging suspected osteomyelitis or septic arthritis in the pediatric population.

Table 14.1. Diagnostic performance characteristics of imaging studies for osteomyelitis in children and adults

	Sensitivity	Specificity
Plain radiograph (32,46,47)	43–75%	75–83%
Radionuclide scintigraphy (36,41,49–53)	73–100% (53–87% in infants)	73–79%
MRI (33,57–64)	82–100%	75–96%

Table 14.1 presents the performance characteristics of imaging studies for osteomyelitis in children and adults.

Imaging Case Studies

Case 1

Young child with fever and limp (Fig 14.2).

Case 2

Child with fever (Fig 14.3).

Case 3

Teenager with right buttock pain and fever (Fig 14.4).

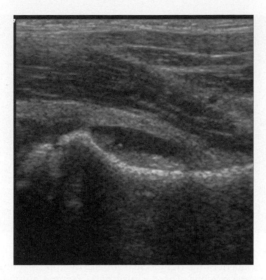

Figure 14.2. Ultrasound depicting hip effusion with synovitis. Frank pus was aspirated from the joint.

Suggested Imaging Protocols

• Plain radiograph: At least two orthogonal views of the body part of interest should be obtained; views of the opposite limb may be useful for comparison to detect subtle changes. Imaging should be performed on all patients suspected of osteomyelitis or septic arthritis to evaluate for destruction, as well as to exclude other pathologies such as tumors or fractures.

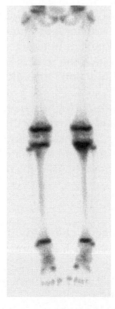

Figure 14.3. Radionuclide bone scan shows abnormal uptake in the proximal left tibial metaphysis that was found to be osteomyelitis. The imaging findings are not specific for osteomyelitis, because neoplasms and trauma could have a similar appearance.

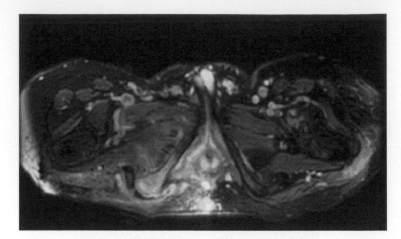

Figure 14.4. Axial MRI of the pelvis after administration of gadolinium shows abnormal enhancement of the right ischial tuberosity and surrounding soft tissues consistent with osteomyelitis. There is also enhancement around the left greater trochanter, consistent with trochanteric bursitis.

- Radionuclide bone scintigraphy: Three-phase radionuclide bone scintigraphy with technetium 99m (Tc-99m)-labeled MDP should be obtained, with planar images during blood flow and soft tissue phases. Planar images of extremities and single photon emission computed tomography (SPECT) images of the axial skeleton during the bone phase should be obtained. This imaging should be used if symptoms are nonlocalizing or if there is a suspicion of polyostotic disease.
- Magnetic resonance imaging: Axial and coronal T1 spin echo, axial and sagittal T2 fast spin echo with fat saturation, coronal short-time inversion recovery (STIR), axial and coronal T1 two-dimensional (2D) spoiled gradient recalled (SPGR) with fat saturation before and after intravenous gadolinium should be obtained. Imaging should be performed if there are localizing symptoms or if the patient fails to respond to antibiotics within 48 hours. Early evaluation with MRI also may be of use if immediate surgery is planned.
- Ultrasound: Linear transducer high-frequency probe (7–12 MHz) imaging should be obtained and compared with that for the opposite joint to assess symmetry. Color or power Doppler assesses for hyperemia. Imaging should be performed to evaluate for joint effusion and joint aspiration. It is most commonly used for the hip joint.

Future Research

- Can the use of emerging whole-body imaging techniques in MRI obviate the need for radionuclide scintigraphy in the evaluation of osteomyelitis?
- Can MRI with gadolinium provide more information than ultrasound in the evaluation of septic arthritis?
- Can findings on imaging (plain film, MRI, ultrasound) predict the likelihood of success of medical therapy alone, and provide early triage to surgical therapy?
- Does positron emission tomography (PET)- CT have a role in the evaluation of osteomyelitis or septic arthritis?

References

1. Waldvogel FA, Medoff G, Swartz MN. N Engl J Med 1970;282(4):198–206.
2. Faden H, Grossi M. Am J Dis Child 1991;145(1):65–69.
3. Kao HC, et al. J Microbiol Immunol Infect 2003;36(4):260–265.
4. Oudjhane K, Azouz EM. Radiol Clin North Am 2001;39(2):251–266.
5. Barton LL, Dunkle LM, Habib FH. Am J Dis Child 1987;141(8):898–900.
6. Azouz EM, Greenspan A, Marton D. Skeletal Radiol 1993;22(1):17–23.
7. Welkon CJ, et al. Pediatr Infect Dis 1986;5(6):669–676.
8. Choi IH, et al. J Bone Joint Surg Am 1990;72(8):1150–1165.
9. Betz RR, et al. J Pediatr Orthop 1990;10(3):365–372.
10. Alderson M, et al. J Bone Joint Surg Br 1986;68(2):268–274.
11. Tice AD, Hoaglund PA, Shoultz DA. J Antimicrob Chemother 2003;51(5): 1261–1268.
12. Jensen AG, et al. J Infect 1997;34(2):113–118.
13. Sonnen GM, Henry NK. Pediatr Clin North Am 1996;43(4):933–947.
14. Asmar BI. Infect Dis Clin North Am 1992;6(1):117–132.
15. Nelson JD. Infect Dis Clin North Am 1990;4(3):513–522.
16. Karwowska A, Davies HD, Jadavji T. Pediatr Infect Dis J 1998;17(11): 1021–1026.
17. Dormans JP, Drummond DS. J Am Acad Orthop Surg 1994;2(6):333–341.
18. Nixon GW. AJR 1978;130(1):123–129.
19. Restrepo SC, Gimenez CR, McCarthy K. Rheum Dis Clin North Am 2003;29(1): 89–109.
20. Matan AJ, Smith JT. Orthopedics 1997;20(7):630–635; quiz 636–637.
21. Caksen H, et al. Pediatr Int 2000;42(5):534–540.
22. Perlman MH, et al. J Pediatr Orthop 2000;20(1):40–43.
23. Wang CL, et al. J Microbiol Immunol Infect 2003;36(1):41–46.
24. Razak M, Nasiruddin J. Med J Malaysia 1998;53(suppl A):86–94.
25. Campagnaro JG, et al. Chir Organi Mov 1992;77(3):233–245.
26. Dagan R. Pediatr Infect Dis J 1993;12(1):88–92.
27. Howard CB, et al. J Bone Joint Surg Br 1994;76(2):311–314.
28. Razak M, Ismail MM, Omar A. Med J Malaysia 1998;53(suppl A):83–85.
29. Khachatourians AG, et al. Clin Orthop 2003;409:186–194.
30. Kocher MS, Zurakowski D, Kasser JR. J Bone Joint Surg Am 1999;81(12): 1662–1670.
31. Zucker MI, Yao L. West J Med 1992;156(3):297–298.
32. Bonakdar-pour A, Gaines VD. Orthop Clin North Am 1983;14(1):21–37.
33. Jaramillo D, et al. AJR 1995;165(2):399–403.
34. Gold R. Pediatr Infect Dis J 1995;14(6):555.
35. Fordham L, Auringer ST, Frush DP. J Pediatr 1998;132(5):906–908.
36. Sullivan DC, et al. Radiology 1980;135(3):731–736.
37. Wald ER, Mirro R, Gartner JC. Clin Pediatr (Phila) 1980;19(9):597–601.
38. Jones DC, Cady RB. J Bone Joint Surg Br 1981;63–B(3):376–378.
39. Berkowitz ID, Wenzel W. Am J Dis Child 1980;134(9):828–830.
40. Handmaker H. Radiology 1980;135(3):787–789.
41. Barron BJ, Dhekne RD. Clin Nucl Med 1984;9(7):392–393.
42. Park HM, Rothschild PA, Kernek CB. AJR 1985;145(5):1079–1084.
43. Stark JE, et al. Radiology 1991;179(3):731–733.
44. Klein DM, et al. Clin Orthop 1997;338:153–159.
45. Capitanio MA, Kirkpatrick JA. AJR Radium Ther Nucl Med, 1970;108(3): 488–496.
46. Kaye JJ. Pediatr Ann 1976;5(1):11–31.
47. Keenan AM, Tindel NL, Alavi A. Arch Intern Med 1989;149(10):2262–2266.
48. Gold R. Pediatr Rev 1991;12(10):292–297.
49. Duszynski DO, et al. Radiology 1975;117(2):337–340.
50. Gelfand MJ, Silberstein EB. JAMA 1977;237(3):245–247.
51. Hankins JH, Flowers WM Jr. J Miss State Med Assoc 1978;19(1):10–12.

52. Nelson HT, Taylor A. Eur J Nucl Med 1980;5(3):267–269.
53. Erasmie U, Hirsch G. Z Kinderchir 1981;32(4):360–366.
54. Ash JM, Gilday DL. J Nucl Med 1980;21(5):417–420.
55. Bressler EL, Conway JJ, Weiss SC. Radiology 1984;152(3):685–688.
56. Handmaker H, Leonards R. Semin Nucl Med 1976;6(1):95–105.
57. Modic MT, et al. Radiol Clin North Am 1986;24(2):247–258.
58. Unger E, et al. AJR 1988;150(3):605–610.
59. Morrison WB, et al. Radiology 1993;189(1):251–257.
60. Fletcher BD, Scoles PV, Nelson AD. Radiology 1984;150(1):57–60.
61. Berquist TH, et al. Magn Reson Imaging 1985;3(3):219–230.
62. Dangman BC, et al. Radiology 1992;182(3):743–747.
63. Mazur JM, et al. J Pediatr Orthop 1995;15(2):144–147.
64. Umans H, Haramati N, Flusser G. Magn Reson Imaging 2000;18(3):255–262.
65. Connolly LP, et al. J Nucl Med 2002;43(10):1310–1316.
66. Lee SK, et al. Radiology 1999;211(2):459–465.
67. Moss SG, et al. Radiology 1998;208(1):43–48.
68. Chao HC, et al. Acta Paediatr Taiwan 1999;40(4):268–270.
69. Chao HC, et al. J Ultrasound Med 1999;18(11):729–734; quiz 735–736.
70. Strouse PJ, DiPietro MA, Adler RS. Radiology 1998;206(3):731–735.
71. Zawin JK, et al. Radiology 1993;187(2):459–463.
72. Lim-Dunham JE, Ben-Ami TE, Yousefzadeh DK. Pediatr Radiol 1995;25(7): 556–559.
73. Espersen F, et al. Rev Infect Dis 1991;13(3):347–358.
74. Speiser JC, et al. Semin Arthritis Rheum 1985;15(2):132–138.
75. Scott RJ, et al. J Pediatr Orthop 1990;10(5):649–652.
76. Le Saux N, et al. BMC Infect Dis 2002;2(1):16.
77. Roine I, et al. Clin Infect Dis 1997;24(5):849–853.
78. Dirschl DR. Orthop Rev 1994;23(4):305–312.
79. McAndrew PT, Clark C. BMJ 1998;316(7125):147.
80. Middleton MS. AJR 1988;151(3):612–613.
81. Snyder RJ, et al. Ostomy Wound Manage 2001;47(1):18–22, 25–30; quiz 31–32.
82. Unal SN, et al. Clin Nucl Med 2001;26(12):1016–1021.
83. Poirier JY, et al. Diabetes Metab 2002;28(6 Pt 1):485–490.
84. Crerand S, et al. J Bone Joint Surg Br 1996;78(1):51–55.
85. Cook TA, et al. Br J Surg 1996;83(2):245–248.
86. Sella EJ, Grosser DM. Clin Podiatr Med Surg 2003;20(4):729–740.
87. Schweitzer ME, Morrison WB. Radiol Clin North Am 2004;42(1):61–71, vi.
88. Craig JG, et al. Radiology 1997;203(3):849–855.
89. Marcus CD, et al. Radiographics 1996;16(6):1337–1348.
90. Morrison WB, et al. Radiology 1995;196(2):557–564.
91. Ledermann HP, Morrison WB, Schweitzer ME. Radiology 2002;223(3):747–755.
92. Croll SD, et al. J Vasc Surg 1996;24(2):266–270.
93. Alcantara AL, Tucker RB, McCarroll KA. Infect Dis Clin North Am 2002; 16(3):713–743, ix–x.
94. Kak V, Chandrasekar PH. Infect Dis Clin North Am 2002;16(3):681–695.
95. Chandrasekar PH, Narula AP. Rev Infect Dis 1986;8(6):904–911.
96. Bonham P. J Wound Ostomy Continence Nurs 2001;28(2):73–88.
97. Sturzenbecher A, et al. Skeletal Radiol 2000;29(8):439–446.
98. Wingstrand H, Egund N, Forsberg L. J Bone Joint Surg Br 1987;69(2):254–256.
99. Zieger MM, Dorr U, Schulz RD. Skeletal Radiol 1987;16(8):607–611.
100. Karchevsky M, et al. AJR 2004;182(1):119–122.
101. Learch TJ, Farooki S. Clin Imaging 2000;24(4):236–242.
102. Graif M, et al. Skeletal Radiol 1999;28(11):616–620.

15

Imaging for Knee and Shoulder Problems

William Hollingworth, Adrian K. Dixon, and John R. Jenner

Imaging of the Knee

   I. What is the role of radiography in patients with an acute knee injury and possible fracture?
      A. Cost-effectiveness analysis
      B. Applicability to children
  II. When should magnetic resonance imaging be used for patients with suspected meniscal or ligamentous knee injuries?
      A. Cost-effectiveness analysis
 III. Is radiography useful in evaluating the osteoarthritic knee?
 IV. Special case: Imaging of the painful prosthesis

Imaging of the Shoulder

  V. When is radiography indicated for patients with acute shoulder pain?
 VI. Which imaging modalities should be used in the diagnosis of soft tissue disorders of the shoulder?

Issues

Key Points

- Knee radiographs of the acutely injured knee in the emergency department are rarely useful for determining therapy except in patients aged 55 or older, or with isolated tenderness of patella, tenderness at the head of fibula, inability to flex the knee 90 degrees, or the inability to bear weight both immediately and in the emergency department for four steps (strong evidence).
- Magnetic resonance imaging (MRI) is an accurate and valuable diagnostic tool for confirming or excluding the presence of meniscal and cruciate ligamentous knee injuries (moderate evidence). If used in selected patients, in whom arthroscopy is probable but not inevitable, MRI can reduce the overall arthroscopy rate and the number of purely diagnostic arthroscopies (moderate evidence).

- There is currently insufficient evidence to demonstrate that the routine use of radiography in patients with suspected chronic osteoarthritic knee pain will alter management or the outcome of patients. However, radiography is required before making decisions regarding knee replacement surgery.
- The use of radiography to evaluate patients with suspected recurrent atraumatic shoulder dislocation is unnecessary in most cases (limited evidence). Furthermore, selective imaging strategies may be able to rationalize the number of prereduction or postreduction radiographs required in suspected first-time or traumatic shoulder dislocations (limited evidence).
- Ultrasound, MRI, and MR arthrography all have high specificity in the diagnosis of full-thickness rotator cuff tears. Therefore, in populations with a moderate prevalence of rotator cuff tears, a positive result on any one of these tests can confirm the diagnosis with a high degree of certainty (moderate evidence). Until further data are available, the choice between these tests will be largely dependent on physician preference and available resources.

Epidemiology of Knee and Shoulder Problems

Approximately 0.3% of the United States population seeks medical care for an acute knee injury each year. These injuries are most frequently seen in young males and are usually precipitated by sports (36%); twisting, bending, or stepping motions (27%); or falls (21%) (1). The annual incidence of traumatic anterior shoulder dislocation is less than 0.02%, most commonly observed in young males with sporting injuries (2,3). Chronic knee and shoulder problems are much more prevalent. One community survey in the United Kingdom found that 19% of adults reported knee pain lasting more than 1 week in the previous month and 16% reported shoulder pain (4). Prevalence in both sexes rose steadily with age, reaching a plateau at about age 65 and was also positively associated with social deprivation. Although the prevalence is high, many people with knee or shoulder pain do not seek medical care (5).

Overall Cost to Society

In the year 2001, knee symptoms and injuries were the primary reason reported by the patient for 1.5 million (1.4%) of all emergency department visits in the United States (6). Furthermore, knee symptoms and injuries led to an estimated 861,000 (1.0%) hospital outpatient department visits and 13.8 million (1.6%) visits to office-based physicians (6,7). Knee problems, therefore, are in the top 15 most frequent reasons for consulting a physician, second only to back pain among musculoskeletal problems. Medical care visits for shoulder problems are slightly less frequent. In total, shoulder symptoms and injury lead to 1.2 million (1.1%) emergency department visits, 425,000 (0.5%) outpatient visits and 8.9 million (1.0%) of office visits (6,7).

For knee and shoulder problems seen in outpatient settings, imaging utilization varies greatly by specialty. A study conducted in the United States observed that orthopedic surgeons requested radiography in 80% of first knee pain consultations and 78% of first shoulder pain consultations, whereas rheumatologists utilized radiography in far fewer knee (45%) and shoulder (36%) cases (8). Orthopedic surgeons were also more likely to refer for MRI of the knee (20% versus 6%) and, to a lesser extent, of the shoulder (4% versus 2%). The direct cost of health care for musculoskeletal problems is about 1% of gross national product in several industrialized countries (9), although we found no convincing estimates of the total societal costs for knee and shoulder problems.

Goals

Among patients who seek medical attention for knee and shoulder problems, the clinician's task is to find the appropriate balance between physical examination, diagnostic imaging, and arthroscopic investigation to achieve accurate diagnosis and initiate cost-effective therapy.

Methodology

Our initial search strategy identified systematic literature reviews of knee and shoulder imaging studies. We searched the Medline database using the PubMed interface for abstracts published between January 1966 and March 2004 with the search words *knee* and *shoulder* and the PubMed designation of a systematic review (systematic [sb]). This strategy identified 203 shoulder and 442 knee abstracts. From this group, we selected several key articles reviewing the role of imaging (10–19). We then searched the articles cited by these systematic reviews to identify the relevant primary studies. For topics where no recent systematic review was available, we selected two seminal articles on the topic and searched for similar work using the related articles PubMed function. Where possible, we obtained and reviewed the full text of all relevant English-language articles identified.

I. What Is the Role of Radiography in Patients with an Acute Knee Injury and Possible Fracture?

Summary of Evidence: Acute knee trauma provides a common diagnostic quandary in accident and emergency departments. Fractures are present in 4% to 12% of patients presenting with knee injuries (20,21), and yet radiography may be requested in excess of 70% of cases (22). Several guidelines are available to help clinicians target imaging at high-risk patients. There is strong evidence (level I) to suggest that the five criteria of the Ottawa knee rule (OKR) are highly sensitive at predicting fractures in adults and moderate evidence (level II) that this rule can be generalized to children older than 5 years of age. Further work is needed to evaluate the impact of the OKR on the cost-effectiveness of medical care.

Supporting Evidence: Several groups have developed clinical decision rules to guide knee radiography requests following trauma in order to save costs and prevent unnecessary radiation (23–26). These decision rules focus variously on patient age, injury mechanism, inability to ambulate, and other clinical signs such as fibula head tenderness. Table 15.1 provides details of four published decision rules. The optimal threshold for radiography requests depends on the trade-off between the clinical and possible legal consequences of a missed fracture compared to the time, cost, and radiation exposure of radiographs. In practice, all of the decision rules place great emphasis on sensitivity at the expense of specificity.

To date, the OKR (25,27) has undergone the most extensive validation. Other decision rules may have greater specificity, but they have not yet been validated by independent investigators. The OKR suggests that radiography should be performed on the acutely injured knee when the patient has one or more of the following criteria: (1) age 55 years or older, (2) isolated tenderness of the patella (no other knee bone tenderness), (3) tenderness of the head of the fibula, (4) inability to flex the knee to 90 degrees, or (5) inability to bear weight both immediately and in the emergency department for four steps. Initial assessment of the interobserver reliability of the OKR suggested excellent agreement between physicians (27); however, more recent work evaluating the agreement between nurses and physicians has been less impressive (20,28,29). These variable results emphasize the need for thorough training and support for clinicians before implementing the OKR.

Table 15.1. Clinical decision rules for radiography of acute knee injury

Rule	Criteria for radiography	% Sensitivity (Ref.)	% Specificity (Ref.)	Validation studies
Ottawa knee rule (25)	• Age 55 or older; or • Isolated tenderness of patella (no other bone tenderness); or • Tenderness at head of fibula; or • Inability to flex 90 degrees; or • Inability to bear weight both immediately and in the emergency department for four steps	99 (10)	49 (10)	20–22,27–35
Pittsburgh rule (24)	• Fall or blunt-trauma and age <12 or >50; or • Fall or blunt trauma and inability to walk four weight-bearing steps in emergency department	99 (21)	60 (21)	21,24,26
Fagan and Davies (23)	Two or more of the following: • Age over 55 years • Effusion • Hemarthrosis • Not able to bear weight in the department (includes touch weight-bearing as non–weight bearing) • History of direct trauma to the knee • Point bony tenderness at the patella, tibial plateau, femoral condyles or the head of fibula	95 (23)	62 (23)	23
Weber et al. (26)	Patient does not need radiograph if: • Able to walk without limping • Twist injury without effusion	100 (26)	34 (26)	26

A recent systematic review found 11 studies evaluating the diagnostic accuracy of the OKR (10). Six of these studies were suitable for inclusion in a meta-analysis, of which four were considered to be of high quality (i.e., consecutive enrollment, universal reference standard, and radiographic assessment of fracture blind to clinical findings). The mean sensitivity of the OKR in these studies was 98.5% and specificity was 48.6%. While this provides strong evidence (level I) that the OKR is sensitive at predicting fracture, it does not prove that it is a cost-effective method of organizing care.

Based on case series, several authors have speculated that adherence to the OKR would reduce the utilization of knee radiography in the emergency department by between 17% and 49% (25,27,30–35). However, these estimates rely on the assumption that clinicians would rigidly follow the OKR and would not be swayed by fears of missed diagnoses or patient expectations of imaging. Only one controlled trial has evaluated whether radiography utilization can be curtailed in practice following the introduction of the OKR (22). Stiell and colleagues (22) enrolled 3907 patients with isolated knee trauma at four hospitals in a prospective, controlled, before-and-after study. In the hospitals where the OKR was introduced, the absolute rate of radiography requests fell by 20.5%. By comparison, there was a minimal (1%) reduction at the control hospitals; this disparity was statistically significant. Furthermore, patients who were not imaged spent less time in the emergency department and had lower follow-up costs than their counterparts who were referred for radiography. Therefore, there is moderate evidence (level II) that the OKR has a beneficial impact.

A. Cost-Effectiveness Analysis

The same research group has also developed a simple cost-benefit decision model comparing the OKR to usual practice (36). The reduced costs of imaging, follow-up care, and days off from work observed after the implementation of the OKR are balanced against the potential for increased malpractice costs. However, in the primary analysis, the model did not quantify any costs that might result from the delayed recovery of patients with fractures falsely diagnosed as normal. The authors conclude that the introduction of the OKR resulted in a modest ($34) saving per patient, but, due to the high volume of minor knee injuries, the total economic impact is large. Because of the high cost of litigation, especially in the U.S., these conclusions were dependent on the exact diagnostic sensitivity of the OKR. If the sensitivity of OKR falls more than 1% below that of usual practice, the conclusions are reversed. Until a broader body of research is available comparing the sensitivity and specificity of OKR to usual practice, we consider that there is limited evidence (level III) to support the hypothesis that the OKR is cost-effective in emergency departments.

In many cases plain radiography is all that is required to allow the clinician to proceed with conservative therapy. If a fracture is seen, there is increasing use of computed tomography (CT) or MRI to determine whether structures such as the tibial plateau are depressed to an extent that warrants surgical elevation. Because there are anecdotal accounts of CT and MRI identifying fractures when plain radiographs are normal, some clinicians seek reassurance from CT/MRI in equivocal cases. Different clinicians have different thresholds for this need for reassurance, and there is little evidence to help in making such decisions. Even when plain radiographs show subtle tibial plateau depression and CT in the coronal or sagittal plane shows 2- to 5-mm depression, clinicians vary in their subsequent management decisions; some may proceed with surgical elevation and some may not. The evidence that patients with a 4-mm depression do significantly better with surgery than without is also scant. However, with increasingly noninvasive techniques now on offer there is a trend toward more imaging being used as a roadmap for intervention.

B. Applicability to Children

The diagnostic performance of the OKR may be altered in the skeletally immature knee due to open growth plates and secondary ossification centers resulting in different injury patterns (37). Additionally, tests such as weight bearing, which rely on considerable patient interaction, may not be as valid in the youngest children. Two case series have studied the applicability of the OKR to children (30,32). In the largest study involving 750 children aged 2 to 16, Bulloch et al. (30) found that the OKR was 100% sensitive [95% confidence interval (CI), 94.9–100%] in predicting the 70 fractures observed and 43% specific (95% CI, 39.1–46.5%). Due to the small numbers of children in the youngest age category, these authors endorsed the OKR in children 5 years of age or over. In a smaller study conducted by Khine et al. (32), the OKR correctly predicted 12 of 13 fractures observed in 234 children aged 2 to 18 years. The one missed injury was a nondisplaced fracture of the proximal tibia in an 8-year-old. In totality, the similarity between these two studies and evaluations conducted in adults provide reassurance that the OKR is valid in children (level II, moderate evidence). However, there is not yet sufficient evidence to demonstrate the cost-effectiveness of the OKR in children.

II. When Should Magnetic Resonance Imaging Be Used for Patients with Suspected Meniscal or Ligamentous Knee Injuries?

Summary of Evidence: Empirical work demonstrates that the utilization of knee MRI among Medicare and Medicaid enrollees increased rapidly by 140% in the early 1990s (38). There is limited evidence (level III) to support the theory that, for some patients, a composite clinical examination performed by an experienced musculoskeletal specialist can bypass the need for MRI by directly identifying patients with cruciate or meniscal injuries amenable to arthroscopic repair. However, there is also moderate evidence (level II) that MRI is a highly accurate method of diagnosing soft tissue knee injuries in patients where the clinical picture is not clear. If MRI is used in patients likely to undergo arthroscopy, there is moderate evidence (level II) indicating that it can substantially reduce the overall arthroscopy rate and limit the number of purely diagnostic arthroscopies without detriment to the patient's quality of life.

Supporting Evidence: The mechanism of injury, clinical history, and physical examination can provide important information on the likelihood of injuries to the menisci and ligaments of the knee. Indeed, some authorities have observed that, with sufficiently experienced clinicians, these methods

have high diagnostic accuracy and might render the use of imaging unnecessary prior to arthroscopy in many cases (39,40). Conversely, others have
argued that MRI is an essential component of the presurgical assessment,
which saves money and reduces referrals for purely diagnostic arthroscopy
(41,42).

Four systematic reviews have summarized the diagnostic accuracy of the
physical examination for suspected injury to the cruciate ligaments and the
menisci (11–14). Each review notes that most diagnostic accuracy studies
interpret the reference standard, usually arthroscopy, without masking the
surgeon to the findings of the physical examination and that, as in many
clinical studies, verification bias (patients with abnormal physical tests
were more likely to undergo the reference standard) was often present.
These biases tend to artificially enhance sensitivity estimates.

Two reviews (11,12) included studies that reported data on composite
clinical examinations without specifying the precise examination maneuvers that were used. In general, these composite examinations resulted in
reasonable sensitivity and specificity for anterior cruciate ligament (82%
and 94%, respectively), posterior cruciate ligament (91% and 98%), and
meniscal (77% and 91%) injuries (12). However, it is very difficult to repli-
cate or generalize these findings given the lack of detail about the individual components of the examination.

To date, the majority of studies have been conducted by musculoskeletal specialists skilled in physical examination techniques. Therefore, these
methods may be less accurate if applied in primary care. Given the
inevitable methodologic flaws in many of these studies, we conclude that
there is limited evidence (level III) that the clinical examination can accurately select patients most likely to benefit from therapeutic arthroscopy.
More high-quality studies of individual physical tests are urgently
required.

The rise in MRI utilization is probably due to increased availability of
equipment and reluctance on the part of physicians to rely solely on the
clinical examination to determine treatment. Furthermore, some legal
judgments have criticized surgeons for operating without full information
about the extent of the lesion(s). However, overreliance on advanced
imaging technology might be counterproductive if MRI is not sufficiently
accurate. In particular, age-related degeneration of the menisci might lead
to false-positive MRI findings and unnecessary surgery (43).

Demographic aspects also play a part: there may be much more reason
for a professional athlete to undergo soft tissue imaging in the acute phase
compared with a middle-aged sedentary person (Fig. 15.1). The advice for
the athlete may be merely to train or not to train. Few surgeons relish intervening in the acute phase when there is a lot of hemorrhage still masking
the operative field. Although MRI may show many unexpected lesions in
the acute phase, the immediate clinical management of the patient rarely
changes (44).

We identified four reviews summarizing the accuracy of MRI compared
to arthroscopy for soft tissue knee injuries (11,15,16,45). All reviewed a
wealth of evidence, albeit from methodologically weak studies in many
instances. The most recent review identified 29 studies conducted between
1991 and 2000 (15). Of these studies, only four (14%) had adequate blinding of the index test (MRI) when conducting arthroscopy, the reference
standard. In addition only 10 (34%) studies clearly avoided verification

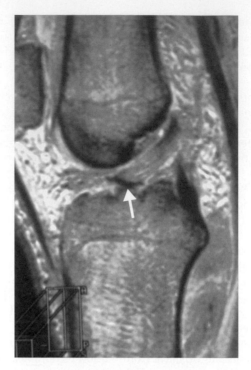

Figure 15.1. Three-dimensional (3D) gradient echo MRI of a soccer player follow-ing recent trauma. The intact anterior cruciate ligament has pulled off a small rind of cortex from the proximal tibia (arrow). Prompt surgery allowed this avulsion fracture, well shown on this preoperative roadmap, to be pinned back promptly. This probably speeded up his return to top-class soccer.

bias. The pooled weighted sensitivity and specificity estimates from this review are reported in Table 15.2. The results suggest that the sensitivity of MRI is consistently lower in lateral meniscal tears than medial meniscal and cruciate injuries; conversely, specificity is higher. One explanation for this finding is that radiologists may have a lower threshold for reporting medial meniscal tears as opposed to lateral tears. Overall, there is moder-ate evidence (level II) that MRI of the knee is a highly accurate method of diagnosing soft tissue knee injuries. In actuality the accuracy of MRI might be higher than the figures indicated in Table 15.2. It is recognized that, while arthroscopy is the only viable reference standard, in particular

Table 15.2. Diagnostic accuracy of MRI for soft tissue knee injuries

Lesion	Pooled weighted sensitivity*	Pooled weighted specificity*	Positive likelihood ratio	Negative likelihood ratio
Medial meniscal tear	93 (92–95)	88 (85–91)	7.75	0.08
Lateral meniscal tear	79 (74–84)	96 (95–97)	19.75	0.22
Anterior cruciate ligament complete tear	94 (92–97)	94 (93–96)	15.67	0.06
Posterior cruciate ligament complete tear	91 (83–99)	99 (99–100)	91.00	0.09

Source: Data extracted from the systematic review of Oei et al. (15).
* Figures in parentheses represent the 95% confidence intervals.

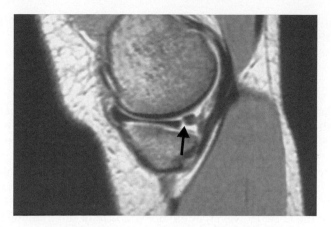

Figure 15.2. A patient with chronic symptoms in the posteromedial aspect of the knee. The 3D gradient echo MRI shows a classical tear at the junction of the middle and posterior thirds of medial meniscus (arrow). Arthroscopy was initially negative. Continuing symptoms led to clinicoradiologic discussion; a second arthroscopy confirmed the tear. [*Source*: From Mackenzie et al. (46), with permission.]

regions of the knee, such as the posterior horn of the medial meniscus, the arthroscopic diagnosis is imperfect, often relying on probing rather than direct visualization of lesions (Fig. 15.2) (46).

Several observational studies have gone beyond the intermediate outcome of diagnostic accuracy to examine whether MRI can decrease the rate of arthroscopy (42,47–53). The estimated reduction in arthroscopy following MRI varies widely. This lack of consensus is not surprising given the range of primary and secondary care settings examined, and varying definitions of what constitutes a purely diagnostic arthroscopy. In perhaps the most detailed study, Vincken et al. (52) performed MRI on 430 consecutive patients who underwent a standardized physical examination performed by an orthopedic surgeon and met *a priori* criteria for arthroscopic surgery. The MRI results indicated that no arthroscopy was required in 209 (49%) patients. Of these patients with negative MRI findings, 93 were randomly selected and received immediate arthroscopy. Ninety-one percent (85/93) of arthroscopies subsequently performed in these patients were purely diagnostic (86%) or had a minor therapeutic procedure (5%) on a lesion that, according to the study protocol, did not require surgical intervention. The remaining 9% (8/93) of negative MRI findings were genuine false negatives overlooking clinically important lesions. Most patients (200/221) with positive MRI findings had subsequent arthroscopy; only 11% (21/200) of these had a purely diagnostic arthroscopy. Based on the large proportion of diagnostic arthroscopies that could have been avoided, these authors concluded that a combination of a clinical examination and MRI was useful in selecting patients for arthroscopy.

A. Cost-Effectiveness Analysis

Two small randomized trials have analyzed the impact of knee MRI on costs and patient quality of life. Both trials were conducted by the same research team (17). The first trial recruited patients attending orthopedic outpatient clinics for whom arthroscopy was contemplated; 118 patients were randomly allocated to MRI or no-MRI prior to the decision to perform arthroscopy. Over the 12 months after randomization, the proportion of patients receiving arthroscopy was statistically significantly lower among patients who were referred for MRI (41% MRI arm versus 71% in the no-MRI arm). This equated to a sizable reduction in surgery costs, but these savings were almost exactly canceled out by the additional costs of the MRI examination itself. This trial found no significant difference in patient quality of life 12 months after randomization, although interpretation is seriously limited by a low response rate.

The second randomized trial recruited patients from a specialist knee clinic assessing patients referred from a hospital emergency department. A total of 120 patients were recruited, all of whom received an MRI examination of the knee. However, in the no-MRI arm of the trial, the imaging results were withheld from patients and clinicians for at least 6 weeks. Unlike the first trial, the arthroscopy rate during 1 year of follow-up was low and was not significantly affected by the availability of MRI findings (30% MRI arm, 24% no-MRI arm). Therefore, in this setting, MRI did not prevent surgery and increased costs. Again, there was no statistically significant effect on patient quality of life at 12 months.

These two trials demonstrate the complexity of judging the cost-effectiveness of MRI for internal derangement of the knee. Routine MRI is not likely to be cost-effective in patients with a low prevalence of soft tissue injuries who are unlikely to receive arthroscopy; this situation might exist in primary care settings (11). Likewise, MRI may not be cost-effective in a subset of patients referred to musculoskeletal specialists who have clear-cut clinical signs of soft tissue injury with a very high probability of requiring therapeutic arthroscopy. However, there is moderate evidence (level II) that MRI can reduce the need for surgery, without increasing costs in many patients who have an intermediate probability of soft tissue injury. The exact threshold at which MRI becomes cost-effective depends on the relative costs of MRI and arthroscopy and the relative scarcity of imaging facilities and musculoskeletal specialists (54–56).

III. Is Radiography Useful in Evaluating the Osteoarthritic Knee?

Summary of Evidence: Radiography is frequently used to assess the extent of disease in the osteoarthritic knee. However, there is poor correlation between imaging findings and patient symptoms. Furthermore, there is currently insufficient evidence (level IV) to support the hypothesis that routine use of radiography in patients with chronic knee pain will improve patient management and quality of life.

Supporting Evidence: For patients with knee pain and locking, the plain radiograph is often regarded as the key investigation to establish the diagnosis and identify/exclude radiopaque loose bodies that may be amenable to arthroscopic removal (57). For patients with chronic knee pain without locking or restriction of movement, the role of radiography is poorly defined. More than 40% of adults aged 40 to 80 years have radiographic evidence of knee osteophytes or joint space narrowing despite reporting no knee pain within the last year (58). Furthermore, a substantial minority (≈35%) of adults in the same age range who do report persistent knee pain have no osteophytes or joint space narrowing on radiography (58), although this proportion diminishes in patients with severely disabling pain (59). Longitudinal studies have also highlighted the weak correlation between radiographic and symptomatic changes over time (60). Therefore, basing management decisions purely on radiographic anomalies risks targeting treatment on innocuous anatomical factors that are not the cause of the patient's joint pain. Despite this, there is evidence that physicians place more emphasis on radiographic rather than clinical signs of osteoarthritis when deciding on the need for an orthopedic referral (61).

In one review of 1153 knee radiographs requested by primary care physicians, most imaging reports (59%) described normal anatomy or degenerative changes (29%) (62). In 20% of patients radiography was used to bolster the case for, or against, referral to a specialist. Other important changes in therapy based on radiography findings were observed in only 3% of cases (62).

In the U.K., the Royal College of Radiologists guidelines recommend that radiography for knee pain without locking or restriction of movement is only indicated in specific circumstances, such as when considering surgery (63). Still, many primary care physicians feel that radiographs are necessary in order to reassure patients, to justify a specialist referral, or for other nondiagnostic reasons (59,61). Therefore, continued use of radiography for patients with chronic knee pain seems inevitable. However, trial data have demonstrated that radiography requests can be reduced by regular educational messages reminding physicians of the limited value of radiography in this setting (64,65).

IV. Special Case: Imaging of the Painful Prosthesis

The potentially infected knee prosthesis is a case where the evidence for the various imaging investigations is rather weak. The patient presents with pain and perhaps instability some months/years after a successful knee replacement. Plain radiography of the total extent of the prosthesis (including the femoral and tibial tips) is performed; interpretation is easier if these images can be compared with those obtained at the postoperative stage, if available; lucency around the stem of the prosthesis may be associated with loosening or infection. Despite software developments to reduce artifacts from the metallic prosthesis, neither CT nor MRI can offer much here. Skeletal scintigraphy can provide evidence of abnormal osteoblastic activity around the prosthesis, which should be more intense in relation to infection than loosening; some centers proceed to white cell scintigraphy, which may help in this distinction. Other centers use arthrography, which may provide a microbiologic sample if there is a large effusion. In any event, there is a wide range of sensitivities and specificities in these tests. Interpretation is also complex because the investigations are often spread out over several weeks. Furthermore there is frequently no gold standard, as the ultimate arbiter, the decision to perform revision surgery, is not undertaken lightly and is ultimately still based on clinical rather than radiologic grounds. At present, there is insufficient evidence (level IV) to recommend any particular imaging approach.

V. When Is Radiography Indicated for Patients with Acute Shoulder Pain?

Summary of Evidence: Conventional teaching advocates both pre- and postreduction radiographs for patients with clinically suspected shoulder dislocation, and survey data confirm that many hospitals follow this recommendation (66). However, more recent research has provided limited evidence (level III) that radiographs are not necessary in most patients with recurrent atraumatic dislocation. Furthermore, there is limited evidence (level III) that the prereduction radiograph may be omitted in traumatic joint dislocations provided that the clinician is confident of the diagnosis. An alternative approach that eliminates the postreduction radiograph in patients with prereduction radiographs demonstrating dislocation and no fracture is also supported by limited evidence (level III). Limited evidence also suggests that, in patients without obvious shoulder deformity, radiography should be targeted at those with bruising or joint swelling, or with a history of fall, pain at rest, or abnormal range of motion. However, more research is needed to validate these guidelines and to provide head-to-head comparisons of selective imaging strategies to demonstrate the relative feasibility and cost-effectiveness of implementation.

Supporting Evidence: Imaging is commonly requested following shoulder trauma. The questions posed differ according to the nature of the injury and the age of the patient. In the elderly, a fracture of the surgical neck of humerus is common after a fall. In the younger patient the clinician may be more worried about possible dislocation, especially in those with recurrent episodes where the chance of recurrent dislocation is high. It is in this precise group of young patients that ionizing radiation should be kept as low as reasonably achievable and requests for imaging kept to a minimum.

A retrospective study conducted in a North American medical center found that radiographs were performed in 59% of emergency department patients with shoulder pain (67). Twenty percent of these radiographs provided therapeutically important information (defined as glenohumeral dislocation, fracture, severe acromioclavicular joint separation, infection, or malignancy).

Hendey (68) has demonstrated that, for patients with suspected recurrent relatively atraumatic dislocation, physicians were certain of the dislocation in more than 90% of cases. In every case this preimaging confidence was justified by radiographic evidence of dislocation without fracture. After reduction of these atraumatic dislocations, physicians were also confident that relocation had been achieved in more than 90% of patients; again this was subsequently radiographically confirmed in all cases. Although this work requires validation, it does provide limited evidence (level III) that radiographs are not routinely indicated in this well-defined recurrent dislocation population.

Opinions differ for suspected traumatic or first-time dislocations. Some have suggested that many postreduction radiographs are not diagnostically or therapeutically useful when the prereduction radiograph demonstrates dislocation without fracture (68–70). In 53 patients with simple dislocation and clinically successful relocation, Hendey reported that all postreduction radiographs confirmed the reduction and found no unsuspected fractures. Others have argued that it is more practical to eliminate the prereduction radiograph when the physician is certain of the clinical diagnosis of dislocation (71). Omitting the prereduction radiograph enables prompt joint relocation, which would, in any case, be the preferred management even if Hill-Sachs lesions, Bankart lesions, or greater tuberosity fractures are later demonstrated on the postreduction radiograph. Shuster et al. (71) estimated that eliminating the prereduction radiograph would remove approximately 30 minutes from the delay between presentation and reduction.

Either of the strategies described above will significantly reduce radiograph utilization at centers that routinely image pre- and postreduction. There is currently insufficient evidence (level IV) to definitively choose between these selective imaging strategies; both have potential drawbacks. In high-energy injury mechanisms, omitting the prereduction radiograph risks an iatrogenic displacement of an unrecognized fracture of the humeral neck during the attempted reduction (72). Conversely, some physicians are reluctant to eliminate the postreduction radiograph for fear of missing a fracture not evident on initial imaging or overlooking a failed reduction (71).

In patients without obvious bone deformity on initial clinical examination, Fraenkel et al. (73) report that only 12% of shoulder radiographs are therapeutically informative (i.e., demonstrating acute fracture, severe acromioclavicular joint separation, dislocation, infection, or malignancy). In a prospective study involving 206 radiographs, they identified two higher-risk patient groups in which radiographs were most likely to be informative: (1) patients with bruising or joint swelling on examination; and (2) patients with a history of fall, pain at rest, or abnormal range of joint motion. In these two groups 32% of radiographs were therapeutically informative. Only one therapeutically informative radiograph, in a patient with a lytic lesion with known multiple myeloma, would have been missed by a strategy limiting radiography to these two groups. Therefore, the authors advise imaging for all patients with a history of cancer that might involve bone. This prediction rule requires external validation and currently provides no more than preliminary and limited evidence (level III) that some emergency department radiographs on painful shoulders could be avoided by careful patient selection.

VI. Which Imaging Modalities Should Be Used in the Diagnosis of Soft Tissue Disorders of the Shoulder?

Summary of Evidence: There is moderate evidence (level II) that both MRI and ultrasound have fairly high sensitivity (>85%) and specificity (>90%) in the diagnosis of full-thickness rotator cuff (RC) tears, and therefore a positive test result is likely to be useful for confirming tears in patients for whom surgery is being considered. The results of ultrasound studies were more variable perhaps reflecting the operator-dependent nature of the technique. The few studies conducted on the accuracy of MR arthrography (MRA) suggest that it may be more accurate than either MRI or ultrasound; however, more data are needed to reinforce the limited evidence (level III) to date. Until these data are available, the choice between ultrasound and MR techniques is likely to be primarily based on physician preference and the availability of imaging equipment and personnel. The sensitivity of all three of these minimally invasive tests for partial-thickness RC tears is relatively poor. This may be due in part to the poorly defined diagnostic criteria for these more subtle lesions. Several studies including a randomized trial have provided strong evidence (level I) that MRI can influence the management of patients with shoulder pain. However, there is insufficient evidence (level IV) demonstrating an eventual benefit to patient quality of life.

Supporting Evidence: Once a patient has developed chronic shoulder problems there are a large number of differential diagnoses, including impingement syndrome, partial- and full-thickness rotator cuff tears, acromioclavicular joint injuries, adhesive capsulitis, glenohumeral arthritis, glenohumeral instability, and other extrinsic conditions (74,75). The delineation between these diagnoses is not always precise, as evidenced by the existence of multiple diagnostic criteria for categorizing chronic shoulder pain and relatively poor interrater reliability in making the diagnosis (76). Despite this complexity, it is thought that most shoulder problems evaluated in primary care stem from subacromial impingement of the RC tendons, leading to degenerative change and, eventually, partial- and full-thickness tears of the soft tissues, particularly in older patients (77,78). Several tests and signs have been promoted in the literature that aim to help the clinician pinpoint the source of the shoulder pain (78). Some authors have claimed that the diagnostic accuracy of these clinical tests is equal to or better than ultrasound and MRI for many soft tissue injuries (75). Limited evidence (level III) indicates that, when performed by experienced clinicians, the composite clinical evaluation is sensitive in predicting RC tears and bursitis and can therefore accurately rule out these diagnoses in patients with negative test findings (79,80). However, a recent systematic review concluded that too few studies had been conducted to enable any firm conclusions to be drawn about the value of any individual clinical tests (18).

If imaging is requested, there is a range of potential imaging options available, perhaps reflecting that no single investigation is perfect (Table 15.3). It might also reflect the fact that the choice of some treatment options remains controversial and not fully evaluated in terms of cost-effectiveness (77).

Conventional arthrography is falling out of favor but it still remains useful for identifying capsulitis (by showing increase of resistance on

Table 15.3. Some of the common radiologic investigations available for shoulder problems

Examination	Radiation	Cost
Plain radiograph AP/axial	+	+
Plain radiographs under fluoroscopy	++	++
Ultrasound	–	+
Arthrography under fluoroscopy	+++	++
CT	+++	++
CT arthrography	+++	+++
MRI	–	+++
MRI indirect arthrography	–	++++
MRI direct arthrography	–	++++

Table 15.4. **Diagnostic accuracy of ultrasound, MRI, and MRA for rotator cuff (RC) tears**

Modality	Lesion	Pooled sensitivity*	Pooled specificity*	Pooled positive likelihood ratio	Pooled negative likelihood ratio
Ultrasound	Full-thickness RC tear	87 (84–89)[†]	96 (49–97)[†]	13.16	0.16[†]
	Partial-thickness RC tear	67 (61–73)[†]	94 (92–96)[†]	8.90[†]	0.36[†]
MRI	Full-thickness RC tear	89 (86–92)	93 (91–95)	10.63[†]	0.16
	Partial-thickness RC tear	44 (36–51)[†]	90 (87–92)[†]	3.99[†]	0.66[†]
MRA	Full-thickness RC tear	95 (82–98)	93 (84–97)	10.05[†]	0.11[†]
	Partial-thickness RC tear	62 (40–80)[†]	92 (83–97)	8.90[†]	0.43[†]

Source: Data extracted from the systematic review of Dinnes et al. (18) The likelihood ratio estimates cannot be derived directly from sensitivity and specificity estimates as Dinnes et al. separately pooled data from the source studies.
* Figures in parentheses represent 95% confidence intervals.
[†] Authors report that significant heterogeneity existed between the results of the source publications.

installation and lymphatic filling). It also provides unequivocal proof of a full-thickness RC tear (by showing direct extension of contrast medium into the subacromial space). However, the anatomical features of the tear are not well demonstrated. Hence the growing interest in alternative imaging techniques.

Ultrasound is a relatively inexpensive but highly operator dependent investigation that can potentially yield exquisite views of the distal rotator cuff. The systematic review by Dinnes et al. (18) identified 38 studies including a total of 2435 patients where the accuracy of ultrasound for RC tears was compared to arthrography, arthroscopy, open surgery, or MRI. These studies were highly heterogeneous, both in the quality of the research design adopted and in their findings. The overall trends from these studies indicate that ultrasound has high specificity for all RC tears, but sensitivity was lower for both full- and particularly partial-thickness tears (Table 15.4). Therefore, in secondary care settings, a patient with positive ultrasound findings is very likely to truly have a RC tear and could be considered a potential surgical candidate. However, ultrasound has several potential diagnostic pitfalls (81) and, unlike MRI, cannot provide an entire anatomical overview of the shoulder.

Magnetic resonance imaging can show most of the relevant anatomical features and can identify a large proportion of RC tears (Fig. 15.3). Indeed an MR roadmap of anatomical features is often required before a surgeon will contemplate surgery; the anatomy of the acromioclavicular joint is well demonstrated and most surgeons now require information about this area before performing decompression (e.g., acromioplasty—one of the commonest shoulder operations). The pooled results of 20 diagnostic accuracy studies indicate that MRI is not substantially more accurate than ultrasound in detecting RC tears (Table 15.4). In fact, a review of 14 studies focusing on partial-thickness tears indicated that the sensitivity of MRI is only 44%, lower than that of ultrasound (18). Few of these studies used fat-suppressed MRI techniques, which might have increased the diagnostic accuracy for partial-thickness tears.

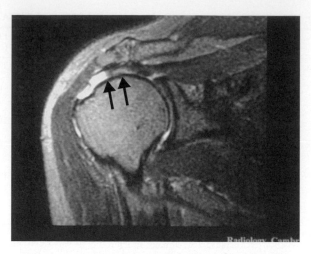

Figure 15.3. Magnetic resonance image of right shoulder. On this fat-suppressed T2-weighted MRI, the high signal intensity defect in the distal supraspinatus tendon provides convincing evidence of a full-thickness rotator cuff tear (arrows). The surgeon can readily assess the degree of retraction, which is essential information before considering repair. Although ultrasound could give some of this information, the full relationship of the damaged frayed tendon with the subacromial region is well demonstrated here.

Direct comparison of the intermodality diagnostic accuracy figures in Table 15.4 may be misleading as the table is based on studies of variable quality. The majority of five studies that conducted head-to-head comparisons of MRI and ultrasound against a common reference standard have concluded that MRI has equal or better accuracy than ultrasonography (82–86). However, taken in aggregate, data from these studies suggest that both the sensitivity and specificity of ultrasound and MRI are similar (18). It is important that imaging findings are closely correlated with the patient's symptoms when selecting management strategies; asymptomatic full-thickness RC tears may be present in one quarter of adults aged 60 or over (87).

One anatomical feature that MR does not demonstrate well is the glenoid labrum. The anatomy of this structure, along with the anterior extent of the anterior joint capsule, is crucial for the surgeon considering strength procedures for anterior instability. Estimates of the sensitivity of MRI without intra-articular contrast range from 55% to 90% (88–92). It has been claimed that MR arthrography (MRA) procedures (indirect or direct) can help clarify the detection of partial RC tears and labral tears (93–97). Nevertheless, it remains difficult, at best, to differentiate normal appearances of the labrum, anatomical variations thereof, and subtle tears (e.g., superior labrum anterior-posterior lesions). The few diagnostic accuracy studies that have been conducted have demonstrated that MRA is a highly sensitive and specific investigation for identifying full-thickness RC tears, but there is currently insufficient evidence (level IV) to support its accuracy for partial-thickness tears (Table 15.4). In some centers CT arthrography is used, especially where access to MR is limited. Although the bone texture is exquisitely demonstrated, CT gives little information about bone edema and the radiation dose has to be justified.

Most of the published literature evaluates the technical performance and diagnostic accuracy of imaging. Less is known concerning whether imaging is actually effective at influencing diagnosis, changing therapy, or improving patients' health. In a review of studies of shoulder MRI, Bearcroft and colleagues (98) found that less than 2% of publications (4/265) addressed the effectiveness of imaging. These studies have collectively demonstrated that MRI and MRA might change therapeutic plans in between 15% and 61% of patients imaged (98,99). This wide range of therapeutic impact probably stems from differences in study methodology and case mix, whereby imaging has most influence in groups of patients with poorly defined symptoms and diagnoses. Furthermore, the presumption that imaging will lead to better treatment selection remains unproven. The sole randomized controlled trial comparing MRI with arthrography demonstrated that 52% of preimaging treatment plans changed following MRI compared to 66% of preimaging treatment plans in the arthrography group (100). However, this trial did not measure patient outcomes; therefore, it is impossible to judge the final benefit of these therapeutic changes. Therefore, we conclude that there is currently insufficient evidence (level IV) to demonstrate that any imaging modality will lead to improved health for patients with suspected soft tissue shoulder injuries.

Despite the limitations in knowledge expressed above, there are now quite robust guidelines designed to help the clinician though the maze of potential investigations (63). At present, there appears to be a split between European practice (18), which emphasizes the value of ultrasound as an inexpensive screening test before more sophisticated evaluation, and North American practice (101), where there is greater reliance on MRI, MRA, and conventional arthrography. However, all of these recommendations are based primarily on consensus opinion.

Suggested Imaging Protocols

- Knee radiography: Anteroposterior (AP) and lateral views often suffice. Following trauma, the lateral is usually obtained as a "shoot-through" to see an effusion and a fluid/fluid level. Depending on the clinical question, tunnel views of the intercondylar notch and skyline views of the patella may be indicated.
- Magnetic resonance imaging of the knee: direct imaging in the three orthogonal planes is desirable. A sensible protocol might include a sagittally acquired 3D gradient echo data set, coronal T1- and T2-weighted images (or dual echo techniques) followed by a fat-suppressed T2-weighted axial series.
- Shoulder radiography: Conventional imaging includes an AP view of the glenohumeral joint, which includes the acromioclavicular joint and either an axial or an oblique view. The axial view may be difficult if the patient cannot fully abduct the arm.
- Ultrasound of the shoulder: This is very highly operator dependent. Increasing use is being made of high-frequency (e.g., 10 to 15 MHz) probes to provide optimal demonstration of tendons.
- Magnetic resonance imaging of the shoulder: Coronal oblique imaging along the plane of the supraspinatus tendon is a key sequence; it can be done by T1- and T2-weighted imaging or by a dual echo technique. Axial

views are essential to see the labrum; T1-weighted views provide good anatomical overview; fat-suppressed T2-weighted images can be very helpful. Many medical centers also use sagittal T1- and T2-weighted images routinely; they provide a good overview of the rotator cuff.

- Magnetic resonance arthrography of the shoulder: This can either be done directly [by instilling dilute gadolinium (Gd) diethylenetriamine pentaacetic acid (DTPA) into the shoulder joint] or indirectly (by giving Gd DTPA intravenously and obtaining images following exercise of the muscles around the joint). There is increasing use of direct MR arthrography.

Future Research

This chapter has summarized the available evidence on the appropriate roles of imaging in knee and shoulder problems. However, in areas where evidence is sparse or where the clinician is in doubt, a comprehensive history and clinical examination remain vital in determining the most appropriate investigation and whether or not imaging is likely to influence diagnosis and treatment. A good clinician should be prepared to disregard imaging guidelines if the patient presents with an unusual clinical picture. For example, a plain radiograph or skeletal scintigraphy, which would not normally be indicated, may reveal a previously unsuspected lesion such as malignancy and help achieve a timely diagnosis. Further research is needed to plug the gaps in the existing literature and to keep evidence up to date. In particular we believe that future research should focus on the following:

- Providing appropriate training for clinicians to implement the Ottawa knee rule while monitoring its impact on the cost-effectiveness of care.
- Defining diagnostic thresholds to ensure the cost-effective use of MRI for meniscal and ligamentous knee injuries in primary and specialist care settings.
- Validating the sensitivity, specificity, and therapeutic impact of clinical prediction rules for radiographic evaluation of patients with shoulder pain in the emergency department.
- Direct comparisons of the diagnostic accuracy of ultrasound, MRI, and MR arthrography for the diagnosis of full- and partial-thickness rotator cuff tears.

References

1. Yawn BP, Amadio P, Harmsen WS, Hill J, Ilstrup D, Gabriel S. J Trauma 2000; 48(4):716–723.
2. Simonet WT, Melton LJ 3rd, Cofield RH, Ilstrup DM. Clin Orthop 1984; 186:186–191.
3. Kroner K, Lind T, Jensen J. Arch Orthop Trauma Surg 1989;108(5):288–290.
4. Urwin M, Symmons D, Allison T, et al. Ann Rheum Dis 1998;57(11):649–655.
5. Picavet HS, Schouten JS. Pain 2003;102(1–2):167–178.
6. National Center for Health Statistics. National Hospital Ambulatory Medical Care Survey: 2001. Hyattsville, MD, 2003.
7. National Center for Health Statistics. National Ambulatory Medical Care Survey: 2001. Hyattsville, MD, 2003.
8. Katz JN, Solomon DH, Schaffer JL, Horsky J, Burdick E, Bates DW. Am J Med 2000;108(1):28–35.

9. Woolf AD, Pfleger B. Bull WHO 2003;81(9):646–656.
10. Bachmann LM, Haberzeth S, Steurer J, ter Riet G. Ann Intern Med 2004;
    140(2):121–124.
11. Jackson JL, O'Malley PG, Kroenke K. Ann Intern Med 2003;139(7):575–588.
12. Solomon DH, Simel DL, Bates DW, Katz JN, Schaffer JL. JAMA 2001;
    286(13):1610–1620.
13. Scholten RJ, Deville WL, Opstelten W, Bijl D, van der Plas CG, Bouter LM.
    J Fam Pract 2001;50(11):938–944.
14. Scholten RJ, Opstelten W, van der Plas CG, Bijl D, Deville WL, Bouter LM.
    J Fam Pract 2003;52(9):689–694.
15. Oei EH, Nikken JJ, Verstijnen AC, Ginai AZ, Myriam Hunink MG. Radiology
    2003;226(3):837–848.
16. Mackenzie R, Palmer CR, Lomas DJ, Dixon AK. Clin Radiol 1996;51(4):251–257.
17. Bryan S, Weatherburn G, Bungay H, et al. Health Technol Assess 2001;
    5(27):1–95.
18. Dinnes J, Loveman E, McIntyre L, Waugh N. Health Technol Assess 2003;
    7(29):iii, 1–166.
19. Schulte-Altedorneburg G, Gebhard M, Wohlgemuth WA, et al. Skeletal Radiol
    2003;32(1):1–12.
20. Matteucci MJ, Roos JA. J Emerg Med 2003;24(2):147–150.
21. Seaberg DC, Yealy DM, Lukens T, Auble T, Mathias S. Ann Emerg Med 1998;
    32(1):8–13.
22. Stiell IG, Wells GA, Hoag RH, Sivilotti ML, Cacciotti TF, Verbeek PR, et al.
    JAMA 1997;278(23):2075–2079.
23. Fagan DJ, Davies S. Injury 2000;31(9):723–727.
24. Seaberg DC, Jackson R. Am J Emerg Med 1994;12(5):541–543.
25. Stiell IG, Greenberg GH, Wells GA, et al. Ann Emerg Med 1995;26(4):405–413.
26. Weber JE, Jackson RE, Peacock WF, Swor RA, Carley R, Larkin GL. Ann Emerg
    Med 1995;26(4):429–433.
27. Stiell IG, Greenberg GH, Wells GA, et al. JAMA 1996;275(8):611–615.
28. Szucs PA, Richman PB, Mandell M. Acad Emerg Med 2001;8(2):112–116.
29. Kec RM, Richman PB, Szucs PA, Mandell M, Eskin B. Acad Emerg Med 2003;
    10(2):146–150.
30. Bulloch B, Neto G, Plint A, et al. Ann Emerg Med 2003;42(1):48–55.
31. Ketelslegers E, Collard X, Vande Berg B, et al. Eur Radiol 2002;12(5):1218–
    1220.
32. Khine H, Dorfman DH, Avner JR. Pediatr Emerg Care 2001;17(6):401–404.
33. Emparanza JI, Aginaga JR. Ann Emerg Med 2001;38(4):364–368.
34. Tigges S, Pitts S, Mukundan S Jr, Morrison D, Olson M, Shahriara A. AJR 1999;
    172(4):1069–1071.
35. Richman PB, McCuskey CF, Nashed A, et al. J Emerg Med 1997;15(4):459–463.
36. Nichol G, Stiell IG, Wells GA, Juergensen LS, Laupacis A. Ann Emerg Med
    1999;34(4 pt 1):438–447.
37. Tepper KB, Ireland ML. Instr Course Lect 2003;52:667–676.
38. Solomon DH, Katz JN, Carrino JA, et al. Med Care 2003;41(5):687–692.
39. O'Shea KJ, Murphy KP, Heekin RD, Herzwurm PJ. Am J Sports Med 1996;
    24(2):164–167.
40. Miller GK. Arthroscopy 1996;12(4):406–413.
41. Suarez-Almazor ME, Kaul P, Kendall CJ, Saunders LD, Johnston DW. Int J
    Technol Assess Health Care 1999;15(2):392–405.
42. Carmichael IW, MacLeod AM, Travlos J. J Bone Joint Surg Br 1997;
    79(4):624–625.
43. Guten GN, Kohn HS, Zoltan DJ. WMJ 2002;101(1):35–38.
44. Odgaard F, Tuxoe J, Joergensen U, et al. Scand J Med Sci Sports 2002;12(3):
    154–162.
45. Rappeport ED, Mehta S, Wieslander SB, Lausten GS, Thomsen HS. Acta Radiol
    1996;37(5):602–609.

46. Mackenzie R, Keene GS, Lomas DJ, Dixon AK. Br J Radiol 1995;68(814): 1045–1051.
47. Bui-Mansfield LT, Youngberg RA, Warme W, Pitcher JD, Nguyen PL. AJR 1997;168(4):913–918.
48. Chissell HR, Allum RL, Keightley A. Ann R Coll Surg Engl 1994;76(1):26–29.
49. Mackenzie R, Dixon AK, Keene GS, Hollingworth W, Lomas DJ, Villar RN. Clin Radiol 1996;51(4):245–250.
50. Ruwe PA, Wright J, Randall RL, Lynch JK, Jokl P, McCarthy S. Radiology 1992; 183(2):335–339.
51. Rappeport ED, Wieslander SB, Stephensen S, Lausten GS, Thomsen HS. Acta Orthop Scand 1997;68(3):277–281.
52. Vincken PW, ter Braak BP, van Erkell AR, et al. Radiology 2002;223(3):739–746.
53. Weinstabl R, Muellner T, Vecsei V, Kainberger F, Kramer M. World J Surg 1997; 21(4):363–368.
54. Sherman PM, Penrod BJ, Lane MJ, Ward JA. Arthroscopy 2002;18(2):201–205.
55. Uppal A, Disler DG, Short WB, McCauley TR, Cooper JA. Radiology 1998; 207(3):633–636.
56. Watura R, Lloyd DC, Chawda S. BMJ 1995;311(7020):1614.
57. Bianchi S, Martinoli C. Radiol Clin North Am 1999;37(4):679–690.
58. Lanyon P, O'Reilly S, Jones A, Doherty M. Ann Rheum Dis 1998;57(10):595–601.
59. Peat G, Croft P, Hay E. Best Pract Res Clin Rheumatol 2001;15(4):527–544.
60. Dieppe PA, Cushnaghan J, Shepstone L. Osteoarthritis Cartilage 1997;5(2): 87–97.
61. Bedson J, Jordan K, Croft P. Ann Rheum Dis 2003;62(5):450–454.
62. Morgan B, Mullick S, Harper WM, Finlay DB. Br J Radiol 1997;70:256–260.
63. RCR Working Party. Making the Best Use of a Department of Clinical Radiology: Guidelines for Doctors, 5th ed. London: Royal College of Radiologists, 2003.
64. Eccles M, Steen N, Grimshaw J, et al. Lancet 2001;357(9266):1406–1409.
65. Ramsay CR, Eccles M, Grimshaw JM, Steen N. Clin Radiol 2003;58(4):319–321.
66. te Slaa RL, Wijffels MP, Marti RK. Eur J Emerg Med 2003;10(1):58–61.
67. Fraenkel L, Lavalley M, Felson D. Am J Emerg Med 1998;16(6):560–563.
68. Hendey GW. Ann Emerg Med 2000;36(2):108–113.
69. Harvey RA, Trabulsy ME, Roe L. Am J Emerg Med 1992;10(2):149–151.
70. Hendey GW, Kinlaw K. Ann Emerg Med 1996;28(4):399–402.
71. Shuster M, Abu-Laban RB, Boyd J. Am J Emerg Med 1999;17(7):653–658.
72. Demirhan M, Akpinar S, Atalar AC, Akman S, Akalin Y. Injury 1998; 29(7):525–528.
73. Fraenkel L, Shearer P, Mitchell P, LaValley M, Feldman J, Felson DT. J Rheumatol 2000;27(1):200–204.
74. Steinfeld R, Valente RM, Stuart MJ. Mayo Clin Proc 1999;74(8):785–794.
75. Brox JI. Best Pract Res Clin Rheumatol 2003;17(1):33–56.
76. de Winter AF, Jans MP, Scholten RJ, Deville W, van Schaardenburg D, Bouter LM. Ann Rheum Dis 1999;58(5):272–277.
77. Speed C, Hazleman B. Clin Evid 2003;9:1372–1387.
78. Stevenson JH, Trojian T. J Fam Pract 2002;51(7):605–611.
79. Litaker D, Pioro M, El Bilbeisi H, Brems J. J Am Geriatr Soc 2000; 48(12):1633–1637.
80. MacDonald PB, Clark P, Sutherland K. J Shoulder Elbow Surg 2000;9(4):299–301.
81. Allen GM, Wilson DJ. Eur J Ultrasound 2001;14(1):3–9.
82. Nelson MC, Leather GP, Nirschl RP, Pettrone FA, Freedman MT. J Bone Joint Surg Am 1991;73(5):707–716.
83. Burk DL Jr, Karasick D, Kurtz AB, et al. AJR 1989;153(1):87–92.
84. Hodler J, Terrier B, von Schulthess GK, Fuchs WA. Clin Radiol 1991; 43(5):323–327.

85. Martin-Hervas C, Romero J, Navas-Acien A, Reboiras JJ, Munuera L. J Shoulder Elbow Surg 2001;10(5):410–415.
86. Swen WA, Jacobs JW, Algra PR, et al. Arthritis Rheum 1999;42(10):2231–2238.
87. Sher JS, Uribe JW, Posada A, Murphy BJ, Zlatkin MB. J Bone Joint Surg Am 1995;77(1):10–15.
88. Zlatkin MB, Hoffman C, Shellock FG. J Magn Reson Imaging 2004; 19(5):623–631.
89. Tung GA, Entzian D, Green A, Brody JM. AJR 2000;174(4):1107–1114.
90. Tuite MJ, Cirillo RL, De Smet AA, Orwin JF. Radiology 2000;215(3):841–845.
91. Shellock FG, Bert JM, Fritts HM, Gundry CR, Easton R, Crues JV 3rd. J Magn Reson Imaging 2001;14(6):763–770.
92. Gusmer PB, Potter HG, Schatz JA, et al. Radiology 1996;200(2):519–524.
93. Waldt S, Burkart A, Lange P, Imhoff AB, Rummeny EJ, Woertler K. AJR 2004; 182(5):1271–1278.
94. Parmar H, Jhankaria B, Maheshwari M, et al. J Postgrad Med 2002;48(4): 270–273; discussion 273–274.
95. Herold T, Hente R, Zorger N, et al. Rofo 2003;175(11):1508–1514.
96. Jee WH, McCauley TR, Katz LD, Matheny JM, Ruwe PA, Daigneault JP. Radiology 2001;218(1):127–132.
97. Bencardino JT, Beltran J, Rosenberg ZS, et al. Radiology 2000;214(1):267–271.
98. Bearcroft PW, Blanchard TK, Dixon AK, Constant CR. Skeletal Radiol 2000; 29(12):673–679.
99. Zanetti M, Jost B, Lustenberger A, Hodler J. Acta Radiol 1999;40(3):296–302.
100. Blanchard TK, Bearcroft PW, Maibaum A, Hazelman BL, Sharma S, Dixon AK. Eur J Radiol 1999;30(1):5–10.
101. Oh CH, Schweitzer ME, Spettell CM. Skeletal Radiol 1999;28(12):670–678.

16

Imaging of Adults with Low Back Pain in the Primary Care Setting

Marla B.K. Sammer and Jeffrey G. Jarvik

Issues

I. What is the role of imaging in patients suspected of having a herniated disk?
   A. Plain radiography
   B. Computed tomography
   C. Magnetic resonance
II. What is the role of imaging in patients with low back pain suspected of having metastatic disease?
   A. Plain radiographs
   B. Computed tomography
   C. Magnetic resonance
   D. Bone scanning and single photon emission computed tomography (SPECT)
   E. Cost-effectiveness analysis
III. What is the role of imaging in patients with back pain suspected of having infection?
   A. Plain radiographs
   B. Computed tomography
   C. Magnetic resonance
   D. Bone scanning and Single Photon Emission Computed Tomography
IV. What is the role of imaging in patients with low back pain suspected of having compression fractures?
   A. Plain radiographs
   B. Computed tomography
   C. Magnetic resonance
   D. Bone scanning and Single Photon Emission Computed Tomography (SPECT)
V. What is the role of imaging in patients with back pain suspected of having ankylosing spondylitis?
   A. Plain radiographs
   B. Computed tomography
   C. Magnetic resonance
   D. Bone scanning and Single Photon Emission Computed Tomography

VI. What is the role of imaging in patients with back pain suspected of having spinal stenosis?
   A. Plain radiographs
   B. Computed tomography
   C. Magnetic resonance
   D. Bone scanning and Single Photon Emission Computed Tomography
VII. What are patients' perceptions of the role of imaging in low back pain?
VIII. What is the role of vertebroplasty for patients with painful osteoporotic compression fractures?

Key Points

- The natural history of low back pain is typically benign; in the absence of "red flags," imaging can safely be limited to a minority of patients with low back pain in the primary care setting (strong evidence).
- Low back pain imaging is often performed to rule out a serious etiology, especially metastases. While the first-line study is plain radiographs, magnetic resonance (MR) is more sensitive. However, initial imaging with MR has not yet proven cost-effective (moderate evidence).
- Many incidental findings are discovered when imaging the lumbar spine, including disk desiccation, anular tears, bulging disks, and herniated disks. Their eventual correlation with back pain is not known. However, while disk bulges and protrusions are common in asymptomatic individuals, extrusions are not (strong evidence).
- Imaging can diagnose surgically treatable causes of radiculopathy (herniated disks and spinal stenosis). However, these are typically not the causes of low back pain and are often incidental findings in asymptomatic individuals; furthermore, the long-term efficacy of corrective surgery for these conditions has not been established (moderate evidence).
- Vertebroplasty is a promising but largely unproven therapy for patients with painful osteoporotic compression fractures. Controlled trials need to be performed to determine its ultimate efficacy (insufficient evidence).

Definition and Pathophysiology

Low back pain (LBP) is a pervasive problem that affects two thirds of adults at some time in their lives. Fortunately, the natural history of LBP is usually benign, and diagnostic imaging can be restricted to a small percentage of LBP sufferers. This chapter reviews the evidence regarding both the diagnostic accuracy of common imaging modalities for several common conditions, and the utility of imaging in patients with LBP in the primary care setting. The most common spine imaging tests are plain x-rays, computed tomography (CT), magnetic resonance (MR), and bone scanning. We do not review other modalities (conventional myelography, diskography, and positron emission tomography), which are usually ordered by specialists prior to surgical intervention. This work is based partly on an article we previously published in the *Annals of Internal Medicine* (1).

Epidemiology and Differential Diagnosis of LBP in Primary Care

Low back pain ranks among the most common reasons for physician visits and is the most common reason for work disability in the United States (2–4). Among those with uncomplicated back pain, it is often impossible to distinguish a precise anatomic cause, and early treatments are generally aimed at symptomatic relief, so a precise anatomic diagnosis is usually both unnecessary and impossible. In fact, a definitive diagnosis is not reached in as many as 85% of patients with LBP (5), and when the etiology cannot be determined it is frequently assumed to result from muscle sprains or strains, ligamentous injuries, and spinal degenerative changes.

Further complicating matters, there are numerous imaging findings in the spines of asymptomatic patients. These include spinal stenosis, mild scoliosis, transitional vertebra, spondylolysis, Schmorl's nodes, spina bifida, and degenerative changes (6). For example, spinal stenosis is present in up to 20% of asymptomatic adults over the age of 60. The relationship of these findings to back pain is questionable because they are equally prevalent among persons with and without pain (7). Steinberg and colleagues (6) studied the radiographs of a large group of male army recruits with and without LBP. While they attempted to find a correlation between numerous variables and LBP (including right and left scoliosis, lordosis, degree of lordosis, vertebral rotation, spina bifida at multiple levels, transitional vertebra, wedge vertebra, degenerative changes, Schmorl's nodes, unilateral spondylolysis, bilateral spondylolysis, spondylolisthesis, spinal canal anteroposterior diameter, interpedicular distance, and intra-apophyso-laminar space), they found an association with only six of the variables. The most statistically significant difference was the presence of right-sided scoliosis (16.8% vs. 5.6% in the control group, $p < .0001$). The study also found lumbarization of S1, wedge vertebra, bilateral spondylolysis, and spondylolisthesis had weaker associations with LBP, with p values up to .04. Since the authors did not have *a priori* hypotheses, their study suffers from the problem of multiple comparisons, limiting the conclusions that can be drawn. Except for right-sided scoliosis, all the other associations must be viewed as exploratory and require independent confirmation.

Still, researchers continue to explore the relationship between possibly incidental findings, especially of intervertebral disk herniation, and the symptoms of back pain. Herniated disks are clearly not the culprit in the vast majority of patients with LBP. Only 2% of persons with LBP actually undergo surgery for a disk herniation (8,9). Moreover, imaging tests identify herniated disks among a large fraction of people without LBP (from 20% to 80%, depending on age, selection, and definition of disk herniation) (Fig. 16.1) (10–12). These asymptomatic herniations appear to be clinically

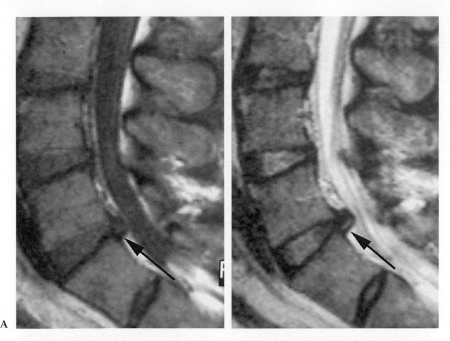

A   B

Figure 16.1. Magnetic resonance (MR) of the lumbar spine in a patient without low back pain (LBP) (rigorously determined for entry into a longitudinal study of people without LBP). T1-weighted (A) and T2-weighted (B) sagittal images demonstrate a moderate sized disk extrusion (arrow) at L5/S1. This is one example of many incidental findings.

unimportant. In a prospective study, our group found that the prevalence of most disk abnormalities, including desiccation, loss of disk height, bulge, anular tear, and protrusion, were not significantly different between asymptomatic subjects with and without a history of prior LBP (12). Boos and colleagues (13) followed asymptomatic individuals with a high rate of disk herniations (73%) for 5 years. They concluded that while the presence of disk abnormalities did not predict future LBP, psychosocial factors, mostly related to occupation, did. Certain imaging findings are likely quite important clinically. Disk extrusions, a subtype of herniation, are much less prevalent than disk protrusions in patients without LBP and are typically considered a clinically important imaging finding (10–12,14).

Imaging is indicated when infection or malignancy is being considered, as well as when patients present with cauda equina syndrome, a true surgical emergency. These serious conditions occur less than 5% of the time in the primary care setting, with only 0.7% of LBP patients having metastatic cancer (with breast, lung, and prostate being the most common primary tumors), 0.01% having spinal infections, and 0.0004% having cauda equina syndrome (15). In their recent retrospective chart review of 2007 lumbar film reports, van den Bosch et al. (16) reported the overall likelihood of finding a serious condition, such as infection or possible tumor at <1%, with no tumors found in patients younger than 55.

Overall Cost to Society

In 1998, health care costs for LBP (inpatient care, office visits, prescription drugs, and emergency room visits) totaled $90.7 billion. This was 2.5% of the national health care expenditure, and did not include physical therapy, chiropractic care, or nursing home care. The data to calculate these figures came from a national database, and included only patients with back disorders, disk disorders, and back injuries, as per International Classification of Diseases (ICD-9) codes. Consequently, a substantial proportion of low-back pain patients, such as those with malignancy, infection, or osteoporotic compression fractures as the primary etiology of pain, were likely excluded from these estimates. Finally, this estimate does not include non-health care expenditures such as workers' compensation, sick leave, and disability, an important consideration since LBP is the largest cause of disability and workers' compensation claims in the United States (17,18).

Goals

There are two major goals in imaging primary care patients with LBP: (1) to exclude serious disease (tumor, infection, or neural tissue compromise requiring decompression), and (2) to find a treatable explanation for the patient's pain.

Methodology

We performed two Medline searchs using PubMed. The first covered the period 1966 to September 2001 and the second, to update the literature search from the original article on which this chapter is based, covered September 2001 to August 2004. For both searches we used the following search terms: (1) *back pain,* (2) *intervertebral disk displacement,* (3) *sciatica,* (4) *spinal stenosis,* and (5) *diagnostic imaging.* We applied the subheadings *diagnosis, radiography,* or *radionuclide imaging* to the first statement. We excluded animal experiments and articles on pediatric patients. We also excluded case reports, review articles, editorials, and non-English-language articles. We included only articles describing plain x-rays, CT, MR (including MR myelography), and bone scanning. In the first search, the total number of citations retrieved was 1468. Two reviewers (J.G.J. and Richard A. Deyo) reviewed all the titles and subsequently the abstracts of 568 articles that appeared pertinent; the full text of 150 articles was then reviewed. At each step, the articles' authors and institutions were masked. Disagreements regarding inclusion of particular articles, which occurred in approximately 15%, were settled by consensus. In the second search, the total number of citations retrieved was 558. Two reviewers (M.B.K.S. and J.G.J.) reviewed all the titles and subsequently the abstracts of 168 articles that appeared pertinent. Finally, we reviewed the full text of 75 articles. Disagreements regarding inclusion of particular articles, which occurred in 12%, were settled by consensus. Only those articles meeting our inclusion criteria were cited for this review.

Because most studies had several potential biases, our estimates of sensitivity and specificity must be considered imprecise. The most common biases were failure to apply a single reference test to all cases; test review bias (study test was reviewed with knowledge of the final diagnosis); diagnosis review bias (determination of final diagnosis was affected by the study test); and spectrum bias (only severe cases of disease were included).

I. What Is the Role of Imaging in Patients Suspected of Having a Herniated Disk?

Summary of Evidence: Radiculopathy is a common and well-accepted indication for imaging; however, it is not an urgent indication, and with 4 to 8 weeks of conservative care, most patients improve. Urgent MR and consultation are needed if the patient has signs or symptoms of possible cauda equina syndrome (bilateral radiculopathy, saddle anesthesia, or urinary retention). Current literature suggests that MR is slightly more sensitive than CT in its ability to detect a herniated disk. Plain radiography has no role in diagnosing herniated disks, though it does, like the other modalities, show degenerative changes that are sometimes associated with herniated disks. Finally, all three methods commonly reveal findings in asymptomatic subjects.

Supporting Evidence

A. Plain Radiography

Because radiographs cannot directly visualize disks or nerve roots, their usefulness is limited. Plain film signs of disk degeneration include disk space narrowing, osteophytes, and end-plate sclerosis. Indirect signs of possible nerve root compromise include facet degeneration as manifested by sclerosis and hypertrophy.

In their recent prospective study examining patients with chronic LBP, Peterson and colleagues (19) considered whether a relationship existed between radiographic lumbar spine degenerative changes and disability or pain severity. They found no link between the severity of lumbar facet degeneration and self-reported pain or disability levels. While they did find a weak link between the number of degenerative disk levels and the severity of degenerative changes at these levels with pain in the week immediately preceding the exam, they found no correlation to pain or disability over the patients' entire pain episode (which in some cases had lasted greater than 5 years) (moderate evidence). Furthermore, in greater than a quarter of the patients, all of whom were considered chronic LBP sufferers, no degenerative changes were evident on their radiographs. Even in those patients with degenerative findings, the severity of degeneration was rated as mild in approximately 50%. Lundin et al. (20) studied athletes for 12 to 13 years and found only a borderline correlation between loss of disk height at baseline and back pain ($P = .06$). However, they found a highly significant correlation between a decrease in disk height over the intervening 12 to 13 years and the development of LBP ($P = .005$) (strong evidence).

B. Computed Tomography

In an often-cited study by Thornbury and colleagues (21), CT had a sensitivity of 88% to 94% for herniated disks and a specificity of 57% to 64%,

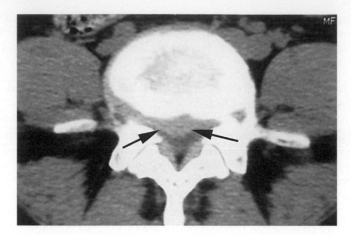

Figure 16.2. Axial computed tomography (CT) image demonstrates a relatively hyperdense focal disk herniation (arrows) outlined by lower density cerebrospinal fluid (CSF) within the spinal canal. This example shows CT's ability to depict disk herniations.

similar to that for MR (Fig. 16.2) (moderate evidence). The area under a receiver operating characteristic (ROC) curve for CT was 0.85–0.86. Diagnosis review bias likely inflated these estimates of accuracy. Interestingly, a study by Jackson et al. (22) arrived at similar estimates of sensitivity and specificity (86% and 60%, respectively) despite the selective use of a surgical reference standard (moderate evidence). Not taken into account in these studies is that herniated disks are commonly present in asymptomatic persons. While likely representing real anatomic abnormalities, these findings are irrelevant for clinical decision making, and thus reduce test specificity (Table 16.1). Finally, while these studies suggest CT is comparable to MR for diagnosing disk disease, an important drawback of CT compared with MR is that with only axial image acquisition, it is more difficult to subcategorize disk herniations into protrusions vs. extrusions (see section below on MR). However, multidetector CTs, with thin-section acquisition allows high-quality sagittal reformations to potentially overcome this limitation.

We did not find any data regarding the accuracy of CT for nerve root impingement. However, because surrounding fat provides natural contrast, CT, as opposed to plain radiography, can accurately depict the foraminal and extraforaminal nerve roots, directly visualizing nerve root displacement or compression. But CT is less effective in evaluating the intrathecal nerve roots (limited evidence) (23).

C. Magnetic Resonance

Magnetic resonance has good sensitivity and variable specificity for disk herniations. Thornbury et al. (21) (moderate evidence) demonstrated a sensitivity for herniated disks of 89% to 100%, but a specificity of only 43% to 57%. The area under the ROC curve was 0.81 to 0.84. In a cohort of 180 patients, Janssen et al. (24) found a sensitivity and specificity of 96% and 97%, respectively. Although this study avoided test review bias, diagnosis

Table 16.1. Studies of lumbar spine imaging in asymptomatic adults

Modality (reference)	Age group description	Prevalence of anatomic conditions				
		Herniated disk	Bulging disk	Degenerated disk	Stenosis	Anular tear
Plain x-rays (108)	14–25 years, high performance athletes n = 143			20%		
Plain x-rays (6)	Army recruits, 18 years old ± 2 months			4% (vs. 5% of sx** pts)		
Myelography (109)	Mean age = 51, referred for posterior-fossa acoustic neuroma, n = 300	31%				
CT (110)	Mean age = 40 <40 years (n = 24) >40 years (n = 27)	20% 27%			0% 3%	
MR (111)	Women mean age = 28 n = 86	9%	44%			
MR (10)	Under age 60 (n = 53) ≥Age 60 (n = 14)	22% 36	54% 79%	46% 93%	1% 21%	
MR (11)	Mean age = 42 n = 98	28%*	52%		7%	14%
MR (12)	Mean age = 36 , matched age + occupation Exposure to pts. having diskectomy, n = 46	76%[†]	51% of disks	85%		
MR (112)	Mean age = 28 n = 41					
MR (113)	Median age = 42 Referred for head or neck imaging, n = 36	33%[‡]	81%	56%		56%
MR (114)	Mean age = 35 n = 60	56–60%	20–28%	72%		19–20%
MR (45)	Mean age = 40 n = 54					24%
MR (14)	Mean = 54 n = 148	38%[§]	64%	91%	10%	38%
MR (13,115)	20–50, unrelated trauma	73% (7% with extrusion)		49%	29%	
MR (14)	Mean age = 54, VA patients	38%	64%	91%	10%	38%
MR (45)	Mean age = 40.1; cohort of prior cervical diskectomy					39%

** sx = symptomatic.
* 64% had disk bulge, protrusion, or extension; only 1% had extrusions.
[†] Nerve root compression in 4%; contact or displacement of nerve root in 22%.
[‡] 0% had extrusions.
[§] 6% had extrusions, 3% had nerve root compromise.
Source: Adapted from Jarvik and Deyo (1), permission pending.

review bias was likely present, with selective application of the surgical reference standard (moderate evidence).

While data regarding sensitivity and specificity of MR for nerve root compromise is lacking, MR has several advantages over CT, including superior soft tissue contrast, multiplanar imaging, and the ability to characterize intrathecal nerve roots (12,25–27). Still unclear is how best to evaluate nerve root compromise. In a prospective evaluation of 96 consecutive lumbar spine MRs, Gorbachova and Terk (28) found no correlation between nerve root sleeve diameter and disk pathology, concluding that measuring the nerve diameter is not clinically useful (strong evidence). Pfirrmann and colleagues (29) devised a reliable grading system for nerve root compromise: 1, normal; 2, nerve root contacted; 3, nerve root displaced; and 4, nerve root compressed. They retrospectively evaluated 500 nerve roots in 250 symptomatic patients, and then compared their MR grading system to a similar surgical scale in the 94 nerve roots that were evaluated operatively. They found that their system correlated well with surgical findings, and that intra- and interobserver reliability for the grading scale was high with kappas of 0.72 to 0.77 for intraobserver, and 0.62 to 0.67 for interobserver (moderate evidence).

Despite the high prevalence of herniated disks (from 20% to 80%, depending on age, selection, and definition of disk herniation) (Table 16.1) (10–12), and evidence of disk degeneration among asymptomatic individuals (on MR 46% to 93%), several studies have attempted to correlate disk disease with disability and pain. In a prospective study of 394 patients, Porchet et al. (30) found that leg pain (but not back pain), disability, and bodily pain (all $p < .005$) were significantly associated with MR disk disease severity. Beattie and colleagues (25) also studied MR abnormalities and their correlation to pain, finding relationships between distal leg pain and both disk extrusions and severe nerve compression ($p < .008$ and $<.005$, respectively). Interestingly, however, in the majority of the participants, they found no MR abnormality that corresponded to the distribution of the patient's pain.

Brant-Zawadzki et al. argued that the distinction between protrusions and extrusions is important because extrusions are rare in asymptomatic subjects (1%), but bulges (52%) and protrusions (27%) are common. In a prospective trial, our group found that extrusions, but not bulges or protrusions, were significantly associated with a history of LBP ($p < .01$) (14). Ahn and colleagues (31), though they did not use the terms *protrusion or extrusion*, agreed that distinguishing the type of herniation is important. Comparing transligamentous herniations (extrusions or migrated extrusions) to protrusions and bulges, they found that patients with transligamentous herniations had slightly better outcomes. In 2001 the North American Spine Society, the American Society of Neuroradiology, and the American Society of Spine Radiology jointly published recommendations regarding the use of a consensus nomenclature for describing disk abnormalities that incorporated these terms (protrusions and extrusions) (32).

In a series of 125 subjects, Brant-Zawadzki et al. (33) looked at the inter- and intraobserver agreement for four categories of disk morphologies (normal, bulge, protrusion, and extrusion). The authors defined a bulge as a circumferential and symmetrical extension of disk material beyond the interspace, while a herniation was a focal or asymmetrical extension of disk material. Protrusions and extrusions are subcategories of herniations. Protrusions are broad based, while extrusions have a "neck" that makes the base against the parent disk narrower than the extruded material itself (Fig. 16.3). Using these definitions for disk morphologies, the interreader kappa was 0.59, indicating moderate agreement. Intraobserver agreement was slightly higher, ranging from 0.69 to 0.72, indicating substantial agreement. Others have obtained comparable degrees of interreader agreement (kappa = 0.59) in cohorts of 34 and 45 patients, respectively (34,35). In a study of the reliability of chiropractors' interpretations, Cooley and colleagues (36) found interexaminer reliability comparable to that of radiologists (kappa = 0.60).

Magnetic resonance myelography (MRM) is a relatively new method that uses heavily T2-weighted three-dimensional (3D) images to provide high contrast between cerebrospinal fluid (CSF) and the cord and nerve roots. Because of the high contrast of CSF, MRM has been used for diagnosing suspected spinal stenosis. However, its role in disk imaging has not been well established. In one prospective evaluation of preoperative candidates with prior diagnoses of disk herniation, Pui and Husen (37) found no difference between the sensitivity and specificity of MRM and conventional MR for diagnosis of disk herniation (strong evidence). Spectrum bias was likely present, since the reference standard, which was applied to all patients, was surgical confirmation. Also, MRM may be useful in the diagnosis of dorsal root pathology. In their prospective study of 83 patients with MR-verified lumbar disk herniation and sciatica, Aoto et al. (38) found that swelling in the dorsal root ganglia at clinically involved lumbar nerve

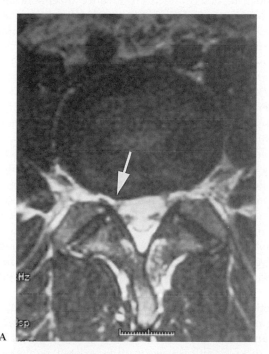

A

Figure 16.3. T2-weighted MR images in two different patients showing a disk protrusion (arrow) (A) vs. disk extrusion (arrows) (B and C). See text for definition. Protrusions are common in asymptomatic individuals and may clinically act as false positives.

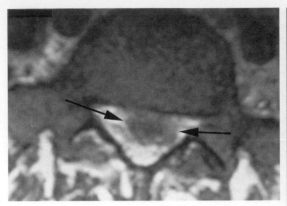

B

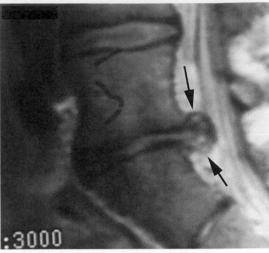

C

Figure 16.3. *Continued*

segments was clearly seen on MRM, and the degree of root swelling correlated with pain severity.

The evidence for the use of gadolinium to detect nerve root enhancement, and thereby increase specificity, is conflicting (39–41) (moderate evidence). Autio and colleagues (42) prospectively studied 63 patients with unilateral sciatica to determine the relevance of enhancement patterns. They found a negative correlation between the duration of symptoms and the extent of enhancement. While they failed to find a correlation between enhancement and multiple clinical symptoms, they did find a significant correlation between percent rim enhancement (greater than 75%) and the presence of an abnormal Achilles reflex, with a sensitivity and specificity of 76% and 82%, respectively (moderate evidence). Currently, gadolinium is usually reserved for the evaluation of postoperative patients. But even in postoperative imaging, its role has recently been challenged. In a prospective study of postdiskectomy patients, Mullin et al. (43) found no significant difference between pre- and postcontrast sensitivity (92–93%) and specificity (97%) for recurrent disk herniation (strong evidence).

Aprill and Bogduk (44) proposed the term *high-intensity zone* (HIZ) to describe the presence of focal high signal in the posterior anulus fibrosus on T2-weighted images (Fig. 16.4). However, over a decade after publication of their manuscript, the clinical importance of anular tears remains uncertain. While some investigators have not found a strong relationship between the presence of an anular tear and either positive diskography (45) (moderate evidence) or clinical symptoms (46) (moderate evidence), others have found a correlation (44,47) (limited evidence and moderate evidence). In a retrospective twin cohort study, Videman and colleagues (48) found that anular tears were present in 15% of their patients and were statistically significantly associated with many of the LBP parameters they studied. The most significant association existed between anular tears and pain intensity in the past year [odds ratio (OR) 2.2, 95% confidence interval (CI) 1.3–3.9) (moderate evidence). Similar associations existed between anular tears and any LBP in the past year, disability from LBP in

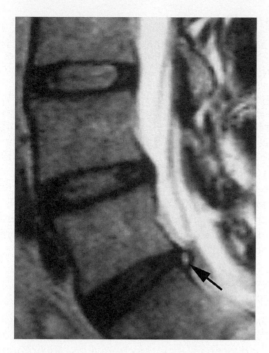

Figure 16.4. Sagittal T2-weighted MR demonstrating high-intensity zone (HIZ) (arrow) in an asymptomatic subject.

the past year, and LBP at the time of the study. But as with other imaging findings, the high prevalence of anular tears in subjects without LBP calls its clinical value into question (14,45).

II. What Is the Role of Imaging in Patients with Low Back Pain Suspected of Having Metastatic Disease?

Summary of Evidence: Both radionuclide studies and MR are sensitive and specific studies for detecting metastases. We did not identify studies supporting the use of CT for detecting bony spinal metastases; however, CT does depict cortical bone well. Plain films are the least sensitive imaging modality for detecting metastases. Nevertheless, current recommendations still advocate using plain films as the initial imaging in selected patients.

Supporting Evidence

A. Plain Radiographs

Radiographs are a specific but relatively insensitive test for detecting metastatic disease. A primary limitation is that 50% of trabecular bone must be lost before a lytic lesion is visible (limited evidence) (49,50). If only lytic or blastic lesions are counted as a positive study, radiographs are 60% sensitive and 99.5% specific for metastatic disease [limited evidence (49,50); strong evidence (51)]. If one includes compression fractures as indicating a positive examination, then sensitivity is improved to 70% but specificity is decreased to 95%.

B. Computed Tomography

We found no adequate data on the accuracy of CT for metastases.

C. Magnetic Resonance

While the sensitivity of MR for metastases is likely high, the variable quality of the available literature makes arrival at a summary estimate difficult. In five studies of patients with metastatic cancer or other infiltrative marrow processes, MR appeared more sensitive than bone scintigraphy. The sensitivity of MR ranged from 83% to 100% and specificity was estimated at 92%. These studies used a combination of biopsy and follow-up imaging as the reference standard. Several biases (selection, sampling, nonuniform application of reference standard, and diagnosis review) likely inflated apparent performance (52–56) (Albra, moderate evidence; Avrahami, moderate evidence; Carroll, moderate evidence; Carmody, limited evidence; and Kosuda, moderate evidence).

D. Bone Scanning and Single Photon Emission Computed Tomography (SPECT)

In seven studies, the sensitivity of radionuclide bone scans for tumor ranged from 74% to 98% (all moderate evidence except for McNeil, which was limited evidence) (57–64). Spectrum bias, incorporation bias, test review bias, and diagnosis review bias were all present and likely inflated the accuracy estimates.

E. Cost-Effectiveness Analysis

Despite advances in imaging over the past decade, there is no compelling evidence to justify substantial deviation from the diagnostic strategy published by the Agency for Health Care Research and Quality (AHRQ) in 1994 (65). These guidelines reflect the growing evidence-based consensus that plain radiography is unnecessary for every patient with back pain because of the low yield of useful findings, potentially misleading results, high dose of gonadal radiation, and interpretation disagreements. However, in patients in whom the pretest probability of a serious underlying condition is elevated (e.g., patients older than the age of 50, patients with a history of a primary cancer, etc.), the combination of radiographs and laboratory tests such as an erythrocyte sedimentation rate (ESR) or CBC is likely the appropriate first step.

Magnetic resonance is clearly a more accurate diagnostic test for detecting tumor than are radiographs; nevertheless, it is not a cost-effective initial option. This is nicely illustrated in the recent paper by Joines et al. (66). Building a decision analytic model to compare strategies for detecting cancer in primary care patients with LBP, they combined information from the history, ESR, and radiographs, and compared this strategy to one that used MR on all patients. They found that to detect a case of cancer, the MR strategy cost approximately 10 times as much as the radiograph strategy ($50,000 vs. $5,300). Even more impressive was that the incremental cost of performing MR on all patients was $625,000 per additional case found. The authors did not attempt to convert cost per case detected into cost per life year saved or cost per quality-adjusted life year (QALY). However, since metastatic cancer presenting with back pain is usually incurable, the life year costs would likely be much greater. Hollingworth and colleagues (67) attempted to further elaborate on Joines et al.'s conclusions by limiting the MR imaging to rapid MR. In a decision model created for a hypothetical cohort of primary care patients referred to exclude cancer as the etiology of their back pain, they also found that there was not enough evidence to advocate routine rapid MR for this purpose. While there was a small increase in quality-adjusted survival (0.00043 QALYs), the incremental cost was large ($296,176). Using rapid MR rather than radiographs, fewer than one new case of cancer was detected per 1000 patients imaged.

III. What Is the Role of Imaging in Patients with Back Pain Suspected of Having Infection?

Summary of Evidence: When infection is suspected, MR is the imaging modality of choice. Its sensitivity and specificity are superior to the alternatives, and the images obtained provide the anatomic information needed for surgical planning.

Supporting Evidence

A. Plain Radiographs

In contrast to metastatic disease, radiographic changes in infection are generally nonspecific. Furthermore, radiographic changes occur relatively late in the disease course. Findings of infection after several weeks include poor cortical definition of the involved end plate with subsequent bony lysis and decreased disk height. A paraspinous soft tissue mass may also be present. In one study, the overall sensitivity of radiographs for osteomyelitis was 82%, and the specificity was 57% (strong evidence) (68).

B. Computed Tomography

We found no adequate data on the accuracy of CT for infection in the lumbar spine.

C. Magnetic Resonance

In the single best-designed study, the sensitivity of MR for infection was 96% and the specificity was 92%, making MR more accurate than radiographs or bone scans (68) (strong evidence). Perhaps more importantly, MR delineates the extent of infection better than other modalities, which is critical to surgical planning.

The characteristic MR appearance of pyogenic spondylitis is diffuse low marrow signal on T1-weighted images and high signal on T2-weighted images (Fig. 16.5). These changes reflect increased extracellular fluid. Although classically two vertebral bodies are involved along with their intervening disk, the early imaging is more variable, occasionally with only one vertebral body being involved (69). The disk itself is high in signal and may herniate through a softened end plate. Gadolinium may increase the specificity of MR, with enhancement of an infected disk and end plates, although rigorous evidence is lacking (70).

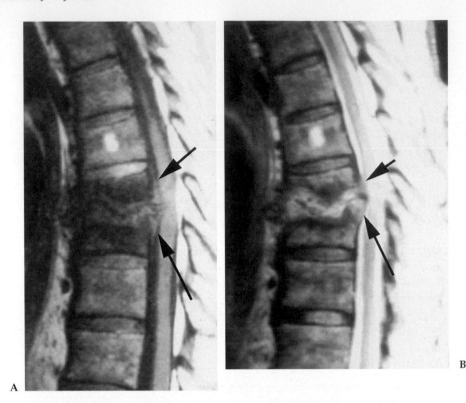

A   B

Figure 16.5. Sagittal MR of the thoracic spine demonstrating characteristic findings of diskitis and osteomyelitis, with virtual obliteration of the intervertebral disk, low signal on T1-weighted (A) and high signal on T2-weighted (B) images adjacent to the destroyed disk. Note the posterior extension of the process into the spinal canal and epidural space, causing compression of the cord (arrows).

We found no studies quantifying the accuracy of MR for epidural abscesses, but because of greater soft tissue contrast, MR should be better able to characterize the extent of an epidural process than CT.

D. Bone Scanning and Single Photon Emission Computed Tomography

In one study investigating bone scanning and infection, the sensitivity was moderately high at 82%, but specificity poor; only 23% (71) (moderate evidence). In the same study, gallium-67 SPECT had a 91% sensitivity and 92% specificity.

IV. What Is the Role of Imaging in Patients with Low Back Pain Suspected of Having Compression Fractures?

Summary of Evidence: There are no good estimates on which imaging modality is best for compression fracture imaging. When differentiation between metastatic and osteoporotic collapse is sought, MR is currently the method of choice.

Supporting Evidence

A. Plain Radiographs

Various biases (diagnosis review bias, test review bias, and selective use of reference standards) make it difficult to provide a summary estimate of the radiographic sensitivity and specificity for acute compression fractures. While radiographs are likely reasonably sensitive, they probably cannot distinguish between acute and chronic compression fractures. Clues that a fracture is old include the presence of osteophytes or vertebral body fusion. Because MR identifies marrow edema or an associated hematoma, and because bone scan evaluates metabolic activity, they provide more useful information regarding fracture acuity (limited evidence) (72).

B. Computed Tomography

We found no adequate data on the accuracy of CT for compression fractures.

C. Magnetic Resonance

We were unable to identify accurate sensitivity and specificity estimates for MR imaging in compression fractures. While there is an abundance of literature on MR and compression fractures, the overwhelming majority of articles focus on differentiating malignant from osteoporotic etiologies.

D. Bone Scanning and Single Photon Emission Computed Tomography

Bone scans are widely used for differentiating acute from older (subacute or chronic) compression fractures. Old fractures should be metabolically inactive, while recent fractures should have high radiotracer uptake (53). We did not identify articles that allowed us to calculate sensitivity and specificity for this condition.

V. What Is the Role of Imaging in Patients with Back Pain Suspected of Having Ankylosing Spondylitis?

Summary of Evidence: There are only a few studies that attempt to determine which imaging modality is best for diagnosing ankylosing spondylitis (AS). Plain radiographs and bone scans with SPECT both have relatively high specificity; specificity on CT and MR is currently not available. Plain radiographs appear to be adequate for initial imaging in a patient suspected of having AS.

Supporting Evidence

A. Plain Radiographs

The characteristic imaging findings in AS are osteitis, syndesmophytes, erosions, and sacroiliac joint erosions, with joint erosions occurring relatively early and being readily detectable by radiography. While the sensitivity of radiographs is poor (45%), the specificity appears high (100%), although in the single study examining this issue, spectrum bias likely inflated both estimates (moderate evidence) (73).

B. Computed Tomography

We found no adequate data on the accuracy of CT for ankylosing spondylitis.

C. Magnetic Resonance

In a small study by Marc et al. (73), MR showed abnormalities in 17 of 31 subjects with spondyloarthropathies yielding a sensitivity of 55%. Specificity could not be determined (73) (moderate evidence).

D. Bone Scanning and Single Photon Emission Computed Tomography

In two studies, bone scan sensitivity ranged from 25% to 85%, with the higher sensitivity achieved by using SPECT (73,74) (both studies moderate evidence). Specificity ranged from 90% to 100%. These studies suffered from a lack of high-quality reference standards and independent interpretations.

VI. What Is the Role of Imaging in Patients with Back Pain Suspected of Having Spinal Stenosis?

Summary of Evidence: Both CT and MR can be used to diagnosis central stenosis. On MR, the radiologists' general impression, rather than a millimeter measurement, is valid.

Supporting Evidence

A. Plain Radiographs

No studies provided good estimates of radiographic accuracy in detecting central stenosis. Since radiographs can only estimate bony canal compromise, the sensitivity for central stenosis is undoubtedly poorer than that of CT or MR, which depict soft tissue structures.

B. Computed Tomography

A meta-analysis by Kent et al. (75) reported CT sensitivity for central stenosis of 70% to 100% and specificity of 80% to 96% (limited evidence). Methodologic quality was variable but generally poor, making pooling of the data impractical. Central stenosis is also common in asymptomatic persons, with a prevalence of 4% to 28% (limited evidence) (76), and thus the specificity of CT for central stenosis, as it is for disk herniations, is likely less than the reported estimates.

C. Magnetic Resonance

In the 1992 meta-analysis by Kent et al. (75) the sensitivity of MR for stenosis was 81% to 97% while specificity ranged from 72% to 100% (limited evidence). Using stricter criteria for false positives, specificity was 93% to 100%.

Of note, two recent studies suggest that the readers' general impression of central stenosis is valid. In a retrospective study comparing electromyogram (EMG) findings to radiologists' MR interpretations, Haig et al. (77) found that the radiologists' subjective sense of central stenosis (normal, mild, moderate, or severe) was statistically significantly correlated with the EMG ($r = .4$, $p < .017$) (moderate evidence). Speciale et al. (78) assessed the intra- and interobserver reliability of physicians for classifying the degree of lumbar stenosis. Two neurosurgeons, two orthopedic spine surgeons, and three radiologists reviewed MRs from patients with a clinical and radiologic diagnosis of lumbar spinal stenosis. While the interobserver reliability was fair among all specialties ($\kappa < 0.26$), it was highest among radiologists (moderate with $\kappa = 0.40$), and considerably lower among the surgeons ($\kappa = 0.21$ for neurosurgeons and $\kappa = 0.15$ for orthopedic surgeons). In concordance with Haig's work, they found that the readers' subjective evaluation of stenosis significantly correlated with the calculated cross-sectional area ($p < .001$).

D. Bone Scanning and Single Photon Emission Computed Tomography

Bone scanning has no role in central stenosis imaging.

VII. What Are Patients' Perceptions of the Role of Imaging in Low Back Pain?

Summary of Evidence: The majority of patients with LBP think imaging is an important part of their care. However, in patients who are imaged, results of satisfaction with care are conflicting and overall not significantly higher than in those who were not imaged. Additionally, when plain radiographs are obtained, outcome is not significantly altered (and in some cases, is worse). But when MR or CT is used early in the workup of LBP, there is a very slight improvement in patient outcome.

Supporting Evidence: While the majority of studies attempt to validate a modality by its diagnostic accuracy, possibly more important is whether the test actually alters patient outcomes. In their recent randomized controlled trial, Kerry et al. (79) studied 659 patients with LBP, randomizing 153 patients to either lumbar spine radiographs or care without imaging, while also studying 506 patients in an observational arm (strong evidence). At 6 weeks and at 1 year, there was no difference between the groups in physical functioning, disability, pain, social functioning, general health, or need for further referrals. However, in the treatment arm at both 6 weeks and 1 year, there was a small improvement in self-reported overall mental health (Table 16.2). In a similar randomized controlled trial of 421 patients, Kendrick and colleagues (80) actually found a slight increase in pain duration, and a decrease in overall functioning in the radiograph group at 3 months, though at 9 months there was no difference between the groups (strong evidence).

  A few studies have attempted to demonstrate how CT and MR relate to outcome. In a large randomized study, Gilbert et al. (81) studied 782 patients, randomizing them to early imaging with CT or MR, or imaging only if a clear indication developed (strong evidence). They found that treatment was not influenced by early imaging. However, while both groups improved from baseline, there was slightly more improvement in the early imaging arm at both 8 ($p = .005$) and 24 ($p = .002$) months. In a subgroup of these patients, Gillan et al. (82) found that while there was an increase in diagnostic confidence in the early imaging group (Table 16.2), imaging did not change diagnostic or therapeutic impact (strong evidence). Our group also performed a randomized controlled trial assigning primary care patients with LBP to receive either lumbar spine radiographs or a rapid lumbar spine MR (83) (strong evidence). We found nearly identical outcomes in the two groups. Vroomen and colleagues (84), however, did find in patients with leg pain, utilizing early MR helped predict the patient's prognosis (strong evidence).

Patient satisfaction and expectations must also be accounted for when developing an imaging strategy. Many patients with LBP believe imaging is important or necessary to their care (85–87). However, there are conflicting results regarding improved satisfaction of care when imaging is actually performed. In their randomized trial using plain radiographs, Kendrick and colleagues (80) discovered that if participants had been given the choice, 80% would have elected to be imaged (strong evidence). They also found that while satisfaction was similar at 3 months in both the imaging and nonimaging groups (Table 16.3), by 9 months the intervention group was slightly more satisfied with their care. In the same cohort, Miller et al. (87) reported that the imaging group had a higher overall satisfaction score at 9 months. In a comparable study, Kerry and colleagues (79) found no difference in early patient satisfaction (strong evidence). They did not provide data for long-term satisfaction. Finally, in our comparison of rapid MR to radiographs, there was no difference in overall patient satisfaction between the two groups, but patients who received an MR were more reassured (83) (strong evidence).

Table 16.2. Patient outcome

Imaging type	Comparison	Difference (95% CI, p)
Plain radiographs		
Kerry et al. 2002 (79)	Radiograph vs. no radiograph 6 weeks 1 year	Mental health −8 (−14 to −1, $p < 0.05$) −8 (−15 to −2, $p < 0.05$)
Kendrick et al. 2001 (80,116)	Radiograph vs. no radiograph Pain at 3 months Disability at 3 months	1.26 (1.0–1.6, $p < 0.04$) −1.90 (CI not provided, $p < 0.05$)
CT/MR		
Gilbert et al. 2004 (81)	Early CT or MR vs. selective delayed 8 months 2 years	Acute LBP score −3.05 (−5.16 to −0.95, $p < 0.005$) −3.62 (−5.92 to −1.32, $p < 0.002$)
Gillan et al. 2001 (82)	Early CT or MR vs. selective delayed Treatment altered Median change in diagnostic confidence	$p = 0.733$ $p = 0.001$
Jarvik et al. 2003 (83)	Early MR vs. plain radiograph Mean back-related disability (Roland) at 12 months	−0.59 (−1.69 to 0.87, $p = 0.53$)
Vroomen et al. 2002 (84)	Prognostic value of MR for sciatic Favorable prognosis, anular rupture Favorable prognosis, nerve root compression Poor prognosis, disk herniation into foramen	$p = 0.02$ $p = 0.03$ $p = 0.004$

Table 16.3. Patient satisfaction

Study	Comparison	Difference (95% CI, p when provided)
Kendrick et al. 2001 (80,116) and Miller et al. 2002 (87)	Radiograph vs. no radiograph Satisfaction at 3 months	−1.50 (CI not provided, $p = 0.13$)
	Satisfaction at 9 months	−2.69 (CI not provided, $p < 0.01$)
Kerry et al. 2002 (79)	Radiograph vs. no radiograph Satisfaction with initial consultation/6 weeks	
	Very satisfied	1.0/1.0
	Satisfied	0.87 (0.40 to 1.9)/0.89 (0.37 to 2.1)
	Indifferent or dissatisfied	0.41 (0.12 to 1.3)/0.54 (0.19 to 1.5)
Jarvik et al. 2003 (83)	Rapid MR vs. radiograph Overall satisfaction at 12 months	0.30 (−0.42 to 0.99)
	Correlation of satisfaction with reassurance at 1, 3, and 12 months.	Pearson correlation coefficients $p < 0.001$ for all

VIII. What Is the Role of Vertebroplasty for Patients with Painful Osteoporotic Compression Fractures?

Summary of Evidence: Percutaneous vertebroplasty, first described by Galibert et al. (88) in 1987, is the injection of polymethylmethacrylate (PMMA) into a painful vertebra, with the intention of stabilizing it, relieving pain, and restoring function. Rarely, serious complications from bone cement leaks can occur. What is unknown is whether vertebroplasty increases the rate of adjacent vertebral fractures (89). Uncontrolled studies indicate that vertebroplasty is a promising therapy for patients with painful osteoporotic compression fractures, but confirmation by controlled trials is needed.

Supporting Evidence: Osteoporotic vertebral compression fractures occur annually in about 700,000 Americans, including 25% of postmenopausal women (90,91) and often produces psychologically and physically devastating pain, as well as an increased risk of death. Although the pain of an acute fracture is usually relieved within several weeks by conservative treatment (bed rest, antiinflammatory and analgesic medications, calcitonin, or external bracing), it occasionally requires narcotics, and even then may persist (92–94).

To date, there have been no published controlled studies of vertebroplasty. Only case series and uncontrolled prospective studies have been published (95–107). As with most new technology assessments, initial reports have been positive and even enthusiastic. However, the lack of controlled data indicates the need for a prospective controlled trial to evaluate the efficacy of this procedure (insufficient evidence).

Table 16.4. Accuracy of imaging for lumbar spine conditions*

	Sensitivity	Specificity	Likelihood ratio +	Likelihood ratio −
X-ray				
Cancer	0.6	0.95–0.995	12–120	0.40–0.42
Infection	0.82	0.57	1.9	0.32
Ankylosing spondylitis	0.26–0.45	1	Not defined	0.55–0.74
CT				
Herniated disk	0.62–0.9	0.7–0.87	2.1–6.9	0.11–0.54
Stenosis	0.9	0.8–0.96	4.5–22	0.10–0.12
MR				
Cancer	0.83–0.93	0.90–0.97	8.3–31	0.07–0.19
Infection	0.96	0.92	12	0.04
Ankylosing spondylitis	0.56			
Herniated disk	0.6–1.0	0.43–0.97	1.1–33	0–0.93
Stenosis	0.9	0.72–1.0	3.2—not defined	0.10–0.14
Radionuclide				
Cancer				
Planar	0.74–0.98	0.64–0.81	3.9	0.32
SPECT	0.87–0.93	0.91–0.93	9.7	0.14
Infection	0.90	0.78	4.1	0.13
Ankylosing spondylitis	0.26	1.0	Not defined	0.74

* Estimated ranges derived from multiple studies. See specific test sections in text for references.
Source: Jarvik and Deyo (1), permission pending.

Overall Modality Accuracy Summary

Table 16.4 summarizes the diagnostic accuracy parameters for each of the four modalities described. The likelihood ratio (LR) summarizes the sensitivity and specificity information in a single number, comparing the probability of having a positive test result in patients with the disease with the probability of a positive test in patients without the disease, or LR+ = (Probability (+test | disease))/(Probability (+ test | no disease)). This is equivalent to (sensitivity/(1 − specificity)). Similarly, the LR for a negative test is ((1 − sensitivity)/specificity). The larger the LR, the better the test is for ruling-in a diagnosis; conversely, the smaller the LR, the better it is for excluding a diagnosis. Likelihood ratios greater than 10 or less than 0.1 are generally thought to be clinically useful. A LR equal to 1 provides no clinically useful information.

Suggested Imaging Protocols

Plain Radiographs

Lateral and anteroposterior (AP) radiographs should be obtained for initial imaging in primary care patients with LBP; recent evidence supports lateral radiographs alone.

Supporting Evidence: The 1994 Agency for Health Care Research and Quality (AHRQ) evidence-based guidelines for the diagnosis and treatment of patients with acute LBP (65) recommend only two views of the lumbar spine be obtained routinely (117,118). More recently, a prospective study by Khoo et al. (119) suggests that a single lateral radiograph may be as effective as the standard two view examination. In 1030 lumbar spine radiographs, the AP film significantly altered the diagnosis in only 1.3% of cases (all cases of possible sacroiliitis or pars defects). More importantly, infection and malignancy were not missed on the lateral film alone. In certain circumstances, other views are important. When compared with AP views alone, oblique films better demonstrate the pars interarticularis in profile to assess for spondylolysis. Flexion-extension films are used to assess instability, and angled views of the sacrum are used to assess sacroiliac joints for ankylosing spondylitis. Limiting the number of views is particularly important to younger females, because the gonadal dose of two views alone are equal to the gonadal radiation of daily chest x-rays for several years (120–122).

Computed Tomography

For routine lumbar spine imaging in the University of Washington health system, we use a multidetector CT with 2.5-mm detector collimation and 2.5-mm intervals at 140 kVp and 200 to 220 mA. If the radiologist determines prior to the study that sagittal and coronal reformats are needed, we scan at 1.25 mm with 1.25-mm intervals.

Supporting Evidence: We found no studies to support specific CT imaging protocols.

Magnetic Resonance

The MR sequences we use for routine lumbar spine imaging in the University of Washington system are as follows:

1. Sagittal T1-weighted 2D spin echo, TR 400/TE minimum, 192 × 256 matrix, 26-cm field of view (FOV), 4-mm slice thickness, and 1-mm skip.
2. Sagittal T2-weighted fast recovery (frFSE) fast spin echo 2D spin echo, TR 4000/TE 110, echo train length (ETL) 25, 224 × 320 matrix, 26-cm FOV, 4-mm slice thickness, and 1-mm skip.
3. Axial T1-weighted 2D spin echo, TR 500/TE minimum, 192 × 256 matrix, 20-cm FOV, 4-mm slice thickness, and 1-mm skip.
4. Axial T2-weighted FSE-XL, TR 4000/TE 102, ETL 12, 192 × 256 matrix, 20-cm FOV, 4-mm slice thickness, and 1-mm skip.

Supporting Evidence: We found no studies to support specific MR imaging protocols.

Future Research

- It is uncertain which imaging findings are the best predictors of surgical benefit in patients undergoing fusion for degenerative disease. Prospective cohort studies and randomized treatment trials could help to determine which imaging variables are key determinants of outcome.
- While compression fractures are readily identified on imaging, their natural history, including identifying which fractures will lead to chronic pain and what their best management is, has not yet been described.
- Both MR and bone scans are highly effective in identifying metastases. Because MR is more costly than bone scans, future studies may compare the cost-effectiveness of each option and may focus on whether patient outcome is changed from use of either method.

- With infection, molecular imaging techniques may eventually be developed that can identify specific organisms based on imaging properties.
- Data on the best imaging technique to diagnose ankylosing spondylitis are sparse. Future studies may determine the role and cost-effectiveness of MR in early diagnosis.
- In patients with spinal stenosis and symptomatic herniated disks, definitive studies to document patient outcomes from surgical intervention are needed.

Acknowledgment: This work is supported in part by grant 1 P60 AR48093 from the National Institute for Arthritis, Musculoskeletal, and Skin Diseases.

References

1. Jarvik JG, Deyo RA. Ann Intern Med 2002;137(7):586–597.
2. Frymoyer JW. N Engl J Med 1988;318:291–300.
3. Barondess JA. Ann Intern Med 1993;119(2):153–160.
4. Salkever DS. DHHS Publication 1985;1–13. PHS Report #86–3343.
5. White AAD, Gordon SL. Spine 1982;7(2):141–149.
6. Steinberg EL, et al. Clin Radiol 2003;58(12):985–989.
7. van Tulder MW, et al. Spine 1997;22(4):427–434.
8. Deyo R, Tsui-Wu Y. Spine 1987;12:264–268.
9. Currey HL, et al. Rheumatol Rehabil 1979;18(2):94–104.
10. Boden SD, et al. J Bone Joint Surg (Am) 1990;72(3):403–408.
11. Jensen MC, et al. N Engl J Med 1994;331(2):69–73.
12. Boos N, et al. Spine 1995;20(24):2613–2625.
13. Boos N, et al. Spine 2000;25(12):1484–1492.
14. Jarvik JJ, et al. Spine 2001;26(10):1158–1166.
15. Deyo RA, Rainville J, Kent DL. JAMA 1992;268(6):760–765.
16. van den Bosch MA, et al. Clin Radiol 2004;59(1):69–76.
17. Luo X, et al. Spine 2004;29(1):79–86.
18. Klein BP, Jensen RC, Sanderson LM. J Occup Med 1984;26:443.
19. Peterson CK, Bolton JE, Wood AR. Spine 2000;25(2):218–223.
20. Lundin O, et al. Scand J Med Sci Sports 2001;11(2):103–109.
21. Thornbury JR, et al. Radiology 1993;186(3):731–738.
22. Jackson RP, et al. Spine 1989;14(12):1362–1367.
23. Wilmink JT. AJNR 1989;10(2):233–248.
24. Janssen ME, et al. Orthopedics 1994;17(2):121–127.
25. Beattie PF, et al. Spine 2000;25(7):819–828.
26. Vroomen PC, de Krom MC, Wilmink JT. J Neurosurg 2000;92(2 suppl):135–411.
27. Rankine JJ, et al. Spine 1998;23(15):1668–1676.
28. Gorbachova TA, Terk MR. Skeletal Radiol 2002;31(9):511–515.
29. Pfirrmann CW, et al. Radiology 2004;230(2):583–588.
30. Porchet F, et al. Neurosurgery 2002;50(6):1253–1259; discussion 1259–1260.
31. Ahn SH, Ahn MW, Byun WM. Spine 2000;25(4):475–480.
32. Fardon DF, Milette PC. Spine 2001;26(5):E93–E113.
33. Brant-Zawadzki MN, et al. Spine 1995;20(11):1257–1263; discussion 1264.
34. Milette PC, et al. Spine 1999;24(1):44–53.
35. Jarvik J, et al. Acad Radiol 1996;528–531.
36. Cooley JR, et al. J Manipulative Physiol Ther 2001;24(5):317–326.
37. Pui MH, Husen YA. Australas Radiol 2000;44(3):281–284.
38. Aota Y, et al. Spine 2001;26(19):2125–2132.
39. Kikkawa I, et al. J Orthop Sci 2001;6(2):101–109.
40. Lane JI, Koeller KK, Atkinson JL. AJNR 1994;15(7):1317–1325.

41. Crisi G, Carpeggiani P, Trevisan C. AJNR 1993;14(6):1379–1392.
42. Autio RA, et al. Spine 2002;27(13):1433–1437.
43. Mullin WJ, et al. Spine 2000;25(12):1493–1499.
44. Aprill C, Bogduk N. Br J Radiol 1992;65(773):361–369.
45. Carragee EJ, Paragioudakis SJ, Khurana S. Spine 2000;25(23):2987–2992.
46. Rankine JJ, et al. Spine 1999;24(18):1913–1919; discussion 1920.
47. Lam KS, Carlin D, Mulholland RC. Eur Spine J 2000;9(1):36–41.
48. Videman T, et al. Spine 2003;28(6):582–588.
49. Sartoris DJ, et al. Radiology 1986;160(3):707–712.
50. Sartoris DJ, et al. Radiology 1986;160(2):479–483.
51. Deyo RA, Diehl AK. J Gen Intern Med 1988;3:230–238.
52. Algra PR, et al. Radiographics 1991;11:219–232.
53. Avrahami E, et al. J Comput Assist Tomogr 1989;13(4):598–602.
54. Carroll KW, Feller JF, Tirman PF. J Magn Reson Imaging 1997;7(2):394–398.
55. Carmody RF, et al. Radiology 1989;173:225.
56. Kosuda S, et al. J Nucl Med 1996;37(6):975–978.
57. McDougall IR, Kriss JP. JAMA 1975;231(1):46–50.
58. Corcoran RJ, et al. Radiology 1976;121(3 pt 1):663–667.
59. Savelli G, et al. Anticancer Res 2000;20(2B):1115–1120.
60. Petren-Mallmin M. Acta Radiol Suppl 1994;391:1–23.
61. McNeil BJ. Semin Nucl Med 1978;8(4):336–345.
62. Jacobson AF. Arch Intern Med 1997;157(1):105–109.
63. Even-Sapir E, et al. Radiology 1993;187(1):193–198.
64. Han LJ, et al. Eur J Nucl Med 1998;25(6):635–638.
65. Bigos S, et al. Acute low back problems in adults. Clinical Practice Guideline No. 14. Rockville, MD: Agency for Health Care Policy and Research, Public Health Service, U.S. Department of Health and Human Services, 1994.
66. Joines JD, et al. J Gen Intern Med 2001;16:14–23.
67. Hollingworth W, et al. J Gen Intern Med 2003;18(4):303–312.
68. Modic M, et al. Radiology 1985;157:157–166.
69. Gillams AR, Chaddha B, Carter AP. AJR 1996;166(4):903–907.
70. Breslau J, et al. AJNR 1999;20(4):670–675.
71. Love C, et al. Clin Nucl Med 2000;25(12):963–977.
72. Yamato M, et al. Radiat Med 1998;16(5):329–334.
73. Marc V, et al. Rev Rheum Engl Ed 1997;64(7–9):465–473.
74. Hanly JG, et al. J Rheumatol 1993;20(12):2062–2068.
75. Kent D, et al. AJR 1992;158:1135–1144.
76. Porter RW, Bewley B. Spine 1994;19(2):173–175.
77. Haig AJ, et al. Spine 2002;27(17):1918–25; discussion 1924–1925.
78. Speciale AC, et al. Spine 2002;27(10):1082–1086.
79. Kerry S, et al. Br J Gen Pract 2002;52(479):469–474.
80. Kendrick D, et al. BMJ 2001;322(7283):400–405.
81. Gilbert FJ, et al. Radiology 2004;231(2):343–351.
82. Gillan MG, et al. Radiology 2001;220(2):393–399.
83. Jarvik JG, et al. JAMA 2003;289(21):2810–2818.
84. Vroomen PC, Wilmink JT, de KM. Neuroradiology 2002;44(1):59–63.
85. Espeland, A, et al. Spine 2001;26(12):1356–1363.
86. Kerry, S, et al. Health Technol Assess 2000;4(20):i–iv, 1–119.
87. Miller, P, et al. Spine 2002;27(20):2291–2297.
88. Galibert, P, et al. Neurochirurgie 1987;33(2):166–168.
89. Kim SH, et al. Acta Radiol 2004;45(4):440–445.
90. Melton LJ 3rd. Spine 1997;22(24 suppl):2S–11S.
91. Riggs BL, Melton LJ 3rd. Bone 1995;17(5 suppl):505S–511S.
92. Gold DT. Bone 1996;18(3 suppl):185S–189S.
93. Kado DM, et al. Arch Intern Med 1999;159(11):1215–1220.
94. Silverman SL. Bone 1992;13(suppl 2):S27–31.

95. McKiernan F, Faciszewski T, Jensen R. J Bone Joint Surg Am 2004; 86–A(12):2600–2606.

96. Legroux-Gerot I, et al. Clin Rheumatol 2004;23(4):310–317.

97. Perez-Higueras A, et al. Neuroradiology 2002;44(11):950–954.

98. Dudeney S, Lieberman I. J Rheumatol 2000;27(10):2526.

99. Jensen ME, Dion JE. Neuroimaging Clin North Am 2000;10(3):547–568.

100. Heini PF, Walchli B, Berlemann U. Eur Spine J 2000;9(5):445–450.

101. Martin JB, et al. Bone 1999;25(2 suppl):11S–15S.

102. Wenger M, Markwalder TM. Acta Neurochir (Wien) 1999;141(6):625–631.

103. Cortet B, et al. J Rheumatol 1999;26(10):2222–2228.

104. Jensen ME, et al. AJNR 1997;18(10):1897–1904.

105. Cotten A, et al. Radiology 1996;200(2):525–530.

106. Weill A, et al. Radiology 1996;199(1):241–247.

107. Gangi A, Kastler BA, Dietemann JL. AJNR 1994;15(1):83–86.

108. Hellstrom M, et al. Acta Radiol 1990;31(2):127–132.

109. Hitselberger WE, Witten RM. J Neurosurg 1968;28(3):204–206.

110. Wiesel S, et al. Spine, 1984. 9:549–551.

111. Weinreb JC, et al. Radiology 1989;170(1 pt 1):125–128.

112. Burns JW, et al. Aviat Space Environ Med 1996;67(9):849–853.

113. Stadnik TW, et al. Radiology 1998;206(1):49–55.

114. Weishaupt D, et al. Radiology 1998;209(3):661–666.

115. Elfering A, et al. Spine 2002;27(2):125–134.

116. Kendrick D, et al. Health Technol Assess 2001;5(30):1–69.

117. Robbins SE, Morse MH. Clin Radiol 1996;51(9):637–638.

118. Scavone JG, Latshaw RF, Weidner WA. AJR 1981;136(4):715–717.

119. Khoo LA, et al. Clin Radiol 2003;58(8):606–609.

120. Hall FM. Radiology 1976;120:443–448.

121. Webster E, Merrill O. N Engl J Med 1957;257:811–819.

122. Antoku S, Russell W. Radiology 1957;101:669–678.

17

Imaging of the Spine in Victims of Trauma

C. Craig Blackmore and Gregory David Avey

Key Points

- Cervical spine imaging is not necessary in subjects with all five of the following: (1) absence of posterior midline tenderness, (2) absence of focal neurologic deficit, (3) normal level of alertness, (4) no evidence of intoxication, and (5) absence of painful distracting injury (strong evidence).
- Computed tomography (CT) scan of the cervical spine is cost-effective as the initial imaging strategy in patients at high probability of fracture (neurologic deficit, head injury, high energy mechanism) who are already to undergo head CT (moderate evidence).

- No adequate data exist on the appropriate cervical spine evaluation in subjects who cannot be examined due to a head injury (insufficient evidence).
- Imaging of the thoracolumbar spine is not necessary in blunt trauma patients with all five of the following: (1) absence of thoracolumbar back pain, (2) absence of thoracolumbar spine tenderness on midline palpation, (3) normal level of alertness, (4) absence of distracting injury, and (5) no evidence of intoxication (moderate evidence).

Definition and Pathophysiology

The majority of spine fractures occur from high-energy trauma such as high-speed motor vehicle accidents and falls from heights (1,2). However, an important minority occur from relatively low-energy mechanisms such as falls from a standing height or low-velocity automobile accidents (3,4).

Epidemiology

Cervical spine fractures occur in approximately 10,000 individuals per year in the United States, most the result of blunt trauma (5,6). Among patients with a fracture, approximately one third will sustain severe neurologic injury (6,7). Unfortunately, fractures of the cervical spine may not be clinically obvious. Patients may be neurologically intact initially, but if not treated appropriately and promptly, progress to severe neurologic compromise (8). Delayed onset of paralysis occurs in up to 15% of missed fractures, and death due to unidentified cervical spine fracture is possible (9,10). Furthermore, the mechanism of injury is also not always useful for excluding cervical spine fracture.

Thoracolumbar spine injury has been estimated to occur in between 2% and 4% of all blunt trauma patients (11,12). These injuries were judged to require treatment in approximately three fourths of those identified (13). Much like cervical spine fractures, a resulting neurologic deficit is noted in approximately one third of those with thoracolumbar injury (14,15). Given the potentially serious consequences of these injuries, it is unsettling to find that studies have noted a significant delay in diagnosis in 11% to 22% of patients with spine fractures (9,16,17).

Overall Cost to Society

There is enormous variability in the practice of cervical spine imaging (18,19), but in most centers, imaging is used liberally. As a result, the yield from cervical spine imaging is low, with only 0.9% to 2.8% of such imaging studies demonstrating injury (20,21). Overall, the total cost of the imaging, evaluation, and care of patients with cervical spine trauma in the United States is an estimated $3.4 billion per year (22). The yield of thoracolumbar imaging is somewhat higher than cervical spine imaging, with positive studies accounting for 7.6% to 9% of blunt trauma thoracolumbar exams (23). The total societal cost of thoracolumbar spine injury has been estimated at $1 billion per year (24).

Goals

The overall goal of initial spine imaging is to detect potentially unstable fractures to enable immobilization or stabilization and prevent development or progression of neurologic injury. Additional imaging studies may be performed to inform prognosis and guide surgical intervention for unstable injuries.

Methodology

A Medline search was performed using PubMed (National Library of Medicine, Bethesda, Maryland) for original research publications discussing the diagnostic performance and effectiveness of imaging strategies in the cervical and thoracolumbar spine. Clinical predictors of cervical and thoracolumbar spine fracture were also included in the literature search. The search for cervical spine–related publications covered the period 1966 to March 2002. The search strategy employed different combinations of the following terms: (1) *cervical spine*, (2) *radiography* or *imaging* or *computed tomography*, and (3) *fracture* or *injury*. The search for thoracolumbar spine–related publications covered the period 1980 to March 2004. The search strategy included the MESH headings (1) *spine* and *diagnosis*, and (2) *imaging* and *trauma*. Additional articles were identified by reviewing the reference lists of relevant papers. This review was limited to human studies and the English-language literature. The authors performed an initial review of the titles and abstracts of the identified articles followed by review of the full text in articles that were relevant.

I. Who Should Undergo Cervical Spine Imaging?

Summary of Evidence: Determination of which blunt trauma subjects should undergo cervical spine imaging, and which should not undergo imaging, is a question that has been studied in detail in literally tens of thousands of subjects. The two major level I (strong evidence) studies, the NEXUS trial (Table 17.1), and the Canadian C-spine rule (Table 17.2) were comprehensive multicenter investigations of this topic. The NEXUS rule (Table 17.1) has undergone extensive validation and demonstrates high sensitivity for detection of fractures. The Canadian C-spine rule (Table 17-2) also has high sensitivity, and potentially higher specificity than the NEXUS. However, neither of these rules has been tested in an implementation trial to determine their impact outside the research setting.

Table 17.1. NEXUS criteria: imaging of the cervical spine is not necessary if all five of the NEXUS criteria are met

1. **Absence of posterior midline tenderness**
2. **Absence of focal neurologic deficit**
3. **Normal level of alertness**
4. **No evidence of intoxication**
5. **Absence of painful distracting injury**

Source: Adapted from Hoffman et al. (29).

Table 17.2. The Canadian C-spine rule

If the following three determinations are made, then imaging is not indicated
1. No high-risk factor, including:
Age >64 years
Dangerous mechanism, including:
Fall from >3 m/5 stairs
Axial load to head (diving)
High-speed motor vehicle accident (60 mph, rollover, ejection)
Bicycle collision
Motorized recreational vehicle
Paresthesias in extremities
2. Low-risk factor is present
Simple rear-end vehicular crash, excluding:
Pushed into oncoming traffic
Hit by bus/large truck
Rollover
Hit by high-speed vehicle
Sitting position in emergency department
Ambulatory at any time
Delayed onset of neck pain
Absence of midline cervical tenderness
3. Able to actively rotate neck (45 degrees left and right)

Source: Adapted from Dickinson et al. (33).

Supporting Evidence: The low yield of cervical imaging has prompted a number of investigators to attempt to identify clinical factors that can be used to predict cervical spine fracture. Early studies of this question were largely level III (limited evidence) investigations consisting of unselected case series. For example, in 1988, Roberge and colleagues (25) studied 467 consecutive subjects who underwent cervical spine radiography and found that subjects with cervical discomfort or tenderness were more likely to have a fracture than those without such symptoms or signs. Additional investigators identified associations between cervical spine fracture and mechanism of injury (26,27), level of consciousness (20,21,27), and intoxication (20,28). However, all of these investigations involved small numbers of subjects with fracture and a single or small number of centers.

A. NEXUS Prediction Rule

The first major cohort investigation of clinical indicators for cervical spine imaging was the National Emergency X-Radiography Utilization Study (NEXUS) (5,29). This was a large Level I study performed at 23 different emergency departments across the United States. The goal of the NEXUS study was to assess the validity of four predetermined clinical criteria for cervical spine injury (Table 17.1). These criteria were (1) altered neurologic function, (2) intoxication, (3) midline posterior bony cervical spine tenderness, and (4) distracting injury. The NEXUS investigators prospectively enrolled over 34,000 patients who underwent radiography of the cervical spine following blunt trauma. Of these, 818 (2.4%) had cervical spine injury. These authors found that the clinical predictors had a sensitivity of 99.6% for clinically significant injury (Table 17.3) (5,29). The authors also reported high interobserver agreement ($\kappa = 0.73$) for the prediction rule (30), and reported that use of the rule would have decreased the overall ordering of cervical radiography by an estimated 12.6% (29).

B. Canadian Cervical Spine Prediction Rule

A second level I clinical prediction rule, the Canadian C-spine rule for radiography (25) was published subsequent to the NEXUS trial, but with a similar objective: to derive a clinical decision rule that is highly sensitive for detecting acute cervical spine injury. The Canadian C-spine rule was a prospective cohort study of 8924 subjects from 10 community and university hospitals in Canada. Excluded were patients who had neurologic impairment, decreased mental status, or penetrating trauma. Like the NEXUS study, the Canadian C-Spine Study was an observational study performed without informed patient consent. However, patients who were eligible for the study but did not undergo radiography were followed up with a structured telephone interview 14 days following their discharge from the emergency department (ED). Thus, any patients who had not undergone radiography, and who had missed fracture would potentially be discovered during the investigation. The Canadian study investigated the predictive ability of 20 factors, and based on the reliability and predictive properties of these factors, developed a prediction rule consisting of three questions. According to the Canadian C-spine rule (Table 17.2), the probability of cervical spine injury is extremely low, and imaging is not indicated if the following three determinations are made: (1) absence of high-risk factor (age >65 years, dangerous mechanism, paresthesias in extremities); (2) presence of a low-risk factor (simple rear-end motor vehicle collision, sitting position in ED, ambulatory at any time since injury, delayed onset of neck pain, or absence of midline cervical C-spine tenderness); or (3) patient is able to actively rotate neck 45 degrees to left and right. The Canadian study group reported sensitivity of 100% and specificity of 42.5% for this clinical prediction rule and also reported that the rate of ordering radiography would be 58.2% of the current rate (Table 17.3) (31).

The Canadian C-spine rule was validated using a prospective cohort study of 8283 patients presenting at the same 10 Canadian community and academic hospitals as the original study (32). The results of this verification trial noted a sensitivity of 99.4% and a specificity of 45.1%, very similar

Table 17.3. Diagnostic performance

Test (reference)		Sensitivity	Specificity	Potential decrease in radiography
C-spine prediction rules				
NEXUS (29)		99.6	12.9	12.6
Canadian C-spine rule (31)		100	42.5	41.8
TL-spine prediction rules				
Holmes et al. (11)		100	3.9	3.7
C-spine imaging				
Radiography (43,45)	Overall	93.9	95.3	N/A
	Low risk		96.4	N/A
	High risk		78.1–89.3	N/A
CT (39,41,42,46)[1]	Overall			
TL-spine imaging		99.0	93.1	N/A
Radiography (60,64)[1]		63.0	94.6	N/A
CT (60–64)		97.8	99.6	N/A

[1] Pooled from these references.
N/A, not applicable.

to the results of the derivation study. It was noted during the course of this study that physicians failed to evaluate neck range of motion, as required by the Canadian C-spine rule, in 10.2% of patients. While virtually all of this group of incompletely evaluated patients underwent cervical spine imaging (98.8%), this group was found to have a lower rate of injury (0.8%) than the cohort as a whole (2.0%).

The data supporting the adoption of one cervical spine prediction rule over the other is limited. Two studies, the validation study for the Canadian C-spine rule and a retrospective analysis of the Canadian C-spine derivation cohort have attempted to compare the NEXUS and Canadian rules (32,33). However, both cohorts excluded those with altered levels of consciousness, effectively eliminating one of the NEXUS criteria. In addition, others have voiced concerns regarding physician familiarity with the various rules, side-by-side comparison, and the definitions of the NEXUS criteria used in these trials (34,35). The choice of clinical prediction rule in a broader clinical context is also unclear, as no trial has examined the impact of implementing these prediction rules outside of the research setting.

C. Applicability to Children

Evidence for who should undergo imaging is less complete in children than in adults. Determination of clinical predictors of injury in pediatric patients is complicated by the decreased incidence of injury in children, requiring a larger sample size for adequate study (36,37). In addition, children may sustain serious cervical cord injuries that are not radiographically apparent (37,38). Among the level I studies, the Canadian clinical prediction rule development study excluded children (31). The NEXUS trial included children, but there were only 30 injuries in patients under age 18, and only four in patients under age 9 (36). Although no pediatric injuries were missed in the NEXUS study, sample size was too small to adequately assess the sensitivity of the prediction rule in this group. Therefore, no adequate evidence exists regarding appropriate criteria for imaging in children.

II. What Cervical Spine Imaging Is Appropriate in High-Risk Patients?

Summary of Evidence: Cervical spine CT is more sensitive than radiography, and more specific in patients at high risk of fracture. But CT has higher direct costs than radiography. However, cost-effectiveness analysis demonstrates that CT is cost-effective, and may actually be cost-saving from the societal perspective in patients at high probability of fracture. Cost savings with CT are from a decreased number of second imaging examinations resulting from inadequate radiograph studies, and to the high cost in dollars and health for the rare fracture missed from radiography that leads to severe neurologic deficit. Radiography remains the most cost-effective imaging option in patients at low probability of injury (Fig 17.1).

Supporting Evidence: There are multiple investigations of radiography accuracy, although most are retrospective, level III (limited evidence) studies (39,40). Further, sensitivity of radiography is dependent on the selected reference standard. Studies incorporating CT as the reference

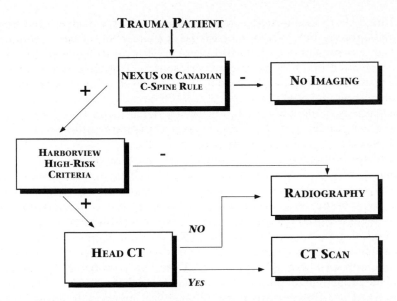

Figure 17.1. Evidence-based decision tree for imaging of the cervical spine in victims of trauma. The NEXUS or Canadian prediction rules are used to select patients for imaging. If imaging is appropriate, the Harborview prediction rule is used to select patients for CT rather than radiography. However, cervical spine CT is only used as the initial imaging strategy in patients who are to undergo head CT. Patients who are not to undergo head CT are imaged with radiography.

standard suggest that radiography misses 23% to 57% of fractures (41,42). However, the clinical relevance of these missed fractures is uncertain. Studies using fractures that become apparent clinically as the reference standard are probably more relevant for clinical practice. No formal meta-analyses of radiograph accuracy exist. However, weighted pooling of the larger studies using a clinical gold standard suggests that radiography is relatively accurate, with a sensitivity of approximately 94% and a specificity of approximately 95% when all trauma patients are considered (Table 17.3) (43).

Cervical radiography has substantial limitations in patients at the highest probability of fracture. Patients involved in high-energy trauma are commonly on backboards, have other injuries, and may be uncooperative. Cervical radiography in this group has been found to be more difficult to perform adequately, resulting in lower specificity, and requiring longer time, more repeat radiographs, and higher costs (44,45). Radiograph specificity ranges from approximately 96% in patients with only minor noncervical injuries, to 89% in patients with head injury, to 78% in patients with head injury and a high-energy mechanism such as motorcycle crash (45). Radiographs are relatively inexpensive, with direct, short-term resource ranging from $34 to $60 (44).

More recently, CT has been proposed as an initial cervical spine evaluation modality in patients who are victims of major trauma. Nuñez and colleagues studied the use of CT in the initial evaluation of trauma patients and demonstrated high sensitivity for fracture (99%) in a large, level II prospective series (moderate evidence) (42). This has been subsequently confirmed by other studies (46,47). Also, CT demonstrated high specificity (93%), even in patients at high-risk of fracture (Table 17.3) (46).

Direct, short-term resource costs of cervical spine CT likely exceed those of radiography, but no comprehensive cost analyses of CT have been published. Assessment of cost of cervical spine CT is difficult as many institutions obtain economies of scale by performing CT of the cervical spine in the same setting as CT of the head (43,47). However, CT may be faster than radiography, and Nuñez and colleagues (42) have suggested that use of CT may decrease patient time in the emergency department. Therefore, CT has higher sensitivity and specificity for cervical spine fracture in high-risk patients, but at potentially higher cost.

The appropriateness of CT as initial cervical spine imaging strategy in patients who are also undergoing head CT has been examined with cost-effectiveness analysis (43). This analysis, taken from the societal perspective, was based on a decision-analysis model, and compared the cost effectiveness of radiography and CT for patients at different probabilities of cervical spine fracture. The cervical spine cost-effectiveness model, taken from the societal perspective, was dependent on radiograph sensitivity, radiograph specificity, CT sensitivity, CT specificity, probability of fracture, and the probability of paralysis or the likelihood that a patient will become paralyzed if a fracture was missed by cervical imaging. In addition, the cost-effectiveness model was dependent on the short-term resource cost of radiography and CT, as well as the cost of the imaging that was induced by the initial strategy, and the cost of any neurologic deficit (paralysis) that developed from missed fracture. Costs were estimated from Medicare reimbursement data, and literature estimates, and the analysis was limited to adults (43).

A. Cost-Effectiveness Analysis

Cost-effectiveness analysis revealed that in patients at high risk (>10%) of cervical spine fracture, CT was actually a dominant strategy, both saving money and improving health through the prevention of paralysis. The cost savings associated with the use of CT was due to fewer inadequate exams, and to the very high medical and financial cost of the rare case of paralysis. The probability of a patient developing paralysis from missed fracture was actually extremely low, as fractures were uncommon, and the sensitivity of imaging was very high. However, the lifetime medical costs of a patient who became paralyzed were high, with estimates ranging from $525,000 to $950,000 (1995 dollars), and not including societal costs such as lost wages. In addition to the cost, there were obvious health consequences of paralysis. The dominance of CT over radiography in these high-probability patients was robust to sensitivity analysis testing of the uncertainty in the estimates. In patients at moderate probability of fracture (4–10%), CT cost more overall than radiography, but with a cost-effectiveness ratio on the order of $25,000 per quality-adjusted life year. In patients at low probability of cervical spine fracture (<4%) CT was clearly not cost-effective, and radiography was the preferred strategy (43).

III. Special Case: Defining Patients at High Fracture Risk

Summary of Evidence: Selection of patients for cost-effective use of cervical spine CT is dependent on probability of fracture. The Harborview high-risk cervical spine criteria have been developed and validated by a single

Table 17.4. Harborview high-risk cervical spine criteria

Presence of any of the following criteria indicates a patient at sufficiently high-risk to warrant initial use of CT to evaluate the cervical spine

1. High-energy injury mechanism
    High-speed (>35mph) motor vehicle or motorcycle accident
    Motor vehicle accident with death at scene
    Fall from height greater than 10 feet

2. High-risk clinical parameter
    Significant head injury, including intracranial hemorrhage or unconscious in emergency department
    Neurologic signs or symptoms referable to the cervical spine
    Pelvic or multiple extremity fractures

Source: Adapted from Hanson et al. (49).

institution level II (moderate evidence) study. Using these criteria, patients can be identified with injury probabilities ranging from 0.2% to 12.8%.

Supporting Evidence: Patients at risk for cervical spine fracture are a heterogeneous group. Some patients have sustained major trauma and will be at high probability of injury, while others will have sustained only minor trauma and will be at low probability of having sustained cervical spine fracture. Given that cost-effectiveness of imaging is dependent on the probability of cervical spine fracture, optimization of imaging in the cervical spine requires stratification of patients into different levels of probability of fracture. This stratification must be based on clinical findings that are apparent when patients are first evaluated in the ED, prior to any imaging.

To identify patients at high probability of fracture, Blackmore and colleagues (48) developed and validated a clinical prediction rule. This level II study employed a case-control study design, in which 160 patients were evaluated at Harborview Medical Center in the years 1994 to 1995 who had cervical spine fracture. Controls were 304 randomly selected adult blunt trauma patients from the same institution. The authors used logistic regression and recursive partitioning to develop a clinical prediction rule, which was then validated internally using the bootstrap technique. Using likelihood ratios from the clinical prediction rule and the known base prevalence of cervical spine fracture in the institution's population, the authors developed a series of fracture probability estimates for patients of different clinical circumstances (48). Although derived retrospectively, this prediction rule was subsequently prospectively validated on a separate patient group at the same institution (Table 17.4) (49). To date, this prediction rule has not been validated at other institutions. A clinical prediction rule has also been developed (but not validated) to evaluate predictors of cervical spine fracture in the elderly. The elderly prediction rule was identical to that in all adults, except that a higher proportion of injured patients were missed by the prediction rule criteria (50).

A. Applicability to Children

Comparison of CT versus radiography has not been well explored in children. The cost-effectiveness analysis of Blackmore and colleagues (43) excluded children, as did the studies of the Harborview high-risk cervical spine criteria (48,49). Further, the lower frequency of injury in children

(36,37) and the increased radiosensitivity of pediatric patients (51) suggest that cost-effectiveness results from adults may not be relevant.

IV. Special Case: The Unconscious Patient

Summary of Evidence: The theoretical risk of radiographically occult unstable ligamentous injury in patients who are unexaminable due to head injury has led to a variety of imaging approaches. There is insufficient evidence to support any particular approach.

Supporting Evidence: Standard radiologic and CT examinations of the cervical spine allow assessment of bony alignment. However, anecdotal reports exist in the literature describing unstable ligamentous injuries without malalignment on imaging (52,53). Accordingly, organizations including the Eastern Association for the Surgery of Trauma recommend additional imaging of the neck soft tissues to exclude unstable ligamentous injury. Proposed imaging approaches include magnetic resonance imaging (MRI), flexion and extension radiography, and fluoroscopy.

To date, there have been no reported level I or level II studies of the accuracy or clinical utility of any of the proposed imaging algorithms. Case-series data suggest that approximately 2% of obtunded patients may have unstable cervical spine injuries not detectable on initial CT or radiography (52,54,55). The clinical significance of these injuries has not been established.

V. Who Should Undergo Thoracolumbar Spine Imaging?

Summary of Evidence: Clinical prediction rules to determine which patients should undergo thoracolumbar spine imaging have been developed but not validated. Although these prediction rules have high sensitivities for detecting thoracolumbar fractures, their low specificities and low positive predictive values would require imaging a large number of patients without thoracolumbar injuries. This drawback limits the clinical utility of these prediction rules (moderate evidence).

Supporting Evidence: Given the relative lack of clarity regarding which blunt trauma patients require thoracolumbar imaging, several level III (limited evidence) studies have examined potential risks for thoracolumbar fracture. These limited studies have identified associations among the risk of thoracolumbar injury and high-speed motor vehicle accident (53,54), fall from a significant height (13,56,57), complaint of back pain (12–14,56,58), elevated injury score (13,56), decreased level of consciousness (14,56–58), and abnormal neurologic exam (14,57).

Two separate clinical predication rules to guide thoracolumbar spine imaging decisions have been validated. The smaller study, conducted by Hsu et al. (59), examined the effect of six clinical criteria on two retrospective groups (59). The first group consisted of a cohort of 100 patients with known thoracolumbar fracture, while the second group consisted of 100 randomly selected multitrauma patients. The criteria evaluated were

Table 17.5. Thoracolumbar spine imaging criteria

1. Thoracolumbar spine pain
2. Thoracolumbar spine tenderness on midline palpation
3. Decreased level of consciousness
4. Abnormal peripheral nerve examination
5. Distracting injury
6. Intoxication

(1) back pain/midline tenderness, (2) local signs of injury, (3) neurologic deficit, (4) cervical spine fracture, (5) distracting injury, and (6) intoxication. The results of this small-scale, retrospective trial found that 100% of the patients in the known thoracolumbar fracture group would have been imaged appropriately using the proposed criteria. This proposed pathway was then tested retrospectively in the group of randomly selected blunt trauma patients, and was found to have a sensitivity of 100%, a specificity of 11.3%, and a negative predictive value of 100%. Implementing these criteria would still require imaging the thoracolumbar spine in 92% of the selected multitrauma patients.

A much larger prospective, single center study by Holmes et al. (11) evaluated similar criteria in 2404 consecutive blunt trauma patients who underwent thoracolumbar imaging (moderate evidence). These clinical criteria were (1) complaints of thoracolumbar spine pain, (2) thoracolumbar spine pain on midline palpation, (3) decreased level of consciousness, (4) abnormal peripheral nerve examination, (5) distracting injury, and (6) intoxication (Table 17.5). This prediction rule was successful in achieving 100% sensitivity for detecting thoracolumbar fracture; however, the specificity was only 3.9%. Due to this low specificity, implementing this prediction rule in this patient population would have decreased the rate of thoracolumbar imaging by merely 4%.

A. Applicability to Children

It is unknown if these clinical prediction rules may be applied to children. The largest study by Holmes et al. (11) did allow the enrollment of children; however, they do not report the actual number of children enrolled. The youngest patient enrolled in the small trial by Hsu et al. (59) was 14 years.

VI. Which Thoracolumbar Imaging Is Appropriate in Blunt Trauma Patients?

Summary of Evidence: Multiple studies have shown that some CT protocols used for imaging the chest and abdominal visceral organs are more sensitive and specific for detecting thoracolumbar spine fracture than conventional radiography. In patients undergoing such scans, conventional radiography may be eliminated (limited evidence). The effect of primary screening with CT scan on cost and radiation exposure has not been thoroughly studied for the thoracolumbar spine.

Supporting Evidence: Multiple level III (limited evidence) studies examine the possibility of eliminating conventional radiography in those patients who are candidates for both conventional thoracolumbar radiographs and CT evaluation of the chest or abdominal viscera; however, many of these trials are hampered by small sample sizes or verification bias (60–64). Studies that combine the results of both CT and conventional radiography as the reference standard suggest that CT has a sensitivity of 78.1% to 97%, while conventional radiographs have a sensitivity of 32.0% to 74% for detecting thoracolumbar fracture (61–63). The clinical importance of thoracolumbar fractures not found with conventional radiography is unknown, as no studies with clinically based outcome measures were located.

A single level III (limited evidence) trial examined the use of CT as an initial evaluation in patients for whom a CT scan is not indicated for other reasons (62). This prospective, single center trial examined 222 trauma patients with both CT and conventional radiographs as initial screening exams. The reported sensitivity was 97% for CT examination and 58% for conventional radiographs. The results of this trial are limited in that only 36 patients were diagnosed with thoracolumbar fracture during the course of the trial.

Future Research

- Studies in both cervical spine and thoracolumbar spine imaging indicate that CT is more sensitive than traditional radiography in detecting fractures. However, the clinical relevance of these fractures is uncertain.
- The applicability of spine injury clinical prediction rules in pediatric patients is unknown. In addition, the sensitivity, specificity, and cost-effectiveness of the various imaging exams in the pediatric population are not well established.
- Clinical prediction rules for imaging of the thoracolumbar spine have been developed, but further research is necessary to validate such approaches. The effect of implementing these rules on cost, cost-effectiveness, and radiation exposure has not been determined.
- Appropriate imaging to detect unstable ligamentous injury, particularly in clinically unexaminable patients remains unresolved.

Take-Home Table and Figure

Suggested Imaging Protocols

- Cervical spine radiography: anteroposterior, open mouth, lateral, swimmer's lateral (optional: 45-degree oblique views with 10-degree cephalad tube angulation).
- Cervical spine CT (multidetector): C0 to T4, detector collimation 1.25 mm. Sagittal reformations: 3-mm intervals, right neuroforamen to left neuroforamen. Coronal reformations: 3-mm intervals, front of vertebral body through spinal canal, C0 to C5 only.
- Thoracolumbar spine radiography: anteroposterior and interval. Swimmer's lateral of cervirothoracic junction if no CT cervical spine.

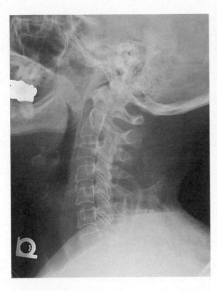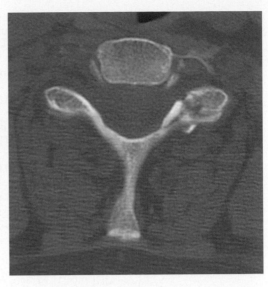

Figure 17.2. Imaging case study. Victim of a motor vehicle accident who met criteria for initial cervical spine imaging with CT scan. A potentially unstable C6–7 facet and pars interarticularis fracture is apparent on CT (A), but may be missed on contemporaneous radiography (B). CT has higher sensitivity for fracture than radiography.

- Thoracolumbar spine CT (reconstructions from trauma abdomen pelvis CT). Axial images at 2.5 mm slice interval and sagittal reformations at 2.5 mm intervals.

References

1. DeVivo MJ, Rutt RD, Black KJ, Go BK, Stover SL. Arch Phys Med Rehabil 1992; 73:424–430 [published erratum appears in Arch Phys Med Rehabil 1992; 73(12):1146].
2. Kalsbeek WD, McLaurin RL, Harris BSd, Miller JD. J Neurosurg 1980;31:S19–31.
3. Lomoschitz F, Blackmore C, Mirza S, Mann F. AJR 2002;178:573–577.
4. Blackmore CC, Ramsey SD, Mann FA, Deyo RA. Radiology 1999;212:117–125.
5. Hoffman J, Wolfson A, Todd K, Mower W. Ann Emerg Med 1998;32:461–469.
6. Bracken MB, Freeman DH, Hellenbrand K. Am J Epidemiol 1981;113:615–622.
7. Fine PR, Kuhlemeier KV, DeVivo MJ, Stover SL. Paraplegia 1979;17:237–250.
8. Rogers WA. J Bone Joint Surg 1957;39–A:341–376.
9. Reid DC, Henderson R, Saboe L, Miller JD. J Trauma 1987;27:980–986.
10. Gerrelts BD, Petersen EU, Mabry J, Petersen SR. J Trauma 1991;31:1622–1626.
11. Holmes JF, Panacek EA, Miller PQ, Lapidis AD, Mower WR. J Emerg Med 2003; 24:1–7.
12. Samuels LE, Kerstein MD. J Trauma 1993;34:85–89.
13. Durham RM, Luchtefeld WB, Wibbenmeyer L, Maxwell P, Shapiro MJ, Mazuski JE. Am J Surg 1995;170:681–684.
14. Meldon SW, Moettus LN. J Trauma 1995;39:1110–1114.
15. Saboe LA, Reid DC, Davis LA, Warren SA, Grace MG. J Trauma 1991;31:43–48.
16. van Beek E, Been H, Ponse K, Mass M. Injury 2000;31:219–223.

17. Dai LY, Yao WF, Cui YM, Zhou Q. J Trauma 2004;56:348–355.
18. Blackmore CC, Mann FA, Nuñez DB. Emerg Radiol 2000;7:142–148.
19. Mirvis SE, Diaconis JN, Chirico PA, Reiner BI, Joslyn JN, Militello P. Radiology 1989;170:831–834.
20. Hoffman JR, Schriger DL, Mower W, Luo JS, Zucker M. Ann Emerg Med 1992; 21:1454–1460.
21. Kreipke DL, Gillespie KR, McCarthy MC, Mail JT, Lappas JC, Broadie TA. J Trauma 1989;29:1438–1439.
22. Berkowitz M. J Emerg Med 1993;1:63–67.
23. Terregino C, Ross S, Lipinski M, Foreman, Hughes R. Emerg Med 1995;26:126–1329.
24. DeVivo MJ, Fine PR, Maetz HM, Stover SL. Arch Neurol 1980;37:707–708.
25. Roberge RJ, Wears RC, Kelly M, et al. J Trauma 1988;28:784–788.
26. Jacobs LM, Schwartz R. Ann Emerg Med 1986;15:44–49.
27. Cadoux CG, White JD, Hedberg MC. Ann Emerg Med 1987;16:738–742.
28. Bachulis BL, Long WB, Hynes GD, Johnson MC. Am J Surg 1987;153:473–478.
29. Hoffman J, Mower W, Wolfson A, Todd K, Zucker M. N Engl J Med 2000;343: 94–99.
30. Mahadevan S, Mower W, Hoffman J, Peeples N, Goldberg W, Sonner R. Ann Emerg Med 1998;31:197–201.
31. Stiell I, Wells G, Vandemheen K, et al. JAMA 2001;286:1841–1848.
32. Stiell IG, Clement CM, McKnight RD, et al. N Engl J Med 2003;349:2510–2518.
33. Dickinson G, Stiell IG, Schull M, Brison R, Clement C, Vandemheen K. Ann Emerg Med 2004;43:507–514.
34. Yealy DM, Auble TE. N Engl J Med 2003;349:2553–2555.
35. Mower WR, Wolfson AB, Hoffman JR, Todd KH. N Engl J Med 2004;350: 1467–1468.
36. Viccellio P, Simon H, Pressman B, Shah M, Mower W, Hoffman J. Pediatrics 2001;108:E20.
37. Kokoska E, Keller M, Rallo M, Weber T. J Pediatr Surg 2001;36:100–105.
38. Finch G, Barnes M. J Pediatr Orthop 1998;18:811–814.
39. Acheson MB, Livingston RR, Richardson ML, Stimac GK. AJR 1987;148:1179–1185.
40. Clark CR, Igram CM, el Khoury GY, Ehara S. Spine 1988;13:742–747.
41. Woodring JH, Lee C. J Trauma 1993;34:32–39.
42. Nuñez DB, Ahmad AA, Coin CG, et al. Emerg Radiol 1994;1:273–278.
43. Blackmore CC, Ramsey SD, Mann FA, Deyo RA. Radiology 1999;212:117–125.
44. Blackmore CC, Zelman WN, Glick ND. Radiology 2001;220:581–587.
45. Blackmore CC, Deyo RA. Emerg Radiol 1997;4:283–286.
46. Hanson JA, Blackmore CC, Mann FA, Wilson AJ. Emerg Radiol 2000;7:31–35.
47. Nuñez DB, Quencer RM. AJR 1998;171:951–957.
48. Blackmore CC, Emerson SS, Mann FA, Koepsell TD. Radiology 1999;211:759–765.
49. Hanson JA, Blackmore CC, Mann FA, Wilson AJ. AJR 2000;174:713–718.
50. Bub L, Blackmore C, Mann F, Lomoschitz F. Radiology 2005;234:143–149.
51. National Research Council. Health effects of exposure to low levels of ionizing radiation: BEIR V. Washington, DC: National Academy Press, 1990.
52. Ajani A, Cooper D, Scheinkestel C, et al. Anaesth Intensive Care 1998;26:487–491.
53. Beirne J, Butler P, Brady F. Int J Oral Maxillofac Surg 1995;24:26–29.
54. Davis JW, Parks SN, Detlefs CL, Williams GG, Williams JL, Smith RW. J Trauma 1995;39:435–438.
55. Sees D, Rodriguez C, Flaherty S, et al. J Trauma 1998;45:768–771.
56. Cooper C, Dunham CM, Rodriguez A. J Trauma 1995;38:692–696.
57. Frankel HL, Rozycki GS, Ochsner MG, Harviel JD, Champion HR. J Trauma 1994;37:673–676.
58. Stanislas MJ, Latham JM, Porter KM, Alpar EK, Stirling AJ. Injury 1998;29:15–18.

59. Hsu JM, Joseph T, Ellis AM. Injury 2003;34:426–433.
60. Gestring ML, Gracias VH, Feliciano MA, et al. J Trauma 2002;53:9–14.
61. Wintermark M, Mouhsine E, Theumann N, et al. Radiology 2003;227:681–689.
62. Hauser CJ, Visvikis G, Hinrichs C, et al. J Trauma 2003;55:228–234; discussion 234–225.
63. Sheridan R, Perlata R, Rhea J, Ptak T, Novelline R. J Trauma 2003;55:665–669.
64. Rhee PM, Bridgeman A, Acosta JA, et al. J Trauma 2002;53:663–667; discussion 667.

18

Imaging of Spine Disorders in Children: Dysraphism and Scoliosis

L. Santiago Medina, Diego Jaramillo, Esperanza Pacheco-Jacome, Martha C. Ballesteros, and Brian E. Grottkau

Issues

Issues of Imaging of Spinal Dysraphism

I. How accurate is imaging in occult spinal dysraphism?
II. Defining risk of occult spinal dysraphism.
III. What is the natural history and role of surgical intervention in occult spinal dysraphism?
IV. What is the cost-effectiveness of imaging in children with occult spinal dysraphism?

Issues of Imaging of Scoliosis

V. How should the radiographic evaluation of scoliosis be performed?
VI. What radiation-induced complications result from radiographic monitoring of scoliosis?
VII. What is the use of magnetic resonance imaging (MRI) for severe idiopathic scoliosis?
VIII. What is the use of MRI for high-risk subgroups of scoliosis?

Key Points

Spinal Dysraphism

- The prevalence of occult spinal dysraphism (OSD) ranges from as low as 0.34% in children with intergluteal dimples to as high as 46% in newborns with cloacal malformation (moderate evidence).
- Magnetic resonance imaging (MRI) and ultrasound have better overall diagnostic performances (i.e., sensitivity and specificity) than plain radiographs (moderate evidence) in children with suspected occult spinal dysraphism.
- Early detection and prompt neurosurgical correction of occult spinal dysraphism may prevent upper urinary tract deterioration, infection of dorsal dermal sinuses, or permanent neurologic damage (moderate and limited evidence).

- Cost-effectiveness analysis suggests that, in newborns with suspected OSD, appropriate selection of patients and diagnostic strategy may increase quality-adjusted life expectancy and decrease cost of medical workup (moderate evidence).

Scoliosis

- Radiographic measurements of scoliosis are reproducible, particularly when the levels of the end plates measured are kept constant (moderate evidence). Unexpected findings on radiographs are unusual (limited evidence).
- Radiographic monitoring of scoliosis results in a clear increase in the radiation-induced cancer risk, particularly to the breast (moderate evidence). It also results in a high dose of radiation to the ovaries and worsens reproductive outcome in females (moderate evidence). Therefore, it is very important to reduce the radiation exposure. Posteroanterior projection greatly reduces exposure, and some digital systems also decrease radiation.
- Minimal tonsillar ectopia (<5 mm) is significantly prevalent in scoliosis and correlates with abnormalities in somatosensory-evoked potentials and with the severity of scoliosis (moderate evidence). Otherwise, a paucity of significant findings on magnetic resonance (MR) images of patients evaluated for idiopathic scoliosis is noted, even in severe cases.
- Unlike adolescent idiopathic scoliosis, juvenile and infantile idiopathic scoliosis and congenital scoliosis have a high incidence of neural axis abnormalities (limited evidence). Increased incidence of neural axis abnormalities has also been seen with atypical idiopathic scoliosis and left (levoconvex) thoracic scoliosis.

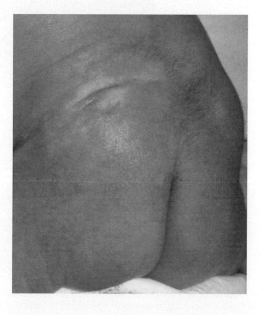

Figure 18.1. Photograph of the lower back reveals skin discoloration, hairy patchy, and dorsal lipoma. (See color insert)

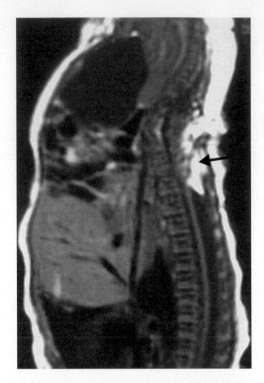

Figure 18.2. Sagittal T1-weighted imaging shows a dorsal lipoma extending into the spinal canal with an associate low lying conus medullaris (arrow).

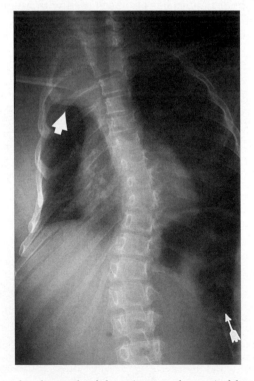

Figure 18.3. Frontal radiograph of the spine reveals atypical levoconvex thoracic scoliosis and right thoracic apical mass (arrow).

Figure 18.4. Coronal T2-weighted image shows a large right neck and chest plexiform neurofibroma (arrow).

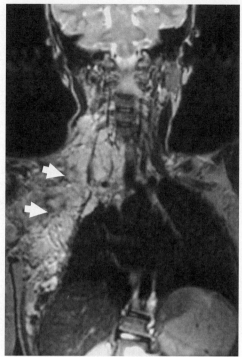

Definition and Pathophysiology

Spinal Dysraphism

Spinal dysraphism is a wide spectrum of congenital anomalies that result from abnormal development of one or more of the midline mesenchymal, bony, and neural elements of the spine (1). This entity can be divided into open and closed spina bifida. Open spina bifida is characterized by a dorsal herniation of all or part of the spinal content without full skin coverage. Open spina bifida entities include meningocele and myelomeningocele. Closed or occult spinal dysraphism (OSD) is characterized by a spinal anomaly covered with skin and hence with no exposed neural tissue (2,3). The OSD spectrum includes dorsal dermal sinus, thickened filum terminale, diastematomyelia, caudal regression syndrome, intradural lipoma, lipomyelocele, lipomyelomeningocele, anterior spinal meningocele and other forms of myelodysplasia (Figs. 18.1 and 18.2).

Scoliosis

Scoliosis is defined as an abnormal spinal curvature most apparent in the coronal plane (4). Scoliosis can be classified as congenital, degenerative, neuromuscular, or idiopathic. Most pediatric cases are idiopathic in nature. Idiopathic scoliosis is further subdivided according to the age at which the disease presents: infantile (birth to 3 years), juvenile (4 to 9 years), and adolescent (10 years and beyond) (5). Congenital scoliosis is caused by vertebral anomalies of embryologic etiology (6). Scoliosis can also be seen in disorders such as neurofibromatosis (Figs. 18.3 and 18.4) and Marfan syndrome (4).

Conus Medullaris Position

Controversy has existed about the normal position of the conus medullaris. The normal level of the conus medullaris was thought to vary with the age of the child (7–9). Additional imaging studies, however, indicate that the normal conus medullaris position can vary from the middle of T11 to the bottom of L2 by age 2 months (7,9) and probably at birth (7,10). Although a spinal cord terminating at these normal levels can be tethered (8), the conus that terminates caudal to the L2-L3 disk space is at much higher of being tethered (7,9,11). Neuroimaging can define the anatomic location of the conus medullaris, but "tethered" is a neurophysiologic concept that requires clinical input (12). Small fibrolipomas in the filum terminale may be seen in untethered cords. Five to six percent of normal individuals can have variable amounts of fat in the filum terminale (13,14).

Epidemiology

Spinal Dysraphism

Three percent of neonates have major central nervous system or systemic malformations (15). Furthermore, 5% to 15% of pediatric neurology hospital admissions are related to cerebrospinal anomalies (16). The incidence of neural tube defects in the United States is 1.2 to 1.7 per 1000 births (17,18). Almost half of neural tube defects are caused by anencephaly (0.6–0.8 per 1000 births), and the majority of the remaining are caused by spinal dysraphism (0.5–0.8 per 1000 births) (17,18). Occult spinal dysraphism is the most prevalent spinal axis malformation (19) and the most common indication for spinal imaging in children (20). Occult spinal dysraphic lesions are commonly associated with urinary tract anomalies (21).

   The clinical spectrum of occult dysraphism is broad, ranging from skin stigmata such as a dimple, sinus tract, hair patch, or hemangioma to motor, bladder, or bowel dysfunction (22–24). About 50% to 80% of occult spinal dysraphic cases exhibit a dermal lesion (25–28). However, 3% to 5% of all normal children have skin dimples (29,30).

Scoliosis

Adolescent idiopathic scoliosis, by far the most common form, has a prevalence between 0.5% (31) and 3% (32,33) and occurs more often in females. In a United Kingdom study of 15,799 children and young adolescents, Stirling and colleagues (31) found that the prevalence ratio of girls to boys was 5.2 [95% confidence interval (CI), 2.9–9.5]. In a study of 26,947 students, Rogala et al. (33) found that for curves ranging from 6 to 10 degrees, the girl-to-boy ratio was 1:1, whereas the ratio was 5.4:1 for curves greater than 20 degrees. The more severe the curve, the greater the predominance of girls over boys. Infantile scoliosis constitutes approximately 8% of idiopathic scoliosis whereas juvenile scoliosis represents 18% (34). Male predominance is seen in infantile scoliosis. Congenital scoliosis is caused by failure of segmentation of formation of spinal elements (4). In a series of 60 cases of congenital scoliosis, Shahcheraghi and Hobbi (6) found that the most common type of anomaly was a hemivertebra (failure of formation), and that the most severe deformity was associated with a unilateral unsegmented bar (failure of segmentation) with a contralateral hemivertebra).

The etiology of adolescent scoliosis remains a mystery; however, some principles are generally agreed on (35):

1. The progression of scoliosis is related to severity and skeletal maturity. The younger the onset and the greater the severity of the curve, the faster the progression. Although previously it was believed that scoliosis remained stable after skeletal maturity was attained, Weinstein and Ponseti (36) demonstrated that 68% of curves worsened after bone maturity.

2. The typical scoliosis curve is not associated with pain or neurologic signs and symptoms. Painful curves, especially if rapidly progressive or if associated with an atypical curve pattern, are frequently caused by underlying diseases (37).

3. Less than 10% of the curves require treatment (35).

Goals

Spinal Dysraphism

In patients with spinal dysraphism, the goal of imaging is to detect early neurosurgical correctable occult dysraphic lesions in order to prevent neurologic damage, upper urinary tract deterioration, and potential infection of the dorsal dermal sinuses.

Scoliosis

In patients with scoliosis, the goal of imaging is to detect and characterize the type of curve and its severity, to track disease progression and monitor changes related to treatment, and to identify those cases in which occult etiologies exist (4).

Methodology

The authors performed a Medline search using Ovid (New York, New York) and PubMed (National Library of Medicine, Bethesda, Maryland) for data relevant to the diagnostic performance and accuracy of both clinical and radiographic examination of patients with occult spinal dysraphism or scoliosis during the period 1966 to August 2003. Animal studies and non–English-language articles were excluded. The titles, abstracts, and full text of the relevant articles were reviewed at each step.

I. How Accurate Is Imaging in Occult Spinal Dysraphism?

Summary of Evidence: Several studies have shown that magnetic resonance imaging (MRI) and ultrasound have better overall diagnostic performances (i.e., sensitivity and specificity) than plain radiographs (moderate evidence) (20,26,38,39). The sensitivity of spinal MRI and ultrasound has been estimated at 95.6% and 86.5%, respectively (31,39). The specificity of spinal MRI and ultrasound has been estimated at 90.9% and 92.9%, respectively (20,39). Conversely, the sensitivity and specificity of plain radiographs have been estimated at 80% and 18%, respectively (26,38).

Table 18.1. Diagnostic performance of imaging test

Variable	Baseline value	95% confidence interval*	Reference
Ultrasound			
Sensitivity	86.5%	75–98%	30,39
Specificity	92.0%	84–100%	30,39
MRI			
Sensitivity	95.6%	89.8–99.7%	20,30
Specificity	90.9%	75.7–98.1%	20,30
Plain radiographs			
Sensitivity	80%	80–100%	26,30,38
Specificity	18%	11–25%	30,38

* 95% confidence intervals were estimated from the available literature.

Supporting Evidence: The diagnostic performance of the imaging tests available is shown in detail in Table 18.1.

II. Defining Risk of Occult Spinal Dysraphism

Summary of Evidence: The prevalence of OSD ranges from as low as 0.34% in children with intergluteal dimples to as high as 46% in newborns with cloacal malformation (moderate evidence). Table 18.2 categorizes the spectrum of occult spinal dysraphism into low-, intermediate-, and high-risk groups.

Supporting Evidence: Children in the low-risk group included those with simple skin dimples as the sole manifestation, or newborns of diabetic mothers. Intergluteal dimples over the sacrococcygeal area rarely extend into the spinal canal (40,41,43). Caudal regression syndrome has been reported in children born to diabetic mothers (42). The prevalence (pretest probability) of a dysraphic lesion among low-risk patients has been estimated at 0.3% to 3.8% (Table 18.2). In the low range (0.3%) are children with low intergluteal dimples while children in the upper range (3.8%) have higher lumbosacral dimples (18,26,31) (moderate and limited evidence).

Children in the intermediate-risk group included those with complex skin stigmata (hairy patch, hemangiomas, lipomas, and well-defined dorsal

Table 18.2. Risk groups for occult spinal dysraphism

Variable	Baseline value	Reference
Low-risk group		
Offspring of diabetic mothers	0.3%	30,64–66
Intergluteal dimples	0.34%	25,30
Lumbosacral dimple	3.8%	29
Intermediate-risk groups		
Low anorectal malformation	27%	67
Intermediate anorectal malformation	33%	67
Complex skin stigmata*	36%	29
High-risk group		
High anorectal malformation	44%	67
Cloacal malformation	46%	21
Cloacal exstrophy	100%	21

* Hemangiomas, hairy patches, and subcutaneous masses.

dermal sinus tracks), or low and intermediate anorectal malformations. The prevalence (pretest probability) of a dysraphic lesion among intermediate-risk patients has been estimated at 27% to 36% (Table 18.2) (moderate evidence). Children in the high-risk group included those with high anorectal malformations, cloacal malformation, and cloacal exstrophy. The prevalence (pretest probability) of a dysraphic lesion among high-risk patients has been estimated at 44% to 100% (Table 18.2) (moderate evidence).

III. What Is the Natural History and Role of Surgical Intervention in Occult Spinal Dysraphism?

Summary of Evidence: Early detection and prompt neurosurgical correction of occult spinal dysraphism may prevent upper urinary tract deterioration, infection of dorsal dermal sinuses, or permanent neurologic damage (44–48) (moderate and limited evidence). Several studies have demonstrated that motor function, urologic symptoms, and urodynamic patterns may be improved, stabilized, or prevented by early surgical intervention in patients with occult spinal dysraphism (49,50) (moderate and limited evidence). The surgical outcome may be better if intervention occurs before the age of 3 years (49–51) (moderate and limited evidence). Spinal neuroimaging, therefore, has the important role of determining the presence or absence of an occult spinal dysraphic lesion so that appropriate surgical treatment can be instituted in a timely manner.

At our institution, occult dysraphic lesions diagnosed in the newborn period are usually operated at age 2 to 3 months. Therefore, if ultrasound is indicated, it is performed in the early newborn and infancy period to avoid a limited sonographic window from posterior element mineralization (52,53). If MRI is required, it is usually performed a few days before surgery.

Supporting Evidence: In the newborn period most children with OSD are neurologically asymptomatic (29). Symptoms from occult spinal dysraphism are often not apparent until the child becomes older and is ambulating (29) (moderate evidence). The most common clinical presentations for occult dysraphic patients later in life include delay in walking, delay in development of sphincter control, asymmetry of the legs or abnormalities of the feet (i.e., pes cavus and pes equinovarus), and pain in the lower extremities or back (44,45,49,54–57).

Several studies have demonstrated improvement of the multiple symptoms associated with occult dysraphism if surgical intervention is performed (49–51) (moderate and limited evidence). However, there are differences in outcome depending on the timing of surgery (51). Using surgical outcome data from the study by Satar and colleagues (51), in the children diagnosed and surgically treated before the age of 3 years, 60% became asymptomatic, 30% were unchanged, and 10% worsened. Conversely, the same study data for the children diagnosed and surgically treated after age 3 years demonstrated that 27% became asymptomatic, 27% improved, 27% were unchanged, and 19% worsened (51).

Dysraphic patients with a central nervous system communicating dorsal dermal sinus (i.e., 10% of all dysraphic patients) are at risk for infection (26). The most dreaded infection is meningitis. Meningitis in the patient with a communicating dorsal dermal sinus may be caused by aggressive gram-negative or anaerobic bacteria (58,59). Meningitis mortality rate in patients with communicating dorsal dermal sinus ranges between 1% and 12% (58–62) (limited evidence).

Severely symptomatic patients with dysraphism are at high risk of upper urinary tract deterioration (30,63). In this population up to 15% may have upper urinary tract deterioration (30,63) and of those with progressive renal damage, 7.5% may develop end-stage renal disease over a 10-year period if undiagnosed (30,63) (limited evidence).

IV. What Is the Cost-Effectiveness of Imaging in Children with Occult Spinal Dysraphism?

Summary of Evidence: Cost-effectiveness analysis suggests that, in newborns with suspected OSD, appropriate selection of patients and diagnostic strategy may increase quality-adjusted life expectancy and decrease cost of medical workup (30).

Supporting Evidence: A cost-effectiveness analysis (CEA) in children with occult spinal dysraphism assessed the clinical and economic consequences of four diagnostic strategies—MRI, ultrasound, plain radiographs, and no imaging with close clinical follow-up—in the evaluation of newborns with suspected occult spinal dysraphism (30).

A decision-analytic Markov model and CEA was performed incorporating (1) pretest or prior probability of disease in three different risk groups, (2) diagnostic tests sensitivity and specificity of diagnostic tests, and (3) morbidity and mortality rates of early versus late diagnosis and treatment of dysraphism. Outcomes were based on quality-adjusted life year (QALY) gained and incremental cost per QALY gained.

Medina and colleagues (30) found that in low-risk children with intergluteal dimple or newborns of diabetic mothers (pretest probability = 0.3% to 0.34%), ultrasound was the most effective strategy with an incremental cost-effectiveness ratio of $55,100 per QALY gained. For children with lumbosacral dimples who have a higher pretest probability of 3.8%, ultrasound was less costly and more effective than MRI, plain radiographs, or no imaging with close clinical follow-up.

In intermediate-risk newborns with low anorectal malformation (pretest probability 27%), ultrasound was more effective and less costly than radiographs and no imaging. However, MRI was more effective than ultrasound at an incremental cost-effectiveness ratio of $1000 per QALY gained. In the high-risk group that included high anorectal malformation, cloacal malformation, and exstrophy (pretest probability 44% to 46%), MRI was actually cost-saving when compared with the other diagnostic strategies.

For the intermediate-risk group, the CEA was sensitive to the costs and diagnostic performances (sensitivity and specificity) of MRI and ultrasound. Lower MRI cost or greater MRI diagnostic performance improved the cost-effectiveness of the MRI strategy, while lower ultrasound cost or greater ultrasound diagnostic performance worsened the cost-effectiveness of the MRI strategy. Therefore, individual or institutional expertise with a specific diagnostic modality (MRI versus ultrasound) may influence the optimal diagnostic strategy.

V. How Should the Radiographic Evaluation of Scoliosis Be Performed?

Summary of Evidence: Radiographic measurements of scoliosis are reproducible, particularly when the levels of the end plates measured are kept constant (moderate evidence). Unexpected findings on radiographs are unusual (limited evidence) (4).

Supporting Evidence: Many articles have addressed the variability in measurement of the Cobb angle in adolescent idiopathic scoliosis. In a 1990 study by Morrissy and colleagues (68), four orthopedic surgeons performed six measurements on 50 frontal radiographs. The 95% CIs were 4.9 degrees, and the variation was greatest when the end-plate vertebrae were not preselected (moderate evidence). Similar variability was noted in the sagittal and coronal planes. Carman and colleagues (69) had five observers perform two measurements on 28 radiographs showing kyphosis or scoliosis and found 95% CIs of 8 degrees for scoliosis and 7 degrees for kyphosis (moderate evidence). A later study (70) comparing manual versus computer-assisted radiographic measurements (24 radiographs, six observers) found a statistically significant difference between the 95% CIs of manual measurements (3.3 degrees) and computer-generated measurements (2.6 degrees).

Variability is greater for congenital scoliosis versus idiopathic scoliosis. Using six observers and 54 radiographs, Loder and colleagues (71) found 95% CIs of 11.8 degrees (moderate evidence).

The contribution of radiologists' reports of scoliosis radiographs to clinical management was studied by Crockett and colleagues (72). These investigators retrospectively reviewed 161 charts and analyzed them for the presence or absence of information about certain key parameters. There was no mention of how the review was done or whether there was any attempt to correct for bias. Radiologists added information in 1.9% of the cases that, although not specified, was not deemed clinically significant (limited evidence) (72).

VI. What Radiation-Induced Complications Result from Radiographic Monitoring of Scoliosis?

Summary of Evidence: Patients with severe scoliosis are monitored with the use of serial radiographs that expose the body to radiation. Radiographic monitoring of scoliosis results in a clear increase in the radiation-induced cancer risk, particularly to the breast (4) (moderate evidence). It also results in a high dose of radiation to the ovaries and worsens reproductive outcome in females (4) (moderate evidence). Therefore, it is very important to reduce the radiation exposure. Posteroanterior projection greatly reduces exposure, and some digital systems also decrease radiation (73).

Supporting Evidence: In 2000 Morin Doody and colleagues (74) published a retrospective cohort study of 5573 female patients with scoliosis diagnosed before the age of 20 years. The average length of follow-up was 40.1 years, with complete follow-up in 89%. The average number of examinations per patient was 24.7 (range, 0–618), and the mean estimated cumulative radiation dose to the breast was 10.8 cGy (range, 0–170). Seventy-seven breast cancer deaths were observed compared with 45.6 expected deaths on the basis of United States mortality rates. Women with scoliosis had a 1.7-fold risk of dying of breast cancer (95% CI, 1.3–2.1) when compared with the general population. The data suggested that radiation was the causative factor, with risk increasing significantly with the number of radiographic exposures and the cumulative radiation dose (moderate evidence). Potential confounding was noted because the severity of disease was related to radiation exposure and reproductive history; patients with more severe disease were less likely to become pregnant and had a greater risk of breast cancer.

In a large retrospective cohort study of 2039 patients, Levy and colleagues (75) found an excess lifetime cancer risk of 1% to 2% (12 to 25 cases per 1000 population) among women (moderate evidence). The same group suggested that supplanting the anteroposterior (AP) view with the posteroanterior (PA) view would result in a three- to sevenfold reduction in cumulative doses to the thyroid gland and the female breast, three- to fourfold reductions in the lifetime risk of breast cancer, and a halving of the lifetime risk of thyroid cancer (76). The same cohort of women was evaluated for adverse reproductive outcomes (77). Of the initial group of 1793 young women evaluated for scoliosis between 1960 and 1979, 1292 women returned questionnaires in 1990. This cohort was compared with a reference group of 1134 women selected randomly from the general population. The adolescent idiopathic scoliosis cohort had a higher risk of spontaneous abortions [odds ratio (OR), 1.35; 95% CI, 1.06–1.73] (moderate evidence). The odds of unsuccessful attempts at pregnancy (OR, 1.33; 95% CI, 0.84–2.13) and of congenital malformations (OR, 1.2; 95% CI, 0.78–1.84) were also higher but not statistically significant (moderate evidence).

Digital radiography seems to reduce radiation exposure. The results are varied (78–80), and the technology is evolving (limited evidence). Studies report an 18-fold reduction with some systems (73) versus an almost twofold increase with others (81).

VII. What Is the Use of Magnetic Resonance Imaging (MRI) for Severe Idiopathic Scoliosis?

Summary of Evidence: There is increasing concern about the association of idiopathic scoliosis with structural abnormalities of the neural axis. Minimal tonsillar ectopia (<5 mm) is significantly prevalent in scoliosis and correlates with abnormalities in somatosensory-evoked potentials and with the severity of scoliosis (4) (moderate evidence). Otherwise, a paucity of significant findings on MRI of patients evaluated for idiopathic scoliosis is noted, even in severe cases (4).

Supporting Evidence: Cheng and colleagues (82) studied 36 healthy control subjects, 135 patients with moderately severe adolescent idiopathic scoliosis (Cobb angle less than 45 degrees), and 29 similar patients with Cobb angles greater than 45 degrees. All of the patients were evaluated prospectively with MRI looking specifically for tonsillar ectopia and with somatosensory-evoked potentials. Tonsillar herniation was found in none of the controls versus four of 135 (3%) and eight of 29 (27.6%) of the two scoliotic groups ($p < .001$) (moderate evidence). Similarly, the percentages of patients with abnormal somatosensory-evoked potentials were 0%, 11.9%, and 27.6%, respectively. There was a significant association between tonsillar ectopia and abnormal somatosensory function ($p < .001$; correlation coefficient, 0.672) (moderate evidence). Tonsillar ectopia was defined as any inferior displacement of the tonsils, and none of the patients had a displacement greater than 5 mm, which is considered the usual threshold for the diagnosis (83–85).

Several studies have addressed the prevalence of MR abnormalities in patients with severe idiopathic scoliosis who are otherwise asymptomatic. Do and colleagues (86) studied a consecutive series of 327 patients with idiopathic scoliosis requiring surgical intervention (average preoperative curve of 57 degrees) but without neurologic findings. The patients, aged 10 to 19 years, were evaluated from the base of the skull to the sacrum. Seven patients had abnormal MRI, including two with syrinx, four with Chiari malformation type I, and one with a fatty vertebral body. None of them required specific treatment for these findings (moderate evidence). In four other cases, equivocal MRI findings necessitated additional workup. In a similar prospective double-blinded study of 140 patients evaluated preoperatively, Winter et al. (87) found four patients with abnormalities, three with Chiari I malformations, and one with a small syrinx, none of whom required treatment. In another study of MRI examinations performed preoperatively, Maiocco et al. (88) found two of 45 patients with syrinx, one requiring decompression (moderate evidence).

To study whether the severity of the curve increased the risk of associated abnormalities, O'Brien et al. (89) performed MR evaluation on 33 consecutive patients with adolescent idiopathic scoliosis and Cobb angles greater than 70 degrees. No neural axis abnormalities were found (limited evidence).

VIII. What Is the Use of MRI for High-Risk Subgroups of Scoliosis?

Summary of Evidence: Unlike adolescent idiopathic scoliosis, juvenile and infantile idiopathic scoliosis and congenital scoliosis have a high incidence of neural axis abnormalities (limited evidence). Increased incidence of neural axis abnormalities have been seen with atypical idiopathic scoliosis and left (levoconvex) thoracic scoliosis (Figs. 18.3 and 18.4) (4) (limited evidence).

Supporting Evidence: Several studies have shown that, with scoliosis types that are different from the typical adolescent idiopathic form, there is a high prevalence of neural abnormalities (4). Of 30 consecutive children with congenital scoliosis studied by Prahinski and colleagues (90), nine had syringomyelia. Of these children, one required release of the tethered cord and one correction of a diastematomyelia (limited evidence). Two studies of prepubertal children suggest a high incidence of neural abnormalities in juvenile and infantile scoliosis. In a study of 26 consecutive children aged less than 11 years, Lewonowski and colleagues (91) found five (19.2%) with abnormalities of the cord. Three required surgical intervention, two with hydromyelia and one with a mass (91) (limited evidence). Gupta and colleagues (92) found that six of 34 patients under 10 years of age studied prospectively had neural axis abnormalities, including two patients with syrinx requiring syringopleural shunting (one with a Chiari I malformation). Other abnormalities included dural ectasia, tethered cord, and a brainstem astrocytoma (limited evidence).

In a retrospective review of 95 patients with idiopathic scoliosis who had been studied for various indications, Schwend and colleagues (93) found that 12 had a syrinx, one a cord astrocytoma, and one dural ectasia (limited evidence). Left thoracic scoliosis was the most important predictor of abnormality (10 abnormalities in 43 patients). Mejia et al. (94) then performed a prospective study (level II) of 29 consecutive patients with idiopathic left thoracic scoliosis, finding only two with syrinx and no other abnormalities (limited evidence). Barnes and colleagues (37) retrospectively analyzed 30 patients with atypical idiopathic scoliosis and found 17 abnormalities in 11 patients, including seven cases of syringohydromyelia and five Chiari I malformations (limited evidence).

Take-Home Data

How Should Physicians Evaluate Newborns with Suspected Occult Spinal Dysraphism?

The decision tree in Figure 18.5 reinforces the primary importance of a careful acquisition of a medical history and performance of a thorough examination in newborns with suspected spinal dysraphism (30). For those patients in the high-risk group, imaging of the spine with MRI is recommended. For those patients in the intermediate-risk group, imaging of the spine with MRI or ultrasound is suggested, while in the low-risk group the strategies of ultrasound or no imaging may be indicated. Selection between

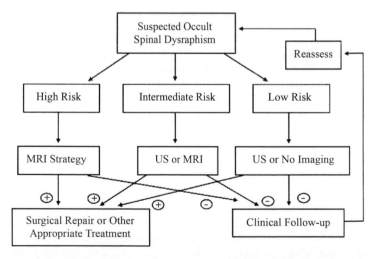

Figure 18.5. Suggested decision tree for use in newborns with suspected occult spinal dysraphism. For those patients in the high-risk group MRI is recommended. For patients in the intermediate-risk group ultrasound (US) or MRI is the strategy of choice, while for the low-risk group ultrasound or no imaging is recommended. For patients with negative imaging studies close clinical follow-up with periodic reassessment is recommended. [*Source:* Medina et al. (30), with permission.]

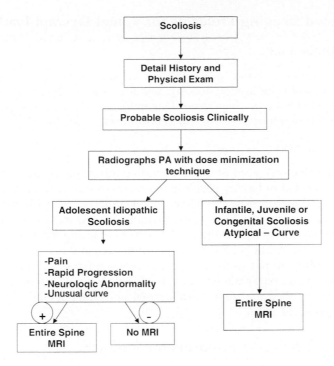

Figure 18.6. Suggested decision tree for use in patients with suspected scoliosis. Decision tree emphasizes importance of clinical history, physical exam, and radiographs in determining the need for MRI.

these two strategies per risk group may be based on individual and institutional diagnostic performance and cost per test. In newborns with suspected occult dysraphism, appropriate selection of patients for imaging based on these risk groups may maximize health outcomes for patients and improve health care resource allocation.

How Should Scoliosis Be Evaluated?

Figure 18.6 summarizes the decision tree for patients with suspected scoliosis.

Imaging Case Study of Spinal Dysraphism

This imaging case study illustrates a child with skin stigmata (Fig. 18.1) who has an occult dysraphic lesion of the intradural lipoma type (Fig. 18.2).

Imaging Case Study of Scoliosis

This imaging case study illustrates a child with atypical levoconvex thoracic scoliosis (Fig. 18.3) who has neurofibromatosis type 1 with underlying plexiform neurofibromas (Fig. 18.4).

Suggested Imaging Protocols for Spinal Dysraphism

Spinal Ultrasound

Spinal ultrasound should be performed in patients before the age of 3 months to avoid the limited acoustic window from mineralization of the posterior elements. An experienced operator should perform the study using a high-frequency, 5- to 15-MHz linear array transducer (52).

Entire Spine MRI

A retrospective case-control study including 101 patients (moderate evidence) suspected of having occult lumbosacral dysraphism demonstrated that conventional three-plane T1-weighted lumbosacral MRI in children and young adults provided better diagnostic information than a fast screening two-plane T1-weighted MRI because of its higher specificity and interobserver agreement (20). T2-weighted images in the axial and sagittal plane are often added to the protocol to assess intrinsic cord abnormalities. Intravenous paramagnetic contrast is not routinely used, unless the patient has a communicating dorsal dermal sinus tract or clinical concerns of underlying infection.

Suggested Imaging Protocols for Scoliosis

Scoliosis Radiographs

Radiographs should be performed only when clinically indicated. Using the posteroanterior projection greatly reduces exposure, and some digital systems also decrease radiation (4,73).

Entire Spine MRI

Patients with scoliosis may represent an imaging challenge. In patients with scoliosis being evaluated with MRI, the entire spine should be covered. Three plain T1- and T2-weighted images should be obtained with different obliquities to optimize imaging information. Another approach is to obtain three-dimensional fast spin echo (FSE) volumetric imaging. Weinberger and colleagues (95) recommend using a TR of 500 ms, TE_{eff} of 21 ms, echo train length (ETL) of 8, 20- to 38-cm field of view, 256×256 in plane matrix, 1-mm sagittal partition thickness, one excitation, and 16 kHz of receive bandwidth. Intravenous paramagnetic contrast is important in the evaluation of intramedullary and extramedullary neoplasm.

Future Research

- Formal cost-effectiveness analysis of imaging in children with scoliosis.
- Further development of low or no radiation imaging techniques for patients with scoliosis.

References

1. Pacheco-Jacome E, Ballesteros MC, Jayakar P, Morrison G, Ragheb J, Medina LS. Neuroimag Clin North Am 2003;13:327–334.

2. Soonawala N, Overweg-Plandsoen WCG, Brouwer OF. Clin Neurol Neurosurg 1999;101:11–14.

3. Tortori-Donati P, Cama A, Rosa ML, Andreussi L, Taccone A. Neuroradiology 1990;31:512–522.

4. Jaramillo D, Poussaint TY, Grottkau BE. Neuroimag Clin North Am 2003;13: 335–341.

5. Oestreich AE, Young LW, Young Poussaint T. Skeletal Radiol 1998;27(11): 591–605.

6. Shahcheraghi GH, Hobbi MH. J Pediatr Orthop 1999;19(6):766–775.

7. DiPietro MA. Radiology 1993;188:149–153.

8. Rowland Hill CA, Gibson PJ. AJNR 1995;16:469–472.

9. Wilson DA, Prince JR. AJNR 1989;10:259–262.

10. Beek FJ, de Vries LS, Gerards LJ, Mali WP. Neuroradiology 1996; 38(suppl):S174–177.

11. Barson AJ. J Anat 1970;106:489–497.

12. Warder DE, Oakes WJ. Neurosurgery 1993;33:374–378.

13. Haworth JC, Zachary RB. Lancet 1955;2:10–14.

14. Milhorat TH, Miller JI. Neurosurgery. In: Avery GB, Fletcher MA, Mhairi GM, eds. Neonatology (4th ed). Philadelphia: JB Lippincott, 1994:1155–1163.

15. Kalter H, Warkany J. Medical progress. N Engl J Med 1983;308:424–431.

16. Bird TD, Hall JG. Neurology 1977;27:1057–1060.

17. Vintzileos AM, Ananth CV, Fisher AJ, et al. Am J Obstet Gynecol 1999; 180(5):1227–1233.

18. Knight GJ, Palomaki GF. Maternal serum alpha-fetoprotein and the detection of open neural tube defects. In: Elias S, Simpson JL, eds. Maternal Serum Screening for Fetal Genetic Disorders. New York: Churchill Livingstone, 1992: 41–58.

19. Egelhoff JC, Prenger EC, Coley BD. The spine. In: Ball W Jr, ed. Pediatric Neuroradiology. Philadelphia: Lippincott-Raven, 1997:717–778.

20. Medina LS, Al-Orfali M, Zurakowski D, Poussaint TY, DiCanzio J, Barnes PD. Radiology 1999;211:767–771.

21. Appignani BA, Jaramillo D, Barnes PD, Poussaint TY. AJR 1994;163:1199–1203.

22. Raghavan N, Barkovich AJ, Edwards M, Norman D. AJR 1989;152:843–852.

23. Brophy JD, Sutton LN, Zimmerman RA, Bury E, Schut L. Neurosurgery 1989;25:336–340.

24. Moufarrij NE, Palmer JM, Hahn JF, Weinstein MA. Neurosurgery 1989;25: 341–346.

25. Milhorat TH, Miller JI. Neurosurgery. In: Avery GB, Fletcher MA, Mhairi GM, eds. Neonatology (4th ed). Philadelphia: JB Lippincott, 1994:1155–1163.

26. Volpe JJ. Neurology of the Newborn, 4th ed. Philadelphia: WB Saunders, 2001.

27. Hoffman HJ, Hendrick EB, Humphreys RP. Childs Brain 1976;2:145–155.

28. Hoffman HJ, Taecholarn C, Hendrick EB, Humphreys RP. J Neurosurg 1985;62:1–8.

29. Kriss VM, Desai NS. AJR 1998;171:1687–1692.

30. Medina LS, Crone K, Kuntz KM. Pediatrics 2001;108:E101.

31. Stirling AJ, Howel D, Millner PA, Sadiq S, Sharples D, Dickson RA. J Bone Joint Surg Am 1996;78(9):1330–1336.

32. Newton PO, Wenger DR. Idiopathic and congenital scoliosis. In: Morrissy RT, Weinstein SL, eds. Lovell & Winter's Pediatric Orthopaedics, 5th ed. Philadelphia: Lippincott Williams & Wilkins, 2000:677–740.

33. Rogala EJ, Drummond DS, Gurr J. J Bone Joint Surg Am 1978;60(2):173–176.

34. Al-Arjani AM, Al-Sebai MW, Al-Khawashki HM, Saadeddin MF. Saudi Med J 2000;21(6):554–557.

35. Weinstein SL. Spine 1999;24(24):2592–2600.

36. Weinstein SL, Ponseti IV. J Bone Joint Surg Am 1983;65(4):447–455.

37. Barnes PD, Brody JD, Jaramillo D, Akbar JU, Emans JB. Radiology 1993; 186(1):247–253.

38. Horton D, Barnes P, Pendleton BD, Polly M. J Okla State Med Assoc 1989; 82:15–19.
39. Rohrschneider WK, Forsting M, Darge K, Tröger J. Radiology 1996;200:383–388.
40. Powell KR, Cherry JD, Hougen TJB, Blinderman EE, Dunn MC. J Pediatr 1975;87:744–750.
41. Byrd SE, Darling CF, McLone DG. Radiol Clin North Am 1991;29:711–752.
42. Estin MD, Cohen AR. Neurosurg Clin North Am 1995;6:377–391.
43. Herman TE, Oser RF, Shackelford GD. Clin Pediatr 1993;32:627–628.
44. Kaplan JO, Quencer RM. Radiology 1980;137:387–391.
45. McLone DG, Naidich TP. The tethered spinal cord. In: McLaurin RL, Schof L, Venes JL, Epstein F, eds. Surgery of the Developing Nervous System. Philadelphia: WB Saunders, 1989:71–96.
46. Yamada S, Iacono RP, Andrade T, Mandybur G, Yamada BS. Neurosurg Clin North Am 1995;6:311–323.
47. Davis PC, Hoffman JC, Ball TI, et al. Radiology 1988;166:679–685.
48. Scatliff JH, Kendall BE, Kingsley DPE, Britton J, Grant DN, Hayward RD. AJNR 1989;10:269–277.
49. Pang D, Wilberger JE. J Neurosurg 1982;57:32–47.
50. Fone PD, Vapnek JM, Litwiller SE, et al. J Urol 1997;157.
51. Satar N, Bauer SB, Shefner J, Kelly MD, Darbey MM. J Urol 1995;154:754–758.
52. Coley BD, Siegel MJ. Spinal ultrasonography. In: Siegel MJ, ed. Pediatric Sonography. Philadelphia: Lippincott Williams & Wilkins, 2002:671–698.
53. Rubin JM, Di Pietro MA, Chandler WF, et al. Radiol Clin North Am 1988; 26:1–27.
54. Page LK. Occult spinal dysraphism and related disorders. In: Wilkins RH, Rengachary SS, eds. Neurosurgery. New York: McGraw-Hill, 1992:2053–2058.
55. Westcott MA, Dynes MC, Remer EM, Donaldson JS, Dias LS. Radiographics 1992;12:1155–1173.
56. Atala A, Bauer SB, Dyro FM, et al. J Urol 1992;148:592–594.
57. Reigel DH, Tchernoukha K, Bazmi B, Kortyna R, Rotenstein D. Pediatr Neurosurg 1994;20:30–42.
58. Law DA, Aronoff SC. Pediatr Infect Dis J 1992;11:968–971.
59. Rogg JM, Benzil DL, Haas RL, Knuckey NW. AJNR 1993;14:1393–1395.
60. DiTullio MV Jr. Surg Neurol 1977;7:351–354.
61. Feigen RD, Cherry JD. Textbook of Pediatric Infectious Diseases, 2nd ed. Philadelphia: WB Saunders, 1987.
62. Givner LB, Baker CJ. Pediatr Infec Dis J 1983;2:385–387.
63. Capitanucci ML, Iacobelli BD, Silveri M, Mosiello G, De Gennaro M. Eur J Pediatr Surg 1996;6(suppl 1):25–26.
64. Mills JL. Teratology 1982;25:385–394.
65. Rusnak SL, Discoll SG. Pediatrics 1965;35:989–995.
66. Becerra JE, Khoury MJ, Cordero JF, Ericson JD. Pediatrics 1990;85:1–9.
67. Long FR, Hunter JV, Mahboubi S, Kalmus A, Templeton JM. Tethered cord and associated vertebral anomalies in children and infants with imperforate anus: evaluation with MR imaging and plain radiography. Radiology 1996;200:3 77–382.
68. Morrissy RT, Goldsmith GS, Hall EC, Kehl D, Cowie GH. J Bone Joint Surg Am 1990;72(3):320–327.
69. Carman DL, Browne RH, Birch JG. J Bone Joint Surg Am 1990;72(3):328–333.
70. Shea KG, Stevens PM, Nelson M, Smith JT, Masters KS, Yandow S. Spine 1998; 23(5):551–555.
71. Loder RT, Urquhart A, Steen H, et al. J Bone Joint Surg Br 1995;77(5):768–770.
72. Crockett HC, Wright JM, Burke S, Boachie-Adjei O. Spine 1999;24(19): 2007–2009; discussion 2010.
73. Kalifa G, Charpak Y, Maccia C, et al. Pediatr Radiol 1998;28(7):557–561.

74. Morin Doody M, Lonstein JE, Stovall M, Hacker DG, Luckyanov N, Land CE. Spine 2000;25(16):2052–2063.

75. Levy AR, Goldberg MS, Hanley JA, Mayo NE, Poitras B. Health Phys 1994; 66(6):621–633.

76. Levy AR, Goldberg MS, Mayo NE, Hanley JA, Poitras B. Spine 1996;21(13): 1540–1547; discussion 1548.

77. Goldberg MS, Mayo NE, Levy AR, Scott SC, Poitras B. Epidemiology 1998;9(3): 271–278.

78. Kalmar JA, Jones JP, Merritt CR. Spine 1994;19(7):818–823.

79. Kling TF Jr, Cohen MJ, Lindseth RE, De Rosa GP. Spine 1990;15(9):880–885.

80. Stringer DA, Cairns RA, Poskitt KJ, Bray H, Milner R, Kennedy B. Pediatr Radiol 1994;24(1):1–5.

81. Geijer H, Beckman K, Jonsson B, Andersson T, Persliden J. Radiology 2001;218(2):402–410.

82. Cheng JC, Guo X, Sher AH, Chan YL, Metreweli C. Spine 1999;24(16):1679–1684.

83. Barkovich AJ, Wippold FJ, Sherman JL, Citrin CM. AJNR 1986;7(5):795–799.

84. Elster AD, Chen MY. Radiology 1992;183(2):347–353.

85. Mikulis DJ, Diaz O, Egglin TK, Sanchez R. Radiology 1992;183(3):725–728.

86. Do T, Fras C, Burke S, Widmann RF, Rawlins B, Boachie-Adjei O. J Bone Joint Surg Am 2001;83–A(4):577–579.

87. Winter RB, Lonstein JE, Heithoff KB, Kirkham JA. Spine 1997;22(8):855–858.

88. Maiocco B, Deeney VF, Coulon R, Parks PF Jr. Spine 1997;22(21):2537–2541.

89. O'Brien MF, Lenke LG, Bridwell KH, Blanke K, Baldus C. Spine 1994; 19(14):1606–1610.

90. Prahinski JR, Polly DW Jr, McHale KA, Ellenbogen RG. J Pediatr Orthop 2000; 20(1):59–63.

91. Lewonowski K, King JD, Nelson MD. Spine 1992;17(6 suppl):S109–116.

92. Gupta P, Lenke LG, Bridwell KH. Spine 1998;23(2):206–210.

93. Schwend RM, Hennrikus W, Hall JE, Emans JB. J Bone Joint Surg Am 1995; 77(1):46–53.

94. Mejia EA, Hennrikus WL, Schwend RM, Emans JB. J Pediatr Orthop 1996; 16(3):354–358.

95. Weinberger E, Murakami J, Shaw D, White K, Radvilas M, Yean C. J Comput Assist Tomogr 1995;19:721–725.

19

Cardiac Evaluation: The Current Status of Outcomes-Based Imaging

Andrew J. Bierhals and Pamela K. Woodard

Issues

I. Does coronary artery calcification scoring predict outcome?
II. Special case: high-risk patients
III. Which patients should undergo coronary angiography?
IV. Which patients should undergo noninvasive imaging of the heart?
V. What is the appropriate use of coronary artery computed tomography and magnetic resonance?

Key Points

- A strong recommendation can be made for initial coronary angiography among high-risk patients and those who are post–myocardial infarction (MI) that was transmural or with ischemic symptoms (strong evidence).
- A strong recommendation can be made for performing a noninvasive imaging examination [e.g., single photon emission computed tomography (SPECT) or stress echo] prior to coronary angiography in low-risk patients and those who have had a non–Q-wave MI (strong evidence).
- Aside from coronary angiography, the appropriate usage of cardiac imaging studies remains unclear, and more research is required to evaluate the outcomes, as well as the cost-effectiveness of the aforementioned modalities (insufficient evidence).
- Coronary artery calcium scoring has been shown in asymptomatic patients to be predictive of coronary artery disease; however, there have been no data to support the position of added predictive value over and above the clinical Framingham model (insufficient evidence).

Definition and Pathophysiology

The etiology of coronary artery disease (CAD) is multifactorial involving both interaction of lifestyle and genetic predispositions. While some factors are not modifiable, those risks that may be altered are often neglected until there evidence of disease. As a result, a multitude of tests and clinical assessment tools have been developed to risk stratify patients in order to direct short- and long-term treatments. The modifiable risk factors (e.g., hypertension, hyperlipidemia, and diabetes) have been on the rise over the past decade (1,2); therefore, a greater urgency has arisen to identify patients with CAD.

Coronary artery disease begins as fatty streaks in the coronary arteries that may begin as early as 3 years of age. The fatty streaks are composed of large cells with intracellular lipids (foam cells) that are located in the subendothelial region. As patients age, the fatty streaks develop into fibrous plaques that narrow the vessel lumen, reducing blood flow. The fibrous plaques over time may calcify, reducing vessel compliance and increasing fragility. This further reduces blood flow and increases the chance of the plaque rupturing, resulting in an acute coronary artery occlusion.

Epidemiology

Coronary artery disease is a nationwide epidemic involving 6.4% of the entire population (3,4) and is the largest cause of mortality, accounting for one in every five deaths (4). This translates into a death rate of 177.8 per 100,000 (based on 2001 estimates) (4). In the United States, over 1.5 million people will have a myocardial infarction, and the majority of the patients will initially present with symptoms in their 50s and 60s.

A large volume of literature has been generated investigating these modalities, but little has focused on the impact the modalities have on the patient outcomes even though there has been a steady increase in the use of costly diagnostic testing and treatment (5). This chapter reviews the literature on the outcomes research of cardiac imaging, and makes recommendations concerning the utilization of the techniques in patient management.

Overall Cost to Society

In the United States, the estimated 2004 cost of heart disease to society is $238 billion, with over half secondary to CAD ($133 billion) (4,6). The cost of heart disease is substantial in comparison to other disease processes, such as cancers ($189 billion) and AIDS ($29 billion) (4,6). The costs of CAD include direct health care of $66 billion, and $67 billion in indirect costs (e.g., loss of productivity secondary to morbidity and mortality) (4,6).

The expenditures for health care are consistently increasing, because of new technologies and the current medicolegal environment. An ever-declining budget results in a need for clinicians to incorporate cost-effective strategies in patient evaluations. However, cost-effective does not mean withholding evaluations or always ordering the seemingly least expensive test, but rather understanding what is most efficient with respect to a specific clinical situation, based on current research. The purpose of this approach is to direct a finite amount of resources and limit costs to society without affecting the quality of health care. This chapter reviews the cost-effectiveness and outcomes of various imaging modalities of heart disease, and makes recommendations concerning these techniques in patient care. Specifically, coronary artery calcification scoring, myocardial SPECT, angiography, stress echocardiography, and cardiac magnetic resonance (MR) and computed tomography (CT) will be evaluated in their potential roles in the evaluation of heart disease.

Goals

The goals of imaging related to CAD are based on the *a priori* risk to the patient. In a low-risk population, the goals of imaging are to identify those with early disease. Subsequently, interventions directed toward risk factors and lifestyle may be initiated in order to reverse disease or halt progression before any long-term effects result. However, risk stratification becomes the goal of cardiac imaging among those patients who are considered high risk. The imaging in the aforementioned population is to determine if any coronary artery intervention (i.e., endovascular or bypass graft) is required over and above medical management.

Methodology

The outcomes and cost-effectiveness literature was evaluated by performing a literature review on Medline from 1999 to 2004 using a keyword search including the terms *calcium scoring and outcomes* and *calcium scoring and cost-effectiveness*. Of the over 2000 reports identified in the literature review, fewer than 50 addressed any issues concerning patient outcomes and not one evaluated cost-effectiveness.

A similar literature review was performed for coronary angiography using Medline. The keyword search from 1999 to 2004 included *coronary angiography and outcomes* and *coronary angiography and cost-effectiveness*. Over 5000 reports were identified, with approximately 100 addressing patient outcomes and 10 evaluating cost-effectiveness.

Lastly, a literature review was performed on Medline from 1999 to 2004 for noninvasive techniques including SPECT, positron emission tomography (PET), echocardiogram, and coronary CT and MR using the same method, as described above. The review yielded over 100 articles addressing patient outcomes and five evaluating cost-effectiveness; however, there were no reports that evaluated either topic for MR or CT angiography.

I. Does Coronary Artery Calcification Scoring Predict Outcome?

Summary of Evidence: Coronary artery calcium scoring has been shown in asymptomatic patients to be predictive of CAD; however, there have been no data to support the position of added predictive value over and above the clinical Framingham model. Therefore, coronary artery calcification scoring cannot be recommended as a screening tool at this time. The lack of cost-effectiveness data necessitates further investigations before a final position can be determined on the utility of calcium scoring (insufficient evidence).

Supporting Evidence: Coronary artery calcium scoring performed by computed tomography (CT) has been utilized in asymptomatic patients to assess their risk of an acute coronary event (7). However, the literature has debated the utility of calcium scoring. Some researchers support its use

(8,9), while others are less enthusiastic concerning the utilization in patient care (10).

Computed tomography calcium scoring, despite conflicting reports, has been shown to be associated with a fourfold increased risk in myocardial infarction and coronary death in a meta-analysis by O'Malley et al. (11) in 2000. The study included nine reports that had a diverse asymptomatic population that was evaluated for coronary artery calcification by electron beam CT. The authors also reported a ninefold increased risk of coronary events (i.e., nonfatal MI, sudden death, or revascularization) among those with a coronary artery calcium score above the median. There is moderate evidence to suggest that coronary artery calcification score is predictive of coronary events.

More recent reports have echoed these results regarding the predictive value of CT calcium scoring. A 2003 study by Shaw et al. (8) developed a multivariate model on a sample of greater than 10,000 asymptomatic individuals incorporating calcium score with typical clinical risk factors (i.e., hypertension, hypercholesterolemia, diabetes, age, and sex) to predict all-cause mortality. The results of the study indicated that calcium score predicted all-cause mortality ($p < .001$) over and above the effects of other risk factors. The study also found that there was a trend with the coronary artery calcium score such that as the calcium burden increased there was a greater risk of all-cause mortality. The relative risk in patients with elevated calcium scores ranged from 1.6 to 4.0 above individuals with the lowest calcium burden; as the calcium burden increased, the risk increased (Fig. 19.1). Based on the results, the authors concluded that calcium scoring of the coronary arteries provides additional information in the prediction of all-cause mortality (8); however, morbidity and mortality secondary to

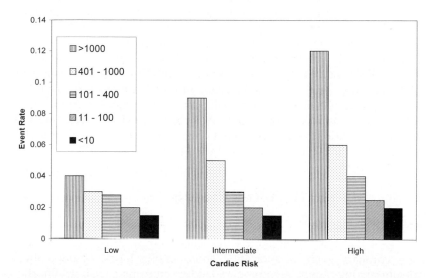

Figure 19.1. Graph shows risk stratification for each category of Framingham risk (from low to high) according to baseline calcium score. Event rate is predicted mortality at 5 years (8). Low risk <0.30 (no risk factors), intermediate risk <0.70 (one to two risk factors), and high risk <0.9 (three or more risk factors) probability of cardiac disease. [*Source:* Shaw et al. (8), with permission from the Radiological Society of North America.]

CAD was not specifically addressed. In addition, the authors did not investigate if the added explanation would have any clinical impact and thus provide information that would have proved clinically important.

Other authors have found similar results in the prediction of mortality from calcium scoring. For example, Arad et al. (12) demonstrated that moderate calcium scores were associated with a 10 times increase in cardiac death or MI. In addition, a small study of 676 subjects demonstrated that coronary artery calcification scores incrementally predicted cardiac events (13). These studies, as with the aforementioned larger sample, were able to show that coronary artery calcification on CT predicted health outcomes (e.g., MI and mortality). But of all the studies that have been evaluated, none has shown any extra value in risk stratification and patient management.

Aside from the earlier described reports, there has been a multitude of similar studies with varying patient population that have reached the same conclusion concerning the ability of coronary artery calcium scoring to predict heart disease and mortality (14–19). Other investigators utilized calcium scoring in conjunction with laboratory tests, such as C-reactive protein to model the mortality of heart disease (20), but no interactive effects were noted, although each independently predicted coronary events and mortality. However, a review of the literature to date has failed to identify any direct data suggesting that calcium scoring has any clinical benefit over the current Framingham risk model (21).

Currently, coronary artery calcium scoring on CT is utilized as a risk stratification tool for CAD. The major proportion of the data to date has shown that calcium scoring can predict CAD as well as mortality related to heart disease among asymptomatic patients. A literature review did not uncover any data that show that calcium scoring adds any additional information over current clinical predictive models in the asymptomatic patient. In addition, there have been no studies specifically evaluating the cost-effectiveness of coronary calcium scoring as a screening tool. As a result, calcium scoring, while predictive of CAD and mortality, has yet to be shown to add any additional information over and above current clinical models. Therefore, at this time there is insufficient data to recommend calcium scoring as a screening or risk stratification tool in the asymptomatic population. However, the dearth of cost-effectiveness data precludes stating that calcium scoring should not be preformed as a screening test. Subsequently, additional cost-effectiveness studies should be instituted to evaluate the role of calcium scoring in the screening for CAD.

II. Special Case: High-Risk Patients

Summary of Evidence: Among high-risk symptomatic populations coronary artery calcium scoring on CT has failed to show any predictive value for a coronary event or mortality. Thus, among high-risk populations calcium scoring cannot be recommended for screening or risk stratification (Insufficient Evidence).

Supporting Evidence: The data in the asymptomatic populations consistently indicated that coronary artery calcium scoring can predict cardiac events and may be helpful in risk stratifying patients. However, the results

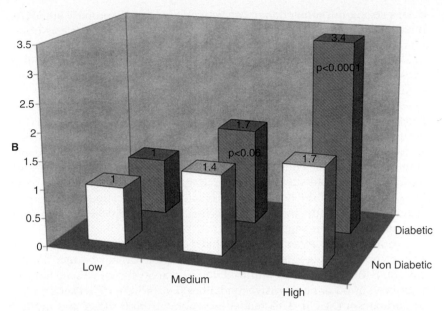

Figure 19.2. A: Relative risks (RRs), stratified by diabetes status, of nonfatal myocardial infarction (MI), or coronary death associated with calcium score risk groups (low, <2.8; medium, 2.8–117.8; high, >117.8). B: RRs, stratified by diabetes status, of nonfatal MI, coronary death, percutaneous transluminal coronary angioplasty (PTCA), coronary artery bypass graft (CABG), or stroke associated with calcium score risk groups (low, <2.8; medium, 2.8–117.8; high, >117.8). [*Source:* From Qu et al. (22).]

in populations with a known risk are not as straightforward. Qu et al. (22) evaluated calcium scoring in a diabetic population. The data showed that when adjusting for other risk factors in a diabetic sample, calcium scores did not predict coronary events, but calcium scoring was predictive among nondiabetics (Fig. 19.2). Although the results have not been as clear among an elderly population that coronary artery calcification is associated with the degree of CAD, some researchers have found that the calcium score has variability among an elderly population, and thus may have the potential to discriminate risk within this group (23). However, other authors have concluded that there is limited utility of using calcium scoring among elderly patients (24,25) because of comorbidities limiting the effect of interventions. Lastly, Detrano et al. (10) concluded that neither clinical risk assessment nor calcium scoring is an accurate predictor of cardiac events in a high-risk population, based on the Framingham model. Currently, there is insufficient evidence to recommend coronary artery calcium scoring in a high-risk population as a means of risk predicting coronary events (insufficient evidence).

III. Which Patients Should Undergo Coronary Angiography?

Summary of Evidence: Coronary angiography has been studied with a greater degree of rigor than the other modalities, with several studies investigating the cost-effectiveness. Based on the large amount of extant data, a strong recommendation can be made for initial coronary angiography among high-risk patients and those who are post-MI that was transmural or with ischemic symptoms. Also, a strong recommendation can be made for performing a noninvasive imaging examination (i.e., SPECT or stress echo) prior to coronary angiography in low-risk patients and those who have had a non–Q-wave MI (Fig. 19.3) (strong evidence).

Supporting Evidence: Over the past 20 years, coronary angiography has been the mainstay in the diagnosis of acute occlusion of the coronary arteries as well as in the quantification of CAD to direct management, whether surgical, medical, or endovascular. Throughout this period, angiography has become the gold standard for the diagnosis of CAD, but unlike other imaging studies of the heart there is greater risk associated with the procedure. Subsequently, the risk and technical factors preclude all patients from undergoing an angiogram.

Several cost-effectiveness models have been proposed to evaluate the role of coronary angiography in the diagnosis of coronary artery disease (26–28). Patterson et al. (27) utilized decision analysis to evaluate angiography versus other noninvasive modalities [i.e., SPECT, PET, exercise electrocardiogram (ECG)]. This model incorporated both direct and indirect costs as well as quality-adjusted life years (QALYs) to evaluate the different diagnostic modalities. The diagnostic evaluations included noninvasive testing followed by angiography (among those with an initial abnormal test) or angiography alone. The results of the study indicate that cost-effectiveness of the diagnostic modality is based on the initial pretest likelihood of disease. The authors found angiography was the most cost-effective modality in those with a high pretest probability ($p > .70$). However, populations with low risk ($p < .70$) noninvasive testing was the most cost-effective with PET > SPECT > exercise ECG. In addition, the authors found that there was little impact on the cost-effectiveness

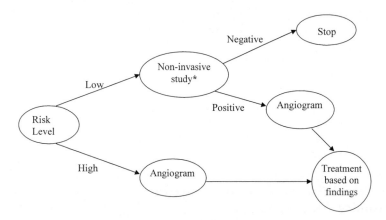

Figure 19.3. The recommended decision tree for the evaluation of CAD based on the patients' initial clinical status. *Noninvasive study can represent SPECT or stress echo depending on the institutional performance characteristics of the imaging study.

from the differing treatment modalities (i.e., surgical, medical, or endovascular). Similar results have been described by Garber and Solomon (28). Their decision analysis demonstrated that while stress echocardiography was the least costly per QALY saved, immediate angiography was an acceptable cost-effective alternative to SPECT and stress echocardiography among patients who are at high risk of cardiac disease. In their model, the relative cost-effectiveness for the modalities remained the same regardless of the patient's age or gender (Fig. 19.4). There is strong evidence to recommend that among low-risk populations a noninvasive cardiac imaging study should be performed prior to coronary angiography (strong evidence).

Coronary angiography seemingly has a specific role in the diagnosis and risk stratification of patients with heart disease and has been shown to be cost-effective in given populations (26–28); however, the data in post-MI populations is not as clear. In a decision analysis by Kuntz et al. (29), the decision analytic model incorporated clinical history and symptoms in the post-MI patient to evaluate the cost-effectiveness of angiography versus medial care. While the authors incorporated clinical elements into the analyses, there was a failure to account for type of MI to address the issue of noninvasive evaluation of cardiac perfusion (e.g., SPECT or stress echo). Based on the model outcomes, angiography was found to be cost-effective in almost all patients in the post-MI setting, and among those at highest risk the cost-effectiveness ratios were less than $50,000 for each QALY saved. Only in those women at low to moderate risk for coronary disease was angiography found not to be cost-effective. Similar results on the patient survival and outcomes have been found in other studies that have included all post-MI patients (30,31), and the largest effects were among the patients with transmural infarctions. There is strong evidence to support the use of angiography in the transmural infarction while those with a nontransmural infarction should undergo a noninvasive study prior to angiography (strong evidence).

Several authors have evaluated low to moderate risk (probability of CAD < .7) subpopulations in the post-MI state to determine the cost-effectiveness and outcomes among those treated with noninvasive image guidance versus immediate angiography. Barnett et al. (32) utilized a randomized controlled trial to evaluate the cost-effectiveness of angiography versus selective angiography (i.e., performing angiography in patients with an abnormal finding on a noninvasive study) in a population with a non–Q-wave MI. The results indicate a conservative management program is more cost-effective than immediate angiography in patients with a non–Q-wave MI. In the acute setting, image-directed angiography resulted in a cost of $14,700 versus $19,200 for immediate angiography and persisted after 2 years of follow-up, at which time there was an approximate $2100 difference in cost. In addition, the conservative group had a better survival (1.86 years) over a 2-year follow-up relative to immediate angiography (1.76 years). Thus, conservative management (i.e., noninvasive image-directed angiography) is the dominant strategy over angiography in the non–Q-wave post-MI patient with resulting lower cost and improved outcome. There is strong evidence to show that noninvasive testing prior to angiography is more cost-effective than angiography alone in patients who have had a nontransmural infarction (strong evidence).

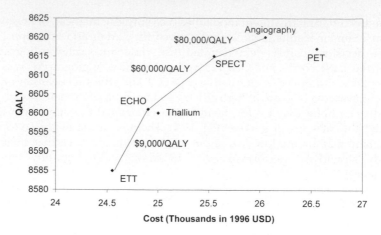

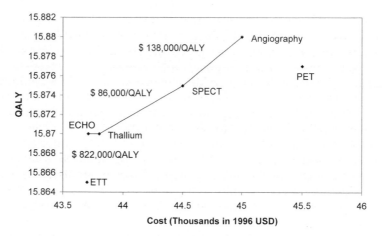

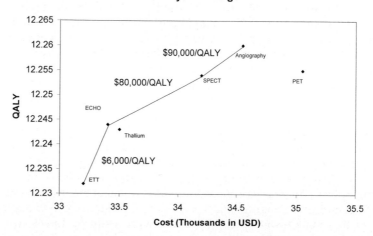

Figure 19.4. A: Cost-effectiveness of tests for coronary artery disease, in thousands of 1996 U.S. dollars per quality-adjusted life year (QALY), for men at 50% pretest risk for disease. B: Cost-effectiveness of tests for coronary artery disease, in thousands of 1996 U.S. dollars per QALY, for women at 50% pretest risk for disease. ECHO, stress echocardiography; ETT, exercise electrocardiography; PET, positron emission tomography; SPECT, single photon emission computed tomography. [*Source:* Garber and Solomon (28).]

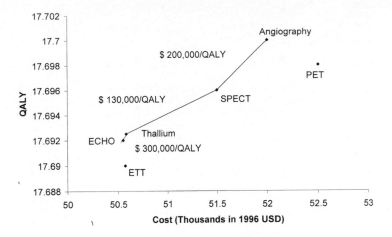

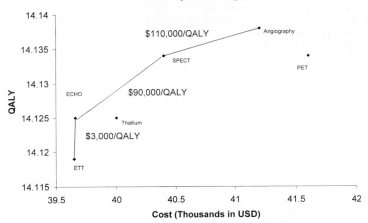

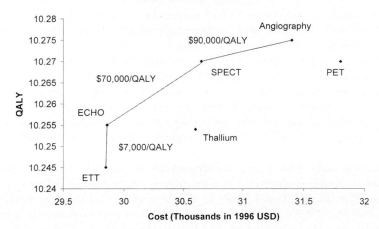

Figure 19.4. *Continued*

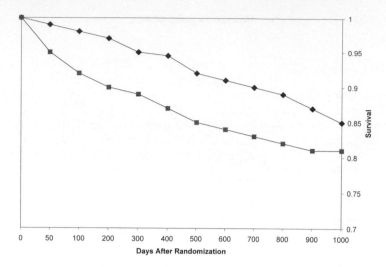

Figure 19.5. Kaplan-Meier analysis of the probability of survival according to strategy group during 12 to 44 months of follow-up. Death from any cause was included in this analysis. The Cox proportional-hazards ratio for the conservative as compared with the invasive strategy was 0.72 (95% confidence interval, 0.51–1.01). [*Source:* Boden et al. (33).]

An earlier report by Boden et al. (33) came to a supporting conclusion regarding patient outcome in the post-MI setting. They evaluated the impact of post-MI angiography in a population with non–Q-wave MIs. Through 2 years of follow-up among the aforementioned patient population (Fig. 19.5), a noninvasive image-directed approach to patient management was found to have a significantly lower mortality and reinfarction rates than those patients who had undergone an initial angiogram in the acute MI state. The findings have been supported by the recommendations of other groups and researchers (34,35).

Coronary angiography has a specific role in the evaluation of heart disease that is based on the patient's clinical history and symptoms. The data support the position that in an asymptomatic population with a low clinical suspicion of heart disease, noninvasive testing should be performed prior to angiography (26–28,36), whereas in situations were there is a high clinical suspicion of CAD, angiography should be the initial test of choice. A similar picture develops in post-MI patients. For instance, individuals who have had a transmural MI or who have clinical signs of ischemia should undergo a coronary angiogram, but those with a non–Q-wave MI without clinical ischemia would best be evaluated by noninvasive imaging (29–35). Therefore, the utilization of coronary angiography is based on the clinical situation and the initial use may not always be the most prudent or cost-effective method to manage patients who are suspected of CAD or recently in the post-MI state.

IV. Which Patients Should Undergo Noninvasive Imaging of the Heart?

Summary of Evidence: There is a moderate amount of support to suggest that stress echo should be recommended prior to coronary angiography in the low-risk patients. However, several authors have suggested that stress echo is highly operator dependent and at times SPECT may be a viable alternative. Both modalities have an acceptable cost-effectiveness profile; as a result, there is insufficient evidence to recommend SPECT over stress echo. More comprehensive cost-effectiveness reports are needed to completely evaluate these modalities (insufficient evidence).

Supporting Evidence: A few cost-effectiveness evaluations have been performed incorporating the aforementioned noninvasive studies that have had some conflicting results. A decision analysis was performed by Kuntz et al. (36) that modeled immediate angiography versus a stepwise approach to angiography. In this situation angiography would be performed only if the initial noninvasive test were positive. The analysis incorporated SPECT, stress echocardiography, and stress electrocardiography. The results indicated that stress echocardiography was more cost-effective than SPECT in the low-risk population with an incremental cost effectiveness ratio of $26,800/QALY versus $27,600/QALY, respectively. Although the model does assume an idealized performance of echocardiography, slight changes in sensitivity of either SPECT or echo affect the results of the model. Thus, decisions concerning the performance of a specific test should be based on the test characteristics at a given institution (36). The model also supported the results of other angiographic studies in which immediate angiography is more cost-effective in the high-risk patient.

Another decision analysis performed by Garber and Solomon (28) included PET in their analyses along with angiography, stress echo, planar thallium, exercise electrocardiography, and SPECT. The results indicated that the initial use of stress echo was the most cost-effective followed by SPECT and angiography (Fig. 19.4). Positron emission tomography was not cost-effective in the diagnosis, resulting in higher cost without improved outcomes. The study also brings to the forefront the idea that there is variability in cost and performance of SPECT and stress echo; subsequently, SPECT may be the initial modality of choice in some regions (28,38).

However, a single study evaluating the cost-effectiveness of SPECT versus exercise electrocardiography was performed to evaluate any additional prognostic value of SPECT (37). The authors found that SPECT provided additional information, which translated into $5500 per level of risk reclassification.

Other researchers have also included PET in decision analysis along with SPECT and angiography (26). The findings of this study contradicted the prior model, such that PET was found to be the most cost-effective modality in diagnosing CAD among low-risk patients (28). Aside from the two prior studies, no other reports were found in the literature review to evaluate the cost-effectiveness of PET in the diagnosis of CAD. Subsequently, there is insufficient evidence to recommend PET in the evaluation of CAD (insufficient evidence).

Similarly, only the previously described studies could be found to evaluate the cost-effectiveness of stress echocardiography (28,36,38). However, several other studies evaluating the cost-effectiveness of SPECT were identified in the literature review. In a small patient sample ($n = 29$), SPECT was found to increase the diagnostic ability in cardiologist who were treating emergency room patients with acute chest pain (39). The study also found a decrease in hospitalizations and a savings of $800 per patient (39), although this study had a small sample size and did not rigorously evaluate cost and outcomes. Lastly, Udelson et al. (40) assessed the effect of SPECT in the evaluation of acute chest pain in the emergency department. There was a lower hospitalization rate among patients without coronary ischemia who had undergone a SPECT in the emergency department (42%) versus usual care (52%). The results suggest that SPECT may have an effect on decision making and possibly lower the costs by reducing hospitalization; however, to date there is insufficient evidence to recommend SPECT in the emergency setting.

In conclusion, multiple decision analyses and randomized studies agree that in a low-risk patient a noninvasive study should be preformed prior to an angiogram. Also, the models seem to support stress echocardiography as the most cost-effective, but also have suggested that SPECT may be as cost-effective depending on the institutional performance. Subsequently, there is little definitive data to use one of these studies over the other. The use of SPECT or echo should be based on the institutional efficacy. Although there is an early suggestion that SPECT may be useful in the emergent chest pain setting for patient triage, there is not enough data at this time to support this position. Lastly, there is conflicting evidence concerning the cost-effectiveness of PET in the diagnosis of CAD and ischemia; more studies are needed to determine the role of PET in the cardiac evaluation (insufficient evidence).

In symptomatic post-MI patients or those at high risk for CAD, coronary angiography is the most cost-effective method to evaluate, diagnose, and plan treatments. However, among those without symptoms, noninvasive modalities (i.e., PET, SPECT, and stress echocardiography) are the more cost-effective means to evaluate heart disease. But the research to date is somewhat unclear as to the utilization of the aforementioned modalities. The current literature is somewhat limited in the cost-effective evaluations of noninvasive studies.

V. What Is the Appropriate Use of Coronary Artery Computed Tomography and Magnetic Resonance?

Summary of Evidence: The newer noninvasive modalities of cardiac MR and CT have a paucity of cost-effectiveness research and outcomes data available at this time and cannot be recommended for the evaluation of ischemic cardiac disease (insufficient evidence).

Supporting Evidence: In the past decade there have been advances in CT and MR in the evaluation of many aspects of the heart and heart disease. The current literature has limited data on the performance of MR and CT with respect to evaluation of the coronary arteries or for assessment of atherosclerosis aside from calcium scoring. However, our literature review found no reports evaluating the cost-effectiveness of either modality.

Huniak et al. (41) performed a decision analysis and developed a model incorporating current initial diagnostic modalities (i.e., SPECT and stress echo) prior to coronary angiography. In addition, coronary MR and CT were also included to determine those cost and performance characteristics necessary for the new modalities to possess in order to be cost-effective. For a new diagnostic study to be more cost-effective than stress echo, a cost of less than $1000 and a sensitivity and specificity greater than 89% and 88%, respectively, should be obtained. The results were similar for replacing SPECT, such that the new imaging study must have a sensitivity and specificity greater than 85% and 80%, respectively. Lastly, as would be expected, a new testing modality required a sensitivity and specificity of 99% to replace angiography (41). While the prior study is a good start in the evaluation of the cost-effectiveness of coronary MR and CT, dedicated studies are required to fully evaluate these aspects of the imaging modalities, in order to have a complete understanding of their role in patient care.

In addition, as opposed to the traditional modalities, cardiac MRI can assess simultaneously a multitude of aspects of the heart and cardiac function. Thus, a modality with such versatility may have higher costs that are offset by evaluating several cardiac dimensions at once, resulting in a greater cost-effective modality. Therefore, studies need to be designed to address cardiac MR's role in a complete heart evaluation encompassing ejection fraction, wall motion, coronary arteries, perfusion, and valvular disease. All of these aspects of cardiac MR have been addressed, but no single study has encompassed all aspects to evaluate cost-effectiveness.

Studies have shown that cardiac perfusion abnormalities can be detected with similar sensitivity and specificity with MR, SPECT, and PET (42–44). Cardiac MRI has been found to comparable to stress echo in the evaluation of wall motion (44,45). In addition, it is better than SPECT in the assessment of myocardial viability as it is of higher resolution and able to differentiate between subendocardial and transmural infarct. Cardiac MR has also been utilized to evaluate the coronary arteries for aberrant vessel course and bypass graft complications, all with a relatively high degree of sensitivity of about 90% (44). Cardiac MR has been found to correlate with Doppler ultrasound findings in the estimation of valvular area size (46,47). Aside from the potential utilization for heart disease, cardiac MR has been shown to have applications for patients with congenital heart disease (48) that assist with surgical planning and medical management. The current cardiac MR data are extremely promising but remain limited and require further investigation regarding a future role in patient care.

Cardiac CT also suffers from a paucity of data evaluating the cost-effectiveness in patient management; as a result, its role in patient care remains unclear. Cardiac CT has made great strides over the past 5 years with the introduction of multidetector scanners, which has improved resolution and speed, allowing for improved performance of multiphase and arterial phase studies. These characteristics do provide some advantage over MR in terms of speed and in the evaluation of stents and patients with pacemakers. But due to the novelty of the modality, the literature remains more limited than that for cardiac MR. Therefore, even before cost-effectiveness studies can be performed, data must be generated on the performance of cardiac CT. Preliminary studies have shown that cardiac CT can evaluate coronary artery stents (49), and others have used cardiac CT to evaluate congenital heart disease (50). Also, preliminary data have been generated in the use of cardiac CT for coronary angiography (51); however, the sample sizes are not substantial enough to generate any accurate assessment of performance.

Recommended Imaging Protocols Based on the Evidence

Cardiac Catheterization

- Selective injection of left coronary artery with at least the projections anteroposterior (AP), left anterior oblique (LAO) cranial, and right anterior oblique (RAO) caudal is the minimum needed to cover the course of the left main anterior descending and circumflex arteries.
- Selective injection of the right coronary artery with at least the projections lateral, RAO, LAO, and LAO cranial are required to evaluate the right coronary artery.

Stress Echo

In a nonpharmacologic stress echocardiogram, the target for an adequate study is similar to that of SPECT or a treadmill test. Failure to meet the stress limits the sensitivity of the examination. The heart rate should reach at least 85% of predicted. However, the study should be terminated if cardiac symptoms arise or there are ECG changes.

Cardiac SPECT

- In the nonpharmacologic stress SPECT, 85% of the maximum heart rate needs to be achieved to prevent limitations in sensitivity.
- Dipyridamole is infused at a rate of 0.6 mg/kg over 4 minutes. Then imaging with thallium 201 begins 10 minutes after infusion. No caffeinated products or xanthines should be taken prior to the study as they will eliminate the effects of dipyridamole. This should not be given to asthmatics as it may precipitate bronchospasm.
- Adenosine is infused intravenously at 140 μg/kg/minute over 4 to 6 minutes. The thallium 201 is injected 3 minutes after infusion. Adenosine is contraindicated in individuals with heart block and bronchospasm.

Future Research

- In the future, cost-effectiveness research should focus on incorporating calcium scoring and clinical risk stratification in the screening for early heart disease. Coronary artery calcification scoring has been shown in the asymptomatic patient to predict a coronary event, but cost-effectiveness has not been adequately evaluated. By evaluating calcium scoring in this manner, a determination can be made concerning the modalities' additional benefits as well as the cost that may be incurred.
- Future research should focus on the potential utilization and outcomes of novel coronary artery imaging modalities, such as CT and MRI. These modalities are promising for the evaluation of coronary arteries in multiple clinical circumstances (52). Prior to any cost-effectiveness studies, an understanding of modality performance characteristics (e.g., sensitivity and specificity) is needed, along with evaluation of the impact on patient management and outcome.

References

1. Hurst W. The Heart, Arteries, and Veins, 10th ed. New York: McGraw-Hill, 2002.
2. CDC/NCHS. National Health and Nutrition Examination Survey III (NHANES III), 1988–1994.
3. American Heart Association. Annual Report. 1996.
4. American Heart Association. Heart Disease and Stroke Statistics—2004 update.
5. Health Resources Utilization Branch, CDC/NCHS. National Hospital Discharge Survey.
6. National Health Expenditures, Amounts, and Average Annual Percent Change, by Type of Expenditure: Selected Calendar Years 1980–2012. cms.hhs.gov.
7. O'Rourke RA, Brundage BH, Froelicher VF, et al., American College of Cardiology. Circulation 2000;102:126–140.
8. Shaw LJ, Raggi P, Schisterman E, Daniel S, Berman DS, Callister TQ. Radiology 2003;228:826–833.
9. Newman AB, Naydeck BL, Sutton-Tyrrell K, Feldman A, Edmundowicz D, Kuller LH. Circulation 2001;104:2679–2684.
10. Detrano RC, Wong ND, Doherty TM, et al. Circulation 1999;99:2633–2638.
11. O'Malley PG, Taylor AJ, Jackson JL, et al. Am J Cardiol 2000;85:945–948.
12. Arad Y, Spadaro LA, Goodman K, Newstein D, Guerci AD. J Am Coll Cardiol 2000;36:1253–1260.
13. Raggi P, Cooil B, Callister TQ. Am Heart J 2001;141:375–382.
14. Detrano RC, Doherty TM, Davies MJ, Stary HC. Curr Probl Cardiol 2000;25:374–402.
15. Raggi P. Herz 2001;26:252–259.
16. Raggi P, Callister TQ, Cooil B, et al. Circulation 2000;101:850–855.
17. Shaw LJ, O'Rourke RA. J Am Coll Cardiol 2000;36:1261–1264.
18. Detrano R, Hsiai T, Wang S, et al. J Am Coll Cardiol 1996;27:285–290.
19. Arad Y, Spadaro LA, Goodman K, et al. Circulation 1996;93:1951–1953.
20. Park R, Detrano R, Xiang M, et al. Circulation 2002;106:2073–2077.
21. Lipid Research Clinics Program. JAMA 1984;251:365–374.
22. Qu W, Le TT, Azen ST, et al. Diabetes Care 2003;26:905–910.
23. Newman AB, Naydeck BL, Sutton-Tyrrell K, Feldman A, Edmundowicz D, Kuller L. Circulation 2001;104:2679–2684.
24. Sangiorgi G, Rumberger JA, Severson A, et al. J Am Coll Cardiol 1998;31:126–133.
25. Janowitz WR, Agatston AS, Kaplan G, et al. Am J Cardiol 1993;72:247–254.
26. Patterson RE, Eisner RL, Horowitz SF. Circulation 1995;91:54–65.
27. Patterson RE, Eng C, Horowitz SF, Gorlin R, Goldstein SR. J Am Coll Cardiol 1984;4:278–289.
28. Garber AM, Solomon NA. Ann Intern Med 1999;130:719–728.
29. Kuntz K, Tsevat J, Goldman L, Weinstein MC. Circulation 1996;94:957–965.
30. FRagmin and Fast Revascularisation during InStability in Coronary artery disease (FRISC II) Investigators. Lancet 1999;354:708–715.
31. Cannon CP, Weintraub WS, Demopoulos LA, et al. N Engl J Med 2001;344:1879–1887.
32. Barnett PG, Chen S, Boden WE, et al. Circulation 2002;105:680–684.
33. Boden W, O'rourke R, Crawford M, et al. N Engl J Med 1998;338:1785–1792.
34. Pepine CJ, Allen HD, Bashore TM, et al. J Am Coll Cardiol 1991;18:1149–1182.
35. Ryan TJ, Anderson JL, Antman EM, et al. J Am Coll Cardiol 1996;28:1328–1428.
36. Kuntz K, Fleischmann KE, Hunick MGM, Douglas PS. Ann Intern Med 1999;130:709–718.
37. Hachamovich R, Berman DS, Kiat H, et al. Circulation 105:823–829.
38. Fleischmann KE, Hunink MG, Kuntz KM, Douglas PS. JAMA 1998;280:913–920.
39. Weissman IA, Dickinson CZ, Dworkin HJ, Oneil WW, Juni JE. Radiology 199:353–357.
40. Udelson JE, Beshansky JR, Ballin DS, et al. JAMA 288:2693–2700.

41. Hunink MGM, Kuntz K, Fleischmann KE, Brady TJ. Ann Intern Med 1999;131: 673–680.
42. Hartnell G, Cerel A, Kamalesh M, et al. AJR 1994;163:1061–1067.
43. Muzik O, Duvernoy C, Beanlands RS, et al. J Am Coll Cardiol 1998;31:534–540.
44. Wagner A, Mahrholdt H, Sechtem U, Kim R, Judd R. Magn Reson Imaging Clin North Am 2003;11:49–66.
45. Baer FM, Voth E, Larosee K, et al. Am J Cardiol 1996;78:415–419.
46. Nishimura T, Yamada N, Itoh A, et al. AJR 1989;153:721–724.
47. Aurigemma G, Reichek N, Schiebler M, et al. Am J Cardiol 1990;66:621–625.
48. Boxt LM, Rozenshtein A. Mag Reson Imaging Clin North Am 2003;11:27–48.
49. Fidler JL, Cheatham JP, Fletcher L, et al. AJR 2000;174:355–359.
50. Choi BW, Park YH, Choi JY, et al. AJR 2001;177:1045–1049.
51. Herzog C, Dogan S, Diebold T, et al. Radiology 2003;229:200–208.
52. Schoepf UJ, Becker CR, Ohnesorge BM, Yucel EK. Radiology 2004;232:18–37.

20

Aorta and Peripheral Vascular Disease

Max P. Rosen

Key Points

- Due to the need for rapid diagnosis of patients with suspected acute aortic rupture or dissection, computed tomographic angiography (CTA) is preferable to magnetic resonance angiography (MRA) (limited evidence).
- Screening with ultrasound for abdominal aortic aneurysm (AAA) among men between the ages of 60 and 74 has been shown to be cost-effective with a mean cost-effectiveness ratio of £28,400 per life year gained (strong evidence).
- Endovascular repair of AAA has been shown to significantly reduce 30-day mortality from repair of AAA rupture. However, the procedural cost of endovascular repair is greater than that for open surgical repair (strong evidence).
- Computed tomographic angiography is preferred to catheter angiography for detection of aortic stent-graft endoleak (moderate evidence).

- Computed tomographic angiography is comparable to MRA for evaluation of peripheral vascular disease and for the preoperative evaluation of renal artery stenosis (moderate evidence).
- The most cost-effective imaging strategy for the evaluation of the living renal donor varies and is dependent on the perspective of the analysis (renal donor or recipient), as well as the specificity of digital subtraction angiography (DSA) (moderate evidence).

Definition, Pathophysiology, and Epidemiology

Imaging of the aorta and peripheral vascular disease poses a unique set of challenges and benefits in medical imaging. For almost all clinical settings, the gold standard is catheter-based angiography. While advances in catheter design and imaging equipment over the past decade have greatly enhanced the field of diagnostic angiography, the basic tenets of the field have changed little in the past 20 years. Thus, there is an extensive body of literature based on catheter-based imaging. With the advent of multidetector CT scans and concurrent advances in MRA, CTA and MRA have become viable alternatives to catheter-based diagnostic angiography. However, unlike any other diagnostic modality, a catheter-based diagnostic study may rapidly be converted to an interventional procedure. Thus, any new modality for imaging the aorta or peripheral vascular disease must be compared to the gold standard of angiography, both for its diagnostic accuracy and for its cost-effectiveness in the context of immediately converting a catheter-based diagnostic study to a therapeutic intervention.

Aortic rupture is usually cased by blunt or penetrating trauma. Aortic dissection can be precipitated by traumatic or nontraumatic causes such as hypertension and aortitis; the latter may be infectious or inflammatory in nature. Aortic aneurysms are caused by a weakening in the aortic wall resulting in either saccular or fusiform dilatation.

While most AAAs are the result of atherosclerosis, they may also have traumatic, infectious, and inflammatory etiologies. In men over the age of 65, ruptured AAAs are responsible for 2.1% of all deaths in England and Wales (1). Approximately 50% of these deaths occur before the patient reaches the hospital. Operative mortality for the 50% of patients with ruptured AAAs who reach the hospital alive is between 30% and 70%.

Peripheral vascular disease is most often caused by hypertension, diabetes, hypercholesterolemia, or cigarette smoking and can be classified as either acute or chronic. Acute limb ischemia (ALI) is defined as a sudden decrease in limb perfusion that may result in threatened viability of the extremity. Chronic manifestations of peripheral arterial disease (PAD) are divided clinically into (1) intermittent claudication and (2) chronic critical limb ischemia.

Overall Cost to Society

Data on the societal cost of imaging for these indications is not available, except for the cost-effectiveness of screening for AAA with ultrasound among men 65 to 74 years of age (see I, below).

Goals

The goals and method of imaging of the aorta and peripheral vascular branches depend on the clinical setting. In the case of suspected traumatic injury or aortic dissection, the goal of imaging is twofold. The most immediate goal is to identify as quickly as possible the patients in need of immediate surgical repair. The secondary goal in this acute setting is to help the surgeon identify the extent of vascular injury and plan the appropriate repair.

The goal of screening asymptomatic patients for AAA is to identify patients with AAA and provide immediate intervention if the size of the AAA at the time of screening warrants repair. For those patients with AAA, the size of which does not warrant immediate repair, the goal of screening is to identify any change in the size of the AAA over time, and to initiate therapy when the rate of expansion of the AAA reaches a threshold that justifies repair.

When vascular insufficiency or ischemia is suspected, the goal of imaging is to identify the level and extent of the stenosis or occlusion. The optimal imaging strategy is somewhat dependent on the most likely method for intervention. If a catheter-based intervention is likely, then a catheter-based imaging study is often warranted as the initial imaging study. On the other hand, if a surgical intervention is likely, then a less invasive initial imaging study such as CTA or MRA may be optimal.

Methodology

PubMed searches for the following index terms were performed from January 2000 to August 2004: *computed tomography (CT) angiography, magnetic resonance (MR), vascular studies, arteries, stenosis* or *occlusion, angiography, comparative studies, aneurysms, aortic, cost-effectiveness,* and *abdominal aortic aneurysms.* Relevant articles in English were obtained and read for appropriateness. The search was limited to articles published in January 2000 or later to ensure that only studies employing current noninvasive technologies would be included. Selected articles published before 2000 and after August 2004 (2) were also included at the time of manuscript review by the book's editors.

I. Aorta: What Are the Appropriate Imaging Studies for Suspected Acute Aortic Dissection or Traumatic Rupture?

Summary of Evidence: Due to the need for rapid diagnosis of patients with suspected acute aortic rupture or dissection (Fig. 20.1), CTA is preferable to MRA. Most modern emergency departments are equipped with helical CT scanners, and unlike MRA, CTA of the entire aorta can be performed in a less than 60 seconds.

Supporting Evidence: Yoshida et al. (3) assessed the sensitivity, specificity, and accuracy of CTA among 57 patients with surgically proven type A dissection who underwent helical CT, and reported 100% sensitivity of helical

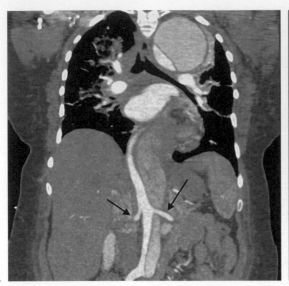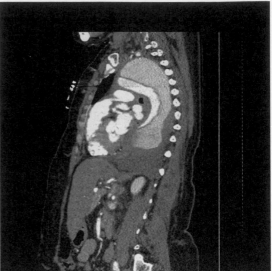

A   B

Figure 20.1. Coronal (A) and sagittal (B) computed tomographic angiography (CTA) demonstrating type B aortic dissection. Both renal arteries are supplied from the true lumen (arrows).

CT to detect aortic dissection in the thoracic aorta. Sensitivity for detection of arch branch vessel involvement was 95% and 83% for detection of pericardial effusion. (The authors explain that the lower sensitivity for detection of pericardial effusion may be due to the delay between CTA and surgery, with the pericardial effusion developing during the delay.) Due to the lack of reported follow-up of the 64 patients in whom the CTA did not show dissection, this study represents limited (level III) evidence. Several other studies support the use of CTA to exclude aortic injury (4,5) but are based on older single detector technology. Although not commonly available in emergency situations, Pereles et al. (6) reported excellent 100% sensitivity for diagnosis of thoracic aortic dissection using true fast imaging with steady-state precision (FISP).

Cost-Effectiveness Analysis: An older paper by Hunink and Bos (7) published in 1995 evaluated the cost-effectiveness of CT compared with plain film chest radiography and immediate angiography in deciding when angiography should be performed in hemodynamically stable patients with suspected aortic injury after blunt chest trauma. This study was performed before the widespread use of multidetector CT, and investigated the use of CT as a triage tool rather than as a definitive diagnostic study. The authors conclude that selecting patients for triage to angiography based on the CT findings yielded higher effectiveness at a lower cost-effectiveness ratio than doing so based on chest radiographs, and that the incremental cost-effectiveness ratio was $242,000 per life saved for the strategy of CT followed by angiography for positive cases.

II. Aorta: What Is the Impact and Cost-Effectiveness of Screening for Abdominal Aortic Aneurysms on Mortality from Abdominal Aortic Aneurysms Rupture?

Summary of Evidence: The Multicenter Aneurysm Screening Study (MASS) (1) investigated the impact of ultrasound screening for AAA in a population of 67,800 men between the ages of 65 and 74 years. The study was a randomized controlled study conducted at four centers in the United Kingdom and provides strong evidence that screening for AAA with ultrasound significantly reduced AAA related deaths.

Supporting Evidence: The MASS group (1) investigated the effect of AAA screening on mortality in men using a randomized controlled trial design of 67,800 men aged 65 to 74 years. Men in whom AAA (>3 cm in diameter) were detected were followed with repeat ultrasound for a mean of 4.1 years. Surgery was considered if the diameter of the AAA was >5.5 cm or if the AAA expanded >1 cm per year, or if symptoms related to the AAA developed. Health-related quality of life was measured using the standardized medical Outcomes Study short-form 36-item survey (SF-36) (8) and the EuroQol EQ-5D (9). The primary outcome measure was mortality related to AAA.

There were 65 (0.19%) AAA-related deaths in the screened group, and 113 (0.33%) in the control group ($p = .0002$) with a 53% risk reduction [(95% confidence interval (CI) 30–64%] among those who underwent screening. Thirty-day mortality following elective surgery was 6% vs. 37% following emergency surgery.

Cost-Effectiveness Analysis: Data from the MASS study (1) were used to estimate the cost-effectiveness of AAA screening using ultrasound over a 4-year period and they provide strong evidence. Costs included in the analysis were costs associated with the initial screening program: clinic staff and study administration, office space, equipment, and costs associated with any follow-up scans. Costs associated with surgery were calculated from the actual costs incurred by the cohort of patients who underwent surgery and any hospital admission during the 12 months after surgery. No costs related to patient death from aneurysm rupture were included if the patient had not been admitted to the hospital for attempted emergency surgery. Cost-effectiveness was measured as survival free from mortality related to AAA for each patient for up to 4 years and was expressed as incremental cost per additional life year gained.

Over 4 years, the mean estimated cost-effectiveness ratio for screening was $51,000 per life year gained, equivalent to $64,600 per quality-adjusted life year (QALY) gained.

III. Aorta: Endovascular vs. Surgical Treatment of Abdominal Aortic Aneurysms: Which Is the Best Choice?

Summary of Evidence: Endovascular treatment of AAA is associated with a significant reduction in 30-day mortality and hospital length of stay, compared to surgical repair. However, the cost of endovascular repair is greater than that of surgical repair, due to the cost of the endograft (strong evidence).

Supporting Evidence: Several recent papers have addressed the clinical effectiveness of endovascular aneurysm repair (EVAR) (10) and calculated the cost-effectiveness of EVAR compared to standard therapy. The short-term (30-day) outcome of patients treated with EVAR has been reported from a prospective registry in which 611 patients were enrolled at 31 centers in the UK (10a). The aneurysm was successfully excluded in 465/611 (76%) of patients. Additional endovascular procedures were required in 71/611 (12%) and additional surgical procedures were required in 30/611 (5%). An additional 32/611 (5%) patients required conversion to open repair. Thirty-day complication rates were as follows: technical, 6%; wound complications, 8%; renal failure, 4%; and other medical complications, 13%. Thirty-day mortality for all patients was 6.6%. For patients considered fit, 30-day mortality was 4% but increased to 18% for unfit patients. Complications of persistent endoleaks and 30-day mortality were significantly greater for AAAs > 6 cm than for AAAs ⩽ 6 cm.

Zeebregts et al. (11) compared the outcome of AAA repair with EVAR ($n = 93$) vs. open surgical repair ($n = 195$) in a nonrandomized prospective trial. All consecutive patients undergoing AAA repair at one institution during a 10-year period were included in the study. Detailed patient characteristics of the two groups were not provided, but the authors state, "The study confirmed that patients were mainly selected on anatomic grounds to undergo either open repair or EVAR." Compared to open surgical repair, patients undergoing EVAR had significantly ($p < .05$) shorter stays in the intensive care unit (ICU); shorter hospital stays; fewer bleeding complications, pulmonary complications, and episodes of multiple organ failure; and lesser 30-day morality.

A randomized controlled trial (EVAR 1 trial) (12), comparing EVAR with open repair, has recently been reported in which 1082 elective patients (age >60 with AAA diameter >5.5 cm) were randomized to receive either EVAR ($n = 543$) or open repair ($n = 39$) at 41 British hospitals. Thirty-day mortality by intention to treat was the outcome reported and was significantly less in the EVAR group, 1.7% (9/531), compared to 4.7% (24/516) in the open group (odds ratio 0.35; 95% CI 0.16–0.77; $p = .009$).

A second, multicenter trial, the Dutch Randomized Endovascular Aneurysm Management (DREAM) trial (13) is also being conducted with 345 patients enrolled. Initial results from 153 patients at 1 year demonstrated cumulative survival of 95% in the EVAR group compared to 89% in the operative group, $p = .21$). The cumulative event-free survival at 12 months was 76% in the EVAR group and 72% in the operative group. Data from all 345 patients analyzed from the point of view of 30-day mortality found that endovascular repair was associated with a lower 30-day mortality, 1.2% (95% CI, 0.1–4.2%), compared to 4.6% (95% CI 2.0–8.9%) for open repair, resulting in a risk ratio of 3.9 (95% CI, 0.9–32.9] (14). The DREAM trial has also reported quality of life (QoL) using the SF-36 and EuroQoL(-)5D questionnaires at regular intervals during the first year (15). From 6 months onward the operative group reported a significantly higher score on the EuroQol EQ-5D than the EVAR group ($p = .045$).

The cost of EVAR has been compared to open repair using data from a retrospective analysis of 131 patients undergoing AAA repair and 49 patients undergoing open repair as part of a U.S. Food and Drug Administration phase II prospective multicenter study (16). Total inpatient hospital costs of EVAR were significantly higher than that of open repair ($19,985 ± $7396 vs. $12,546 ± $5944, p = .0001). The cost of the Endograft ($10,400) accounted for 52% of the total cost of EVAR.

Cost-Effectiveness Analysis: While the expected robust cost-effectiveness data from the EVAR 1 and EVAR 2 trials has not yet been published, moderate data calculating the cost per hospital day saved of EVAR vs. open repair from a single institution in which seven patients underwent EVAR and 31 patients underwent open repair have been reported (17). The mean total cost for EVAR ($14,967) was significantly greater than that for open repair ($4823) ($p$ = .004), even though the mean length of stay for the EVAR group (2.09 days) was significantly less than the mean length of stay for the open repair group (4.45 days) (p = .009). The cost of the Endograft accounted for 57% of the total cost of EVAR. The cost of reducing the hospital stay by 1 day by performing EVAR was $1,604.

IV. Peripheral Vascular Disease: What Are the Appropriate Noninvasive Imaging Studies for Patients with Suspected Peripheral Vascular Disease?

Magnetic resonance angiography and CT angiography are the most commonly used noninvasive imaging studies in peripheral vascular disease.

A. Magnetic Resonance Angiography

Summary of Evidence: Numerous studies compare various MRA techniques with catheter angiography for evaluation of patients with suspected peripheral vascular disease (PVD). However, almost all of these studies provide only limited evidence in support of MRA. Many studies are retrospective and suffer from selection bias. Further complicating the analysis is a lack of standardization in the reporting of arterial segments.

Supporting Evidence: Several studies compare the sensitivity and specificity of MRA with digital subtraction angiography (DSA). However, synthesizing these studies into a comprehensive summary is difficult, due to heterogeneous patient populations, disparate reporting methods, and variations in MRA technique. For example, among patients with known or suspected PVD, Loewe et al. (18) reported positive and negative predictive values for overall stenosis detection of 91.2% and 97.3%, respectively. However, when nondiagnostic segments were included, the positive and negative predictive values decreased to 89.9% and 95.9%, respectively. Binkert et al. (19) compared the diagnostic accuracy of dedicated calf MRA vs. standard bolus-chase MRA with catheter angiography and found that dedicated calf studies were superior to standard bolus-chase MRA, 81.5% vs. 67.8% (reader 1) and 79.1% vs. 63.4% (reader 2). Among patients with symptoms and signs of aortoiliac occlusion, MRA has been shown to yield sensitivity of 87.5% and specificity of 100% for diagnosing aortic occlusion, compared to catheter angiography (20). In a retrospective study of 45 patients with lower-limb ischemia at high risk for catheter angiography, none of 28 who subsequently underwent above-knee surgical reconstruction required complementary catheter angiography. However, in seven of 10 patients who underwent below-knee surgical reconstruction, pre- or intraoperative catheter angiography was required (21). Khilnani et al. (22) retrospectively compared the concordance of three readers' selection of inflow and outflow segments for preoperative treatment planning with MRA and catheter angiography and found that the mean percentage of agreement between MRA and catheter angiography ranged from 91% to 97%.

B. Computed Tomography Angiography

Summary of Evidence: There is limited evidence supporting the diagnostic accuracy of CTA for the evaluation of patients with suspected PVD. Compared to MRA, there is less variability in CTA protocols and techniques, which reduces some of the variability in study design. The current literature reports diagnostic performance of four-row multidetector CT (MDCT), which is currently being replaced by up to 32- to 64-row MDCT.

Supporting Evidence: An initial study of the technical feasibility of MDCT for the evaluation of lower extremity arterial inflow and runoff was published in 2001 (23). The study evaluated patients with symptomatic lower extremity arterial occlusive ($n = 19$) or aneurysmal disease ($n = 5$). Indications for CTA among the 19 patients with suspected occlusive disease included calf or thigh claudication, nonhealing foot ulcers, or gangrene. Eighteen of the 24 patients underwent conventional angiography within 3 months of the CTA. The authors reported the degree of arterial enhancement and the number of arterial segments analyzable with CTA. As the scope of this study was limited to technical issues, sensitivity and specificity were not reported.

A more clinically relevant paper was published in 2004 by Romano et al. (24) in which they compared the diagnostic accuracy of four-row multidetector CTA (MDCTA) with DSA in patients with peripheral occlusive disease. Forty-two patients underwent MDCTA and DSA within 5 days. Images were blindly interpreted by two radiologists. The overall sensitivity and specificity of MDCTA, compared to DSA, was 93% and 95%, respectively. Positive and negative predictive values were 90% and 97%, respectively. The accuracy of MDCT for each anatomic segment is provided in Table 20.1.

Normal arterial segments and 100% occluded segments were correctly identified in all cases by MDCT. Almost all cases in which the degree of arterial segment stenosis was misinterpreted were in the calf; 58% of mis-

Table 20.1. Accuracy of multidetector computed tomography (MDCT), compared to digital subtraction angiography (DSA), according to anatomic segment (24)

	Sensitivity	Specificity	PPV	NPV	Diagnostic accuracy
Aortoiliac	95	99	99	97	98
Femoropopliteal	94	97	96	97	97
Infrapopliteal	85	92	74	96	89

PPV, positive predictive value; NPV, negative predictive value.

interpreted stenotic segments were false positives and 42% were false negative. Interobserver agreement (κ) for DSA and MDCT were 0.817 and 0.802, respectively, and for MDCT vs. DSA were 0.835 and 0.857 for reader 1 and reader 2, respectively.

Cost-Effectiveness Analysis: None available.

V. Special Case: Evaluation of Abdominal Aortic Aneurysms Graft Endoleak

Summary of Evidence: Immediate complications of endoluminal stent-graft placement for treatment of AAA include perigraft leaks (Fig. 20.2), occlusion of aortic branches, stent-graft collapse, incomplete stent-graft deployment, and graft thrombosis. Of these complications, perigraft leak is the most common. Endoleaks are classified according to their origin: type I, incomplete attachment; type II, retrograde filling; type III, device degeneration or junctional dehiscence; type IV, transient graft porosity; and type V, continued expansion of the aneurysm without detectable endoleak (endotension) (25). Type I, II, and III endoleaks are often amenable to treatment with a secondary endovascular procedure, whereas type V endoleaks must be corrected with surgical repair. Compared with catheter angiography, CTA has much greater sensitivity and specificity in detecting endoleaks and is the preferred method for imaging a patient with suspected endoleak. However, if an endoleak is detected during CTA, and the etiology of the endoleak is not demonstrated, in a 2004 case report of two patients (14), MR angiography identified the cause of an endoleak that was

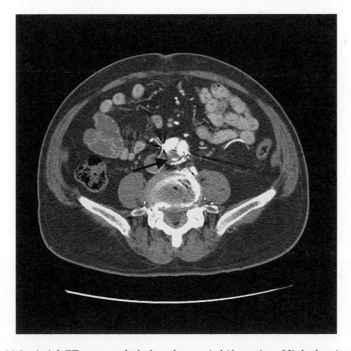

Figure 20.2. Axial CT scan cephalad to the aortic bifurcation. High density within the posterior aspect of the aorta represents an endoleak (arrow).

not detectable by CTA (limited evidence). The data provided from this single study provides moderate evidence in support of CTA as the modality of choice for evaluating patients with suspected endograft leak.

Supporting Evidence: Amerding et al. (26) conducted a retrospective, blinded study comparing the sensitivity and specificity of CTA and catheter angiography in detecting immediate complications of endoluminal stent-graft placement for treatment of AAA. The most common complication, perigraft leak, was observed in 20/46 (43%) of patients. All patients underwent both CTA and conventional angiography and each modality was reviewed by three independent reviewers. The reference standard interpretation was developed by consensus of a CT radiologist and the primary angiographer. Mean sensitivity and specificity for detecting perigraft leaks were 63% (range, 60–70%) and 77% (range, 58–100%) for catheter angiography and 92% (range, 80–100%) and 90% (range, 85–92%) for CTA. The mean κ value for interpretation of catheter angiography was 0.41 (range, 0.27–0.63) and 0.81 (range, 0.73–0.91) for CTA. Wicky et al. (25) reported two cases in which the cause of an endoleak was not detected on CTA, but was detected on MRA.

Cost-Effectiveness Analysis: Not available.

VI. Special Case: Evaluation of the Renal Donor

Summary of Evidence: Several studies reported the sensitivity and specificity of CTA and MRA in identifying anatomic variations and arterial stenosis or occlusion, which are needed prior to selecting a donor kidney from a living donor. However, these studies only provide limited evidence, as most studies lack a gold standard (i.e., surgical confirmation of the anatomy of the kidney that was not chosen as the donor). The majority of these studies simply report the interobserver agreement between two preoperative imaging modalities. However, using existing data from the literature, Liem et al. (27) evaluated the cost-effectiveness of several imaging strategies for the preoperative evaluation of living renal donors.

Supporting Evidence: Halpern et al. (28) compared CTA and MRA in the preoperative evaluation of living renal donors in which 35 donors underwent preoperative assessment with both CTA and gadolinium-enhanced MRA. Both CTA and MRA studies were evaluated by two independent reviewers and the following data were recorded: number and size of renal arteries found on each side, presence of arterial stenosis or a proximal arterial branch, and the anatomy of renal veins and ureters. Forty-one patients initially enrolled in the study, but only six underwent CTA. Surgical correlation with the transplanted kidney was available for 18 kidneys. The κ value for interobserver agreement for MRA was 0.74 and for CTA was 0.73, and for agreement between MRA and CTA was 0.74. Among the 18 kidneys for which surgical correlation was available, one proximal arterial branch to a left kidney was missed at both CTA and MRA, and two very small (<1 mm) accessory arteries suggested at CTA were not found at nephrectomy.

Rankin et al. (29) reported the correlation between CTA or gadolinium-enhanced MRA with findings at nephrectomy for living related kidney donors. Unlike the study of Halpern et al. (28), patients underwent either CTA or MRA. Both CTA and MRA were 100% sensitive in identifying the main renal arteries and renal veins; CTA visualized 37/40 arteries identified at surgery for a detection rate of 93%, and MRA visualized 18/20 arteries identified at surgery, for a detection rate of 90%.

Cost-Effectiveness Analysis: Liem et al. (27) reported a decision- and cost-effectiveness for the evaluation of living renal donors. Their conclusion depends on the perspective (donor vs. recipient) and on the specificity of DSA. For the donor, MRA dominated all other strategies (DSA, CTA, DSA with MRA, MRA with CTA, no testing and transplantation always performed, and no testing and no transplantation performed). For the recipient, DSA and DSA with MRA performed the same day both dominated all other strategies. For both donor and recipient (combined results) DSA dominated all other strategies. If the specificity of DSA was less than 99% for detection of renal disease, MRA with CTA performed the same day was superior. The authors point out the limitations of their study, which include that their model was based on multiple data sources, some of which may be subject to publication bias. Imaging protocols for each of the techniques varied among transplant centers. In addition, all cost data utilized in the analysis was obtained from their own center.

VII. Special Case: Evaluation of Renal Artery Stenosis

Summary of Evidence: There is no statistical difference between three-dimensional (3D) MRA and multidetector row CTA in the detection of hemodynamically significant renal artery stenosis identified in the current literature.

Supporting Evidence: Willmann et al. (30) reported the diagnostic performance of MRA compared with DSA in the detection of hemodynamically renal artery stenosis in 46 patients. Two independent readers participated in the study. The sensitivity for readers one and two were 86% (95% CI, 64–100%) and 100% (95% CI, 99–100%), respectively, and the specificity was 100% (95% CI, 99–100%) and 100% (95% CI, 95–100%), respectively. Stueckle et al. (31) reported the performance of CTA compared to DSA for identification of renal artery aneurysms, low- and high-grade renal artery stenosis, and renal artery occlusion. Data were reported for axial, 3D volume reconstruction (VR) and multiplanar imaging (MPI) CTA techniques. Compared to DSA, MPI achieved the greatest sensitivity (100%) and specificity (100%) for detection of low- and high-grade renal artery stenosis, as well as arterial occlusion.

Cost-Effectiveness Analysis: None available.

Take-Home Table

Table 20.2. Take-home table: questions and answers

Question	Answer	Level of evidence
What is the appropriate imaging study for suspected aortic injury?	CT angiography	Limited
Is screening for AAA with ultrasound cost-effective?	The MASS (1) study has shown a significant reduction in mortality from AAA among patents who underwent ultrasound screening. The mean cost-effectiveness ratio for screening was £28,400 per life-year gained.	Strong
Endovascular vs. surgical repair of AAA—what is the best choice?	Endovascular repair of AAA has been shown to be associated with a significant reduction in mortality when compared with open surgical repair. However, the cost of endovascular repair is greater than that of open repair, mainly due to the cost of the stent-graft.	Strong
What is the appropriate noninvasive imaging study for suspected peripheral vascular disease (PVD)?	Studies of CTA and MRA for PVD are limited to reporting the sensitivity and specificity of CTA and MRA compared to catheter angiography.	Limited
What is the best way to evaluate the patient with suspected AAA endograft leak?	CTA is preferred to catheter angiography, with MRA reserved for cases in which the cause of the endoleak is not evident on CTA.	Moderate
What is the best noninvasive imaging study for evaluation of the renal donor?	The most cost-effective imaging strategy varies and is dependent on the perspective of the analysis (renal donor or recipient), as well as the specificity of digital subtraction angiography (DSA).	Moderate
What is best noninvasive imaging study for evaluation of renal artery stenosis?	CTA and MRA are comparable. MRA is preferred for the patients with impaired renal function.	Moderate

Future Research

The following studies are needed to further define the cost-effectiveness of imaging of the aorta and peripheral vascular disease:

- Impact of CTA and MRA on treatment planning for patients with suspected peripheral vascular disease.
- Impact of CTA and MRA on outcome for patients evaluated for suspected renal artery stenosis.
- Standardization of CTA and MRA techniques to allow for more direct comparison of studies performed at different institutions.

Acknowledgment: Dr. Bertrand Janne contributed to the definition and pathophysiology of peripheral vascular disease.

References

1. Multicenter Aneurysm Screening Study group. Lancet 2002;360:1531–1539.
2. Olin JW, Kaufman JA, Bluemke DA, et al. Circulation 2004;109:2626–2633.
3. Yoshida S, Akiba H, Tamakawa M, et al. Radiology 2003;228:430–435.
4. Dyer DS, Moore EE, Mestek MF, et al. Radiology 1999;213:195–202.
5. Fabian TC, Davis KA, Gavant ML, et al. Ann Surg 1998;227:666–676.
6. Pereles FS, McCarthy RM, Baskaran V, et al. Radiology 2002;223:270–274.
7. Hunink MG, Bos JJ. AJR 1995;165:27–36.
8. Ware Jr JE, Sherbourne CD. Med Care 1992;30:473–483.
9. Rabin R, de Charro F. Ann Med 2001;33:337–343.
10. Brown LC, Epstein D, Manca A, Beard JD, Powel JT, Greenhalgh RM. Eur J Vasc Endovasc Surg 2004;27:372–381.
10a. Thomas SM, Gaines PA, Beard JD. Short-term (30 day) outcome of endovascular treatment of abdominal aortic aneurysm: Results from the prospective registry of endovascular treatment of abdominal aortic aneurysms (RETA). Eur J Vasc Endovas Surg 2001;21:57–64.
11. Zeebregts CJ, Geelkerken RH,van der Palen J, Huisman AAB, de Smit P, van Det RJ. Br J Surg 2004;91:563–568.
12. The EVAR trial participants. Lancet 2004;364:843–848.
13. Prinssen M, Buskens E, Blankensteijn JD. J Cardiovasc Surg (Torino) 2002;43: 379–384.
14. Prinssen M, Verhoeven ELG, Buth J, et al. N Engl J Med 2004;351:1607–1618.
15. Prinssen M, Buskens E, Blankensteijn JD, on behalf of the DREAM trial participants. Eur J Vasc Endovasc Surg 2004;27:121–127.
16. Sternbergh WC, Money SR. J Vasc Surg 2000;31:237–244.
17. Forbes TL, DeRose G, Kribs S, Harris KA. Can J Surg 2002;45:420–424.
18. Loewe C, Schoder M, Rand T, et al. AJR 2002;179:1013–1021.
19. Binkert CA, Baker PD, Petersen BD, Szumowski J, Kaufman JA. Radiology 2004;232:860–866.
20. Torreggiani WC, Varghese J, Haslam P, McGrath F, Munk PL, Lee MJ. Clin Radiol 2002;57:625–632.
21. Brillet PY, Vayssairat V, Tassart M, et al. J Vasc Intervent Radiol 2002;14: 1139–1145.
22. Khilnani NM, Winchester PA, Prince MR, et al. Radiology 2002;224:63–74.
23. Rubin GD, Schmidt AJ, Logan RT, Sofilos MC. Radiology 2001;221:146 158.
24. Romano M, Mainenti PP, Imbriaco M, et al. Eur J Radiol 2004;50:303–308.
25. Wicky S, Fan CM, Geller SC, Greenfield A, Santilli J, Waltman AC. AJR 2003; 181:736–738.
26. Armerding MD, Rubin GD, Beaulieu CF, et al. Radiology 2000;215:138–146.
27. Liem YS, Kock MCJM, Ijzermans JNM, Weimar W, Visser K, Hunink MGM. Radiology 2003;226:53–62.
28. Halpern EJ, Mitchell DG, Wechsler RJ, Outwater EK, Moritz MJ, Wilson GA. Radiology 2000;216:434–439.
29. Rankin SC, Jan W, Koffman CG. AJT 2001;177:349–355.
30. Willmann JK, Wildermuth S, Pfamatter T, et al. Radiology 2003;226:798–811.
31. Stueckle CA, Haegele KF, Jendreck M, et al. Australas Radiol 2004;48:142–147.

21

Imaging of the Cervical Carotid Artery for Atherosclerotic Stenosis

Alex M. Barrocas and Colin P. Derdeyn

Key Points

- At present, carotid imaging is performed to identify the presence and measure the degree of atherosclerotic stenosis, in order to select appropriate candidates for surgical endarterectomy (strong evidence). Several different imaging strategies may be employed in symptomatic patients:
- Catheter angiography (CA) may be used for this purpose (strong evidence).
- Doppler ultrasound (DUS), magnetic resonance angiography (MRA), and computed tomographic angiography (CTA), or some combination, if adequately validated, may be used to screen patients (those with less than 50% stenosis) prior to catheter angiography (moderate evidence).
- Doppler ultrasound, MRA, and CTA, or some combination, if adequately validated, may be used to identify patients with severe

stenosis (greater than 80%) for surgical endarterectomy (moderate evidence).

- Screening of asymptomatic patients with noninvasive methods and highly specific thresholds may be cost-effective in certain high-risk populations, such as patients with known atherosclerotic disease in other circulations or the presence of bruit over the carotid artery on physical examination (moderate evidence).
- More information regarding the safety and efficacy of angioplasty and stenting relative to surgical endarterectomy is expected in the near future. As treatment may be incorporated into the diagnostic catheter angiographic procedure, these recommendations may be revised.
- Physiologic imaging tools identify higher-risk subgroups in patients with atherosclerotic carotid stenosis and occlusion (strong evidence).
- The use of these physiologic imaging tools to improve guide therapy and improve outcome is unproven (insufficient evidence). A randomized clinical trial is underway for surgical revascularization of carotid occlusion in patients selected by positron emission tomography (PET).

Definition and Pathophysiology

Extracranial carotid bifurcation atherosclerotic disease is associated with ischemic stroke. The bifurcation of the common carotid artery into internal and external carotid arteries is a preferred site for the development of atherosclerotic plaque. Several biomechanical and physiologic factors are involved in the formation of atheroma at this location (1). As the atherosclerotic plaque builds, it can lead to ischemic stroke via two interrelated mechanisms: embolism and hemodynamic impairment. Embolism of plaque debris or thrombus that develops in or on the plaque may break free and lodge in a distal artery of the brain. Embolism likely accounts for the majority of stroke that occurs in association with carotid atherosclerotic disease. The second mechanism is that of low flow (2). Depending on the adequacy of collateral flow, primarily determined by the status of the circle of Willis, severe stenosis may limit the flow of blood to the distal cerebral hemisphere. Significant hemodynamic impairment due to severe stenosis or occlusion at the carotid bifurcation is an independent predictor of stroke, likely due to synergistic effects with embolic events. Primary hemodynamic or low-flow stroke may also occur, but is uncommon relative to primary embolic or synergistic embolic and hemodynamic mechanisms.

At present, only the degree of luminal diameter narrowing as measured by catheter angiography has been proven as a predictor of outcome in large-scale clinical trials of intervention versus medical therapy (3,4). Many other features of atherosclerotic plaque, including length of stenosis, cross-sectional area reduction, blood flow velocity, and plaque ulceration or irregularity have been associated with higher risks of stroke on medical treatment, but none has been proven in randomized clinical trials as predictors of stroke risk.

Epidemiology

First-ever or recurrent ischemic stroke affects approximately 750,000 people in North America annually (5). A larger number of patients present with transient ischemic attacks (TIA), rather than a completed stroke. Associated carotid bifurcation disease is involved in 20% to 30% of patients with these neurologic symptoms (6). Clinical trials of surgical endarterectomy in symptomatic patients (TIA and stroke) with severe stenosis (measured by catheter angiography) have shown substantial benefit for secondary stroke prevention over medical therapy (7). The issue of carotid imaging is relevant both for this population, for the purpose of secondary stroke prevention, as well as for patients with asymptomatic carotid stenosis. Asymptomatic carotid stenosis is present in up to 20% of patients with prior myocardial infarction or peripheral vascular disease.

Overall Cost to Society

In 1999 the American Heart Association (AHA) estimated the total economic burden for stroke to be $51 billion. The large majority of this cost is for acute and long-term care after stroke. Consequently, even expensive diagnostic evaluation and expensive treatments aimed at primary or secondary stroke prevention are often cost-effective. For example, a recent analysis found that screening patients with complete occlusion of the carotid artery with a PET study of cerebral blood flow and oxygen use followed by selective extracranial to intracranial arterial bypass for those patients with severe hemodynamic impairment would be cost-effective (8).

Goals of Carotid Imaging

The overall goal of carotid imaging is identifying appropriate candidates for surgical or endovascular revascularization. Patients with insignificant degrees of stenosis are treated medically. Imaging must detect, localize, and accurately measure the degree of stenosis in order to accomplish this goal.

Methodology

PubMed (National Library of Medicine, Bethesda, Maryland) was used to search for original research publications investigating the diagnostic performance and effectiveness of imaging strategies for the extracranial carotid artery bifurcation. The search included the period 1966 to June 2004. Search terms included combinations of the following key words: *carotid, stenosis, imaging, ultrasound, angiography, magnetic resonance, computed tomography, stroke,* and *ischemia.* Additional articles were identified from the reference lists of these papers. The review was limited to human studies and English-language literature. Abstracts and titles of articles were reviewed for relevance to this topic. Relevant articles were reviewed in full.

I. What Is the Imaging Modality of Choice in Symptomatic Carotid Stenosis?

Summary of Evidence: At present, carotid imaging is performed to identify the presence and measure the degree of atherosclerotic stenosis, in order to select appropriate candidates for surgical endarterectomy (strong evidence). Several different imaging strategies may be employed in symptomatic patients:

- Catheter angiography (CA) can be used for this purpose (strong evidence).
- Doppler ultrasound (DUS), magnetic resonance angiography (MRA), and computed tomographic angiography (CTA), or some combination, if adequately validated at the local institution with quality assurance data, may be used to screen patients for those with less than 50% stenosis prior to catheter angiography (moderate evidence).
- Doppler ultrasound or MRA, alone or in combination, if adequately validated locally, may be used to identify patients for surgical endarterectomy (limited evidence).
- Doppler ultrasound or MRA can be used both to screen for patients with less than 50% stenosis and reliably identify patients with severe, >80% stenosis. Catheter angiography is used to investigate the degree of stenosis for the remaining patients (moderate evidence).

Supporting Evidence: Patients presenting with focal ischemic symptoms, either ocular or cerebral, or permanent or temporary, are considered symptomatic. High-grade carotid stenosis is common in patients with anterior circulation ischemic symptoms (6,9). Carotid endarterectomy is highly effective in reducing stroke risk in patients with ≥70% stenosis. This has been established by two large multicenter randomized trials of endarterectomy versus best medical therapy (level I, strong evidence) (3,4). The decision for surgery for patients with 50% to 69% stenosis should consider other risk factors, as the benefit is not dramatic. Males, patients with recent symptoms, and cerebral rather than ocular ischemic symptoms have greater benefit with surgery.

Both the North American Symptomatic Carotid Endarterectomy Trial (NASCET) and the European Carotid Surgery Trial (ECST) used catheter angiography to select patients for surgery (3,4). The degree of stenosis by deciles was correlated with surgical benefit in both studies. The use of catheter angiography, therefore, has been correlated to clinical outcome in a way that no other noninvasive imaging modality has been or will be validated (level I, strong evidence).

The use of noninvasive screening tools to reduce or eliminate the need for catheter angiography has been extensively investigated. These imaging tools have the advantage of reducing costs and risk to patients due to catheter angiography, but at the expense of both overestimating stenosis and subjecting patient's to unnecessary operation and surgical risk, as well as underestimating stenosis and subjecting the patient to an increased risk of stroke from their underlying disease. Sound validation of these different modalities against catheter angiography with local quality assurance data is imperative (10).

Doppler ultrasound (DUS) is the most widely employed and most heavily investigated of these methods. Magnetic resonance angiography (MRA) is another commonly used technique. Newer MRA methods, such as contrast-enhanced first-pass methods may be better than time-of-flight techniques, but have fewer validation studies. Computed tomographic angiography (CTA) is also emerging, but very few validation studies have been done.

The noninvasive imaging strategies can be divided into three broad categories. First, patients with a very low likelihood of surgically significant disease can be screened out prior to angiography. This strategy has the strongest support behind it. Using a highly sensitive threshold, DUS can very reliably identify patients with less than 50% stenosis (level II, moderate evidence). Magnetic resonance angiography can also be used for this purpose (level II, moderate evidence). The data for CTA is emerging (level III, limited evidence).

The second strategy is to use noninvasive tools entirely. Doppler ultrasound or MRA alone or in some combination have all been advocated and are in common use. The data supporting this strategy are limited, given the wide margin for error between angiography and these methods for any given individual. Cost-effectiveness analyses of this and other strategies is discussed below.

The third strategy is to use noninvasive imaging to identify patients with less than 50% stenosis and those with very high-grade stenosis (level II, moderate evidence). Catheter angiography is reserved for those patients with estimated stenoses between 50% and 80% stenosis. All modalities can reliably identify these patients with high-grade stenosis.

The results of cost-effectiveness analyses of these different strategies are variable (8,11,12). Critical and variable local data that have profound impact on these models are the local rate of stroke with angiography, the accuracy of local DUS or MRA studies, and surgical complication rates. Different imaging strategies may be the most cost-effective at different institutions, depending on these local factors.

Finally, the advent of carotid angioplasty and stenting adds a new wrinkle in that accurate imaging and intervention can be performed during the same procedure. One randomized trial supports the use of angioplasty and stenting over endarterectomy in patients at high risk for surgery (13). The benefit of angioplasty and stenting in patients who are good surgical candidates remains to be established. For these patients, screening with a noninvasive modality, followed by angiography and treatment at that time, would be reasonable.

A. Catheter Angiography

Imaging of the cervical carotid artery in TIA or stroke victims (i.e., symptomatic) is entirely focused on determination of the degree of stenosis. This single parameter predicted outcome in two large, randomized, multicenter trials (14,15). In the NASCET (3,15), symptomatic patients included patients with TIA, amaurosis fugax, or stroke. Patients with ≥70% carotid stenosis, determined angiographically (Fig. 21.1), had a 2-year cumulative risk of ipsilateral stroke of 9% (including perioperative morbidity and mortality of 5.8%), compared to best medical treatment 2-year cumulative risk of 26%.

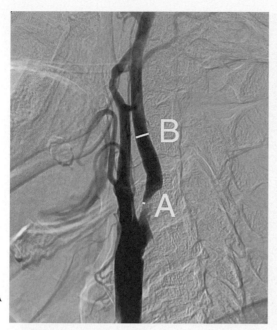
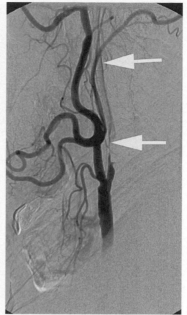

A

B

Figure 21.1. Selective arterial angiograms of carotid bifurcation showing 85% stenosis without near occlusion by the NASCET method of measurement (A) and near occlusion (severe stenosis with narrowing of the distal ICA) (B). To calculate the degree of stenosis, the lumen diameter at the point of maximum stenosis (point A) was measured as the numerator in NASCET. The lumen diameter of the distal ICA (point B) is used as the denominator. The percent stenosis is calculated as (1 − A/B)*100. In near occlusion (Fig. 21.1B) the denominator (B in Fig. 21.1A) is artifactually low.

For fatal or severe stroke, again in patients with ≥70% carotid stenosis, the surgical arm had a 2-year cumulative risk of 2.5% (including perioperative morbidity and mortality of 2.1%), whereas the medical group had a 2-year cumulative risk of 13.1%. In patients who had 50% to 69% stenosis there was an absolute risk reduction of 6.5% over 5 years, but only if the 30-day postoperative morbidity and mortality does not exceed 2%. For those patients who had less than 50% stenosis, the risk of stroke was the same as in the medicine arm. There were no significant differences between the reanalyzed results of the ECST and the results of the NASCET (16).

B. Magnetic Resonance Angiography

The bulk of the validation literature has been for time-of-flight techniques (17). Fewer studies have evaluated the use of contrast-enhanced methods. Nederkoorn et al. (18) critically reviewed the recent literature (including both MRA techniques) from 1994 through 2003 and found a pooled sensitivity and specificity of time-of-flight MRA for the detection of greater than 70% stenosis of 95% [95% confidence interval (CI), 92–97] and 90% (95% CI, 86–93), respectively, and a sensitivity and specificity for the identification of complete occlusion of 98% (95% CI, 94–100) and 100% (95% CI, 99–100), respectively (Fig. 21.2).

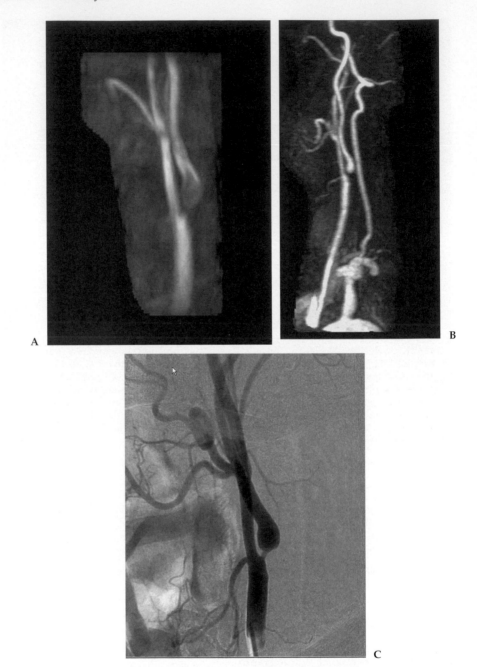

Figure 21.2. A: Time-of-flight MRA in a patient with recent transient ischemic attack shows a long segment of flow-gap, consistent with turbulent flow and suggesting high-grade stenosis. B: The contrast-enhanced (CE) MRA depicts the lumen better than the time-of-flight method, but a segment of flow gap remains. C: Catheter angiography shows an 80% stenosis. This case illustrates the reliability of MRA, particularly CE-MRA to accurately identify severe stenosis. With less severe, but clinically relevant stenosis (50% to 70%), the wide error range for MRA makes it less reliable for individual patients.

Butz et al. (19) used the care-bolus technique combined with a nearly real-time two-dimensional (2D) FLASH (fast low-angle shot) sequence and a 3D FLASH with elliptical centric view order for the angiographic pulse time to report a sensitivity of 96% and a specificity of 90% for carotid stenosis of ≥70%. Randoux et al. (20) prospectively studied dynamic 3D gadolinium-enhanced MRA with digital subtraction angiography (DSA) and concluded that there was a tendency to overestimate the degree of ostial stenosis. Many authors report the use of multiple overlapping thin-slab acquisition (MOTSA) to directly measure stenosis of the carotid artery (12,21–23). Development of first-pass contrast-enhanced MRA resulted in more rapid image acquisitions that are physiologically more similar to those of DSA with the advantage of being less prone to motion artifacts than standard time-of-flight MRA. Hathout et al. (24) presented their institution's 4-year retrospective study of all carotid arteries with stenosis from 10% to 90% diagnosed angiographically and compared to 3D gadolinium-enhanced MRA. They found a linear relationship between DSA and contrast-enhanced MRA, with a Spearman rank correlation coefficient of 0.82, $p < .001$, with increasing severity of stenosis correlating angiographically. However, MRA was less reliable at predicting the degree of stenosis in the individual patient. There were wide confidence intervals and the addition of ultrasound peak systolic velocity did not improve the predictive accuracy. They recommended use of MRA as a screening tool: patients with 50% or less stenosis treated medically, those with >80% treated surgically, and those in between evaluated with angiography. Older studies show the continuing improvement of sensitivity and specificity of this technique over time with modifications of technique and reduction of signal-to-noise ratios, but none has the validation of large numbers of patients and clinical correlation such as NASCET (25–33).

C. Computer Tomography Angiography

Koelemay et al. (34) reviewed data from 28 studies published between 1990 and 2003, using single-slice scanners. Eight of the 28 studies were considered to be methodologically sound, with blinded review of images and reduction of other sources of bias. The pooled sensitivity and specificity of CTA for the detection of 70% stenosis was 85% (95% CI, 79–89%) and 93% (95% CI, 89–96%), respectively. For detection of complete occlusion, the sensitivity and specificity was 97% (95% CI, 93–99%) and 99% (95% CI, 98–100%), respectively.

The advent of multirow detector machines has expanded the vascular imaging capabilities of CT scanners. There are very few reports with the newer hardware. Zhang et al. (35) have demonstrated that the interfering factors such as ulcerations, calcifications, and adjacent vessels can be circumvented by manually correcting the automated stenosis recognition software. This improved the correlation between CTA and DSA from 0.69 to 0.81. Prokop et al. (36) expand on the thinnest possible section collimation, multislice scanning, to image from the aortic arch through the intracranial vessels. They derive a pooled sensitivity of 95% and specificity of 98% for the detection of >70% stenoses (including single-slice techniques). The Carotide-Angiographic par Resonance Magnétigue-Echographic-Doppler-Angiosce (CARMEDAS) multicenter study (37) compared the concordance rates of contrast-enhanced MRA, DUS, and

CTA prospectively in 150 patients for symptomatic stenoses ≥50% and ≥70% and for asymptomatic stenoses ≥60%, for occlusion. Using CTA alone resulted in the misclassification of the stenosis in 11 of 64 cases.

D. Doppler Ultrasound

The performance of DUS can be highly variable (Fig. 21.3) (38). In a pooled meta-analysis of studies published since 1994, Nederkoorn et al. (18) reported a sensitivity and specificity of DUS for the detection of greater than 70% stenosis of 86% (95% CI, 84–89) and 87% (95% CI, 84–90), respectively, and a sensitivity and specificity for the identification of complete occlusion of 96% (95% CI, 94–98) and 100% (95% CI, 99–100), respectively. These numbers may reflect several biases, including publication bias. A better, real-world estimate, of DUS may have been from the NASCET investigators (39). In this analysis, they reviewed the DUS and catheter angiographic findings in 1011 symptomatic patients screened for inclusion in NASCET. As all patients were considered for inclusion, verification bias was minimal. The sensitivities and specificities of DUS for the identification of 70% stenosis ranged from 0.65 to 0.71. The risk of stroke at 18 months declined sharply as the degree of angiographically defined stenosis declined from 99% to 70%. No pattern of decline was apparent on the basis of the ultrasonographic data. The authors concluded that DUS could be used as a screening tool to exclude patients with no carotid artery disease from further testing.

Furthermore, different criteria are often better correlated with angiography in different laboratories. For example, in a study by Alexandrov et al. (40), peak systolic velocity was more accurate in one lab, while the use of ratios was more accurate in another. Because performance differs substantially among devices, validation of local vascular laboratories is

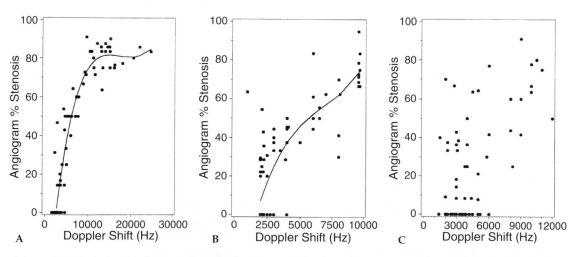

Figure 21.3. Relationship between Doppler frequency/velocity and percent stenosis by angiography for three specific devices: one with a device with a "strong" relationship (A), one with a "moderate" relationship (B), and one with a "poor" relationship (C) (38). This was a validation study performed as part of the Asymptomatic Carotid Surgery Study.

required. With validation, ultrasound performance can be sufficient for the reliable identification of patients with no significant stenosis and of those with severe stenosis (39). As with MRA, the wide confidence limits for degree of stenosis in individual patients limit the ability of this modality to accurately classify patients at the cut-points for clinical decision making (i.e., 70% stenosis). Without quality control, many ultrasound machines are not adequate to accurately predict the degree of carotid stenosis and should not be the only test to decide whether surgery is warranted.

II. What Is the Imaging Modality of Choice in Asymptomatic Carotid Stenosis?

Summary of Evidence: The benefit of surgery in patients with asymptomatic carotid stenosis is marginal. Two large randomized trials have found a 1% absolute annual risk reduction for surgery, compared to best medical therapy. Whether treatment should be pursued will depend on many factors, including patient age and gender (no definite benefit for women). In one of these two studies, restricted to highly selected, relatively healthy asymptomatic patients, 20% of the patients were dead at 5 years, many due to vascular disease.

Imaging of asymptomatic patients is necessarily a screening issue. The low risk of stroke in medically treated patients and the small risk reduction with surgery remove the harsh penalties for false-negative or false-positive noninvasive studies that are incurred in symptomatic patients. Well-validated DUS or MRA laboratories may be used for this purpose (level II, moderate evidence). The critical factors for screening are well-validated noninvasive methods and documented low surgical complication rates.

Supporting Evidence: Two randomized controlled trials show that patients with 60% to 99% ipsilateral carotid stenosis have slight risk reduction with surgery (1% annual absolute risk reduction with surgical complication rates less than 2%). Unlike symptomatic patients, no relationship between degree of stenosis and surgical benefit was found. The Asymptomatic Carotid Atherosclerosis Study (ACAS) (41) had 1662 randomized patients with 60% to 99% diameter asymptomatic stenosis (NASCET measurements). The actuarial estimated 5-year risk of an ipsilateral stroke or operative stroke or death was 5.1% in the surgery group vs. 11.0% in the no-surgery group—a relative risk reduction of about 50% or an absolute risk reduction of 5.9%. If the other (i.e., contralateral) strokes are added in, the absolute risk reduction hardly changes at 5.1%, which is not surprising because one would not expect surgery to influence such strokes. The risk of surgical or angiographic stroke or death was 2.3%. Operating on 85 patients might prevent about one stroke per year, or, if the patients did not die of a cardiac death first, operating on about 17 patients might prevent one stroke in 5 years. However, because only half the strokes were disabling, their absolute risk reduction was 2.6%, which about doubles the numbers of patients needed to treat to prevent one disabling stroke compared with any other stroke. Subgroup analyses should no benefit in women.

The Asymptomatic Carotid Surgery Trial (ACST) (42) yielded similar results. Surgical morbidity and mortality was 3.1%. The absolute risk reduction at 5 years was 5.4%. With good medical care, patients face only a 2% annual stroke rate, which falls below 1% after successful carotid endarterectomy. However, the benefits exceed the risks only if the 30-day postoperative morbidity and mortality remain low; otherwise there is no benefit.

A. Cost-Effectiveness Analysis

Screening of asymptomatic patients with noninvasive methods and highly specific thresholds may be cost-effective in certain high-risk populations, such as patients with known atherosclerotic disease in other circulations or the presence of bruit over the carotid artery on physical examination. Different studies addressing the cost-effectiveness of screening asymptomatic carotid stenosis resulted in divergent conclusions (43). The critical factor in whether intervention is effective is the surgical complication rates. A one-time screening program of a population with a high prevalence (20%) of $\geq$60% stenosis cost $35 130 per incremental quality-adjusted life year (QALY) gained. Decreased surgical benefit (less than 1% annual stroke risk reduction with surgery) or increased annual discount rate resulted in screening being detrimental, resulting in lost QALYs. Annual screening cost $457,773 per incremental QALY gained. In a low-prevalence (4%) population, one-time screening cost $52,588 per QALY gained, while annual screening was detrimental (44).

III. What Is the Role of Carotid Angioplasty and Stenting?

Summary of Evidence: More information regarding the safety and efficacy of angioplasty and stenting relative to surgical endarterectomy is expected in the near future. As treatment may be incorporated into the diagnostic catheter angiographic procedure, these recommendations may be revised.

At present, angioplasty and stenting is accepted as a reasonable therapy for patients with severe stenosis and recent ischemic symptoms who are not good surgical candidates (level II, moderate evidence). Patients who are good surgical candidates should be treated surgically or within clinical trials of stenting versus endarterectomy. Noninvasive screening of symptomatic but surgically ineligible patients for possible carotid stenosis should be done prior to angioplasty and stenting (level II, moderate evidence). The benefit of angioplasty and stenting for asymptomatic patients is unproven (level IV, insufficient evidence).

Supporting Evidence: One randomized controlled study of angioplasty versus carotid endarterectomy in symptomatic patients has been published, the Carotid and Vertebral Artery Transluminal Angioplasty Study (CAVATAS) (45). All patients had recent ischemic symptoms and high-grade stenosis by catheter angiography. The 30-day major stroke and death rates were similar, as was the outcome at 1 year. Limitations of this study include a higher surgical complication rate than NASCET, long-term follow-up for only 3 years, and dated endovascular devices.

A second randomized study has been recently published (13). Enroll-ment was limited to patients considered to be at high risk for complica-tions of surgery. Inclusion criteria included age greater than 80 years, congestive heart failure, chronic obstructive pulmonary disease, prior sur-gical endarterectomy, and local radiation therapy. Both symptomatic and asymptomatic patients were included. Subgroup analyses for presence or absence of ischemic symptoms did not achieve statistical significance. Thirty-day and 1-year outcomes were significantly better in the angio-plasty group. A major issue raised by this study is whether these patients would have done better with medical therapy alone.

IV. What Is the Role of Physiologic Imaging in Carotid Stenosis and Occlusion?

Summary of Evidence: Physiologic imaging studies that identify compen-satory hemodynamic mechanisms for low perfusion pressure have been shown to be powerful predictors of subsequent stroke in patients with symptomatic carotid stenosis or occlusion using some, but not all, physio-logic imaging methods. The best evidence is for measurements of the oxygen extraction fraction (OEF) with PET and breath-holding transcranial Doppler studies (level I, strong evidence). There is moderate evidence (level II) supporting the use of stable xenon CT and single photon emis-sion computed tomography (SPECT) methods. At present, however, the use of this information to guide therapy has not been proven to change outcome (level III, limited evidence). The two patient populations in whom these tools are likely to become important are those with symptomatic complete carotid occlusion and those with asymptomatic carotid stenosis.

Supporting Evidence

A. Methods of Hemodynamic Assessment

A completely occluded carotid artery often has no effect on the pressure in the arteries of the brain beyond the occlusion. In some patients, the circle of Willis or pial collateral branches are sufficient to maintain normal arte-rial pressure and, consequently, normal cerebral blood flow. In other patients, the pressure in the arteries of the brain beyond the occlusion will decrease. There are two compensatory mechanisms by which the brain can maintain normal oxygen metabolism, and thereby normal neurologic function, when arterial pressure falls. First, in autoregulation, blood flow can be maintained by reducing vascular resistance. Second, as flow is reduced passively as a function of pressure and exceeded autoregulatory capacity, the brain can increase the amount of oxygen extracted from the blood.

Single measurements of cerebral blood flow (CBF) alone do not ade-quately assess cerebral hemodynamic status. First, normal values may be found when perfusion pressure is reduced, but CBF is maintained by autoregulatory vasodilation. Second, CBF may be low when perfusion pressure is normal. This can occur when the metabolic demands of the tissue are low. Reduced flow due to reduced metabolic demand may not cause confusion when low regional CBF is measured in areas of frank tissue infarction. However, blood flow can also be reduced in normal, uninfarcted, tissue due to the destruction of normal afferent or efferent fibers by a remote lesion as well (46).

Three basic strategies have been developed to assess regional cerebral hemodynamic status noninvasively (2). The normal compensatory responses of the brain and its vasculature to reduced perfusion pressure, as outlined above, are assumed to be present. The first two strategies are used to indirectly identify the presence and degree of autoregulatory vasodilation. The third relies on direct measurements of the OEF.

The first strategy relies on paired blood flow measurements with the initial measurement obtained at rest and the second measurement obtained following a cerebral vasodilatory stimulus. Hypercapnia, acetazolamide, and physiologic tasks such as hand movement have been used as vasodilatory stimuli. Normally, each will result in a robust increase in CBF. If the CBF response is muted or absent, preexisting autoregulatory cerebral vasodilation due to reduced cerebral perfusion pressure is inferred. Quantitative or qualitative (relative) measurements of CBF can be made using a variety of methods, including xenon 133 by inhalation or intravenous injection, SPECT, stable xenon computed tomography (Xe-CT), PET, and magnetic resonance imaging (MRI). Changes in the velocity of blood in the middle cerebral artery trunk or internal carotid artery can be measured with transcranial Doppler (TCD) and MRI. The blood flow or blood velocity responses to these vasodilatory stimuli have been categorized into several grades of hemodynamic impairment: (1) reduced augmentation (relative to the contralateral hemisphere or normal controls); (2) absent augmentation (same value as baseline); and (3) paradoxical reduction in regional blood flow compared to baseline measurement. This final category, also called the "steal" phenomenon, can only be identified with quantitative CBF techniques.

The second strategy uses the measurement of regional cerebral blood volume (CBV), alone or in combination with measurements of CBF, in the resting brain in order to detect the presence of autoregulatory vasodilation. The CBV/CBF ratio (or, inversely, the CBF/CBV ratio), mathematically equivalent to the vascular mean transit time, may be more sensitive than CBV alone for the identification of autoregulatory vasodilation. Quantitative regional measurements of CBV and CBF can be made with PET or SPECT. Magnetic resonance techniques for the quantitative measurement of CBV have been developed. Patients are identified as abnormal with these techniques based on comparison of absolute quantitative values or hemispheric ratios of quantitative values to the range observed in normal control subjects.

The third strategy relies on direct measurements of OEF to identify patients with increased oxygen extraction. At present, regional measurements of OEF can be made only with PET using O-15–labeled radiotracers. Both absolute values and side-to-side ratios of quantitative and relative OEF have been used for the determination of abnormal from normal.

B. Association with Stroke Risk

Complete occlusion of the carotid artery is found in up to 15% of patients with carotid territory TIAs or strokes (9). The risk of subsequent stroke in this population is high, approximately 5% to 7% per year (47). No preventive therapy has been proven effective. A randomized trial of extracranial to intracranial arterial bypass, the EC/IC bypass trial, found no benefit with bypass compared to medical therapy (48). One limitation of this study was that there was no method of hemodynamic assessment: a large percentage of the patients included in this study may have had normal flow due to circle of Willis and other sources of collateral flow and therefore nothing to gain from an extra-anatomic bypass (49). The presence of severe hemodynamic impairment has since been proven to be an independent and powerful predictor of stroke in patients with carotid occlusion (2,50).

As these methods are inferential and indirect, correlation with outcome is required (2). At present, the strongest evidence is for PET measurements of OEF and TCD measurements of cerebrovascular reserve (level I, strong evidence). The St. Louis Carotid Occlusion Study was a blinded, prospective study of 81 patients with symptomatic carotid occlusion that also specifically assessed the impact of other risk factors (50). The risk of all stroke and ipsilateral ischemic stroke in symptomatic subjects with increased OEF was significantly higher than in those with normal OEF (log rank $p = .005$ and $p = .004$, respectively). Univariate and multivariate analysis of 17 baseline stroke risk factors confirmed the independence of this relationship. The age-adjusted relative risk conferred by increased OEF was 6.0 (95% CI 1.7–21.6) for all stroke and 7.3 (95% CI 1.6–33.4) for ipsilateral ischemic stroke. Similar data were reported by a study by Yamauchi et al. (51). Based on these data, a randomized trial of extracranial to intracranial arterial bypass in patients with increased OEF has been funded and is under way.

Several investigators have studied the association of paired flow techniques with stroke risk. Six found an association with stroke risk and three found none. Two of the six positive studies used a TCD method (breath-holding) and provided level I (strong evidence) for patients with complete carotid occlusion and patients with asymptomatic carotid stenosis (52,53). Vernieri et al. (54) enrolled 104 patients with complete carotid occlusion and followed them for a median period of 24 months. The blood velocity response to 30 seconds of breath-holding was measured by TCD on study entry. Baseline stroke risk factors were assessed. The threshold for an abnormal TCD was set prospectively. Eighteen patients suffered a stroke during the follow-up period. Age and abnormal TCD response were independent risk factors for subsequent stroke.

Klieser and Widder (55) reported an association between abnormal blood velocity responses to hypercapnia (by TCD) and the risk of subsequent stroke in 85 patients with carotid occlusion. Both symptomatic and asymptomatic patients were included. The risk of contralateral stroke in the patients with a diminished or exhausted CO_2 reactivity was increased, which suggests that the groups were not matched for other stroke risk factors, which were not evaluated. A subsequent study by these same authors reported the outcome of 86 patients with carotid occlusion (56). A much lower risk of stroke was observed in this second study and the number of asymptomatic patients was not reported.

Yonas and coworkers (57) reported an association of the steal phenomena (reduced blood flow by Xe-CT) after acetazolamide and subsequent stroke. This study included patients with high-grade carotid stenosis and patients with carotid occlusion. The hemodynamic data of patients with subsequent stroke was analyzed retrospectively in order to establish threshold values for the categorization of high- and low-risk groups. These authors subsequently repeated the analysis with an additional 27 patients (58). The hemodynamic criteria used to establish high- and low-risk groups were different from the prior analysis. Three of the five new strokes that occurred did so in patients who would not have met criteria for the first study and the definition of clinical outcome included contralateral stroke. Only two of these five new strokes were in the hemodynamically compromised territory of the occluded vessel.

Three studies have failed to find an association of a paired flow technique and stroke risk (59–61). The largest and most methodologically sound study was reported by Yokota and colleagues (60). They prospectively evaluated 105 symptomatic patients with mixed lesions [unilateral occlusion or severe stenosis (>75% in diameter) of the internal carotid artery (ICA) or proximal middle cerebral artery (MCA)] with a SPECT study of relative cerebral blood flow using ^{123}I iodoamphetamine (IMP) and measurement of cerebrovascular reactivity using acetazolamide. Other stroke risk factors were prospectively assessed. Thirteen strokes occurred during a median follow-up of 2.7 years: seven strokes occurred in 39 patients with abnormal hemodynamics and six in the 39 patients with normal hemodynamics. The investigators were not blind to the results of the hemodynamic study. A relatively large number of patients ($n = 16$) were censored from the study because of subsequent cerebrovascular surgery and a significant number of patients ($n = 11$) were lost to follow-up.

C. Cost-Effectiveness Analysis

Cost-effectiveness analysis suggests that the use of these physiologic tools, even expensive ones such as PET, would be cost-effective for patients with symptomatic carotid artery occlusion, provided there is a benefit with surgical bypass (8). The costs of acute and long-term care for stroke victims greatly exceeds the costs of diagnostic workup and surgery.

In addition to patients with complete carotid occlusion, another promising application for hemodynamic assessment is in asymptomatic carotid stenosis. The prevalence of hemodynamic impairment in patients with asymptomatic carotid occlusive disease is very low (53,62). This low prevalence may account in part for the low risk of stroke with medical treatment, and consequently, the marginal benefit with revascularization. The presence of hemodynamic impairment may be a powerful predictor of subsequent stroke in this population (53,62). This is one area of research with enormous clinical implications: if a subgroup of asymptomatic patients at high risk due to hemodynamic factors could be identified, it would be possible to target surgical or endovascular treatment at those most likely to benefit.

Only one study has been performed in this population, to date. Silvestrini et al. (53) performed a prospective, blinded longitudinal study of 94 patients with asymptomatic carotid artery stenosis of at least 70% followed for a mean of 28.5 months. Breath-holding TCD was performed on entry, as well as the assessment of other stroke risk factors. An abnormal TCD study was shown to be a powerful and independent risk factor for subsequent stroke.

Take-Home Tables

Table 21.1. Suggested algorithm for imaging symptomatic patients (39,63)

1. Screening ultrasound, CTA, or MRA (after establishing accuracy of local laboratory versus angiography) to exclude patients with less than 50% stenosis from further evaluation for carotid stenosis
   a. Patients with less than 50% stenosis treated medically

2. Subsequent imaging decisions are based on the accuracy of local noninvasive tests for the presence of occlusion and for severe stenosis
   a. If not reliable for severe stenosis or occlusion, all patients with suspected stenosis greater than 50% or occlusion should undergo angiography
   b. If noninvasive tests are reliable for the identification of greater than 80% stenosis, then these patients go to surgery and patients with suspected 50% to 80% stenosis or occlusion go to angiography

Table 21.2. Suggested algorithm for imaging asymptomatic patients

If surgical complication rates (stroke and death) for asymptomatic patients are less than 2%, and the patient is a male in relatively good health with a life-expectancy of least 5 years, then a screening ultrasound, CTA, or MRA with highly specific threshold for greater than 60% stenosis, followed by surgery if positive may be reasonable.

Table 21.3. Suggested algorithm for imaging patients with carotid occlusion

If noninvasive screening tool is documented as accurate for complete occlusion, then no further imaging is necessary for asymptomatic patients. The risk for stroke with a missed high-grade asymptomatic stenosis is so low that the risk of angiography is not worth the benefit. There is no increased risk of stroke with higher degrees of stenosis in asymptomatic patients. If the patient is symptomatic, the diagnosis should be confirmed by angiography, as a missed high-grade stenosis has a very high chance of causing a future stroke.

Protocols Based on the Evidence

Carotid Angiography

The key is to obtain measurements of linear diameter reduction using selective carotid artery injections. For ICA lesions, the point of maximal stenosis is measured and expressed as a percentage of the normal distal internal carotid artery diameter (64). For eccentric stenoses, the maximal degree of stenosis in any projection is reported. If there is evidence of collapse of the ICA due to low flow, the denominator will be artifactually reduced. By convention this is termed "near occlusion," and the degree of stenosis is not reported. These procedures are optimally performed using a biplane digital subtraction unit. An arch injection is useful to evaluate for origin stenosis and arch morphology. Selective carotid injections are obtained in magnified anteroposterior (AP) and lateral projections with orthogonal oblique views, if necessary. If a complete occlusion is encountered, be certain to perform a long run in the neck run to look for string, as well as to assess external to internal collaterals. Subclavian or vertebral injections to assess for collateral flow are also useful.

Doppler Ultrasound

Five- or 7.5-MHz linear array transducers are generally used. The following measurements must be acquired: the highest angle-adjusted peak systolic velocity in the common, proximal, and distal ICAs, and at the point of maximal stenosis. Angle adjustment for Doppler measurements is based on flow direction by color Doppler. End-diastolic velocity measurements are also at these levels. Ratios of these velocities should be calculated. No one specific protocol or value can be recommended to use as a threshold for degree of stenosis. The optimal thresholds for different degrees of stenosis must be determined at each laboratory versus angiography.

Contrast-Enhanced Magnetic Resonance Angiography

A three-dimensional subtracted gradient-recalled echo sequence and turbo FLASH sequence (4/1.6, 25-degree flip angle, 120 × 256 matrix) is generally used. A total of 20 mL of MR contrast is injected by a power injector at approximately 3 cc/sec. Some clinicians use a timing bolus followed by a saline flush to estimate the optimal time for the contrast-enhanced scan. Others generate up to three postgadolinium runs and select the one with the best arterial visualization for subtraction.

Computed Tomographic Angiography

Helical CT acquisitions for coverage of the arch to the circle of Willis generally employ 3-mm helical beam collimation with a 3 mm/sec table speed, 12-cm scan field of view from the origin of the great vessels through the circle of Willis, 140 kV, mA 240, and 90 mL of nonionic contrast media injected at 3 mL/sec by a power injector. A 25-second delay between injection and scan start is employed.

References

1. Malek AM, Alper SL, Izumo S. JAMA 1999;282(21):2035–2042.
2. Derdeyn CP, Grubb RL Jr, Powers WJ. Neurology 1999;53(2):251.
3. North American Symptomatic Carotid Endarterectomy Trial Collaborators. N Engl J Med 1991;325(7):445–453.
4. Rothwell PM, Gutnikov SA, Warlow CP. Stroke 2003;34(2):514–523.
5. Kissela B, et al. Stroke 2001;32(6):1285–1290.
6. Bogousslavsky J, et al. Arch Neurol 1986;43(3):223–228.
7. Rothwell PM, et al. Lancet 2003;361(9352):107–116.
8. Derdeyn CP, et al. J Nucl Med 2000;41(5):800–807.
9. Mead GE, et al. Br J Surg 1997;84(7):990–992.
10. Howard G, Chambless LE, Baker WH. A multicenter validation study of Doppler ultrasound versus angiography. J Stroke Cerebrovasc Dis 1991;1:166–173.
11. Buskens E, et al. Radiology 2004;233:101–112.
12. Kent KC, et al. JAMA 1995;274(11):888–893.
13. Yadav JS, et al. N Engl J Med 2004;351:1493–1501.
14. Carotid Surgery Trialists' Collaborative Group. Lancet 1998;351(9113):1379–1387.
15. Barnett HJM, et al. N Engl J Med 1998;339(20):1415–1425.

16. Morgenstern L, et al. Neurology 1997;48(4):911–915.
17. Kallmes D, et al. AJNR 1996;17(8):1501–1506.
18. Nederkoorn PJ, van der Graaf Y, Hunink MGM. Stroke 2003;34(5):1324–1331.
19. Butz B, et al. Acta Radiol 2004;45(2):164–170.
20. Randoux B, et al. Radiology 2003;229(3):697–702.
21. DeMarco JK, Huston J III, Bernstein MA. AJR 2004;183(3):787–793.
22. Nederkoorn PJ, et al. Stroke 2002;33(8):2003–2008.
23. Huston J, et al. AJNR 1998;19(2):309–315.
24. Hathout GM, Duh MJ, El-Saden SM. AJNR 2003;24(9):1747–1756.
25. Alvarez-Linera J, et al. AJNR 2003;24(5):1012–1019.
26. Sundgren PC, et al. Neuroradiology 2002;44(7):592–599.
27. Remonda L, et al. AJNR 2002;23(2):213–219.
28. Randoux B, et al. Radiology 2001;220(1):179–185.
29. Serfaty JM, et al. AJR 2000;175(2):455–463.
30. Sardanelli F, et al. J Comput Assist Tomogr 1999;23(2):208–215.
31. Slosman F, et al. AJR 1998;170(2):489–495.
32. Remonda L, Heid O, Schroth G. Radiology 1998;209(1):95–102.
33. Leclerc X, et al. AJNR 1998;19(8):1405–1413.
34. Koelemay MJW, et al. Stroke 2004;35(10):2306–2312.
35. Zhang Z, et al. Eur Radiol 2004;14(4):665–672.
36. Prokop M, Waaijer A, Kreuzer S. Jbr-Btr 2004;87(1):23–29.
37. Nonent M, et al. Stroke 2004;35(3):682–686.
38. Howard G, et al. Stroke 1996;27(11):1951–1957.
39. Eliasziw M, et al. Stroke 1995;26(10):1747–1752.
40. Alexandrov AV, et al. Stroke 1997;28(2):339–342.
41. Executive Committee for the Asymptomatic Carotid Atherosclerosis Study. JAMA 1995;273(18):1421–1428.
42. Halliday A, et al. Lancet 2004;363(9420):1491–1502.
43. Holloway RG, et al. Stroke 1999;30(7):1340–1349.
44. Derdeyn CP, Powers WJ. Stroke 1996;27(11):1944–1950.
45. CAVATAS Investigators. Lancet 2001;357(9270):1729–1737.
46. Feeney DM, Baron JC. Stroke 1986;17:817–830.
47. Klijn CJM, et al. Stroke 1997;28:2084–2093.
48. The EC/IC Bypass Study Group. N Engl J Med 1985;313:1191–2000.
49. Ausman Jr, Diaz FG. Critique of the extracranial-intracranial bypass study. Surg Neurol 1986;26:218–221.
50. Grubb RL Jr, et al. JAMA 1998;280(12):1055–1060.
51. Yamauchi H, et al. J Nucl Med 1999;40:1992–1998.
52. Vernieri F, et al. Stroke 1999;30:593–598.
53. Silvestrini M, et al. JAMA 2000;283(16):2122–2127.
54. Vernieri F, et al. Stroke 2001;32:1552–1558.
55. Kleiser B, Widder N. Stroke 1992;23:171–174.
56. Widder B, Kleiser B, Krapf H. Stroke 1994;25:1963–1967.
57. Yonas H, et al. J Neurosurg 1993;79:483–489.
58. Webster MW, et al. J Vasc Surg 1995;21:338–345.
59. Powers WJ, Tempel LW, Grubb RL Jr. Ann Neurol 1989;25:325–330.
60. Yokota C, et al. Stroke 1998;29:1743–1744.
61. Hasegawa Y, et al. Stroke 1997;28:242.
62. Powers WJ, et al. Neurology 2000;54:878–882.
63. Derdeyn CP, et al. Radiology 1995;197(3):635–643.
64. Fox AJ. Radiology 1993;186(2):316–318.

22

Imaging in the Evaluation of Pulmonary Embolism

Krishna Juluru and John Eng

Issues

I. What is the performance of various imaging modalities in the evaluation of pulmonary embolism?
   A. Modality 1: angiography
   B. Modality 2: nuclear ventilation-perfusion imaging
   C. Modality 3: computed tomography pulmonary angiography (scanners with fewer than four detectors)
   D. Modality 4: multidetector computed tomography
   E. Modality 5: electron beam computed tomography
   F. Modality 6: magnetic resonance angiography
   G. Modality 7: ultrasound of lung and pleura
   H. Method 8: echocardiography
   I. Modality 9: chest radiography
II. How can imaging modalities be combined in the diagnosis of pulmonary embolism?

Key Points

- When using a clinical outcome reference standards, angiography, VQ scan, non–multidetector computed tomography (MDCT) pulmonary angiography, MDCT pulmonary angiography, and electron beam computed tomography (EBCT), are all associated with negative predictive values of 94% or greater for diagnosing pulmonary embolism (PE).
- Differences in negative predictive values of non-MDCT in diagnosis of PE between studies using an imaging reference standard and studies using clinical outcome reference standard may be due to clinically insignificant pulmonary emboli at the subsegmental level.
- The performance of magnetic resonance angiography (MRA) in evaluation of PE has not been adequately studied.
- The performances of ultrasound of the lung and pleura, echocardiography, and plain radiographs are insufficient to justify the use of these modalities in the primary evaluation of PE.

■ Several pathways in the diagnosis of PE have been described using combinations of imaging modalities, clinical exam, and laboratory data. These pathways are equally effective with respect to clinical outcome, but differ in imaging utilization and may differ in safety.

Definition and Pathophysiology

Pulmonary emboli originate from blood clots in the venous system, blood clots in the right side of the heart, neoplasms invading the venous system, and other substances such as air, bone marrow fat, and amniotic fluid. Over 90% of pulmonary emboli originate from clots in the deep veins of the lower extremities. Major risk factors include advanced age, recent surgery, immobilization, malignancy, obesity, cigarette smoking, congestive heart failure, and history of deep venous thrombosis (1).

Epidemiology

The incidence of PE has been estimated to be 0.2 to 0.6 per 1000 per year (2,3) with an estimated mortality rate of 11% to 15% (1).

Overall Cost to Society

Estimating the economic impact of PE is difficult since the overall incidence of this disease is hard to ascertain. However, in one well-defined group of patients at risk for developing deep venous thrombosis (DVT), patients who have undergone total hip replacement surgery, the average discounted lifetime cost of long-term DVT complications has been estimated to be $3069 per patient, of which $333 is attributed to PE (4).

Goals

The goal of imaging is to identify evidence of clot in the pulmonary arterial system. Identification of any clot generally results in treatment with anticoagulant therapy.

Methodology

The medical literature was searched using PubMed (National Library of Medicine, Bethesda, Maryland) for original research publications that address the use of various imaging modalities in the evaluation of PE. The search parameters were *pulmonary embolism AND (CT OR ultrasound OR sonography OR echo OR nuclear OR ventilation perfusion OR MRI OR angiography OR imaging OR radiography) AND (evaluation OR diagnosis OR diagnostic)*. The search covered the period 1990 to April 2004 and was limited to human studies in the English language. Relevant articles from the search were entered into a database and classified into the following categories: (1) article type (systematic review vs. primary literature), (2) subject of evaluation (diagnostic imaging vs. diagnostic pathway), (3) imaging modality (if applicable), and (4) diagnostic reference standard (imaging vs. clinical outcome). The authors then rated the articles based on the quality of evidence.

Comment

It is important to recognize the limitations of studies reporting clinical outcomes in patients who receive diagnostic testing for pulmonary embolism. These studies can only report negative predictive values and rates of false negative results. The number of false negatives is the number of patients initially diagnosed as not having PE but who later return within a specified period of time with PE symptoms and imaging findings. This value is also known as the recurrence rate. Studies using clinical outcome as a reference standard did not follow patients initially diagnosed with PE, as these patients were treated. Therefore, positive predictive values and rates of false-positive results could not be determined.

I. What Is the Performance of Various Imaging Modalities in the Evaluation of Pulmonary Embolism?

A. Modality 1: Angiography

Summary of Evidence: Pulmonary angiography has traditionally been considered the gold standard diagnostic test in the evaluation of PE. Consequently, the major articles that evaluated the accuracy of pulmonary angiography itself have used clinical outcome as a reference standard. The risk of recurrent PE following negative pulmonary angiography is low, even though interobserver agreement is relatively low for subsegmental pulmonary arteries (5).

Supporting Evidence: One major level I (strong evidence) systematic review and three major level II (moderate evidence) primary studies were identified in our search that evaluated pulmonary angiography against a clinical outcome reference standard. Van Beek et al. (6) performed a systematic review of the literature from 1965 to 1999 for prospective studies of untreated patients with suspected PE and negative pulmonary angiograms who were followed-up for a minimum of 3 months. Eight articles were selected on the strength of the study design, comprising a total study population of 1050 patients with negative pulmonary angiograms. Of these, 51 patients were lost to follow-up, 15 patients had nonfatal PE during the follow-up period, and three patients had fatal pulmonary embolism. In the worst-case scenario, if all patients who were lost to follow-up died from fatal PE, the recurrence rate of PE would have been 6.3% [95% confidence interval (CI), 4–7%]. In the best-case scenario, if all patients who were lost to follow-up did not have PE in the follow-up period, the recurrence rate of PE would have been 1.6% (95% CI, 1.0–2.6%). The study's authors note that the three oldest studies in the review, performed between 1978 and 1988, accounted for the majority of cases of recurrent PE as well the majority of cases that were lost to follow-up, and they argue that the lower recurrence rate in the more recent studies may be due to improvements in imaging technology. Excluding the three oldest studies from the analysis, the overall recurrence rate of PE drops to 5.4% in the worst-case scenario.

Of the three major primary articles identified in our search (5,7,8) (all level II), one article by Nilsson et al. (5) was not included in the van Beek analysis. In this study, 269 consecutive patients with clinical suspicion for PE were evaluated. Ninety-nine patients (37%) were excluded because of disease other than PE, refusal to participate, being too ill to participate, unavailability of diagnostic catheterization, contraindication to pulmonary angiography, or inadequate completion of protocol. The remaining 170 patients all underwent pulmonary angiography regardless of scintigraphic findings, and all had 6-month follow-up. Three of 119 patients (2.5%) with negative angiograms were later determined to have PE.

Our search identified no major studies that evaluated conventional angiography against an imaging reference standard.

B. Modality 2: Nuclear Ventilation-Perfusion Imaging

Summary of Evidence: Using imaging reference standards, the sensitivity of normal VQ scan is 98% and the specificity of a high-probability VQ scan is 97%. By both imaging and clinical outcome reference standards, negative predictive values of a normal scan range between 96% and 100%, while positive predictive values of high-probability scans range between 86% and 88%. A VQ scan with a normal result can be used to safely withhold anticoagulation in a patient suspected of PE, and a high probability scan can be used to justify treatment. A high percentage of patients have indeterminate probability, so nondiagnostic scans limit the usefulness of this modality.

Supporting Evidence: One major level II (moderate evidence) study used an imaging reference, though applied nonuniformly, to evaluate the performance of VQ scanning. The 1990 Prospective Investigation of Pulmonary Embolism Diagnosis (PIOPED) study (9) established the convention of reporting VQ scans as normal, low probability, indeterminate, or high probability; 931 patients with a PE prevalence of 27% were studied prospectively, with 731 obtaining both a VQ scan and diagnostic pulmonary angiogram. Based on patients who obtained a pulmonary angiogram, this study established the sensitivity and negative predictive values of a normal VQ scan as 98% and 96%, respectively. The specificity and positive predictive values of a high-probability scan were 97% and 87%, respectively. Of note, 150 patients who had low-probability or normal VQ scans either did not obtain an angiogram or had angiograms with uncertain interpretations. These patients were followed clinically for 1 year, with none experiencing recurrent symptoms of PE. A frequently cited deficit of the PIOPED reporting criteria is that 39% of patients fell into an intermediate probability category, of whom 30% were positive for PE.

Level II (moderate evidence) studies by Hull et al. (10) and van Beek et al. (11) both addressed the risk of withholding anticoagulation in patients with normal perfusion scans in a total of 628 patients who were followed for a minimum of 3 months. Only one of these patients (0.2%) developed symptomatic PE, establishing a negative predictive value of nearly 100%. A level III (limited evidence) study by Rajendran and Jacobson (12) found the 6-month mortality of low-probability lung scans due to PE to be 0%.

However, it is not clear whether anticoagulation was withheld in patients with low-probability scans in this study.

One systematic review by van Beek et al. (13) reported negative and positive predictive values of 99.7% and 88%, respectively.

C. Modality 3: Computed Tomography Pulmonary Angiography (Scanners with Fewer than Four Detectors)

Summary of Evidence: Computed tomography pulmonary angiography (CTPA) is increasingly being used for the diagnosis of PE. Level I (strong evidence) studies using a clinical outcome reference standard find rates of PE recurrence to be 0% to 6%, with negative predictive values of 94% to 100%. Studies using a conventional pulmonary angiography reference standard find broad variations in sensitivities, specificities, and positive and negative predictive values, likely due to variations in detection of subsegmental emboli. Despite these variations, there is strong evidence to show that it is safe to withhold anticoagulation in patients with negative CTPA.

Supporting Evidence: A systematic review of all published literature from 1966 to 2003 (Eng et al., in press) identified eight primary prospective levels I to II (strong to moderate evidence) studies in which all subjects underwent both CTPA and conventional angiography, the latter being considered the reference standard. Among the eight primary studies, the sensitivities ranged from 45% to 100%, and specificities ranged from 78% to 100%.

Nine major studies were found in our search that evaluated the negative predictive value of CTPA using clinical outcomes. One prospective level I (strong evidence) study with a total PE prevalence of 25% followed 378 patients with negative CTPA for 3 months (14). No patients were lost to follow-up, none were anticoagulated during the follow-up period, and no patients were excluded for other reasons. Four of the 378 patients developed PE (recurrence rate = 1%, negative predictive value = 99%). In all studies, recurrence rates ranged from 0% to 6%, and negative predictive values ranged from 94% to 100%. The study with the highest recurrence rate and lowest negative predictive value (level II) followed 81 hospitalized patients from cardiology and pulmonary wards with a PE prevalence of 38%, a majority of whom (82%) had underlying cardiorespiratory disease (15).

D. Modality 4: Multidetector Computed Tomography

Summary of Evidence: Multidetector computed tomography, with higher image acquisition rates than non-MDCT scanners, reduces the rate of respiratory and motion artifacts, particularly in sections obtained during the end of the scan when patients may not be able to maintain apnea, and improves overall spatial resolution. Limited evidence in clinical outcome studies demonstrates that the recurrence rate in patients with MDCT findings negative for PE is 1%, with a negative predictive value of 99%. Although definitive evidence is still forthcoming, it is reasonable to assume the performance of MDCT is at least as good as that of non-MDCT. It is safe, therefore, to withhold anticoagulation in patients with negative MDCT findings.

Supporting Evidence: There have been no major direct comparisons of conventional CTPA with MDCT. While we expect MDCT to be more sensitive for clots, negative predictive values cannot be much improved beyond the 94% to 100% achievable by conventional CTPA with clinical outcome as a reference standard. It is possible that subsegmental clots missed by conventional CTPA may have no clinical significance. The benefit of MDCT over non-MDCT appears to be the reduction in the number of patients with inconclusive scan results.

Two prospective level III (limited evidence) studies were identified in our search evaluating MDCT against a clinical outcome reference standard (16,17). The studies evaluated a total of 236 patients, with PE prevalence of 18% to 19%. Patients were referred for MDCT scanning by clinicians who also had the option to choose other imaging modalities (e.g., nuclear imaging), thus introducing potential selection bias. Both studies reported a PE recurrence rate of 1% and negative predictive value of 99%. In comparison to non-MDCT scan, MDCT scans had fewer respiratory and cardiac motion artifacts, higher rates of interpretation down to subsegmental arterial levels, and fewer inconclusive results (17).

In our search, there were no major systematic reviews of MDCT or articles that evaluated MDCT against an imaging reference standard. A multicenter clinical trial, the PIOPED II sponsored by the National Heart, Lung, and Blood Institute, is currently obtaining data to assess the efficacy of multidetector CT (among other tests) in patients suspected of having acute PE (18).

E. Modality 5: Electron Beam Computed Tomography

Summary of Evidence: Electron beam computed tomography has undergone limited evaluation in the detection of PE, probably because this technology is not widely available. One major level I (strong evidence) study using clinical outcome as a reference standard has shown that it is safe to withhold anticoagulation in patients with negative EBCT findings. When using conventional pulmonary angiography as a reference standard, EBCT has sensitivities and specificities similar to those of CTPA.

Supporting Evidence: A level I (strong evidence) study by Swensen et al. (19) evaluated 993 patients with a PE prevalence of 34% who had negative EBCT findings and were not anticoagulated. At 3-month follow-up, seven patients developed PE or died from PE. No history was available in 19 patients who were known to have lived by the 3-month follow-up period. Recurrence of PE therefore ranged from 0.7% (7/993) to 2.6% [(7 + 19)/993].

One major level III (limited evidence) study evaluated EBCT against a pulmonary angiography reference standard (20). Sixty consecutive patients who had already been referred for conventional pulmonary angiography were imaged with EBCT. In this population with a PE prevalence of 38%, the sensitivity, specificity, and positive predictive and negative predictive values were 65%, 97%, 93%, and 82%, respectively.

There have been no major systematic reviews evaluating EBCT.

F. Modality 6: Magnetic Resonance Angiography

Summary of Evidence: Magnetic resonance angiography has undergone limited evaluation, predominantly in populations referred for conventional pulmonary angiography. There is incomplete evidence to suggest that MRA can be used as the primary imaging modality in the evaluation of PE.

Supporting Evidence: In four level III (limited evidence) studies, patients were selected from a population referred for conventional pulmonary angiography. The oldest study in 1994 (21), with a PE prevalence of 52%, reported problems with identification of pulmonary emboli at the segmental levels. Sensitivity and specificity of MRA in this study were 83% and 100%, respectively. In the remaining three studies performed between 1997 and 2002 (22–24) with PE prevalences ranging from 25% to 36%, problems with identification of PE occurred mostly at the subsegmental levels. Sensitivities and specificities ranged from 77% to 100% and 95% to 98%, respectively. All three studies had at least two readers with interobserver agreement ranging from 57% to 91%, with lower values again noted mostly at subsegmental levels.

In our search, there were no major systematic reviews of MRA, and there were no major studies that evaluated MRA against a clinical outcome reference standard.

G. Modality 7: Ultrasound of Lung and Pleura

Summary of Evidence: Evidence on the use of transthoracic ultrasound imaging of the lung and pleura to diagnose PE is limited. The available data show that this method does not have adequate sensitivity or specificity for the detection sof PE.

Supporting Evidence: One major level II (moderate evidence) study was identified in our search that used ultrasound imaging of the lung and pleura for evaluation of suspected PE against an imaging reference standard (25). Ultrasound diagnosis of PE was made by the identification of (1) wedge-shaped hypoechoic homogeneous pleural-based lesions, or (2) sharply outlined pleural-based lesions with central hyperechoic reflection. Final diagnosis was established by a combination of nuclear lung imaging, clinical probability, CT, lower extremity Doppler ultrasound, and conventional angiography. In this study with a PE prevalence of 42%, the sensitivity, specificity, positive predictive, and negative predictive values were 71%, 77%, 69%, and 79%, respectively.

There were no major systematic reviews of ultrasound in our search, and there were no major studies that evaluated ultrasound against a clinical outcome reference.

H. Method 8: Echocardiography

Summary of Evidence: Studies on the use of transthoracic echocardiography (TTE) have employed various criteria in the evaluation of pulmonary embolism. These include tricuspid regurgitation, right ventricular dilatation, right ventricular dyskinesis, right-sided cardiac thrombus, and flattening of the interventricular septum. Combinations of these criteria have yielded inadequate sensitivities and variable specificities.

Data on the effectiveness of transesophageal echocardiography (TEE) for direct pulmonary thrombus visualization is limited, and this modality also suffers from poor sensitivity and specificity. The limited data on both TTE and TEE show that both modalities are inadequate as a primary imaging modality in the evaluation of PE.

Supporting Evidence: Two level II studies (moderate evidence) and one level III (limited evidence) study were identified in our search that utilized TTE for the diagnosis of PE against an imaging reference standard (26–28). Miniati et al. (28) studied a group of 110 patients with a PE prevalence of 39%. All patients had TTE followed by VQ scan. Conventional angiography was performed when the VQ scan was not normal. Echocardiographic criteria for diagnosis of PE included enlarged right ventricle, tricuspid regurgitation, or right ventricular hypokinesis. Sensitivity, specificity, and positive and negative predictive values were 56%, 90%, 77%, and 76%, respectively. Sensitivities in the other studies ranged from 19% to 52%, and specificities from 87% to 100%.

A level III (limited evidence) study by Steiner et al. (29) utilized TEE and TTE for diagnosis of PE in 35 patients with a PE prevalence of 63%, using helical CT as a reference standard. Pulmonary embolism was diagnosed by visualization of thrombus in the main pulmonary artery, dilatation of the right ventricle or pulmonary artery, tricuspid regurgitation, or abnormal motion of the interventricular septum. Sensitivity, specificity, and positive and negative predictive values were 59%, 77%, 81%, and 53%, respectively.

There were no major systematic reviews of echocardiography in our search, and there were no major studies that evaluated echocardiography against a clinical outcome reference standard.

I. Modality 9: Chest Radiography

Summary of Evidence: There is limited evidence on the use of chest radiography in the evaluation of PE. Various chest radiographic findings are associated with poor sensitivity and only modest specificity. Chest radiography should not be the primary modality in PE evaluation.

Supporting Evidence: In one major level II (moderate evidence) study by Worsley et al. (30), 1063 patients from the PIOPED group who underwent both diagnostic angiography and chest radiography were retrospectively evaluated. Radiographic signs evaluated included prominent central artery (Fleischner sign), enlarged hilum, enlarged mediastinum, pulmonary edema, chronic obstructive pulmonary disease (COPD), oligemia (Westermark sign), vascular redistribution, pleural-based areas of increased opacity (Hampton hump), pleural effusion, and elevated diaphragm. The highest sensitivity obtained was 36% for pleural effusion, and the highest specificity obtained was 96% for COPD. Combinations of the signs were not assessed.

There were no major systematic reviews of chest radiography in our search, and there were no major studies that evaluated chest radiography against a clinical outcome reference standard.

II. How Can Imaging Modalities Be Combined in the Diagnosis of Pulmonary Embolism?

Summary of Evidence: Various proposed strategies have employed combinations of clinical exams, serum D-dimer measurement, lower extremity ultrasound, CTPA, VQ imaging, venography, impedance plethysmography, and conventional pulmonary angiography in the diagnosis of PE. Despite the heterogeneity in test utilization, recurrence rates for venous thromboembolism (VTE) in patients determined to be negative for PE were less than 2% in all major strategies identified. Safety, cost-effectiveness, and availability of resources may help to further differentiate these algorithms, and these issues require further investigation.

Supporting Evidence: Nearly all of the pathway articles identified in our search employed clinical pretest probability in the diagnostic algorithm. We excluded those articles in which clinical pretest probability was not explicitly defined. All six of the major studies identified included a 3-month follow-up on patients who were determined to be negative for PE by the algorithm (31–36), and all had recurrence rates of VTE of less that 2%, although in one study (33), the high percentage of patients who were lost to follow-up may make the reported recurrence rate unreliable. One algorithm by Kruip et al. (34) employed only clinical exam, D-dimer, and lower extremity ultrasound, but with a notably high conventional angiography rate of 63%. Another study by Hull et al. (36) published in 1994 is also less than ideal because it relied on impedance plethysmography, a diagnostic modality that is no longer widely available.

A level I (strong evidence) study by Wells et al. (31) deserves special mention because it most effectively limited the number of patients receiving intravenous contrast, thereby reducing the overall risk of contrast-induced renal insufficiency. The study included 1252 patients with a PE prevalence of 15% who presented with symptoms of PE, had no contraindications to contrast media, and had an expected survival of greater than 3 months. Following clinical assessment, all patients received VQ scans, followed by single or serial lower extremity ultrasound exams (Fig. 22.1). Lower extremity venography or conventional pulmonary angiography was performed in only 2% of patients. Although this algorithm limited the number of contrast examinations, it did so at the expense of a high number of lower extremity ultrasound examinations. An estimated 3093 lower extremity ultrasounds were performed on 1252 patients in this study (2.5 ultrasounds per patient). At most 19 patients (including 13 who were lost to follow-up) out of 1070 who were not anticoagulated by the algorithm developed VTE, equal to a recurrence rate of 1.8%.

A more recent level I (strong evidence) study by Perrier et al. (32) placed greater emphasis on D-dimer measurement and CTPA (D-dimer measurements were not performed in the Wells algorithm). This study involved 965 patients (PE prevalence of 24%) with suspected PE who had no contraindications to CT and who could be followed for 3 months. Following clinical probability assessment (Table 22.1), serum D-dimer was obtained in all patients, and a value less than $500\,\mu g/L$ excluded PE. None of these patients had recurrent VTE on 3-month follow-up. The remaining patients received combinations of venous ultrasound, CTPA, and conventional angiography. Sixty-two percent of patients obtained a contrast study (compared to 2% in the Wells algorithm), and complications from contrast administration were not discussed. However, ultrasound examinations were performed in only 71% of patients (compared to 2.5 ultrasounds per patient in the Wells algorithm). At most 10 patients (including three who were lost to follow-up) out of 685 who were not anticoagulated developed VTE, equivalent to a recurrence rate of 1.5%.

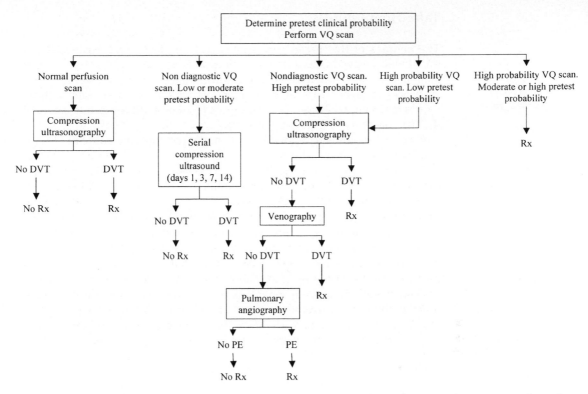

Figure 22.1. Clinical pathway proposed by Wells et al. [*Source:* Wells et al. (31), with permission from the *Annals of Internal Medicine*.]

Table 22.1. Criteria for evaluating the clinical probability of pulmonary embolism (PE) according to Perrier et al. (32)

Variable	Score
Previous PE or deep vein thrombosis	+2
Heart rate >100 beats per minute	+1
Recent surgery	+3
Age (years)	
60–79	+1
≥80	+2
PaCO$_2$	
<4.8 kPa (36 mm Hg)	+2
4.8–5.19 kPa (36–38.9 mm Hg)	+1
PaO$_2$	
<6.5 kPa (48.7 mm Hg)	+4
6.5–7.99 kPa (48.7–59.9 mm Hg)	+3
8–9.49 kPa (60–71.2 mm Hg)	+2
9.5–10.99 kPa (71.3–82.4 mm Hg)	+1
Chest radiograph	
Platelike atelectasis	+1
Elevated hemidiaphragm	+1

Clinical probability according to total score: low, 0 to 4 points; intermediate, 5 to 8 points; high, 9 or more points.

Take-Home Points

The findings of this review are summarized in Table 22.2. Note that the sensitivities, specificities, and positive and negative predictive values shown in the table are derived from studies that range from level I (strong evidence) to level III (limited evidence). Therefore, comparison of these values between imaging modalities must be done with caution because of the heterogeneity in evidence strength.

All of the diagnostic algorithms for suspected PE were associated with similar performances. The algorithm developed by Wells et al. (31) (Fig. 22.1) most effectively limited the use of intravenous contrast. However, the high number of ultrasound examinations and the use of serial compression ultrasound up to 2 weeks following initial presentation challenge the practicality of this approach. Furthermore, although the algorithm may be effective in diagnosing pulmonary embolism, alternative etiologies of the presenting symptoms are more often discovered with CT.

In Figure 22.2, we suggest an algorithm that is a modification of that proposed by Perrier et al. (32). The Perrier et al. algorithm makes use of enzyme-linked immunosorbent assay (ELISA) D-dimer as an initial screen, followed by lower extremity venous ultrasound in all patients with positive D-dimer values. Studies have shown that DVT is unlikely in the absence of the clinical features noted in Table 22.3 (37). In our algorithm,

Table 22.2. Summary of representative performance of various imaging modalities in detection of pulmonary embolism

| Modality | Imaging reference studies | | | | Clinical outcome reference studies |
	Sn (%)	Sp (%)	PPV (%)	NPV (%)	NPV (%)
Angiography	—	—	—	—	95[1]
Nuclear ventilation-perfusion imaging	98[2]	97[3]	86–88[3]	96–100[2]	99.8
Non–multidetector CT pulmonary angiogram	45–100	78–100	60–100	60–100	94–100
Multidetector CT pulmonary angiogram	—	—	—	—	99
Electron beam CT	—	—	—	—	97
MR angiography	—	—	—	—	—
Ultrasound of lung and pleura	71	77	69	79	—
Echocardiography	56	90	77	76	—
Plain film	36[4]	92[5]	38[6]	76[7]	—

[1] Excludes three of the oldest studies, performed between 1978 and 1988.
[2] For a normal scan.
[3] For high-probability scan.
[4] Highest sensitivity obtained using pleural effusion.
[5] Highest specificity obtained using oligemia.
[6] Highest positive predictive value obtained, using oligemia.
[7] Highest negative predictive value obtained, using oligemia, pleural-based areas of increased opacity, pleural effusion, or elevated diaphragm.
Sn, sensitivity; Sp, specificity; PPV, positive predictive value; NPV, negative predictive value.

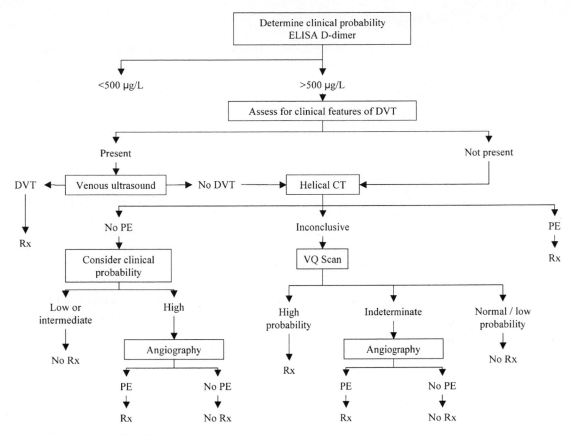

Figure 22.2. Suggested algorithm for evaluation of pulmonary embolism. Refer to Table 22.1 for method of determining clinical probability and Table 23.3 for clinical features of DVT.

we propose that only patients with clinical features of DVT undergo venous ultrasound, followed by CTPA when venous ultrasound is negative. In the absence of clinical features of DVT, we propose that patients immediately undergo CTPA. The remainder of the investigation matches the Perrier et al. algorithm. We feel this approach provides rapid diagnosis of PE and offers the opportunity to identify alternative etiologies for the patients' symptoms through use of chest CT. Overall cost-effectiveness and safety need further study.

Table 22.3. Clinical features of deep venous thrombosis according to Wells et al. (37)

Active cancer (treatment ongoing or within previous 6 months or palliative)
Paralysis, paresis, or recent plaster immobilization of the lower extremities
Recently bedridden for more than 3 days or major surgery within 4 weeks
Localized tenderness along the distribution of the deep venous system
Entire leg swollen
Calf swelling by more than 3 cm when compared with the asymptomatic leg
  (measured 10 cm below tibial tuberosity)
Pitting edema (greater in the symptomatic leg)
Collateral superficial veins (nonvaricose)

Imaging Case Studies

These cases highlight the advantages and limitations of the different imaging modalities.

Case 1

History
A 20-year-old woman with sickle cell trait was diagnosed with right popliteal vein thrombosis. She presents with shortness of breath, fever, and bilateral leg pain.

Imaging
Multiple planar perfusion images demonstrate decreased perfusion to the left lung (Fig. 22.3A). Ventilation images demonstrate normal ventilation to both lungs (Fig. 22.3B). These findings suggest central left-sided pulmonary emboli or a mass compressing the left main pulmonary artery. The CTPA demonstrates bilateral pulmonary emboli (Fig. 22.3C).

Discussion
This case demonstrates an instance in which both nuclear ventilation-perfusion imaging and CTPA detected evidence of pulmonary emboli necessitating treatment. However, it is notable that CTPA detected emboli in the right lung, where perfusion imaging was interpreted as normal.

Case 2

History
A 41-year-old woman has an extensive vascular history and DVT in both lower extremities. She presents with pleuritic chest pain and shortness of breath.

Imaging
Multiple planar perfusion images demonstrate heterogeneous activity throughout both lungs with large perfusion defects in the basal segments of both lower lobes (Fig. 22.4A). Additional small perfusion defects are seen in the right and left apices. The perfusion defects in the lower lobes do not correspond to any defects in ventilation imaging (not shown). These findings led to an interpretation of a high probability for pulmonary embolism. Findings on perfusion imaging also include abnormal activity in the liver, raising the suspicion for collateral circulation and vascular shunting. The CTPA demonstrates occlusion of the superior vena cava (Fig. 22.4B) and multiple collateral vessels around the liver (Fig. 22.4C). No pulmonary emboli were identified on CTPA.

Discussion
This case demonstrates an instance in which nuclear ventilation-perfusion imaging findings and CTPA findings are discordant. The CTPA detected occlusion of the superior vena cava with collateral vessels around the liver that were suggested by VQ scanning. The patient received anticoagulation therapy based on VQ findings without further imaging.

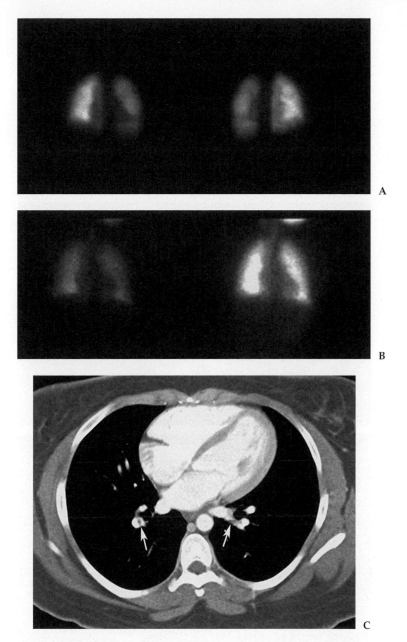

Figure 22.3. A: Anterior and posterior technetium 99m (Tc-99m) macroaggregated albumin (MAA) planar perfusion images demonstrate decreased perfusion to the left lung. B: Anterior single-breath and equilibrium-phase ^{133}Xe ventilation images in same patient demonstrate normal ventilation to both lungs. In combination with perfusion imaging, these findings led to an interpretation of high probability for pulmonary embolism. C: The CTPA demonstrates filling defects in right and left pulmonary arteries (arrows) consistent with pulmonary emboli.

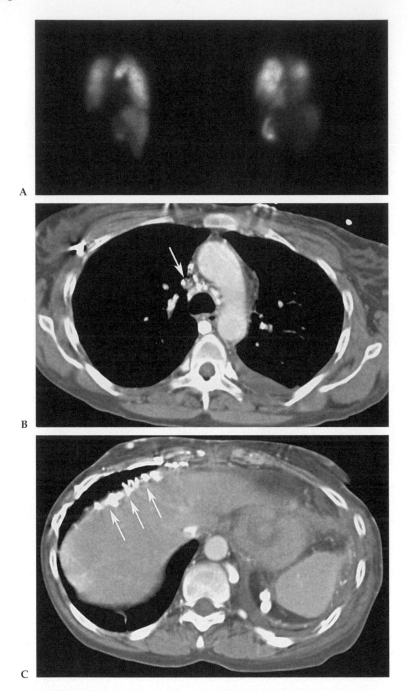

Figure 22.4. A: Right and left posterior oblique Tc-99m MAA planar perfusion images demonstrate heterogeneous activity in both lungs with large perfusion defects in the basal segments of both lower lobes. Additional perfusion defects are seen in the apices. Ventilation imaging (not shown) demonstrated no corresponding defects, which led to an interpretation of high probability for pulmonary embolism. There is abnormal activity in the liver, suggesting collateral circulation and vascular shunting. B: The CTPA in the same patient demonstrates occlusion of the superior vena cava (arrow). In discordance with the VQ scan findings, no evidence of PE was identified on CTPA. C: CTPA in the same patient demonstrates multiple perihepatic collateral vessels (arrows), explaining the abnormal liver activity present in the perfusion scan.

Protocols Based on the Evidence

The following protocols are employed at Johns Hopkins Hospital based on a literature review and clinical experience.

A. Ventilation/Perfusion Imaging

Ventilation imaging is performed prior to perfusion. After the patient takes one or two normal breaths through a mask, 10 to 30 mCi (370–1110 MBq) of ^{133}Xe gas is introduced into the mask at end expiration. Images are obtained in anterior and posterior projections on a 128×128 matrix using a parallel-hole collimator centered at 80 keV. A single breath image is first obtained for 100,000 counts. Equilibrium images are obtained for 300,000 counts after the patient breathes normally in the closed system for 3 minutes. After obtaining three 5-second pre-washout images, the system is placed in washout phase, and twelve 5-second washout images are obtained, followed by four 1-minute delayed washout images.

Perfusion imaging is performed after intravenous injection of 4 mCi (111 MBq) of technetium 99m Tc-99m macroaggregated albumin (MAA). Images are obtained in the posterior, right and left posterior oblique, right and left lateral, right and left anterior oblique, and anterior projections. All images are obtained for a minimum of 600,000 counts on a 256×256 matrix using a parallel hole collimator centered at 140 keV.

B. Computed Tomography Pulmonary Angiography

Computed tomography pulmonary angiography (CTPA) is performed with an intravenous injection of 100 to 120 cc nonionic iodinated contrast agent at a rate of 3 to 4 cc/sec. The scan is performed from the lung apices to bases after a 23- to 28-second delay at 120 kV, 0.5-second rotation time, and 1- to 2-mm slice thickness. The mA·s varies according to scanner manufacturer.

Acknowledgments: The authors would like to give special thanks to Marge Sturgill and Christine Simmons for helping to obtain the many references used in writing this paper.

Future Research

- Assess the clinical significance of subsegmental emboli.
- Determine the performance of CTPA in the detection of PE, with attention to the benefits of MDCT over non-MDCT and safety. The PIOPED II study will address some of these important questions.
- Determine the performance and role of MRA in detection of PE.
- Further develop diagnostic algorithms that can adequately exclude PE while being safe and cost-effective.
- Clarify the role of imaging relative to other types of diagnostic tests.

References

1. Goldhaber SZ. Semin Vasc Med 2001;1:139–146.
2. Anderson FA, Wheeler HB, Goldberg RJ, et al. Arch Intern Med 1991;151: 933–938.

3. Oger E. Throm Haemost 2000;83:657–660.
4. Caprini JA, Botteman MF, Stephens JM, et al. Value Health 2003;6:59–74.
5. Nilsson T, Turen J, Billstrom A, Mare K, Carlsson A, Nyman U. Eur Radiol 1999; 9(2):276–280.
6. van Beek EJ, Brouwerst EM, Song B, Stein PD, Oudkerk M. Clin Radiol 2001; 56(10):838–842.
7. van Beek EJ, Reekers JA, Batchelor DA, Brandjes DP, Buller HR. Eur Radiol 1996; 6(4):415–419.
8. van Rooij WJ, den Heeten GJ, Sluzewski M. Radiology 1995;195(3):793–797.
9. The PIOPED Investigators. JAMA 1990;263(20):2753–2759.
10. Hull RD, Raskob GE, Coates G, Panju AA. Chest 1990;97(1):23–26.
11. van Beek EJ, Kuyer PM, Schenk BE, Brandjes DP, ten Cate JW, Buller HR. Chest 1995;108(1):170–173.
12. Rajendran JG, Jacobson AF. Arch Intern Med 1999;159(4):349–352.
13. van Beek EJ, Brouwers EM, Song B, Bongaerts AH, Oudkerk M. Clin Appl Thromb Hemost 2001;7(2):87–92.
14. van Strijen MJ, de Monye W, Schiereck J, et al. Ann Intern Med 2003; 138(4):307–314.
15. Bourriot K, Couffinhal T, Bernard V, Montaudon M, Bonnet J, Laurent F. Chest 2003;123(2):359–365.
16. Kavanagh EC, O'Hare A, Hargaden G, Murray JG. AJR 2004;182(2):499–504.
17. Remy-Jardin M, Tillie-Leblond I, Szapiro D, et al. Eur Radiol 2002;12(8):1971–1978.
18. Gottschalk A, Stein PD, Goodman LR, Sostman HD. Semin Nucl Med 2002; 32:173–182.
19. Swensen SJ, Sheedy PF 2nd, Ryu JH, et al. Mayo Clin Proc 2002;77(2):130–138.
20. Teigen CL, Maus TP, Sheedy PF 2nd, et al. Radiology 1995;194(2):313–319.
21. Loubeyre P, Revel D, Douek P, et al. AJR 1994;162(5):1035–1039.
22. Meaney JF, Weg JG, Chenevert TL, Stafford-Johnson D, Hamilton BH, Prince MR. N Engl J Med 1997;336(20):1422–1427.
23. Gupta A, Frazer CK, Ferguson JM, et al. Radiology 1999;210(2):353–359.
24. Oudkerk M, van Beek EJ, Wielopolski P, et al. Lancet 2002;359(9318):1643–1647.
25. Mohn K, Quiot JJ, Nonent M, et al. J Ultrasound Med 2003;22(7):673–678; quiz 680–681.
26. Bova C, Greco F, Misuraca G, et al. Am J Emerg Med 2003;21(3):180–183.
27. Kurzyna M, Torbicki A, Pruszczyk P, et al. Am J Cardiol 2002;90(5):507–511.
28. Miniati M, Monti S, Pratali L, et al. Am J Med 2001;110(7):528–535.
29. Steiner P, Lund GK, Debatin JF, et al. AJR 1996;167(4):931–936.
30. Worsley DF, Alavi A, Aronchick JM, Chen JT, Greenspan RH, Ravin CE. Radiology 1993;189(1):133–136.
31. Wells PS, Ginsberg JS, Anderson DR, et al. Ann Intern Med 1998;129(12):997–1005.
32. Perrier A, Roy PM, Aujesky D, et al. Am J Med 2004;116(5):291–299.
33. Lorut C, Ghossains M, Horellou MH, Achkar A, Fretault J, Laaban JP. Am J Respir Crit Care Med 2000;162(4 pt 1):1413–1418.
34. Kruip MJ, Slob MJ, Schijen JH, van der Heul C, Buller HR. Arch Intern Med 2002;162(14):1631–1635.
35. Leclercq MG, Lutisan JG, van Marwijk Kooy M, et al. Thromb Haemost 2003; 89(1):97–103.
36. Hull RD, Raskob GE, Ginsberg JS, et al. Arch Intern Med 1994;154(3):289–297.
37. Wells PS, Anderson DR, Bormanis J, et al. Lancet 1997;350(9094):1795–1798.

23

Imaging of the Solitary Pulmonary Nodule

Anil Kumar Attili and Ella A. Kazerooni

Key Points

- Further evaluation of a solitary pulmonary nodule (SPN) incidentally detected on chest radiography is not needed when either of the following two criteria (moderate evidence) are met:
  - Nodule is stable in size for at least 2 years when compared to prior chest radiographs.
  - There is a benign pattern of calcification demonstrated on chest radiography.
- Further evaluation of a pulmonary nodule showing a benign pattern of calcification, fat, or stability for 2 years or more on thin-section computed tomography (CT) is not needed (moderate evidence).

- In the absence of benign calcification, fat, or documented radiographic stability for at least 2 years, the choice of subsequent imaging strategy to differentiate between benign and malignant nodules is critically dependent on the pretest probability of malignancy.
  - Computed tomography should be the initial test for most patients with radiographically indeterminate pulmonary nodules (moderate evidence).
  - 18-Fluorodeoxyglucose positron emission tomography ([18]FDG-PET) has a high sensitivity and specificity for malignancy (strong evidence), and is most cost-effective when used selectively in patients where the CT findings and pretest probability of malignancy are discordant.
- The use of multidetector CT (MDCT) scanners with improved spatial resolution for lung cancer screening has led to the increased detection of small (<1 cm) pulmonary nodules. Nodules are categorized on CT as (1) solid, (2) part-solid (mixed solid and ground-glass attenuation), or (3) non-solid (pure ground-glass attenuation).
- The imaging strategy for the further evaluation of small solid pulmonary nodules in the absence of a known primary malignancy is based on nodule diameter (moderate evidence).
  - For solid nodules 4 to 10 mm in diameter, a strategy of careful observation with serial thin-section CT scanning is recommended at 6, 12, and 24 months. In patients with a known primary neoplasm, initial reevaluation at 3 months is recommended.
  - For solid nodules larger than 10 mm in diameter, further evaluation with [18]FDG-PET, percutaneous needle biopsy, or video-assisted thoracoscopic surgery (VATS) is recommended.
- Part-solid nodules (solid and ground-glass components) and non-solid nodules (pure ground glass) detected at lung cancer screening have a higher likelihood of malignancy than solid nodules; therefore, tissue sampling (percutaneous CT-guided biopsy or VATS) is recommended (moderate evidence). For nodules less than 1 cm where this may not be possible, close serial CT evaluation at 3-month intervals in recommended.

Definition and Pathophysiology

Fleischner Society nomenclature defines nodule as "any pulmonary or pleural lesion represented in a radiograph by a sharply defined, discrete, nearly circular opacity 2 to 30 mm in diameter" and should always be qualified with respect to "size, location, border characteristics, number and opacity." A mass is defined as any similar lesion "that is greater than 30 mm in diameter (without regard to contour, border characteristics, or homogeneity), but explicitly shown or presumed to be extended in all three dimensions" (1). The differential diagnosis for an SPN is extensive, as listed in Table 23.1.

Epidemiology

An SPN may be found on 0.09% to 0.20% of all chest radiographs (2,3). With the advent of CT scanning and screening for lung cancer, the discovery of SPNs has increased. From lung cancer screening studies, 23% to

Table 23.1. Differential diagnosis of a solitary pulmonary nodule

Neoplastic	*Malignant*	Primary bronchogenic carcinoma
		Pulmonary lymphoma
		Carcinoid tumor
		Metastasis
		Chondrosarcoma
		Pulmonary blastoma
		Hemangiopericytoma
		Epithelioid hemangioendothelioma
	Benign	Hamartoma
		Chondroma
		Teratoma
		Hemangioma
		Lipoma
		Leiomyoma
		Endometriosis
		Neurofibroma and neurilemmoma
		Benign clear cell tumor
		Chemodectoma
Infectious		Granuloma (tuberculosis, histoplasmosis)
		Parasites (hydatid)
		Round pneumonia
		Lung abscess
Inflammatory		Rheumatoid arthritis
		Wegener's granulomatosis
		Sarcoidosis
		Intrapulmonary lymph node
		Inflammatory pseudotumor (synonym: plasma cell granuloma)
Vascular		Arteriovenous malformation
		Hematoma
		Pulmonary infarct
Developmental		Bronchial atresia
		Bronchogenic cyst
		Sequestration

51% of cigarette smokers over 50 years of age will have at least one SPN detected on screening CT (4,5). The reported incidence of malignancy in SPNs varies from 5% to 69% (6–9). This wide range in part depends on the modality used for detection and the characteristics of the patient population studied. Compared to chest x-ray (CXR), low-dose helical CT detects three to four times more nodules, the majority of which are benign (5,10). Large-scale screening studies with CXR report a 5% to 10% incidence of malignancy in SPNs, versus less than 1% rate of malignancy in CT screening trials (5). In comparison, the incidence of malignancy in SPNs taken from series of surgically resected nodules is higher, due to selection bias and the high pretest probability of cancer in patients undergoing surgery (8,9,11). For nonselected adult populations, a new SPN on CXR has a 20% to 40% likelihood of being malignant (12–14). Infectious granulomas are responsible for approximately 80% of benign SPNs, and hamartomas approximately 10% (15,16).

Overall Cost to Society

See Chapter 4 for the overall cost of lung cancer to society. A review of the literature reveals no information on the cost of evaluation of SPNs. In many ways, this subject is a moving target. As more nodules are detected with evolving MDCT scanners using thinner and thinner collimation, there are more and more nodules to evaluate. The majority of these nodules are too small to evaluate with PET scan or biopsy, leaving them to serial CT follow-up for at least 2 years to document stability as an indicator of benign biologic behavior. Needless to say, detecting and then following more nodules increases the total cost to society.

Goals

The goal for the imaging evaluation of an SPN is to accurately distinguish benign nodules from malignant nodules, enabling resection of malignant nodules without undue delay and avoiding exploratory thoracotomy, percutaneous biopsy, or additional testing such as CT or PET scanning, for patients with benign nodules.

Methodology

A Medline search was performed using PubMed (National Library of Medicine, Bethesda, Maryland) for original research publications discussing the diagnostic performance and effectiveness of imaging strategies in the evaluation of an SPN. The search covered the period 1966 to May 2004. The search terms were also entered into a Google search. The search strategy employed different combinations of the following subject headings and terms: (1) *coin lesion, pulmonary,* or *solitary pulmonary nodule*; (2) *lung neoplasms* or *lung cancer*; (3) *mass screening* or *lung cancer screening*; (4) *costs* and *cost analysis*; (5) *cost-benefit analysis,* (6) *socioeconomic factors,* (7) *incidence,* (8) *radiography* or *imaging* or *tomography, x-ray computed* or *tomography, emission-computed* or *tomography, emission-computed, single-photon* or *magnetic resonance imaging.* Additional articles were identified by reviewing the reference list of relevant papers. The review was limited to the English-language literature. The authors performed an initial review of the titles and abstracts of the identified articles followed by review of the full text in articles that were identified.

I. Who Should Undergo Imaging?

Summary of Evidence: Pulmonary nodules are commonly discovered incidentally on chest radiographs or CT examinations. There are four imaging findings that are highly predictive of benignity. If one or more of these four features is identified, no further diagnostic evaluation is required. If there is doubt on CXR about the presence of these findings, CT should be performed for better anatomic resolution.

1. Nodule calcification on CXR or CT that is either central, diffuse, popcorn or laminar (concentric rings) (Fig. 23.1).
2. Fat within a nodule on CT is highly specific for hamartoma (Fig. 23.2).
3. A feeding artery and draining vein indicate an arteriovenous malformation.
4. A pleural-based opacity with in-curving bronchovascular bundles associated with adjacent pleural thickening or effusion is a characteristic of rounded atelectasis (comet tail sign).

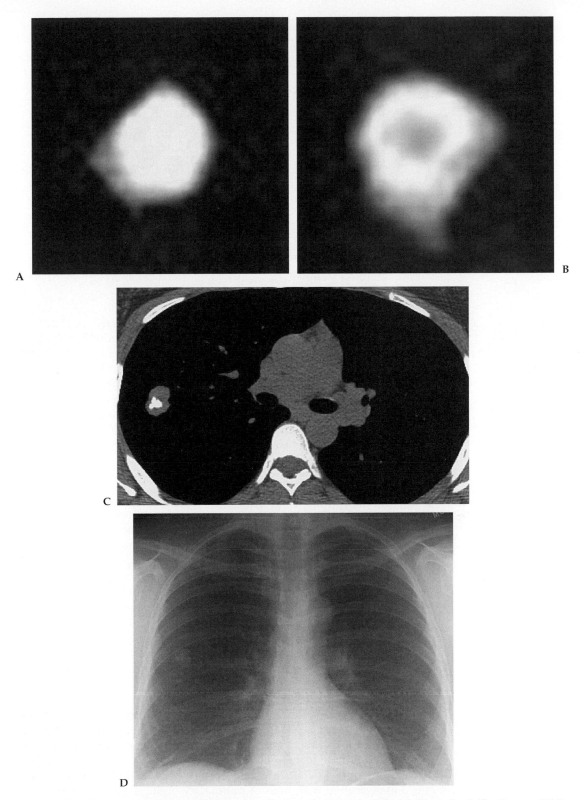

Figure 23.1. Benign patterns of calcification in solitary pulmonary nodules. A: Central calcification on CT. B: Target or concentric calcification on CT. C: Popcorn pattern in a hamartoma on CT. D: Chest x-ray.

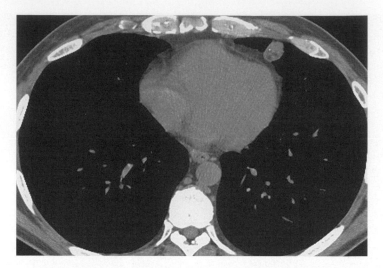

Figure 23.2. Hamartoma with both calcification and fat on CT.

Stability on CXRs for 2 years or more has been considered an indicator of benignity. This is based on retrospective case series in which surgical resection was performed. A recent reevaluation of the original data shows that the 2-year stability criterion on CXR has a predictive value of only 65% for benignity, limiting the use of this criterion; 10% to 20% of small or subtle lesions interpreted as possible SPNs on CXRs do not actually represent SPNs, but rather lesions in the ribs, pleura, or chest wall or artifacts. When there is doubt about the presence of a nodule on CXR, further imaging is required.

Supporting Evidence

A. Nodule Stability in Size

An imperative step in determining the significance of an SPN is determining how long the nodule has been present. The widely accepted radiographic criterion for identifying nodules as benign is stability for 2 years or more. The evidence on which this is based was reanalyzed by Yankelevitz and Henschke (17), who traced the concept to articles by Good and Wilson (18). These include retrospective reviews of 1355 patients who underwent surgical lung resection between 1940 and 1951. Using no growth on chest radiographs has only a 65% positive predictive value for benignity, with sensitivity of 40% and specificity of 72%. In view of these retrospective studies and bias only for nodules undergoing resection in the pre-CT era, this constitutes only limited evidence for 2 years or longer stability in size as a marker of benignity.

Fundamental to nodule stability is the concept of tumor doubling time. Collins et al. (19) advanced the theory of exponential tumor growth from a single cell, providing a methodology for predicting growth rates of human tumors that were previously evaluated only in animal models (20,21). Nathan et al. (22), in a level II (moderate evidence) study, determined malignant growth rates of pulmonary nodules using Collins exponential equations; their predictions were verified in several subsequent using CXR studies (23–25). Malignant nodules had a volume doubling time of 30 to 490 days. Lesions that doubled more rapidly were usually infection, and nodules with a slower doubling time are usually benign. Two-year stability implies a doubling time of well more than 730 days (26). Using the stability criterion assumes nodule diameter can be accurately measured on CXR; however, the limit of detectable change in size with CXR is 3 to 5 mm; smaller changes are better evaluated with thin-section CT, with a 0.3-mm lower limit of resolution. However, even using thin-section CT, human observers measuring small nodules (<5 mm) are prone to inter- and intraobserver variation (27).

Recently, calculating volumetric tumor growth rate from serial CT examinations has been investigated in a small number of retrospective level II (moderate evidence) studies (28,29). Volumetric CT measurements are highly accurate for determining lung nodule volume, and useful to evaluate growth rate of small nodules by calculating nodule doubling time (30). Winer-Muram et al. (28) in a level II (moderate evidence) retrospective study evaluated CT volumetric growth of untreated stage I lung cancers in 50 patients. The median doubling time was 181 days (ranging from unchanged to 32 days). Of note, 11 lung cancers (22%) had a doubling time of 465 days or more. A wide variability in tumor doubling times was also demonstrated by Aoki et al. (31) in a retrospective level II (moderate evidence) CT study of peripheral lung adenocarcinomas. The group of nodules appearing as focal ground-glass opacity grew slowly (doubling time mean 2.4 years, range 42 to 1486 days), while the group of solid nodules grew more quickly (doubling time mean 0.7 years, range 124 to 402 days).

Stability as an indicator of a benign process precluding further evaluation requires accurate measurement of growth using reproducible high-resolution imaging techniques. The CXR dictum of 2-year stability indicating a benign process should be used with caution. Every effort should be made to obtain prior comparison examinations, preferably from at least 2 years earlier. Stability of a nodule for 2 years on thin-section CT may be a more reasonable guideline for predicting benignity.

B. Nodule Morphology: Calcification

Several morphologic features can be used to indicate benignity with a high degree of specificity. The first is identifying a benign pattern of calcification. In an early case series of 156 SPNs surgically resected between 1940 and 1951, Good et al. (32) found no calcification on chest radiographs in any of the malignant lesions. Subsequently, O'Keefe et al. (33), in a 1957 level II (moderate evidence) study, performed careful analysis of the specimen radiographs from 207 resected pulmonary nodules. Calcification was found histologically in 49.6% of the benign nodules and 13.9% of the malignant nodules. The patterns of diffuse, central, laminated, and popcorn calcification were only found in the benign pulmonary nodules. Eccentric calcifications were found both in malignant (Fig. 23.3) and benign nodules (34). Calcification in primary bronchogenic carcinomas is usually amorphous or stippled (35,36). A later large case series demonstrated a popcorn pattern of calcification in one third of hamartomas.

Berger et al. (37) in a level II (moderate evidence) study evaluated the effectiveness of standard chest radiographs for detecting calcification in

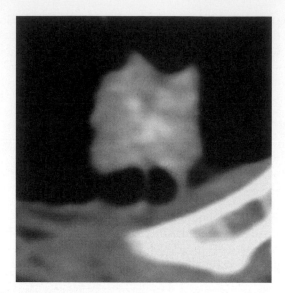

Figure 23.3. Indeterminate pattern of calcification for malignancy in a solitary pulmonary nodule in a histologically proven carcinoid tumor.

SPNs, using thin-section CT (1.5- to 3-mm slice thickness) as the reference standard. Chest radiographs were 50% sensitive and 87% specific for detecting any calcification, with a positive predictive value of 93%. The overall ability of CXR to detect calcification of any kind in SPNs is low. The superiority of CT for detecting calcification that is occult on CXR has been shown in several subsequent level II (moderate evidence) studies (8,38,39). These will be discussed further in the following section.

Without documentation of radiographic stability for a noncalcified pulmonary nodule detected on CXR, there should be a very low threshold for recommending further imaging with CT for these indeterminate pulmonary nodules.

C. Nodule Morphology: Fat

For nodules detected incidentally on CT, the additional finding of intranodular fat is a highly specific indicator of a hamartoma, a benign lung tumor. Fat may be found on CT in up to 50% of pulmonary hamartomas, and when present negates the need for further evaluation. In a prospective level II (moderate evidence) study of 47 hamartomas (31 pathology proven, 16 presumed by serial follow-up CT examinations) with thin-section CT, the correct diagnosis of hamartoma could be made based on the detection of fat alone in 18 nodules, and by the presence of fat and calcification in 12 nodules; together, this represented 69% of the hamartomas studied (40).

D. Nodule Morphology: Feeding Artery and Draining Vein

The third morphologic feature that indicates a benign nodule with a high degree of specificity is the presence of a feeding artery and a draining vein. While occasionally seen on chest radiographs, it is more easily seen on contrast-enhanced CT, and is a very reliable indicator of an arteriovenous malformation (41). No further noninvasive imaging to prove this diagnosis is required (strong evidence).

E. Nodule Morphology: Rounded Atelectasis

Rounded atelectasis is atelectasis of a peripheral part of the lung due to pleural adhesions and fibrosis, causing deformation of the lung and inward bending of adjacent bronchi and blood vessels, known as the "comet tail sign." It occurs in a variety of pleural abnormalities, but is typically associated with asbestos exposure and asbestos-related pleural plaques. In one series, 86% of cases were associated with asbestos exposure (42). To suggest the diagnosis of rounded atelectasis on thin-section CT, the opacity should be (1) round or oval in shape, (2) subpleural in location, (3) associated with curving of pulmonary vessels or bronchi into the edge of the lesion (comet tail sign), and (4) associated with ipsilateral pleural abnormality either effusion or pleural thickening.

Rounded atelectasis may show significant enhancement after the injection of intravenous contrast agents (43). If the criteria for rounded atelectasis listed above are met, a confident diagnosis can usually be made (42). No further invasive imaging is necessary (moderate evidence). However, if there is any question about the findings, follow-up serial CT examinations are recommended.

F. Applicability to Children

The evidence to determine who should undergo imaging is less complete in children than in adults. The vast majority of pulmonary nodules and masses in children are benign. Pneumonia may present as a spherical nodule or mass in children, referred to as round pneumonia. Clinical features and prompt response to antibiotic treatment serve to differentiate round pneumonia from malignancy (44). Most pediatric nodular disease is granulomatous in origin (45). Infections and congenital lesions in children together outnumber neoplastic lesions. Pulmonary metastases in children are most often secondary to Wilms' tumor, followed in frequency by sarcomas (45). Primary pulmonary malignancy is rare.

II. Which Imaging Is Appropriate?

Summary of Evidence: Management strategies for an SPN are highly dependent on the pretest probability of malignancy. The strategies include observation, resection, and biopsy. A CT should be the initial test in most patients with a new radiographically detected indeterminate SPN. Advances in technology have improved the ability to differentiate benign and malignant nodules using nodule perfusion and metabolic characteristics, as can be evaluated with intravenous contrast enhanced CT, [18]FDG-PET, and single photon emission computed tomography (SPECT); [18]FDG-PET should be selectively used when the pretest probability and CT probability of malignancy are discordant. If the pretest probability of malignancy after CT is high, [18]FDG-PET is not cost-effective. Recommendations for the use of CT, PET, watchful waiting, transthoracic needle biopsy, and surgery in the evaluation of an indeterminate SPN are shown in Table 23.2. The diagnostic algorithm for the SPN is detailed in Figure 23.4.

Supporting Evidence: The limited ability of CXR to distinguish between benign and malignant SPNs has prompted development of CT-based techniques for noninvasive assessment. Computed tomography is more accurate than CXR in determining where an abnormality is located in the lungs, and if it is in the lung, CT optimally evaluates the morphologic characteristics of the nodule. Several different CT techniques for the evaluation of SPNs have been described including, thin-section CT, CT densitometry, dual-energy CT, and CT nodule enhancement studies.

A. Computed Tomography Densitometry

In the mid-1980s the use of a representative CT number and a reference phantom, known as CT densitometry, was applied to CT to improve its accuracy for the detection of calcification. A large multi-institutional level II (moderate evidence) study of 384 visibly noncalcified nodules on conventional thick-section nonhelical CT used CT nodule densitometry with 264 Hounsfield units (HU) or more to classify a nodule as benign (9). In

Table 23.2. Recommendations for the use of computed tomography, positron emission tomography, watchful waiting, transthoracic needle biopsy, and surgery in the evaluation of an indeterminate solitary pulmonary nodule.

Intervention	Indications
CT	When pretest probability is <90%
[18]FDG-PET	• When pretest probability is low (10–50%) and CT results are indeterminate (possibly malignant) • When pretest probability is high (77–89%) and CT results are benign • When surgical risk is high, pretest probability is low to intermediate (65%), and CT results are possibly malignant • When CT results suggest a benign cause and the probability of nondiagnostic biopsy is high, or the patient is uncomfortable with a strategy of watchful waiting
Watchful waiting	• In patients with very small, radiographically indeterminate nodules (<10 mm in diameter) • When the pretest probability is very low (<2%) or when pretest probability is low (<15%) and [18]FDG-PET results are negative • When pretest probability is low (<35%) and CT results are benign • When needle biopsy is nondiagnostic in patients who have benign findings on CT or negative findings on [18]FDG-PET
Percutaneous transthoracic needle aspiration/biopsy	• When [18]FDG-PET results are positive and surgical risk or aversion to the risk of surgery is high • When pretest probability is low (20–45%) and [18]FDG-PET results are negative • When pretest probability is intermediate (30–70%) and CT results are benign
Surgery	• When pretest probability is high and CT results are indeterminate (possibly malignant) • When [18]FDG -PET results are positive • As the initial intervention when pretest probability is very high (>90%)

Source: Adapted from Gould et al. (86), with permission.

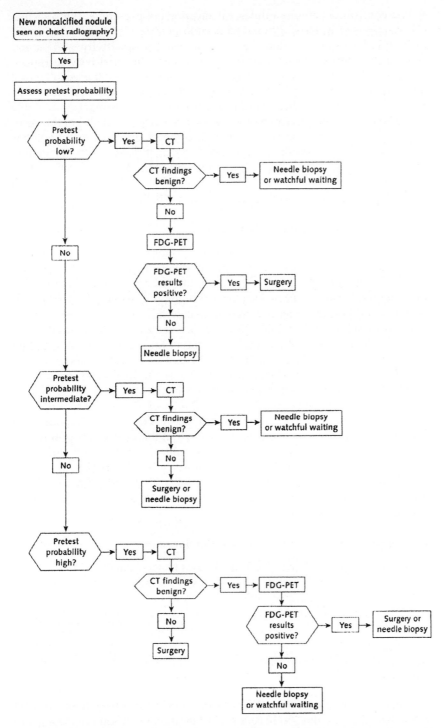

Figure 23.4. Suggested algorithm for clinical management of patients with SPNs and average risk of surgical complications. [*Source*: Gould et al. (86), with permission.]

the 118 confirmed benign nodules, calcification not present on thick-section CT was present in an additional 65 nodules, either visibly ($n = 28$) on CT or by CT densitometry alone ($n = 37$), yielding a sensitivity of 55% and specificity of 99% for identifying benign nodules. The sensitivity and specificity of this technique for benign disease depends on the cutoff point above which benign nodules are diagnosed and scanner calibration. The results of different studies using this technique are summarized in Table 23.3. The overall sensitivity (50–63%) and specificity (78–100%) of this technique for benign disease is variable, not optimal, and this technique has fallen out of favor. While a high specificity of 99% to 100% for benign disease has been reported using this technique in study samples with a high prevalence of malignancy (8,9,38), lower specificity, 78%, is reported when the prevalence of malignancy is lower (46).

B. Thin-Section Computed Tomography

Visual inspection of thin-section CT images is more accurate than CXR for identifying calcification in pulmonary nodules. Thin-section CT enables more accurate differentiation of benign from malignant nodules through a more detailed assessment of nodule morphology. However, the application of different criteria for identifying malignancy, as illustrated by the studies detailed in below and in Table 23.4, yields different sensitivity and specificity for identifying malignancy. For example, Takanashi et al. (47) studied thin-section CT for the evaluation of SPNs. This level II (moderate evidence) prospective study demonstrated 56% sensitivity and 93% specificity for identifying malignancy. Seemann et al. (48) in a level I (strong evidence) prospective study achieved a higher sensitivity of 91% at the sacrifice of a lower specificity of 57% by applying different criteria. In both studies the prevalence of malignancy was higher (53–78%) than a general population of indeterminate SPNs detected on radiography. In a comparative prospective level I (strong evidence) study of thin-section CT versus helical CT at 8-mm collimation, malignant SPNs were identified with 88% sensitivity and 60.9% specificity on helical CT, versus 91.4% sensitivity and 56.5% specificity on thin-section CT (49).

C. Computed Tomography Contrast Enhancement

Dynamic contrast-enhanced CT uses nodule vascularity to distinguish between benign and malignant nodules. Malignancies are thought to enhance more than benign nodules due to tumor neovascularity. In a multi-institutional level II (moderate evidence) prospective study, the absence of significant lung nodule enhancement ($\leq 15\,HU$) on a CT enhancement study was strongly predictive of benignity (50). On nonenhanced, thin-section CT, the 356 solid, relatively spherical nodules studied measured 5 to 40 mm in diameter, and were homogeneously of soft tissue attenuation without visible calcification or fat on CT. The CT images at 3-mm collimation were obtained before and at 1, 2, 3, and 4 minutes after intravenous contrast administration. Of the 356 nodules, 171 (48%) were malignant. Malignant nodules enhanced a median of 38.1 HU (range 14.0 to 165.3 HU), while granulomas and benign neoplasms enhanced a median of 10 HU (range −20 to 96 HU; $p < .001$). Using 15 HU or more of enhancement from baseline as the threshold, the technique was 98% sensitive and 58% specific for identifying malignancy, with a negative predictive value of 96%. The

Table 23.3. Investigations of computed tomography densitometry for the evaluation of solitary pulmonary nodules

Study, year (reference)	No. of subjects	No. of nodules or masses	Lesion diameter (cm)	Prevalence of malignancy (%)	Reference test	Definition of a positive test	Sensitivity for benign disease (%)	Specificity for benign disease (%)
Zerhouni et al., 1986 (9)	384	295	<6.0	60	Tissue diagnosis 207; observation >18–30 months in 195	Greater than reference phantom	55	99
Siegelman et al., 1986 (8)	720	634	Any size (564 nodules >3.0)	56	Tissue diagnosis 367; observation >2 years in 195; NS in 72	>164 HU; <2.5 cm with smooth edge	63	100
Proto et al., 1985 (38)	218	177	0.6–4.5	54	Observation 15–24 months 14; tissue diagnosis 111; observation >22 months 52; calcification on chest radiographs in 14	>200 HU	54	99
Khan et al., 1991 (46)	75	62	Any size (59 nodules <2.0)	15	Tissue diagnosis in 20; observation >2 years in 42	NS	58	78

NS, not specified.

Table 23.4. Investigations of thin-section CT for the evaluation of solitary pulmonary nodules

Study, year (reference)	No. of subjects	No. of lung nodules	Prevalence of malignancy	Reference test	Definition of a positive result (malignancy)	Sensitivity for malignancy (%)	Specificity for malignancy (%)
Takanashi et al., 1995 (47)	60	60	53	Bronchoscopy or surgery	Three or more of the following: irregular margin, spiculation, convergence, air bronchogram, >3 vessels involved	56 (18/32)	93 (26/28)
Seemann et al., 1999 (92)	104	104	78	Surgical resection	Any one of the following: pleural retraction or thickening, bronchus sign, vessel sign, ground glass, spiculation with or with extension to visceral pleura	91 (74/81)	57 (13/23)

Table 23.5. Studies of dynamic computed tomography lung nodule enhancement

Study, year (reference)	No. of nodules or masses	Prevalence of malignancy (%)	Reference test	Definition of a positive test (malignancy)	Sensitivity for malignancy (%)	Specificity for malignancy (%)
Swensen et al., 2000 (50)	356	48	Tissue diagnosis 237 Observation 119	Enhancement ≥15 HU	98	58
Yamashita et al., 1995 (93)	32	56	Surgical resection or biopsy	Enhancement ≥20 HU	100	93
Potente et al., 1997 (94)	40	25	68	Thoracotomy 18 Needle biopsy 6	100	75

results of this prospective study corroborate earlier, smaller case series, as summarized in Table 23.5 (50–52).

Several potential practical limitations exist to the widespread clinical application of the CT nodule enhancement technique. Nodules less than 5 mm do not fulfill the selection criteria used for the published studies. They are too small to reliably place a region of interest to measure attenuation and are difficult to consistently use due to differences in depth of a patient respiration. However, advances in multidetector CT technology with submillimeter collimation and isotropic resolution in the z-axis may lower this size threshold in the future. The imaging protocol and nodule selected for evaluation, as described above, should be carefully followed to obtain similar results. The technique should be preformed only on nodules that are relatively homogeneous in attenuation and without evidence of fat, calcification, cavitation, or necrosis on thin-section CT images. Patients considered for this technique must be able to perform repeated, reproducible breath holds. Finally, while the absence of significant enhancement is strongly predictive of benignity (high negative predictive value for malignancy), a significant number of benign nodules enhance above threshold. These nodules remain suspicious for malignancy after a CT enhancement study, and require further radiologic evaluation or tissue diagnosis.

D. Dual-Energy Computed Tomography

This technique is based on increased photon absorption by calcium as the beam energy is decreased, resulting in an increase in the CT attenuation number of calcified nodules imaged at 80 kVp compared to 140 kVp. Despite initial reports in level III studies (53,54), a multicenter prospective level II (moderate evidence) study demonstrated the technique to be unreliable for distinguishing between benign and malignant nodules (3-mm-collimation CT at 140 kVp and 80 kVp; 157 noncalcified, relatively spherical, solid, 5- to 40-mm-diameter nodules without visible calcification or fat) (55). The median increase in nodule mean CT number from 140 kVp to 80 kVp was 2 HU for benign nodules and 3 HU for malignant nodules, not significantly different.

E. Positron Emission Tomography

The uptake of ^{18}FDG is used to measure glucose metabolism on PET. Pulmonary malignancies demonstrate higher ^{18}FDG uptake than normal lung parenchyma and benign nodules, due to their increased metabolic activity (Fig. 23.5). In a multicenter prospective level I (strong evidence) investigation of ^{18}FDG-PET of 89 lung nodules, 92% sensitivity and 90% specificity for malignancy was reported, using a standardized uptake value (SUV) of ≥2.5 as the criterion for malignancy (56). All patients in this study had newly identified indeterminate SPNs on chest radiographs or CT, with pathology (either by surgical resection or biopsy) as the reference test. Several other studies confirm the high sensitivity and moderately high specificity of ^{18}FDG–PET for identifying malignancy in pulmonary nodules (56–68). A summary of several investigations is presented (Table 23.6). In a meta-analysis of 13 studies using ^{18}FDG-PET for the evaluation of CT indeterminate SPNs, Gould et al. reported mean 93.9% sensitivity (98% median) and 85.5% specificity (83.3% median) for identifying malignancy

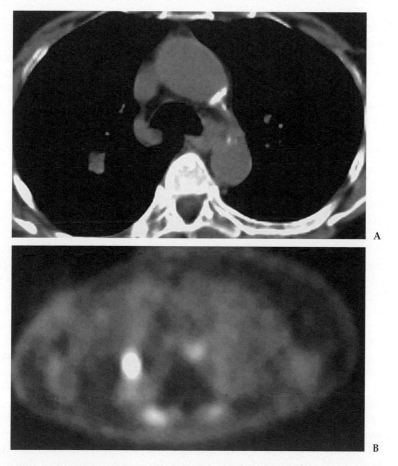

A

B

Figure 23.5. Concordant CT and PET scans for bronchogenic cancer in a 60-year-old woman. At resection this was a squamous cell carcinoma. A: A 1.6-cm indeterminate noncalcified right upper lobe nodule on CT. B: Corresponding ^{18}FDG-PET image shows increased radiotracer uptake corresponding to the nodule.

Table 23.6. Selected investigations of [18]FDG-PET for the evaluation of solitary pulmonary nodules

Study, year (reference)	No. of nodules or masses	Lesion diameter (cm)	Prevalence of malignancy (%)	Reference test	Sensitivity for malignancy (%)	Specificity for malignancy (%)
Lowe et al., 1998 (56)	89	0.7–4.0	66	Needle biopsy or open lung biopsy	92	90
Prauer et al., 1998 (68)	54	0.3–3.0	57	Surgery	90	83
Gupta et al., 1998 (66)	19	1.0–3.5	63	Needle biopsy 10 Thoracotomy 8 Bronchoscopy 1	100	100
Dewan et al., 1997 (65)	52	<3	65	Thoracotomy 36 Needle biopsy 9 Bronchoscopy 3 Mediastinoscopy 3 Observation 1	95	87

(56,58–63,65–70). A summary receiver operating characteristic (ROC) curve based on the meta-analysis is shown in Figure 23.6.

Limited spatial resolution for nodules less than 8 to 10 mm in diameter may result in false-negative results for malignancy (56). False-negative results may also occur with carcinoid tumors and bronchoalveolar carcinoma (71,72). False-positive results may occur with inflammatory and infectious lesions, such as tuberculous and fungal granulomas (56).

F. Single Photon Emission Computed Tomography

Pulmonary nodules can be evaluated using single photon emission computed tomography (SPECT), and [18]FDG, [201]thallium, or the somatostatin analogue [99]technetium deptreotide; SPECT imaging is considerably less expensive and more widely available than PET. A prospective level I (strong evidence) study of [18]FDG-SPECT to evaluate indeterminate lung nodules reported 100% sensitivity and 90% specificity for malignancy for nodules 2 cm or larger in diameter, but only 50% sensitivity and 94% specificity for nodules 1 to 2 cm diameter (73). Similar to PET, the sensitivity for SPECT is dependent on nodule size; however, the lower limit of nodule size that can reliably be evaluated with SPECT is larger than PET. A retrospective level II (moderate evidence) study by Higashi et al. (74) compared [18]FDG-PET and [201]thallium SPECT in the evaluation of 33 patients with histologically proven lung cancer; [18]FDG-PET was significantly more sensitive than [201]thallium SPECT for the detection of malignancy in nodules less than 2 cm in diameter (85.7% vs. 14.3%). The sensitivity in nodules greater than 2 cm was not significantly different. In addition, [18]FDG-PET detected mediastinal lymph node metastases not detected on [201]thallium SPECT (three of four lymph nodes on PET versus one of four on SPECT).

Deptreotide is a somatostatin analogue that can be complexed to [99m]technetium (^{99m}Tc deptreotide) for optimal imaging properties. Blum and colleagues (75) demonstrated 99.6% sensitivity and 73% specificity for identifying malignancy in SPNs using ^{99m}Tc deptreotide in a multicenter level I (strong evidence) prospective series. The study subjects were 114

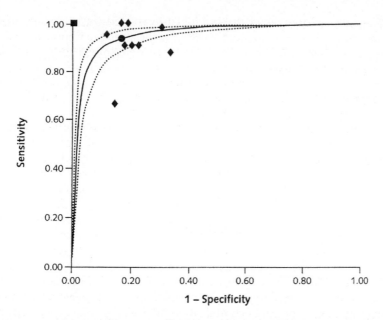

Figure 23.6. Summary receiver operating characteristic (ROC) curve for [18]FDG-PET. The ROC curves illustrate the trade-off between sensitivity and specificity as the threshold that defines a positive test result varies from most stringent to less stringent. The ROC curve for [18]FDG-PET is shown with 95% confidence intervals (dotted lines). Black diamonds represent individual study estimates of sensitivity and specificity. Four studies reported perfect sensitivity and specificity (black square). The point on the summary ROC curve that corresponds to the median specificity reported in 13 studies of [18]FDG-PET for pulmonary nodule diagnosis is shown (black circle). At this point, sensitivity and specificity were 94.2% and 83.3%, respectively. [*Source:* Gould et al. (86), with permission.]

patients with indeterminate pulmonary nodules (no benign pattern of calcification; no demonstrable radiologic stability for the prior 2 years), 30 years of age or more with nodules ranging from 0.8 to 6.0 cm in diameter (mean 2.8 ± 1.6 cm); 88 patients had malignant nodules. [99m]Technetium deptreotide scintigraphy correctly identified 85 of 88 of the malignancies (sensitivity 96.6%). The three false-negative results were adenocarcinomas (one colon cancer metastasis and two primary lung cancers), ranging in diameter from 1.1 to 2.0 cm. There were seven false-positive results, including six granulomas and one hamartoma (specificity 73.1%). The sensitivity and diagnostic accuracy of ^{99m}Tc depreotide compare favorably with that of [18]FDG-PET for differentiating between benign and malignant nodules, with a lower projected cost for ^{99m}Tc depreotide than [18]FDG-PET, and therefore a more favorable cost-benefit analysis (76).

G. Percutaneous Needle Biopsy

There have been numerous investigations of CT-guided percutaneous transthoracic needle biopsy of pulmonary nodules (61,77–84). A prospective randomized level I (strong evidence) study of immediate cytologic evaluation versus offsite cytology demonstrated significantly greater diagnostic accuracy using immediate cytologic evaluation without a significant increase in complication rates (80). Adequate samples were obtained in

100% of procedures when the cytologist evaluated the adequacy of the sample immediately, compared to 88% in the group without immediate cytologic assessment. If the onsite cytologist determined the sample was inadequate, additional aspiration was performed without requiring an additional procedure at a later date. With immediate cytologic evaluation, 99% sensitivity and 100% specificity for malignancy was obtained, versus 90% and 96%, respectively, without it.

Computed tomography–guided percutaneous fine-needle aspiration biopsy of small pulmonary lesions less than or equal to 1 cm has been reported with diagnostic accuracy rates approaching that of larger nodules (85). In a retrospective level II (moderate evidence) study of 61 patients with pulmonary nodules 1 cm or smaller, adequate samples were obtained in 77% of patients. Overall 82% sensitivity and 100% specificity were reported for malignancy in 57 patients; four patients were not included in the analysis due to lack of follow-up. Results for 0.8- to 1.0-cm lesions were significantly better than for 0.5- to 0.7-cm lesions (sensitivity 88% versus 50%; $p = .013$). The percentage of nondiagnostic percutaneous lung biopsies ranges from 4% to 40% in various series. This wide variation reflects no differences in technique, study population, and prevalence of malignancy. The most important complication of imaging-guided percutaneous lung biopsy is pneumothorax, with a 20% to 30% incidence, and a chest tube rate of 5% or less. In a small retrospective level II (moderate evidence) study comparing [18]FDG-PET with percutaneous needle aspiration biopsy for the evaluation of pulmonary nodules, [18]FDG-PET was more sensitive for malignancy (100% vs. 81%), while transthoracic needle aspiration was more specific (100% vs. 78%) (61).

H. Cost-Effectiveness

The cost-effectiveness of management strategies for SPNs was evaluated by Gould et al. (86) in an analysis taken from a societal perspective. The decision-analysis model compared the cost-effectiveness of 40 clinically plausible combinations of five diagnostic interventions (CT, [18]FDG-PET, percutaneous needle biopsy, surgery, and watchful waiting) for the evaluation of a newly identified 2-cm noncalcified pulmonary nodules on a CXR in adults with no known extrathoracic malignancy who were hypothetically 62 years of age. Strategies that did and did not include [18]FDG-PET were specifically compared. The CT sensitivity and specificity for malignancy used were 96.5% and 55.8%, respectively, and for [18]FDG-PET the values were 94.2% and 83.3%, respectively. A logistic regression model using three clinical characteristics (age, cigarette smoking, and history of cancer) and three radiologic characteristics (diameter, spiculation, and upper lobe location) was used to stratify patients into three categories of pretest probability of malignancy. A separate analysis was performed for patients with low (10–50%), intermediate (51–76%), and high (77–90%) pretest probabilities of malignancy. A final diagnosis was established at surgery or after 24 months of observation with serial CXRs. In the watchful waiting strategy, serial CXRs were obtained at 1, 2, 4, and 6 months from baseline and every 3 months thereafter; a nodule that had no growth after 24 months was considered benign. The accuracy and complications of diagnostic tests were estimated from meta-analysis and a literature review. Cost estimates were derived from Medicare reimbursements. The effectiveness and cost-effectiveness of management strategies depended critically on the pretest probability of malignancy, and to a lesser extent on the patients risk for experiencing surgical complications, as listed in Table 23.2. An algorithm for clinical management of patients with a new non-calcified SPN and average risk of surgical complications based on the analysis by Gould et al. (86) is shown in Figure 23.4. The selective use of [18]FDG-PET was the most cost-effective when the pretest probability of malignancy and CT findings were discordant, or in patients with an inter-mediate pretest probability of malignancy who were at high risk for surgical complications. In most other circumstances, CT-based strategies resulted in similar quality-adjusted life years and lower cost. The only cir-cumstance in which CT was not the first test of choice was when the pretest probability of malignancy was extremely high, defined as greater than 90%. In summary, CT should be the initial test in the management of most SPNs. It is relatively inexpensive, noninvasive, and highly specific for identify-ing some benign nodules.

- In patients with a low pretest probability of malignancy (10–50%), [18]FDG-PET should be used selectively when the CT results are indeter-minate for malignancy.
  - For an indeterminate SPN on CT coupled with a positive [18]FDG-PET result, surgery is highly cost-effective, and slightly more effective than performing percutaneous needle biopsy before surgery.
  - For an indeterminate SPN on CT coupled with a negative [18]FDG-PET result, percutaneous needle biopsy is more effective than observation alone due to the possibility of a false-negative [18]FDG-PET result that may potentially lead to a delayed diagnosis of malignancy and missed opportunity for curative surgery.
  - When CT results are benign, observation or needle biopsy were rec-ommended; however, the definition of a benign nodule on CT is stated to be "negative for malignancy" and the imaging characteristics attrib-uted to a benign nodule on CT were not further specified.
- In patients with an intermediate pretest probability of malignancy (51–76%):
  - Surgery or percutaneous needle biopsy was recommended when CT results are possibly malignant.
  - Needle biopsy or observation was recommended when CT results are benign.
  - More aggressive use of surgery and needle biopsy resulted in slightly better health outcomes and slightly higher costs. The choice between more or less aggressive approaches should depend on factors such as the risk for surgical complications, expected yield of needle biopsy, and patient preference.
  - Percutaneous needle biopsy is warranted in patients with a con-traindication to surgical resection, such as severe lung or cardiovas-cular disease, or in the setting of a known extrapulmonary malignancy.
- In patients with high pretest probability of malignancy (77–90%):
  - Surgery was recommended when CT results are possibly malignant, and there are no surgical contradictions.
  - [18]FDG-PET was recommended when CT results are benign; if [18]FDG-PET is positive, surgery is recommended. When [18]FDG-PET results are negative, percutaneous needle biopsy was marginally more effective than watchful waiting.

The results of this study support and extend the findings of others. In a decision analysis Cummings et al. (87) also found that the choice of evaluation strategy depended on the pretest probability of malignancy. Watchful waiting was preferred over biopsy when the pretest probability of cancer was less than 3%. Surgery was preferred over biopsy when the probability of cancer was greater than 68%. This study did not evaluate PET or cost-effectiveness. To examine the potential role of contrast-enhanced dynamic CT, Gould et al. (86) evaluated six additional strategies for dynamic CT when noncontrast CT indicated a possible malignancy. The use of contrast-enhanced dynamic CT was most cost-effective when used selectively in patients with a low-to-intermediate pretest probability of malignancy with a possibly malignant result on noncontrast CT.

III. Special Case: Estimating the Probability of Malignancy in Solitary Pulmonary Nodules

Summary of Evidence: The effectiveness and cost-effectiveness of management strategies for evaluation of SPNs is highly dependent on the pretest probability of malignancy. Bayesian analysis and multivariate logistic regression models can be used to predict the likelihood of malignancy for a given nodule, and perform equal to or better than expert human readers of imaging tests. Using Bayesian analysis, [18]FDG-PET as a single test is a better predictor of malignancy in SPNs than standard CT criteria.

Supporting Evidence: Given that the cost-effectiveness of imaging a SPN is dependent on the pretest probability of malignancy, optimum use of imaging requires stratification of subjects by their probability of malignancy. Bayesian analysis uses likelihood ratios (LRs) for radiologic findings and clinical features to estimate the probability of cancer (pCa) (13,88). The LR for a given characteristic is derived as follows:

$$LR = \frac{\text{Number of malignant nodules with feature}}{\text{Number of benign nodules with feature}}$$

An LR of 1 indicates a 50% chance of malignancy. An LR of less than 1 favors a benign lesion, whereas an LR greater than 1 favors malignancy. Likelihood ratios for various clinical and radiologic features of SPNs derived from the literature are presented in Table 23.7 (88). The odds of malignancy are calculated as below. The LR prior is the likelihood of malignancy in all nodules based on the local prevalence of malignancy.

$$\text{Odds of malignancy} = LR \text{ prior} \times LR \text{ size} \times LR \text{ edge} \times LR \text{ etc.}$$

The probability of malignancy is calculated as follows below.

$$\text{Probability of malignancy} = \frac{\text{odds of malignancy}}{(1 + \text{odds of malignancy})}$$

The probability of malignancy for a nodule can be calculated using Bayesian analysis at www.chestx-ray.com. Gurney et al. (13) in a level II (moderate evidence) study showed that readers using Bayesian analysis performed significantly better at identifying malignancy than expert readers alone, classifying fewer malignant nodules as benign when presented with the same clinical and radiological data.

Table 23.7. Likelihood ratios (LRs) for malignancy
in solitary pulmonary nodules (88)

Feature or characteristic	LR
>70 years of age	4.16
30–39 years of age	0.24
Current cigarette smoker	2.27
Never smoked	0.19
Growth rate 7–465 days	3.40
Growth rate <7 days	0
Growth rate >465 days	0.01
Spiculated margin	5.54
Smooth margin	0.30
Upper/middle lobe location	1.22
Lower lobe location	0.66
Size >3 cm	5.23
Size <1 cm	0.52
Previous malignancy	4.95

Swensen's group (89) initially developed and then internally validated a clinical prediction model to estimate the probability of malignancy in SPNs. This level II (moderate evidence) retrospective study used a cohort of 629 patients with 4- to 30-mm indeterminate SPNs newly discovered on chest radiographs. Using multivariate logistic regression analysis a clinical prediction model was developed from a random sample of two thirds of the patients, then tested on the remaining third. Three clinical features (age, cigarette-smoking status, and history of cancer diagnosed more than 5 years ago) and three radiologic characteristics (diameter, spiculation, and upper lobe location) were identified as independent predictors of malignancy. A further level II (moderate evidence) study by the same investigators comparing the performance of the clinical prediction model to physician estimates of malignancy demonstrated no statistically significant differences (2).

Dewan et al. (65) compared Bayesian analysis to the results of ^{18}FDG-PET scans in a level II (moderate evidence) retrospective study. Fifty-two patients with noncalcified, solid nodules less than 3 cm in size were studied. The probability of malignancy was calculated using standard criteria (patient age, history of prior malignancy, smoking history, and nodule size and border), and compared to the probability of malignancy based on the ^{18}FDG-PET scan, with histology as the reference test. The LR for malignancy in a SPN was 7.11 with an abnormal ^{18}FDG-PET scan compared to 0.06 with a normal ^{18}FDG-PET scan. The LRs for malignancy were higher with an abnormal ^{18}FDG-PET scan compared to most LRs for age, size, history of previous malignancy, smoking history, and nodule edge in the literature. Receiver operating characteristic curves (ROC) were drawn to compare the standard criteria using Bayesian analysis, standard criteria plus ^{18}FDG-PET, and ^{18}FDG-PET alone. Analysis of the ROC curves revealed that ^{18}FDG-PET alone had the highest sensitivity and specificity at different levels of probability of cancer, the standard criteria the least, and the standard criteria plus ^{18}FDG-PET was intermediate; ^{18}FDG-PET as a single test had the highest percentage of nodules correctly classified as malignant or benign and was a better predictor of malignancy in SPNs than Bayesian analysis.

IV. Special Case: Solitary Pulmonary Nodule in a Patient with a Known Extrapulmonary Malignancy

An SPN in a patient with an existing extrapulmonary malignancy warrants special consideration, as it is often detected on staging, follow-up chest radiographs, or CT. The etiology of these nodules is important in determining the appropriate therapy and in differentiating a new lung cancer from a pulmonary metastasis or nodule of another etiology, such as infection.

In a level II (moderate evidence) retrospective study, Quint et al. (90) demonstrated that the likelihood of primary lung malignancy in such nodules depends on the histologic characteristics of the extrapulmonary neoplasm and the patient's cigarette smoking history. The medical records of 149 patients with an extrapulmonary malignancy and a SPN at chest CT were reviewed. The histologic characteristics of the nodule were correlated with the extrapulmonary malignancy, patient age, and cigarette smoking history. Patients with carcinomas of the head and neck, bladder, breast, cervix, bile ducts, esophagus, ovary, prostate, or stomach were more likely to have primary bronchogenic carcinoma than lung metastasis (ratio 8.3:1 for patients with head and neck cancers; 3.2:1 for all other malignancies combined). Patients with carcinomas of the salivary glands, adrenal gland, colon, parotid gland, kidney, thyroid gland, thymus, or uterus had fairly even odds of having bronchogenic carcinoma or pulmonary metastasis (ratio 1:1.2). Patients with melanoma, sarcoma, or testicular carcinoma were more likely to have a solitary metastasis than bronchogenic carcinoma (ratio 2.5:1). The results of this study were similar to an earlier study performed by Cahan et al. (91) in the pre-CT era. The authors analyzed thoracotomy results obtained for 35 years in over 800 patients with a history of cancer, and obtained similar odds ratios for bronchogenic carcinoma versus solitary pulmonary metastases in different primary malignancies, based on conventional radiographic detection of the SPN.

Future Research

- Computer-aided diagnosis (CAD) both to assist with nodule detection on CXR and CT and to distinguish benign from malignant SPNs is under development, with some programs currently available for use. Their role in practice and effectiveness in clinical practice are currently unknown. While preliminary results are promising, further studies are necessary prior to the use of CAD schemes in actual clinical situations.
- Imaging techniques combined with patient biomarker evaluation from blood, sputum or urine samples may help guide which patients need more aggressive, serial follow-up examinations and which patients do not.

References

1. Tuddenham WJ. AJR 1984;143:509–517.
2. Earnest F, Ryu JH, Miller GM, et al. Radiology 1999;211:137.
3. Holin SM, Dwork RE, Glaser S, Rikli AE, Stocklen JB. Am Rev Tuberc 1959;79: 427–439.
4. Swensen SJ, Jett JR, Sloan JA, et al. Am J Respir Crit Care Med 2002;165:508–513.
5. Henschke CI, McCauley DI, Yankelevitz DF, et al. Lancet 1999;354:99–105.
6. Comstock GW, Vaughan RH, Montgomery G. N Engl J Med 1956;254:1018–1022.

7. Stelle JD. J Thorac Cardiovasc Surg 1963;46:21–39.
8. Siegelman SS, Khouri NF, Leo FP, Fishman EK, Braverman RM, Zerhouni EA. Radiology 1986;160:307–312.
9. Zerhouni EA, Stitik FP, Siegelman SS, et al. Radiology 1986;160:319–327.
10. Kaneko M, Eguchi K, Ohmatsu H, et al. Radiology 1996;201:798–802.
11. Steele JD. J Thorac Cardiovasc Surg 1963;46:21–39.
12. Yankelevitz DF. Semin Ultrasound CT MR 2000;21:95–96.
13. Gurney JW, Lyddon DM, McKay JA. Radiology 1993;186:415–422.
14. Bateson EM. Clin Radiol 1965;16:51–65.
15. Ray JFd, Lawton BR, Magnin GE, et al. Chest 1976;70:332–336.
16. Higgins GA, Shields TW, Keehn RJ. Arch Surg 1975;110:570–575.
17. Yankelevitz DF, Henschke CI. AJR 1997;168:325–328.
18. Good CA, Wilson TW. The solitary circumscribed pulmonary nodule; study of seven hundred five cases encountered roentgenologically in a period of three and one-half years. J Am Med Assoc 1958;166(3):210–215.
19. Collins VP, Loeffler RK, Tivey H. AJR 1956;76:988–1000.
20. Brues AM WA, Andervant HB. Proc Soc Exp Biol Med 1939;43:375–377.
21. Mottram J. J Pathol 1935;40:407–414.
22. Nathan MH, Collins VP, Adams RA. Radiology 1962;79:221–232.
23. Steele JD, Buell P. J Thorac Cardiovasc Surg 1973;65:140–151.
24. Geddes DM. Br J Dis Chest 1979;73:1–17.
25. Weiss W. Am Rev Respir Dis 1971;103:198–208.
26. Lillington GA. Dis Mon 1991;37:271–318.
27. Wormanns D, Diederich S, Lentschig MG, Winter F, Heindel W. Eur Radiol 2000;10:710–713.
28. Winer-Muram HT, Jennings SG, Tarver RD, et al. Radiology 2002;223:798–805.
29. Henschke CI, Yankelevitz D, Westcott J, et al. ACR Appropriateness Criteria. Radiology 2000;215S:607–609.
30. Yankelevitz DF, Reeves AP, Kostis WJ, Zhao B, Henschke CI. Radiology 2000;217:251–256.
31. Aoki T, Nakata H, Watanabe H, et al. AJR 2000;174:763–768.
32. Good CA, Hood RT Jr, Mc D Jr. AJR 1953;70:543–554.
33. O'Keefe ME, Good CA, McDonald JR. AJR 1957;77:1023–1033.
34. Bateson EM, Abbott EK. Clin Radiol 1960;11:232–247.
35. Stewart JG, MacMahon H, Vyborny CJ, Pollak ER. AJR 1987;148:29–30.
36. Mahoney MC, Shipley RT, Corcoran HL, Dickson BA. AJR 1990;154:255–258.
37. Berger WG, Erly WK, Krupinski EA, Standen JR, Stern RG. AJR 2001;176:201–204.
38. Proto AV, Thomas SR. Radiology 1985;156:149–153.
39. Zerhouni EA, Boukadoum M, Siddiky MA, et al. Radiology 1983;149:767–773.
40. Siegelman SS, Khouri NF, Scott WW Jr, et al. Radiology 1986;160:313–317.
41. Remy J, Remy-Jardin M, Wattinne L, Deffontaines C. Radiology 1992;182:809–816.
42. Hillerdal G. Chest 1989;95(4):313–317.
43. Westcott JH, Volpe JP. Radiology 1991;181(P):182.
44. Rose RW, Ward BH. Radiology 1973;106:179–182.
45. Eggli KD. Radiol Clin North Am 1993;31:651–666.
46. Khan A, Herman PG, Vorwerk P, Stevens P, Rojas KA, Graver M. Radiology 1991;179:477–481.
47. Takanashi N, Nobe Y, Asoh H, Yano T, Ichinose Y. Lung Cancer 1995;13:105–112.
48. Seemann MD, Staebler A, Beinert T, et al. Eur Radiol 1999;9:409–417.
49. Seemann MD, Seemann O, Luboldt W, et al. Lung Cancer 2000;29:105–124.
50. Swensen SJ, Viggiano RW, Midthun DE, et al. Radiology 2000;214:73–80.
51. Potente G, Iacari V, Caimi M. Comput Med Imaging Graph 1997;21:39–46.
52. Yamashita K, Matsunobe S, Takahashi R, et al. Radiology 1995;196:401–408.
53. Bhalla M, Shepard JA, Nakamura K, Kazerooni EA. J Comput Assist Tomogr 1995;19:44–47.

54. Higashi Y, Nakamura H, Matsumoto T, Nakanishi T. J Thorac Imaging 1994;9: 31–34.
55. Swensen SJ, Yamashita K, McCollough CH, et al. Radiology 2000;214:81–85.
56. Lowe VJ, Fletcher JW, Gobar L, et al. J Clin Oncol 1998;16:1075–1084.
57. Abe Y, Matsuzawa T, Fujiwara T, et al. Int J Radiat Oncol Biol Phys 1990;19: 1005–1010.
58. Gupta NC, Frank AR, Dewan NA, et al. Radiology 1992;184:441–444.
59. Dewan NA, Gupta NC, Redepenning LS, Phalen JJ, Frick MP. Chest 1993;104: 997–1002.
60. Patz EF Jr, Lowe VJ, Hoffman JM, et al. Radiology 1993;188:487–490.
61. Dewan NA, Reeb SD, Gupta NC, Gobar LS, Scott WJ. Chest 1995;108:441–446.
62. Duhaylongsod FG, Lowe VJ, Patz EF Jr, Vaughn AL, Coleman RE, Wolfe WG. J Thorac Cardiovasc Surg 1995;110:130–139; discussion 139–140.
63. Duhaylongsod FG, Lowe VJ, Patz EF Jr, Vaughn AL, Coleman RE, Wolfe WG. Ann Thorac Surg 1995;60:1348–1352.
64. Gupta NC, Maloof J, Gunel E. J Nucl Med 1996;37:943–948.
65. Dewan NA, Shehan CJ, Reeb SD, Gobar LS, Scott WJ, Ryschon K. Chest 1997; 112:416–422.
66. Gupta N, Gill H, Graeber G, Bishop H, Hurst J, Stephens T. Chest 1998; 114:1105–1111.
67. Orino K, Kawamura M, Hatazawa J, Suzuki I, Sazawa Y. Jpn J Thorac Cardio-vasc Surg 1998;46:1267–1274.
68. Prauer HW, Weber WA, Romer W, Treumann T, Ziegler SI, Schwaiger M. Br J Surg 1998;85:1506–1511.
69. Kubota K, Matsuzawa T, Fujiwara T, et al. J Nucl Med 1990;31:1927–1932.
70. Gupta NC, Maloof J, Gunel E. J Nucl Med 1996;37:943–948.
71. Erasmus JJ, McAdams HP, Patz EF Jr, Coleman RE, Ahuja V, Goodman PC. AJR 1998;170:1369–1373.
72. Higashi K, Ueda Y, Seki H, et al. J Nucl Med 1998;39:1016–1020.
73. Mastin ST, Drane WE, Harman EM, Fenton JJ, Quesenberry L. Chest 1999;115: 1012–1017.
74. Higashi K, Nishikawa T, Seki H, et al. J Nucl Med 1998;39:9–15.
75. Blum J, Handmaker H, Lister-James J, Rinne N. Chest 2000;117:1232–1238.
76. Gambhir SS, Handmaker H. J Nucl Med 1999;41(S):57P.
77. van Sonnenberg E, Casola G, Ho M, et al. Radiology 1988;167:457–461.
78. Garcia Rio F, Diaz Lobato S, Pino JM, et al. Acta Radiol 1994;35:478–480.
79. Li H, Boiselle PM, Shepard JO, Trotman-Dickenson B, McLoud TC. AJR 1996; 167:105–109.
80. Santambrogio L, Nosotti M, Bellaviti N, Pavoni G, Radice F, Caputo V. Chest 1997;112:423–425.
81. Westcott JL, Rao N, Colley DP. Radiology 1997;202:97–103.
82. Yankelevitz DF, Henschke CI, Koizumi JH, Altorki NK, Libby D. Clin Imaging 1997;21:107–110.
83. Hayashi N, Sakai T, Kitagawa M, et al. AJR 1998;170:329–331.
84. Laurent F, Latrabe V, Vergier B, Montaudon M, Vernejoux JM, Dubrez J. Clin Radiol 2000;55:281–287.
85. Wallace MJ, Krishnamurthy S, Broemeling LD, et al. Radiology 2002;225: 823–828.
86. Gould MK, Sanders GD, Barnett PG, et al. Ann Intern Med 2003;138:724–735.
87. Cummings SR, Lillington GA, Richard RJ. Am Rev Respir Dis 1986;134:453–460.
88. Gurney JW. Radiology 1993;186:405–413.
89. Hartman TE, Tazelaar HD, Swensen SJ, Muller NL. Radiographics 1997;17:377–390.
90. Quint LE, Park CH, Iannettoni MD. Radiology 2000;217:257–261.
91. Cahan WG, Shah JP, Castro EB. Ann Surg 1978;187:241–244.
92. Seemann MD, Beinert T, Dienemann H, et al. Eur J Med Res 1996;1:371–376.
93. Yamashita K, Matsunobe S, Tsuda T, et al. Radiology 1995;194:399–405.
94. Potente G, Guerrisi R, Iacari V, et al. Radiol Med 1997;94:182–188.

24

Blunt Injuries to the Thorax and Abdomen

Frederick A. Mann

Issues

I. What imaging is appropriate for patients with blunt trauma to the chest?
   A. Chest wall
   B. Pleura and lung
   C. Diaphragm
II. What imaging is appropriate for patients with blunt trauma to the abdomen?
   A. Spleen and liver injuries
   B. Bowel and mesentery injuries
III. What is the optimal imaging approach in patients suspected of having retroperitoneal injury?

Key Points

- Conventional radiography remains the appropriate initial screening evaluation of the chest in patients with major trauma. Computed tomography (CT) is appropriate for the definitive evaluation of abnormalities identified on initial radiography.
- Clinical evidence of hemodynamic instability or ongoing blood loss is the strongest indicator for operative intervention in the abdomen. Among patients with such indication of ongoing hemorrhage, transabdominal ultrasound and diagnostic peritoneal lavage (DPL) are diagnostically equivalent in identifying patients with intraperitoneal hemorrhage from solid organ injury.
- Computed tomography has high sensitivity for surgically important injuries of the liver and spleen, but CT grading of injury shows poor correlation with outcome.
- In patients with clinical suspicion of retroperitoneal injury, CT is the diagnostic procedure of choice.
- Computed tomography is the preferred imaging modality for identification of hollow viscus injury, although DPL may have higher sensitivity at the expense of lower specificity.

Definition and Pathophysiology

Thoracic trauma is responsible for approximately 25% of trauma deaths in North America. Since death from thoracic trauma commonly occurs after presentation to the hospital, many of these deaths are presumed to be preventable with prompt and appropriate treatment. Important injuries leading to rapid death in trauma include aortic rupture, massive hemothorax, pericardial tamponade, and tension pneumothorax. Pulmonary contusion, myocardial contusion, tracheobronchial injury, and diaphragmatic rupture may also be fatal if not recognized and treated emergently. Fewer than 10% of chest injuries require thoracotomy for treatment (1).

In the abdomen, blunt trauma may result in compression or shear injury to the viscera, leading to hemorrhage and peritonitis. Among patients who undergo laparotomy for blunt trauma, the spleen, and liver are the most frequently injured organs. Because of the large potential space of the peritoneum, large volumes of hemorrhage can occur without tamponade, and exsanguination may occur rapidly from arterial and large venous injuries in the organ parenchyma.

Mechanisms of hollow viscus or mesenteric injury include direct blow to the abdomen (handlebars, kicks, motor vehicle accident), and seatbelt injury, especially when associated with distraction-type spine injury. The spectrum of hollow viscus injuries (HVIs) include wall contusions, serosal injuries ("deserosalization"), perforations and transection, and mesenteric rents and hematomas. When mural disruption occurs in the proximal gastrointestinal tract (stomach through proximal jejunum), leakage of alimentary tract contents into the peritoneum induces acute chemical peritonitis and related clinical findings. Distal small bowel and colon spillage tends to present later as peritoneal sepsis. Delays in diagnosis are associated with complicated clinical courses and increased mortality. Serial physical examination evaluation alone may be associated with delay in diagnosis in individuals who have concomitant distracting injuries, such as femur fractures.

Among retroperitoneal injuries, in adults the duodenum and pancreas are rarely injured in isolation. However, children and adolescents may sustain isolated duodenal, or duodenal and pancreatic, injuries, especially from bicycle handlebar goring mechanisms. Pancreatic injuries range from contusions, lacerations, fractures, and duodenal-pancreatic disjunctions. In adults, injuries to the main pancreatic duct and combined pancreatoduodenal injuries necessitate intervention and are often associated with complicated treatment courses. In children, aggressive and early treatment remains controversial, and treatment directed at complications is more common.

Epidemiology

Injuries are the leading cause of death of individuals between the ages of 1 and 44 in the United States. In the 15 to 24 age group, injuries account for 78% of all deaths. Because trauma deaths tend to occur in younger individuals, there is a great burden on society in terms of years of life lost and lost lifetime earnings (2).

Motor vehicle accidents account for approximately half of unintentional injury deaths, followed by falls. Injury death rates are higher in the elderly population (over age 70), as well as in individuals in their early 20s. Males also have higher death rates than females (3).

Overall Cost to Society

Discounting lifetime earnings at 6%, the total lifetime cost of injuries that occurred in the year 1985 in the United States was estimated by Rice and colleagues (4) to be $150 billion. This is more than the cost of cancer, heart disease, and stroke combined. Despite this, the U.S. federal government spends only approximately a tenth as much money on injury research as on cancer research.

Goals

The goals of imaging in chest and abdominal trauma are twofold. Initial imaging must allow for rapid identification of life-threatening injuries to enable treatment of the injuries in the initial hour after presentation of the patient to the hospital. Secondary imaging provides a detailed evaluation of all injuries potentially leading to morbidity and mortality, including appropriate staging of these injuries.

Search Criteria

The literature review was based on combinations of the following terms: *imaging* and (*injury* or *wounds, nonpenetrating*) and *1990–2004* and (*chest wall, rib, pleura, scapulothoracic, hemothorax, pneumothorax, diaphragm, abdominal injuries, intestine-small, mesentery, spleen,* or *liver*) or (*lung* or *pulmonary* and *contusion* or *laceration*), and (*radiography* OR *tomography, x-ray computed*) and with this limit: *not case reports*. Studies that consisted of case series, case reports, and expert opinion after review were not included. Included were both English-language and non-English-language articles.

I. What Imaging Is Appropriate for Patients with Blunt Trauma to the Chest?

Summary of Evidence: Radiography remains the most appropriate initial imaging evaluation for blunt trauma to the chest. Radiography has high sensitivity for clinically important disease. Additional imaging, usually with CT or computed tomographic angiography (CTA) is often necessary to adequately evaluate abnormalities identified on conventional radiography (moderate evidence).

Supporting Evidence

A. Chest Wall

With the exception of medicolegal documentation purposes necessary for nonaccidental trauma, information necessary for recognition and treatment planning for important chest wall injuries may be achieved with conventional radiography. While bone scintigraphy is considerably more sensitive to the detection of rib fractures in the subacute setting, among polytrauma victims it plays little or no role in treatment planning or an independent role in prognosis. While CT is an important adjunctive test in the evaluation of blunt chest trauma, it is less sensitive in the detection of rib fractures than conventional radiography. Where medicolegal documentation is necessary, such as in the evaluation of nonaccidental trauma, bone scintigraphy, ultrasound, and CT may provide additional evidence of characteristic injury to support the diagnosis. (5–23).

When conventional radiography or clinical examination suggests the presence of scapulothoracic dissociation (closed forequarter amputation), angiography (CTA or catheter angiography) may be used to exclude the presence of the rare intrathoracic pseudoaneurysm of the subclavian or proximal axillary artery, whose intrapleural rupture may be catastrophic (24–29).

B. Pleura and Lung

Computed tomography is more sensitive in the detection of pneumothoraces than conventional radiography. However, the consequences of pneumothoraces that are occult to conventional radiography are generally benign, except when positive pressure ventilation is part of the management of the patient's pulmonary injury (including patients going emergently to the operating theater). Computed tomography is more sensitive in detecting lung hernias through muscular or osseous chest wall disruption, and better characterizes their need for surgical treatment (lung hernias with narrow necks are more likely to experience pulmonary infarctions than those with broad based necks). Computed tomography is also more accurate at assessing the size of hemothoraces. Hemothoraces exceeding 300 to 500 mL are more likely to be associated with delayed pulmonary complications, such as incarcerated lung and empyema (30–34).

In similar fashion, conventional radiography generally provides sufficient information for the diagnosis of pulmonary contusions and lacerations and their therapy. However, quantitative assessment of the volume of lung involved with pulmonary contusion may predict the likelihood of development of acute respiratory distress syndrome and delayed pneumonia (>20% and 30% of lung volume, respectively). Computed tomography is far more sensitive to the detection of pulmonary lacerations. However, there is no current evidence that earlier or more thorough detection of pulmonary laceration effects patient outcome. Certain CT findings, such as subpleural lucency associated with peripheral pulmonary opacity, facilitate confident diagnosis of contusion and distinguishing it from more common causes of pulmonary opacity in trauma (such aspiration and passive atelectasis). Disruption of the aerodigestive tract often leads to pneumomediastinum, and may be associated with mediastinal hematoma. Blunt injury to the esophagus usually occurs in the upper third of the esophagus and may be suggested by CT. However, esophagography and esophagoscopy remain the standard diagnostic modalities for detection and treatment planning. Tracheobronchial injuries may be suggested by massive pneumomediastinum and persistent air leak associated with pneumothorax, and may be directly imaged by CT. However, bronchoscopy remains the principal diagnostic tool in the acute and emergent setting (35–60).

Conventional radiography remains the primary survey for mediastinal abnormalities in blunt polytrauma of the chest. Where the cardiomediastinal silhouette is normal for a patient's age and sex, acute traumatic aortic injuries can be reliably excluded by conventional chest radiography. However, a large minority of patients who are subsequently shown to have normal aortic and great vessels do not show normal cardiomediastinal silhouettes by conventional radiography for various reasons, including low lung volumes, pulmonary or pleural opacities obscuring mediastinal margins, etc. In this setting, CT has largely supplanted catheter angiography in the evaluation of the aorta and its great vessels for acute traumatic injury, particularly when performed as CT angiography (61–63). Detailed discussion of aortic injury is included in Chapter 20.

C. Diaphragm

An high-index of suspicion for diaphragmatic ruptures is warranted in appropriate clinical circumstances (lateral impact crashes, especially when left-sided), because fewer than one third of cases present with classical findings (up to 40% of left-sided and less than 15% of right-sided ruptures) and 10–15% will have a false-negative DPL. Delayed diagnoses are not uncommon (10% to 15% greater than 24-hour delay), especially if the commonly associated intrathoracic (~90%) and intraabdominal (~60%) injuries require endotracheal intubation and positive-pressure ventilation. Conventional radiography (chest radiographs with enteral tube placement; fluoroscopy) is abnormal in 60% to 90% of individuals with acute traumatic diaphragmatic rupture, but most findings are nonspecific (hemothorax, atelectasis, etc.). In unselected series, CT accuracy was equivalent, but not clearly superior to conventional radiographic techniques. At CT, the so-called dependent viscera sign (intraabdominal contents abutting the posterior thoracic wall where the scan level is in the upper third of the liver or spleen) and "collar" sign (narrowed waist of an herniated intraabdominal organ at the site of diaphragm rupture) are nearly 100% specific. Other findings, such as the discontinuous and thickened diaphragm signs, show intermediate sensitivity and specificity (40% to 75%). Among reported series in which magnetic resonance imaging (MRI) depicted no diaphragmatic disruptions, no delayed diagnoses have been reported (64–78).

II. What Imaging Is Appropriate for Patients with Blunt Trauma to the Abdomen?

Summary of Evidence: Computed tomography is the imaging modality of choice for evaluation of the abdomen in trauma patients (moderate evidence). However, clinical status is a more reliable predictor of requirement for operative intervention than imaging (moderate evidence). Ultrasonography is of insufficient sensitivity to allow exclusion of intraabdominal organ injury and hemoperitoneum (moderate evidence) (Fig. 24.1).

Supporting Evidence

A. Spleen and Liver Injuries

Hemodynamic status and evidence of ongoing blood loss are the strongest indicators of the need for intervention for injury to the spleen and liver,

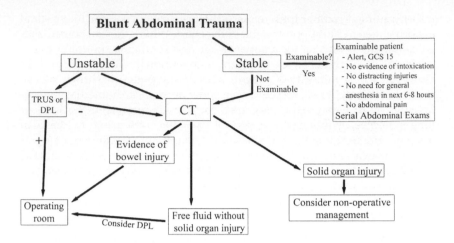

Figure 24.1. Flowchart of abdominal imaging protocol at Harborview Medical Center. The differentiation between hemodynamically stable and unstable is a continuum. With faster multidetector CT scanners and better trauma center design with on-site scanners mitigating the need for patient transport, less stable patients are now safe for CT. Nonoperative management of solid organ injury is preferred, but decision making is affected by hemodynamic stability and presence of arterial extravasation on CT. DPL, diagnostic peritoneal lavage; TUS, trauma ultrasound of the peritoneal space; GCS, Glasgow Coma Scale.

because the most common and life-threatening complication from abdominal trauma is surgically treatable hemorrhage. Among hemodynamically unstable patients that are not taken immediately to the operating suite, transabdominal ultrasound and DPL are diagnostically equivalent in selecting patients whose hemodynamic instability is due to intraperitoneal hemorrhage from solid organ (79–81).

Meta-analyses by Stengel and colleagues (82,83) investigated the accuracy and positive and negative predictive values for the use of trauma ultrasound for the identification of hemoperitoneum. Ultrasound had relatively high specificity for intraperitoneal hemorrhage, indicating high reliability if hemoperitoneum was identified. However, the sensitivity of ultrasound for intraperitoneal fluid was relatively low, with a negative likelihood ratio of only 0.24. At the prevalence of injury encountered in major trauma centers, the posttest probability of disease following negative ultrasound was too high to exclude important injury. Subanalysis of pediatric patients revealed similar results. Accordingly, observation or CT following negative ultrasonography is warranted (strong evidence) (82–84).

Among hemodynamically stable patients, nonoperative management may be guided by information gleaned from adjunctive diagnostic tests and serial physical examination. Computed tomography shows a sensitivity in the middle to high 90s to the detection of surgically important injuries of the liver and spleen. However, CT grading of liver and spleen injuries shows generally poor correlation with the specific outcome of individual cases. Active hemorrhage detected by CT commonly leads to endovascular or surgical interventions in most patients where bleeding was focal [intraparenchymal: pseudoaneurysms vs. arteriovenous (AV) fistula], diffuse (intraperitoneal), or seen in multiple locations (most common with pelvic ring fractures). Extravasated contrast presents as relatively discrete contrast collections that increase or "pool" on delayed imaging, and show measures within 10 to 20 Hounsfield units (HU) of contrast density of an adjacent major artery or aorta. At this time, contrast-enhanced CT does not reliably distinguish between pseudoaneurysms (>70% believed to progress to rupture) and AV fistulae (natural history is uncertain). Although not specifically studied, a clear trend is present in the literature for increasing proportions of blunt trauma patients to show extravasation when multi-detector CT was used with higher injection rates (>2.5 cc per second) (85–92).

The likelihood of surgical intervention increases with the detection of multiple injuries (e.g., spleen and left kidney, left lobe of the liver and pancreas). In addition, liver lacerations that involve the hilum, particularly those associated with partial stripping of the gallbladder, may be benefit from repeat scanning or ultrasound, cholescintigraphy, or direct cholangiography to detect possible biliary complications. Liver lacerations involving the hepatic veins, especially when associated with large regions (>10 cm) of focal hypoperfusion, are thought to reflect retrohepatic vena caval injuries and are strongly predictive of surgically evident bleeding necessitating interventions (91–93).

Among patients who have otherwise uncomplicated postinjury courses (e.g., absent increasing abdominal pain, falling hematocrit, clinical features of intraabdominal sepsis, etc.), serial CT scans do not appear to be useful in altering therapy or determining the time for return to full activities, particularly in the pediatric population. Nonetheless, if serial follow-up imaging is believed indicated in specific cases, ultrasound is a more cost-effective alternative than CT (94–96).

B. Bowel and Mesentery Injuries

Controversy persist regarding the optimum and most cost-effective means of evaluating victims of blunt-force trauma perceived to be at risk for otherwise occult HVI. Diagnostic peritoneal lavage may be a more sensitive test than CT for isolated HVI (sensitivity >97% vs. sensitivity 90–93%), albeit with lower specificity (~50–60% vs. 95%), even with intravenous contrast enhancement, thin sections, and multidetector technologies. Nonetheless, less than 5% of surgically important blunt-force HVIs occurring in adults are found in the absence of other, often more obvious and clinically immediate, intraabdominal injuries. Conventional radiography, ultrasound, and MRI have limited or no role in the routine diagnosis of bowel injuries (97–106).

Computed tomography, especially with appropriately timed data acquisition relative to intravenous contrast administration, is the currently preferred imaging modality, especially when performed with multidetector equipment at slice thickness of 5 mm or less. However, CT performed without oral or intravenous contrast enhancement may show intramural hematoma as focal, asymmetric hyperdensity within bowel thickened wall with adjacent mesenteric edema ("misty mesentery"). Although the role of oral contrast remains hotly contested, larger case series have failed to show a clinical advantage to its use, which may relate to failed opacification of the postduodenal small bowel in ~40% of patients 30 minutes following gastrointestinal contrast administration (107–109).

Numerous findings have been described: bowel wall thickening with or without dilation, bowel wall discontinuity, pathologic enhancement of bowel wall, mesenteric hematoma with adjacent bowel wall thickening, interloop (intramesenteric) fluid with abnormal adjacent bowel, extraluminal air or extravasation of alimentary positive contrast, acute abdominal wall hernias with bowel content, and active vascular extravasation from bowel. Bowel contusion may be suggested on intravenous contrast-enhanced CT by focal or multifocal bowel thickening and mural enhancement (sensitivity ~60%), and oral contrast (positive or negative) may help in appreciation of wall thickening. In contrast, diffuse bowel wall thickening and enhancement, especially associated with slit-like infrahepatic inferior vena cava and hypodense and contracted spleen, suggests underresuscitation and so-called hypoperfusion syndrome. While clear demonstration of spillage of positive alimentary contrast is essentially pathognomonic for bowel perforation, apparent bowel wall discontinuity has a sensitivity of ~60% and specificity of ~95% (110,111). Almost all reports show that free intraabdominal gas is very strongly suggestive of bowel perforation or transaction (sensitivity ~40%; most reports provide a specificity of ~100%). One unrepeated report found ~60% false-positive diagnoses based on CT-demonstrated pneumoperitoneum (112).

III. What Is the Optimal Imaging Approach in Patients Suspected of Having Retroperitoneal Injury?

Summary of Evidence: In general, retroperitoneal injuries must be suspected based on clinical history and physical examination findings, and laboratory tests (e.g., hematuria) (strong evidence). In adults, CT is currently the diagnostic procedure of choice, as neither trauma ultrasound nor DPL adequately assess the retroperitoneum (moderate evidence). In children, ultrasound may be useful to exclude surgically significant renal injury (color Doppler) (limited evidence). On occasion, conventional radiographic procedures (upper gastrointestinal positive-contrast fluoroscopy, intravenous or retrograde pyelography) may be helpful in secondary or follow-up evaluations of individuals known to have sustained injuries to the duodenum and upper urinary tracts, respectively.

Supporting Evidence: Compared to its performance at detecting acute injuries to intraperitoneal solid organ injury, CT is relatively insensitive to acute pancreatic injuries, even severe injuries completely disrupting the main pancreatic duct or panceaticoduodenal junction (sensitivities <80%). Direct signs include a fracture plane traversing the neck, body, or tail of the pancreas, or separation of the duodenum from the head of the pancreas. Indirect findings on intravenous contrast-enhanced CT include heterogeneous enhancement of the pancreatic parenchyma, and fluid around the pancreas, especially when combined with fluid in the lesser sac. Fluid posterior to the pancreas, where it may separate the pancreas from the splenic vein, is nonspecific, especially when seen with diffuse anterior pararenal fluid collections, where it likely represents suffusions from aggressive resuscitation with crystalloid fluids. Definitive diagnosis and staging of main pancreatic duct injuries requires intraoperative, endoscopic, or magnetic resonance (MR) cholangiopancreatography. However, MR cholangiopancreatography may be less reliable in the acute than subacute setting (113–120).

Renal parenchymal injuries are more common, both as isolated retroperitoneal and as combined retro- and intraperitoneal injuries. Treatment choices are strongly guided by patients' hemodynamic status, and active arterial extravasation is commonly amenable to endovascular therapies. Interventions are more often required when the collecting systems or ureters are injured, especially when portions of the kidney appear devitalized and where renal injuries are combined with other intraabdominal injuries, such as liver, spleen, pancreas or bowel lacerations.

Even where trauma ultrasound or DPL are negative, contrast-enhanced CT is indicated for the presence of posttraumatic gross hematuria (all age groups), and microscopic hematuria (>50 red blood cells per high-powered field, 3+ on urine dip) in children (regardless of their hemodynamic status) and in adults who have any documented systolic hypotension (<90 mm Hg). Signs or symptoms (flank ecchymosis or pain) of retroperitoneal injury warrant imaging evaluation, even among victims of low-energy trauma, because up to 5% to 8% of surgically important renal injuries do not show any hematuria and preexisting renal abnormalities (e.g., congenital ureteropelvic junction stenosis, horseshoe kidney) have a much greater propensity for injury, and at least one third of such injured kidneys require intervention (121–123).

Dynamic, contrast-enhanced CT ideally evaluates vascular (vascular pedicle injuries including dissection, pseudoaneurysms, and AV fistulae), parenchymal (parenchymal lacerations), and pyelographic (lacerations involving the collecting system, and ureteropelvic junction disruptions) physiologic phases. When low- or iso-osmolar intravenous contrast agents are employed, imaging during the late parenchymal phase and following an additional 5- to 10-minute delay shows or strongly suggests the presence of essentially all important upper urinary tract injuries. However, the classic finding for renal infarct, the so-called cortical rim sign, may take 8 hours or longer to develop following renal artery occlusion. Other findings, such as retrograde filling of the renal vein, suggest an acute arterial disruption as cause for nonopacification of the kidney. Indirect intravenous contrast-enhanced CT findings of upper urinary tract injury include perinephric stranding and hematoma, and heterogeneous parenchymal enhancement. Medial perinephric hematomas, especially when large and extending into the root of the mesentery, are associated with renovascular and ureteropelvic junction (UPJ) injuries. Otherwise, the location of perinephric hematoma poorly correlates with the severity of parenchymal injury or the need to intervene. However, larger perinephric hematomas tend to be associated with more severe injuries. Direct intravenous contrast-enhanced CT findings of renal injury include parenchymal lacerations and extravasation, either vascular or urinary, and both of these extravasations may necessitate intervention or follow-up imaging. Although the frequency, timing, and optimum methods for follow-up examination remain subjects of debate, repeat contrast-enhanced CT or MR examinations 2 to 4 days following acute injury may guide selection of patients for early nonmedical interventions. In children, the initial assessment of severity of blunt renal injury (advancing grade) does not correlate with ultimate renal function or renal-related late complications (such as hypertension). However, advanced grades of renal injury do show morphologic changes on delayed follow-up. In adults, large subcapsular hematomas can be associated with subsequent renin-induced hypertension (Page kidney), and differential renal function is commonly associated with more advanced grades of renal injury (124–136).

Bladder ruptures may be intra- or extraperitoneal, or a combination of both. Almost all extraperitoneal bladder ruptures are associated with high-energy osseous disruptions of the pelvic ring. Although most intraperitoneal ruptures are also associated with high-energy osseous disruptions of the pelvis, the overdistended bladder (due to prostatism, etc.) rising out of the true pelvis may be subjected to direct blunt-force impact and rupture. Hematuria associated with pelvic ring fractures, especially if perivesical hematoma or bladder wall thickening is present, warrants positive-contrast cystography, which should not be considered adequate to exclude injury unless intravesical pressure is at least $40\,cmH_2O$ (137).

With the advent of CT, adrenal injuries are now recognized as the most common retroperitoneal injury. The right is injured much more often than the left, and bilateral adrenal hemorrhage is relatively rare. An association exists between apparent right adrenal hemorrhage and liver lacerations involving the bare area. Despite their frequency (0.5–5%), adrenal hemorrhages very rarely require treatment: embolization for large, active extravasations associated with ongoing hemodynamic consequences, and adrenocortical replacement therapy for hypoadrenalism as a very infrequent sequel to bilateral adrenal hemorrhage. Computed tomography findings include irregular, globular enlargement of the gland, typically measuring 40 to 70 HU. However, definite distinction from extant nontraumatic adrenal pathology may require targeted follow-up CT, ultrasound, or MRI (138,139).

Imaging Case Studies

Case 1

A 56-year-old male passenger was ejected in an high-speed rollover motor vehicle accident (Fig. 24.2), sustaining left lower rib fractures (not shown) with associated pulmonary contusion, and left diaphragmatic rupture with gastric herniation.

Case 2

A 43-year-old woman sustained severe polytrauma (including adrenal, liver, gallbladder, and renal lacerations) in a 20-foot fall onto concrete (Fig. 24.3).

Future Research

- Development of imaging modalities or imaging-based criteria that enable identification of subjects who require surgical rather than non-surgical treatment for their injuries.
- Improvement in intravenous contrast agents to enable simultaneous imaging of arterial, venous, and organ parenchymal structures.
- Development of imaging equipment and procedures that enable rapid, accurate cross-sectional imaging of injured patients without transport or disruption of resuscitation efforts.
- Incorporation of imaging into injury-site triage to enable appropriate direction of patients within the trauma system.

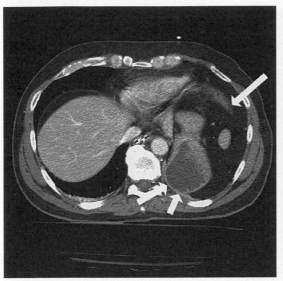
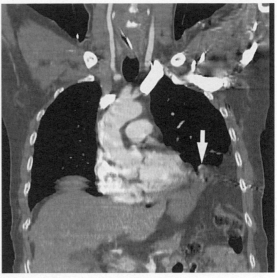

Figure 24.2. A: Axial intravenous contrast-enhanced CT shows a discontinuous and thickened left hemidiaphragm at the 2 o'clock position (arrow), through which the stomach has herniated and abuts posterior chest wall ("dependent viscera" sign) (double arrows). B: Coronal CT reformation shows the free edge of the lacerated diaphragm (arrow) with omentum and stomach herniated into the chest.

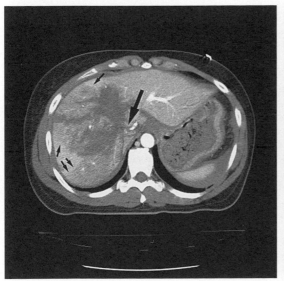
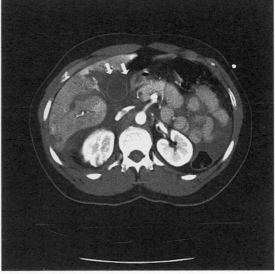

Figure 24.3. A: Axial intravenous contrast-enhanced CT shows complex liver laceration extending to the inferior vena cava (IVC) through the course of the right hepatic vein (large arrow). Note geographic pattern of lesser enhancement involving most of the right lobe of liver (small arrows), which strong suggests disruption of the hepatic vein and may be associated with retrohepatic vena caval injury. B: Axial intravenous contrast-enhanced CT shows complex liver laceration extending into gallbladder fossa, absent enhancement of the gallbladder wall (11 to 2 o'clock positions) suggestive of gallbladder rupture (arrows), and separation of gallbladder from liver, compatible with partial avulsion.

Suggested Imaging Protocols

Trauma Computed Tomography of the Abdomen and Pelvis

Imaging protocols for CT of the abdomen and pelvis in trauma remain in flux as newer scanners are developed with higher numbers of detectors. In general, we scan from the dome of the diaphragm to the pelvic floor with a detector collimation of 2.5 mm. Images are reconstructed at 5-mm intervals for viewing on the workstation. Bone images may be reconstructed at 2.5-mm intervals for the bony pelvis and spine as indicated, with coronal and sagittal reformations. We use 150 cc of nonionic intravenous contrast and scan after a delay of 60 seconds. No oral contrast is used.

Trauma Ultrasound

Scanning is performed on a 3.5- to 5-MHz transducer depending on body habitus. Images are obtained prior to placement of the Foley catheter to preserve some fluid in the bladder. Otherwise, fluid may be inserted via the Foley. Transverse and sagittal images are obtained of the pelvis through the bladder window followed by transverse images of the bilateral upper quadrants and pericolic gutters. The pericardium is also visualized via a subxiphoid and/or left parasternal approach.

References

1. American College of Surgeons. Advanced Trauma Life Support Student Course Manual. Chicago: American College of Surgeons, 1997.
2. National Center for Health Statistics. Monthly Vital Statistics Report 1990; 39:22–25.
3. Baker SP, O'Neill B, Ginsburg MJ, Li G. The Injury Fact Book. New York: Oxford University Press, 1992.
4. Rice DP, MacKenzie EJ, et al. Cost of Injury in the United States: A Report to Congress. Baltimore: Johns Hopkins University, 1989.
5. Kleinman PK, O'Connor B, Nimkin K, et al. Pediatr Radiol 2002;32:896–901.
6. Kleinman PK, Nimkin K, Spevak MR, et al. AJR 1996;167:893–896.
7. Mandelstam SA, Cook D, Fitzgerald M, Ditchfield MR. Arch Dis Child 2003;88:387–390; discussion 387–390.
8. Carty H, Pierce A. Eur Radiol 2002;12:2919–2925.
9. Fuhrman CR, Britton CA, Bender T, et al. AJR 2002;179:1551–1553.
10. Alkadhi H, Wildermuth S, Marincek B, Boehm T. J Comput Assist Tomogr 2004; 28:378–385.
11. Ludwig K, Schulke C, Diederich S, et al. Radiology 2003;227:163–168.
12. Herron JM, Bender TM, Campbell WL, Sumkin JH, Rockette HE, Gur D. Radiology 2000;215:169–174.
13. Omert L, Yeaney WW, Protetch J. Am Surg 2001;67:660–664.
14. Park SH, Song HH, Han JH, et al. Invest Radiol 1994;29:54–58.
15. Gupta A, Jamshidi M, Rubin JR. Cardiovasc Surg 1997;5:48–53.
16. Jelly LM, Evans DR, Easty MJ, Coats TJ, Chan O. Radiographics 2000;20(Spec. No.):S251–259; discussion S260–252.
17. Kara M, Dikmen E, Erdal HH, Simsir I, Kara SA. Eur J Cardiothorac Surg 2003;24:608–613.
18. Calculli L, Papa S, Spagnol A, et al. Radiol Med (Torino) 1995;90:208–211.
19. Erhan Y, Solak I, Kocabas S, Sozbilen M, Kumanlioglu K, Moral AR. Ulus Travma Derg 2001;7:242–245.

20. LaBan MM, Siegel CB, Schutz LK, Taylor RS. Arch Phys Med Rehabil 1994; 75:353–354.
21. Wippermann B, Schmidt U, Nerlich M. Unfallchirurg 1991;94:231–235.
22. Niitsu M, Takeda T. J Comput Assist Tomogr 2003;27:469–474.
23. Ciraulo DL, Elliott D, Mitchell KA, Rodriguez A. J Am Coll Surg 1994; 178:466–470.
24. Lee L, Miller TT, Schultz E, Toledano B. Am J Orthop 1998;27:699–702.
25. Lange RH, Noel SH. J Orthop Trauma 1993;7:361–366.
26. Francois B, Desachy A, Cornu E, Ostyn E, Niquet L, Vignon P. J Trauma 1998; 44:217–219.
27. Zelle BA, Pape HC, Gerich TG, Garapati R, Ceylan B, Krettek C. J Bone Joint Surg Am 2004;86–A:2–8.
28. Sampson LN, Britton JC, Eldrup-Jorgensen J, Clark DE, Rosenberg JM, Bredenberg CE. J Vasc Surg 1993;17:1083–1088; discussion 1088–1089.
29. Lahoda LU, Kreklau B, Gekle C, Muhr G. Unfallchirurg 1998;101:791–795.
30. Teh J, Firth M, Sharma A, Wilson A, Reznek R, Chan O. Clin Radiol 2003; 58:482–486.
31. Abboud PA, Kendall J. J Emerg Med 2003;25:181–184.
32. Chen SC, Markmann JF, Kauder DR, Schwab CW. J Trauma 1997;42:86–89.
33. Sugimoto K, Asari Y, Hirata M, Imai H, Ohwada T. Injury 1998;29:380–382.
34. Shkrum MJ, Green RN, Shum DT. J Forensic Sci 1991;36:410–421.
35. Tyburski JG, Collinge JD, Wilson RF, Eachempati SR. J Trauma 1999;46:833–838.
36. Donnelly LF, Klosterman LA. Radiology 1997;204:385–387.
37. Liman ST, Kuzucu A, Tastepe AI, Ulasan GN, Topcu S. Eur J Cardiothorac Surg 2003;23:374–378.
38. Miller PR, Croce MA, Kilgo PD, Scott J, Fabian TC. Am Surg 2002;68:845–850; discussion 850–841.
39. Hoegerle S, Benzing A, Nitzsche EU, et al. Nuklearmedizin 2001;40:44–50.
40. Hogerle S, Brautigam P, Benzing A, et al. Nuklearmedizin 1997;36:137–141.
41. Holmes JF, Sokolove PE, Brant WE, Kuppermann N. Ann Emerg Med 2002; 39:492–499.
42. Thaete FL, Fuhrman CR, Oliver JH, et al. AJR 1994;162:575–581.
43. Antonelli M, Moro ML, Capelli O, et al. Chest 1994;105:224–228.
44. Kiev J, Kerstein MD. Surg Gynecol Obstet 1992;175:249–253.
45. Le Corre A, Genevois A, Hellot MF, Veber B, Dureuil B. Ann Fr Anesth Reanim 2001;20:23–27.
46. Miller PR, Croce MA, Bee TK, et al. J Trauma 2001;51:223–228; discussion 229–230.
47. Putensen C, Waibel U, Koller W, Putensen-Himmer G, Beck E, Benzer H. Anaesthesist 1990;39:530–534.
48. Adegboye VO, Ladipo JK, Brimmo IA, Adebo AO. Afr J Med Med Sci 2002; 31:315–320.
49. Bokhari F, Brakenridge S, Nagy K, et al. J Trauma 2002;53:1135–1138.
50. Trupka A, Kierse R, Waydhas C, et al. Unfallchirurg 1997;100:469–476.
51. Shiau YC, Liu FY, Tsai JJ, Wang JJ, Ho ST, Kao A. Ann Nucl Med 2003; 17:435–438.
52. Gonzalez RP, Falimirski ME. Am Surg 1999;65:711–713; discussion 714.
53. Helm M, Hauke J, Esser M, Lampl L, Bock KH. Chirurg 1997;68:606–612.
54. Hyre CE, Cikrit DF, Lalka SG, Sawchuk AP, Dalsing MC. J Vasc Surg 1998; 27:880–884; discussion 884–885.
55. Karaaslan T, Meuli R, Androux R, Duvoisin B, Hessler C, Schnyder P. J Trauma 1995;39:1081–1086.
56. Litmanovitz I, Dolfin T, Arnon S, et al. J Perinat Med 2000;28:158–160.
57. Marts B, Durham R, Shapiro M, et al. Am J Surg 1994;168:688–692.
58. Marzi I, Risse N, Wiercinski A, Rose S, Mutschler W. Langenbecks Arch Chir Suppl Kongressbd 1996;113:928–930.

59. von Oettingen G, Bergholt B, Ostergaard L, Jensen LC, Gyldensted C, Astrup J. Neuroradiology 2000;42:168–173.
60. Walz M, Muhr G. Unfallchirurg 1990;93:359–363.
61. Trupka AW, Trautwein K, Waydhas C, Nast-Kolb D, Pfeiffer KJ, Schweiberer L. Zentralbl Chir 1997;122:666–673.
62. Ho RT, Blackmore CC, et al. Emerg Radiol 2002;9:183–187.
63. Hunink MGM, Bos JJ. AJR 1995;165:27–36.
64. Boulanger BR, Milzman DP, Rosati C, Rodriguez A. J Trauma 1993;35:255–260.
65. Chen JC, Wilson SE. Am Surg 1991;57:810–815.
66. Gelman R, Mirvis SE, Gens D. AJR 1991;156:51–57.
67. Guth AA, Pachter HL, Kim U. Am J Surg 1995;170:5–9.
68. Ilgenfritz FM, Stewart DE. Am Surg 1992;58:334–338; discussion 338–339.
69. Karnak I, Senocak ME, Tanyel FC, Buyukpamukcu N. Surg Today 2001;31:5–11.
70. Leung JC, Nance ML, Schwab CW, Miller WT Jr. J Thorac Imaging 1999; 14:126–129.
71. Murray JG, Caoili E, Gruden JF, Evans SJ, Halvorsen RA Jr, Mackersie RC. AJR 1996;166:1035–1039.
72. Nau T, Seitz H, Mousavi M, Vecsei V. Surg Endosc 2001;15:992–996.
73. Rodriguez-Morales G, Rodriguez A, Shatney CH. J Trauma 1986;26:438–444.
74. Scaglione M, Pinto F, Grassi R, et al. Radiol Med (Torino) 2000;99:16–50.
75. Shanmuganathan K, Mirvis SE, White CS, Pomerantz SM. AJR 1996; 167:397–402.
76. Shapiro MJ, Heiberg E, Durham RM, Luchtefeld W, Mazuski JE. Clin Radiol 1996;51:27–30.
77. Voeller GR, Reisser JR, Fabian TC, Kudsk K, Mangiante EC. Am Surg 1990; 56:28–31.
78. Worthy SA, Kang EY, Hartman TE, Kwong JS, Mayo JR, Muller NL. Radiology 1995;194:885–888.
79. Mehall JR, Ennis JS, Saltzman DA, et al. J Am Coll Surg 2001;193:347–353.
80. Stylianos S. J Pediatr Surg 2002;37:453–456.
81. Leinwand MJ, Atkinson CC, Mooney DP. J Pediatr Surg 2004;39:487–490; discussion 487–490.
82. Stengel D, Bauwens K, et al. Br J Surg 2001;88:901–912.
83. Stengel D, Bauwens K, et al. Zentralbl Chir 2003;128:1027–1037 German.
84. Sirlin CB, Brown MA, Andrade-Barreto OA, et al. Radiology 2004;230:661–668.
85. Stengel D, Bauwens K, Sehouli J, Nantke J, Ekkernkamp A. J Trauma 2001; 51:37–43.
86. Barquist ES, Pizano LR, Feuer W, et al. J Trauma 2004;56:334–338.
87. Al-Shanafey S, Giacomantonio M, Jackson R. Pediatr Surg Int 2001;17:365–368.
88. Zabolotny B, Hancock BJ, Postuma R, Wiseman N. Can J Surg 2002;45:358–362.
89. Lutz N, Mahboubi S, Nance ML, Stafford PW. J Pediatr Surg 2004;39:491–494.
90. Catalano O, Lobianco R, Sandomenico F, Siani A. J Ultrasound Med 2003;22:467–477.
91. Willmann JK, Roos JE, Platz A, et al. AJR 2002;179:437–444.
92. Weishaupt D, Hetzer FH, Ruehm SG, Patak MA, Schmidt M, Debatin JF. Eur Radiol 2000;10:1958–1964.
93. Pilleul F, Billaud Y, Gautier G, et al. Gastrointest Endosc 2004;59:818–822.
94. Huebner S, Reed MH. Pediatr Radiol 2001;31:852–855.
95. Lyass S, Sela T, Lebensart PD, Muggia-Sullam M. Isr Med Assoc J 2001; 3:731–733.
96. Rovin JD, Alford BA, McIlhenny TJ, Burns RC, Rodgers BM, McGahren ED. Am Surg 2001;67:127–130.
97. Albanese CT, Meza MP, Gardner MJ, Smith SD, Rowe MI, Lynch JM. J Trauma 1996;40:417–421.
98. Kloppel R, Brock D, Kosling S, Bennek J, Hormann D. Aktuelle Radiol 1997; 7:19–22.
99. Graham JS, Wong AL. J Pediatr Surg 1996;31:754–756.

100. Hickey NA, Ryan MF, Hamilton PA, Bloom C, Murphy JP, Brenneman F. Can Assoc Radiol J 2002;53:153–159.
101. Jamieson DH, Babyn PS, Pearl R. Pediatr Radiol 1996;26:188–194.
102. Ruf C, Kohlberger E, Ruf G, Farthmann EH. Langenbecks Arch Chir Suppl Kongressbd 1997;114:1244–1246.
103. Sivit CJ, Eichelberger MR, Taylor GA. AJR 1994;163:1195–1198.
104. Sivit CJ, Taylor GA, Bulas DI, Kushner DC, Potter BM, Eichelberger MR. Radiology 1992;182:723–726.
105. Sivit CJ, Taylor GA, Newman KD, et al. AJR 1991;157:111–114.
106. Butela ST, Federle MP, et al. AJR 2001;176:129–135.
107. Shankar KR, Lloyd DA, Kitteringham L, Carty HM. Br J Surg 1999;86: 1073–1077.
108. Allen TL, Mueller MT, Bonk RT, Harker CP, Duffy OH, Stevens MH. J Trauma 2004;56:314–322.
109. Federle MP, Yagan N, Peitzman AB, Krugh J. Radiology 1997;205:91–93.
110. Breen DJ, Janzen DL, Zwirewich CV, Nagy AG. J Comput Assist Tomogr 1997; 21:706–712.
111. Brody JM, Leighton DB, Murphy BL, et al. Radiographics 2000;20:1525–1536; discussion 1536–1527.
112. Kane NM, Francis IR, Burney RE, Wheatley MJ, Ellis JH, Korobkin M. Invest Radiol 1991;26:574–578.
113. Jobst MA, Canty TG, Sr., Lynch FP. J Pediatr Surg 1999;34:818–823; discussion 823–814.
114. Soto JA, Alvarez O, Munera F, Yepes NL, Sepulveda ME, Perez JM. AJR 2001; 176:175–178.
115. Fulcher AS, Turner MA, Yelon JA, et al. J Trauma 2000;48:1001–1007.
116. Bigattini D, Boverie JH, Dondelinger RF. Eur Radiol 1999;9:244–249.
117. Porter JM, Singh Y. Am J Emerg Med 1998;16:225–227.
118. Coppola V, Vallone G, Verrengia D, et al. Radiol Med (Torino) 1997;94:335–340.
119. Sivit CJ, Eichelberger MR. AJR 1995;165:921–924.
120. Reaney SM, Parker MS, Mirvis SE, Bundschuh CV, Luebbert PD, Vingan HL. Clin Radiol 1995;50:834–838.
121. Bschleipfer T, Kallieris D, Hallscheidt P, Hauck EW, Weidner W, Pust RA. J Urol 2003;170:2475–2479.
122. Mayor B, Gudinchet F, Wicky S, Reinberg O, Schnyder P. Pediatr Radiol 1995;25:214–218.
123. Brandes SB, McAninch JW. J Trauma 1999;47:643–649; discussion 649–650.
124. Moudouni SM, Patard JJ, Manunta A, Guiraud P, Guille F, Lobel B. BJU Int 2001;87:290–294.
125. Rathaus V, Pomeranz A, Shapiro-Feinberg M, Zissin R. Emerg Radiol 2004; 10:190–192.
126. Toutouzas KG, Karaiskakis M, Kaminski A, Velmahos GC. Am Surg 2002; 68:1097–1103.
127. Perez-Brayfield MR, Gatti JM, Smith EA, et al. J Urol 2002;167:2543–2546; discussion 2546–2547.
128. Nguyen MM, Das S. Urology 2002;59:762–766; discussion 766–767.
129. Pietrera P, Badachi Y, Liard A, Dacher JN. J Radiol 2001;82:833–838.
130. Ku JH, Jeon YS, Kim ME, Lee NK, Park YH. Int J Urol 2001;8:261–267.
131. Blankenship JC, Gavant ML, Cox CE, Chauhan RD, Gingrich JR. World J Surg 2001;25:1561–1564.
132. Sebastia MC, Rodriguez-Dobao M, Quiroga S, Pallisa E, Martinez-Rodriguez M, Alvarez-Castells A. Eur Radiol 1999;9:611–615.
133. McGahan JP, Richards JR, Jones CD, Gerscovich EO. J Ultrasound Med 1999; 18:207–213; quiz 215–216.
134. Perry MJ, Porte ME, Urwin GH. J R Coll Surg Edinb 1997;42:420–422.
135. Mulligan JM, Cagiannos I, Collins JP, Millward SF. J Urol 1998;159:67–70.

136. Kawashima A, Sandler CM, Corriere JN Jr, Rodgers BM, Goldman SM. Radiology 1997;205:487–492.
137. Deck AJ, Shaves S, Talner L, Porter JR. World J Surg 2001;25:1592–1596.
138. Stawicki SP, Hoey BA, Grossman MD, Anderson HL 3rd, Reed JF 3rd. Curr Surg 2003;60:431–436.
139. Schwarz M, Horev G, Freud E, et al. Isr Med Assoc J 2000;2:132–134.

25

Imaging in Acute Abdominal Pain

C. Craig Blackmore, Tina A. Chang, and Gregory David Avey

Given the broad range of diagnoses that may cause acute abdominal pain, several important diseases are examined in other chapters in this book. Guidelines regarding the imaging of ureteral calculi, ectopic pregnancy, hepatobiliary disease, and vascular disease can be found in their respective chapters. Other frequent etiologies of acute abdominal pain are discussed in this chapter as individual entities.

Issues of Imaging of Appendicitis

 I. What is the accuracy of imaging for diagnosing acute appendicitis in adults?
 II. What is the accuracy of imaging for diagnosing acute appendicitis in children?

Issues of Imaging of Small Bowel Obstruction

 III. What is the accuracy of imaging for diagnosing small bowel obstruction?
 IV. What is the accuracy of computed tomography for detecting small bowel ischemia?

Issues of Imaging of Diverticulitis

 V. What is the accuracy of imaging for acute colonic diverticulitis?
 VI. What is the accuracy of computed tomography in predicting the success of conservative management in patients with suspected acute colonic diverticulitis?

Issues

- Computed tomography (CT) examination of adult patients has high sensitivity and specificity for acute appendicitis and is superior to graded compression ultrasound (moderate evidence).

Key Points

457

- In pediatric patients, ultrasound has high sensitivity and specificity for acute appendicitis and is preferred over CT due to absence of ionizing radiation (moderate evidence).
- Computed tomography has high negative predictive value for ischemic bowel in subjects with small bowel obstruction (moderate evidence).
- Computed tomography has high accuracy for detection of colonic diverticulitis (moderate evidence), but the effect on patient management and outcome has not been established (limited evidence).

Definition and Pathophysiology

The term *acute abdomen* is defined as significant abdominal pain that develops over a course of hours (1,2). The list of potential diagnoses is broad and encompasses potentially serious as well as relatively innocuous conditions (3). The initial presenting pain is often vague and diffuse, reflecting the visceral innervation of the abdominal organs (4). These factors can make achieving an accurate clinical diagnosis difficult. For example, one series collected before the advent of graded compression ultrasound or helical CT demonstrated a change from the initial diagnosis to discharge diagnosis in 55% of patients admitted for abdominal pain (5).

Appendicitis is defined as inflammation of the vermiform appendix, usually caused by obstruction of the appendiceal lumen (6). Obstruction leads to bacterial overgrowth and an increase in intraluminal pressure, which in turn causes a decrease in mural perfusion. The resulting inflammation and decrease in vascular perfusion can lead to gangrene and perforation, with possible complications including diffuse peritonitis or localized periappendiceal abscess formation (7–9).

The causes of small bowel obstruction are quite varied, with intraabdominal adhesions, external and internal hernias, and neoplasms underlying the obstruction in the majority of patients (10). Other less common causes include volvulus, intussusception, inflammatory strictures, gallstones, feces, and bezoars. Mechanistically, the ischemic pathology of small bowel obstruction is thought to occur in a similar order as appendicitis, that is, obstruction, bowel wall edema and interluminal fluid accumulation, followed by a decrease in vascular perfusion, potentially causing ischemia and perforation (9). Progression to perforation does not occur in all patients presenting with small bowel obstruction, and the majority of patients with proximal, nonischemic obstruction due to adhesions successfully resolve with nonoperative management (10–12). Additionally, after each operation for small bowel obstruction due to adhesions there is an increasing risk of future episodes, with a recurrence rate of 81% after four such operations (13).

Three interdependent states have traditionally been defined in the study of diverticular disease: the prediverticular state, diverticulosis, and diverticulitis (14). The general term *diverticular disease* and the term *diverticulosis* refer to the presence of uninflamed diverticula, whereas the term *diverticulitis* describes the variety of inflammatory conditions associated with these lesions (15). Diverticulitis originates from both increased interluminal pressure and inherent weakness in the colonic wall near the areas of penetration of the vasa recta (15,16). Epidemiologic studies suggest that a diet low in fiber presents an increased risk of formation of diverticuli in the sigmoid colon (17). Diverticulitis is thought to result from obstruction of diverticuli, resulting in inflammation and eventual microabscess formation (15). Severity of diverticulitis has been categorized by Hinchey et al. (18) into four categories: stage I, microabscess formation; stage II, larger abscess collections; stage III, peritonitis; and stage IV, fecal peritonitis (18).

Epidemiology

Over 7 million patients with acute abdominal pain present to an emergency department (ED) every year, making up 4% to 6% of all ED visits (19–21). Upon discharge, 25% to 41% remain without a specific etiology for their abdominal pain (21,22). These patients with undifferentiated abdominal pain typically have a benign course and a reassuring prognosis (23,24). However, several life-threatening causes of abdominal pain have a high incidence of missed diagnosis, including ruptured aortic aneurysm, appendicitis, ectopic pregnancy, and myocardial infarction (25). Table 25.1 lists the most prevalent diagnoses in patients with acute abdominal pain.

Acute appendicitis represents a relatively common condition, with an estimated lifetime incidence of 9% in males and 7% in females, and is most common in those between 10 and 19 years of age (26,27). The overall rate of perforation is between 19% and 35.5%, with the risk proportionally greater in the pediatric and elderly populations (27,28).

The Health Care Utilization Project, a weighted sample of hospital discharge data, estimated that there were 197,000 discharges with a primary diagnosis of intestinal obstruction in 2001 (29). Intraabdominal adhesions are the most common cause of small bowel obstruction in the United States, accounting for 60% of the total incidence of obstruction (30). A previous

Table 25.1. Common diagnoses in patients presenting to the emergency department with acute abdominal pain

Rank number	Diagnosis	Percent
1	Undiagnosed abdominal pain	25.1
2	Nausea/vomiting	9.8
3	Unspecified	9.0
4	Cystitis	6.7
5	Gastritis	5.3
6	Pancreatitis	3.9
7	Cholecystitis	3.6
8	Pelvic inflammatory disease	3.4
9	Constipation	3.3
10	Musculoskeletal	2.9
11	Ureteral calculus	2.8
12	Ovarian cyst	1.9
13	Dysmenorrhea	1.9
14	Bowel obstruction	1.6
15	GI ulcer	1.5
16	Cardiac	1.5
17	Hernia	1.4
18	Pyelonephritis	1.4
19	Appendicitis	1.4
20	Vaginitis/cervicitis	1.3

Source: Adapted from Powers and Guertler (21).

abdominal operation was noted in 91% of those diagnosed with small bowel obstruction due to adhesions, with colorectal, gynecologic, and appendectomy accounting for the majority of the antecedent operations (12). Neoplasms, hernias, and Crohn's disease cause 20%, 10%, and 5%, respectively, of the small bowel obstructions in the industrialized world (30).

The presence of diverticuli increases with age in Western societies, with a prevalence of 80% in patients over 85 years of age (15). However, only 10% to 35% of patients with diverticular disease develop diverticulitis (31), and of these only 14% to 25% require operative management (32–35).

Overall Cost to Society

Limited data are available to assess the societal cost of patients presenting with acute abdominal pain. One study has noted that the acute abdominal pain is the most prevalent diagnosis among those whose insurance claims are denied following an ED visit, a group whose average patient charge totaled $1107 (36). When the previously noted 7 million annual ED visits for acute abdominal pain are considered, it is clear that acute abdominal pain has a significant financial impact on the health care system.

Comprehensive societal cost data for patients with suspected acute appendicitis is also lacking. However, a recent analysis of the Nationwide Inpatient Sample of the Health Care Utilization Project by Flum and Koepsell (37) estimated that there were 261,134 yearly hospitalizations due to suspected acute appendicitis. These admissions accrued an average hospital charge of $10,584, yielding an estimated national total of $2.76 billion in hospital charges alone. In this same analysis, the authors estimated the national cost of negative appendectomy at $741.5 million.

The literature regarding small bowel obstruction and cost is largely limited to estimates of hospitalization costs. One study found that the cost of the average total charges for small bowel obstruction to be $23,900, with the average surgery patient acquiring charges of $37,000, and the average nonoperative patient acquiring charges of $4,800 (38). The aggregate national charge estimated by the Health Care Utilization Project found that an estimated $4.6 billion in charges were accrued by patients discharged with a major diagnosis of bowel obstruction.

No epidemiologic studies explicitly examining the cost and incidence of diverticulitis were identified in the literature, nor were any such data cited in the identified relevant articles. However, the significant and increasing incidence of diverticular disease with age and the estimated 20% rate of diverticulitis in those with diverticular disease suggest that diverticular disease is a considerable source of health care expenditure. Data from the Health Care Utilization Project, a weighted nationwide inpatient sample, estimated that 196,125 patients were discharged with a primary diagnosis of diverticulitis in 2002, with estimated hospital charges of $3.9 billion (29).

Goals

The main goals of imaging in the setting of acute abdominal pain are to help identify the etiology of the pain and to exclude the possibility of a life-threatening condition. The secondary goal is to determine which patients with acute abdominal pain require surgical intervention.

Methodology

Adult Appendicitis

A recent evidence-based review of the role of CT and graded compression ultrasound in the diagnosis of acute appendicitis was performed by Terasawa (39). In this review, a literature search was performed of English- and non–English-language articles from 1966 to December 2003 using Medline and Embase. Searches used the MeSH terms *appendicitis* or *appendix, ultrasonography, tomography, x-ray computed, sensitivity and specificity, diagnostic use,* and *diagnosis.* Free text search terms were *appendicitis* and *appendix.* In the Embase search, terms included *appendicitis–diagnosis, radiodiagnosis, computer-assisted tomography, echography,* and *diagnostic imaging.* The bibliographies of relevant articles were searched for other potentially relevant articles. Studies were included if they were prospective evaluations of CT or graded compression ultrasound in patients 14 years or older, with outcomes measured by surgical, pathologic, or clinical follow-up.

Pediatric Appendicitis

A literature search was performed of English-language articles from 1966 to June 2004, using the Medline database and the MeSH terms *appendicitis* and *diagnostic imaging* and *child, appendicitis* and *diagnostic imaging* and *adolescent, appendicitis* and *child–preschool* and *diagnostic imaging,* and *appendicitis* and *infant* and *diagnostic imaging.* The bibliographies of relevant articles were searched for other potentially relevant articles. Studies were included if they were prospective evaluations of CT or graded compression ultrasound in patients 18 years or younger, with outcomes measured by surgical, pathologic, or clinical follow-up.

Imaging in Small Bowel Obstruction

A literature search was performed of English-language articles from 1996 to July 15, 2004, using the Medline database and the MeSH terms *diagnostic imaging* and *intestinal obstruction,* as well as *intestinal obstruction,* or the plain text term *small bowel obstruction* paired with the terms *CT, computed tomography, ultrasound, abdominal film, KUB, MRI,* and *magnetic resonance imaging.* Inclusion criteria incorporated prospective studies of imaging in the setting of the evaluation of patients with suspected acute small bowel obstruction. To be eligible for inclusion, studies were required to use some combination of clinical, surgical, or pathologic follow-up to determine the presence of small bowel obstruction.

Imaging in Acute Diverticular Disease

A literature search was performed of English-language articles from 1996 to July 15, 2004, using the Medline database and the MeSH terms *diverticulitis* and *colonic* or the plain text term *diverticulitis* and the MeSH term *diagnostic imaging,* or the plain text terms *CT, computed tomography, ultrasound, sonography, radiography, MRI,* or *magnetic resonance imaging.* Identified works were included if they were prospective studies of imaging in the setting of the evaluation of patients with suspected acute diverticulitis. To be eligible for inclusion studies were required to use some combination of imaging, clinical, surgical, or pathologic follow-up in the determination of the presence of diverticulitis. Studies that enrolled only patients with positive imaging exams or that used imaging alone in the determination of the presence of diverticulitis were excluded.

I. What Is the Accuracy of Imaging for Diagnosing Acute Appendicitis in Adults?

Summary of Evidence: Computed tomography examination of adult patients has high sensitivity and specificity for acute appendicitis and is superior to graded compression ultrasound (moderate evidence) (Table 25.2).

It is unclear if the increased use of CT has decreased the rate of negative appendectomies (limited evidence).

Supporting Evidence: A recent meta-analysis by Terasawa (39) found 22 prospective trials of graded compression ultrasound or CT in adult and adolescent patients with suspected acute appendicitis. This meta-analysis identified 12 studies of CT in adult and adolescent patients, and demonstrated a combined sensitivity of 94% [95% confidence interval (CI), 91–95%], a combined specificity of 95% (95% CI, 93–96%), a combined positive likelihood ratio of 13.3 (95% CI, 9.9–17.9), and a combined negative likelihood ratio of 0.09 (95% CI, 0.07–0.12). When these test specifications are applied to a population with the mean prevalence of appendicitis found in the trials examined by Terasawa (48%), the positive predictive value is 92% (range, 67% to 98%), and the negative predictive value is 92% (range, 76% to 99%). The sensitivity and specificity of CT were homogeneous in these identified studies despite heterogeneous patient populations, differing prevalence of appendicitis, and varying contrast protocols.

There were 14 studies of graded compression ultrasound that met inclusion criteria in the Terasawa study. There was significant heterogeneity in the outcome of the trials, requiring the use of a random effects model to combine study results. The summary sensitivity of ultrasound in adult and adolescent patients was 86% (95% CI, 78–84%), the summary specificity is 81% (95% CI, 78–84%), the summary positive likelihood ratio was 5.8 (95% CI, 9.4–22.2), and the summary negative likelihood ratio was 0.19 (95% CI, 0.13–0.27). The positive predictive value of graded compression ultrasound was 84% (range, 46% to 95%), and the negative predictive value was 85% (range, 60% to 97%).

Several limitations were identified regarding imaging's efficacy in diagnosing adult and adolescent acute appendicitis. All studies reviewed by Terasawa demonstrated differential reference standard bias, in that the imaging test results determined which subjects underwent appendectomy and which had clinical follow-up as the reference standard. Since the diagnostic test influenced the choice of reference standard, there is the possibility that the sensitivity and specificity for imaging were overestimated (40). In addition, some relatively novel ultrasound techniques, such as color Doppler were excluded from analysis.

Whether imaging decreases the rate of negative appendectomy is controversial. Some studies have suggested that the use of imaging decreases the rate of negative appendectomy, avoids unnecessary hospitalization, and reduces cost (41–45). However, other investigators have reported that imaging has not decreased the rate of negative appendectomy at the population level (46–49). It is unclear if this disparity in results is due to differing patient populations, a decrease in the performance of imaging outside of research settings, lack of fundamental efficacy of the imaging test, or slow diffusion of effective imaging protocols outside of the research setting.

A single prospective study examines the direct cost effect of implementing CT examination in patients with suspected acute appendicitis from the hospital's institutional perspective. This study, by Rao et al. (50), examined the direct costs of CT imaging and the subsequent therapy compared with the direct costs of the projected therapy prior to performing the CT scan in a group of 100 consecutive patients. The cost of hospital admission and the cost of removing a normal appendix were determined from a hospital cost database specific to the study institution. The authors found that the subsequent reduction in negative appendectomies and decreased days spent in the hospital decreased direct costs by $447 per patient. Without a better understanding of the effect of imaging on patient outcome, it is difficult to predict the cost-effectiveness of imaging in adult patients with suspected acute appendicitis (Insufficient evidence).

II. What Is the Accuracy of Imaging for Diagnosing Acute Appendicitis in Children?

Summary of Evidence: Graded compression ultrasound is highly sensitive and specific in detecting acute appendicitis in the pediatric population (moderate evidence) (Table 25.2).

A protocol of graded compression ultrasound followed by CT examination in equivocal cases has a higher sensitivity but lower specificity than ultrasound alone in detecting acute appendicitis in the pediatric population because of increased false positives (moderate evidence) (Table 25.2).

There is conflicting evidence regarding the effect of imaging on the rate of negative appendectomy (limited evidence).

Supporting Evidence: Eight eligible prospective trials examining ultrasound in pediatric patients suspected of acute appendicitis were identified in the literature (51–59). All trials used either pathologic examination of the appendix following appendectomy or clinical follow-up as the outcome measure. These trials represent a total of 6404 patients, with the prevalence of appendicitis in the studies ranging from 9% to 47% (pooled weighted mean prevalence 17%). The sensitivity of graded compression ultrasound ranged from 86% to 94%, with a combined pooled sensitivity of 91% (95% CI, 89–93%). The specificity ranged from 89% to 99%, with a combined pooled specificity of 97% (95% CI, 95–99%). At the combined prevalence of appendicitis found in these trials, the positive predictive value was 87% (range, 82% to 98%), and the negative predictive value was 98% (range, 92% to 99%). The positive likelihood ratio was 32.9 (95% CI, 26.3–61.2), whereas the negative likelihood ratio was 0.09 (95% CI, 0.08–0.11).

A single consecutive prospective trial that utilized CT exam as the primary imaging exam in a pediatric population was identified (60). This trial of 75 children with equivocal or atypical signs of appendicitis was designed to compare the resident and attending physician interpretations of limited CT exams in children with suspected appendicitis. The prevalence of appendicitis identified by pathologic examination following surgery or clinical follow-up was 25%. The diagnostic sensitivity of attending physicians was 95%, and the specificity was 98%. This yielded a positive predictive value of 94% and a negative predicative value of 98.3%. These data are similar to other, retrospective, evaluations of CT in the pediatric population (45,61), and correlate with a nonconsecutive prospective study of CT (60). However, the limited number of children in this trial and the lack of a direct comparison to graded compression ultrasound preclude definitive comparison of CT versus ultrasound as the primary imaging exam in the pediatric population.

The desire to increase the accuracy of imaging yet limit the radiation exposure has led investigators to examine combinations of CT and graded compression ultrasound exam. Two prospective studies examined the combination of graded compression ultrasound as the initial imaging, followed by CT study if the ultrasound exam was equivocal or failed to match the clinical presentation (62,63). Another randomized trial compared CT and ultrasound versus ultrasound alone in a pediatric population (59). These trials enrolled 585 patients, and had a prevalence of appendicitis ranging from 23% to 43%, with a pooled prevalence of 39%. The sensitivity of these protocols varied from 77% to 97%, with a pooled sensitivity of 95% (95% CI, 83–100%). The range of specificity was 89% to 99%, with a pooled result of 93% (95% CI, 87–97%). As would be expected, these protocols demonstrated a greater sensitivity when the combined ultrasound followed by CT test results were considered than when the same series of ultrasound data was considered alone. This increased sensitivity, however, was achieved with the drawback of a lower overall specificity. The single randomized trial demonstrated similar results, with CT and ultrasound combined demonstrating a higher sensitivity than ultrasound alone; however, the sensitivities of the two groups were not found to be statistically different (59). The positive and negative predictive values at the pooled prevalence of appendicitis were 97% (range, 87% to 96%) and 88% (range, 93% to 99%), respectively. The positive likelihood ratio of CT followed by graded ultrasound was found to be 13.03, with a negative likelihood ratio of 0.06.

As with the studies of imaging in adult appendicitis, the trials examining imaging and pediatric appendicitis suffer from a number of potential limitations, including the use of different reference standards with the choice of reference standard determined by the imaging result. Thus, the sensitivity and specificity for imaging may be falsely inflated (40). In addition, many included trials conducted imaging only after explicitly excluding patients with a typical disease presentation who underwent immediate appendectomy (51–53,57,60,63,64). Since the diagnosis of "typical" appendicitis is made by individual clinical judgment, the resulting study populations may not be strictly comparable.

As with imaging of appendicitis in adults, there has been conflicting data regarding the effect of imaging on the rate of finding a normal appendix by pathology following appendectomy. Some retrospective studies have found a decrease in the rate of negative appendectomy (41,65,66). Other studies, however, come to the opposite conclusion (67–70). All of these retrospective examinations were potentially limited by sample bias and verification bias. Given these conflicting results, it is unclear if the impact of imaging on the rate of negative appendectomies can be adequately determined outside of the performance of a randomized trial.

The data examining the cost impact of imaging in pediatric patients with suspected appendicitis are limited. A single prospective cohort trial has examined the cost of a protocol of ultrasound followed by CT exam if indicated (65). This trial, from the hospital point of view, was conducted using the same cohort of 139 patients as was used to determine the overall sensitivity of the protocol (63). This trial found that the overall cost was decreased by $565 per patient using the protocol. However, this calculation assumes that the decrease in negative appendectomy can be replicated outside of the research setting. As has been noted previously, there is not a consensus that imaging has decreased the rate of negative appendectomies.

III. What Is the Accuracy of Imaging for Diagnosing Small Bowel Obstruction?

Summary of Evidence: Computed tomography and ultrasound have higher sensitivity and specificity than conventional plain film abdominal imaging for diagnosing small bowel obstruction (moderate evidence) (Table 25.3).

Computed tomography has a higher sensitivity in the detection of small bowel obstruction than ultrasound examination (limited evidence) (Table 25.3).

Supporting Evidence: Four identified series, representing 199 patients, have prospectively examined the efficacy of conventional abdominal imaging in comparison to another imaging modality (38,71–73). No prospective trials examining conventional radiography outside of a comparison study were identified. The pooled sensitivity and specificity of conventional radiography were 65% (95% CI, 42–88%) and 75% (95% CI, 58–92%), respectively. If the prevalence of small bowel obstruction in those referred to imaging is similar to the pooled prevalence found in this review (68%), the positive predictive value of conventional radiography is 85% and the negative predictive value is 50%. In direct comparison trials, conventional plain film examination was found to be less sensitive and specific in the diagnosis of small bowel obstruction than ultrasound (38,71) or magnetic resonance imaging (MRI) (72). When directly compared to CT examination, conventional radiography was found to be both less specific and less sensitive in one study (71), and to have similar specificity, but lower sensitivity in another (73).

The reliability of ultrasound examination of patients with suspected small bowel obstruction has been examined in at least four prospective trials, representing 306 total exams (38,71,74,75). The pooled sensitivity and specificity of ultrasound examination were 92% (95% CI, 87–96%) and 95% (95% CI, 87–100%), respectively. These test characteristics, evaluated with a prevalence of obstruction of 68%, yield a positive predictive value of 98% and a negative predicative value of 84%.

A single, small ($n = 32$) prospective trial has compared ultrasound examination to CT for evaluation of this patient population, and found that ultrasound has lower sensitivity than CT exam in detecting bowel obstruction (71). This study did not find any difference in specificity between ultrasound and CT; however, this work was limited in that only two of 32 patients were not diagnosed with bowel obstruction.

The test characteristics of CT examination have the most prospective data in this area, with a total of seven studies representing 365 patients identified in the literature (71,72,76–80). The sensitivity of CT exam ranged from 71% to 100%, with a pooled sensitivity of 94% (95% CI, 86–100%). The specificity of CT exam was found to range from 57% to 100%, with a pooled result of 78% (95% CI, 63–93%). In a population referred for radiologic imaging with a prevalence of small bowel obstruction of 68%, this would result in a positive predictive value of 90% and a negative predictive value of 86%.

Two small investigatory studies have examined the possibility of utilizing specialized MRI protocols to detect small bowel obstruction (72,80). These two trials, with a total sample size of 51 patients, suggest that MRI has a high sensitivity (range, 93% to 95%) and a high specificity (100%). One study found that MRI had a higher sensitivity and specificity than CT exam; however, this trial was limited in that only 16 patients underwent both radiographic examinations (80).

All of the studies of imaging in patients with suspected small bowel obstruction demonstrate some common limitations. There is potential verification bias, as the imaging exams had a direct impact on the type of outcome verification that the patient was likely to receive. In addition, sample sizes were uniformly small in the eligible studies, with no study enrolling over 100 patients.

IV. What Is the Accuracy of Computed Tomography for Detecting Small Bowel Ischemia?

Summary of Evidence: Computed tomography examination of patients with suspected small bowel is highly sensitive and specific in detecting small bowel ischemia (moderate evidence) (Table 25.3).

Supporting Evidence: Detecting small bowel ischemia is important due to changes in the management of patients with suspected small bowel obstruction. While surgical tradition has dictated "never let the sun set or rise" on a small bowel obstruction, studies have suggested that up to 69% of patients may be safely observed and managed nonoperatively (81–83). The determination of bowel strangulation or ischemia is important in candidates for nonoperative management, as bowel ischemia is considered an indication for initial operative management. However, patient history, physical signs, and laboratory data are neither sufficiently sensitive nor specific to satisfactorily separate patients with and without small bowel ischemia (84,85).

Computed tomography signs such as increased or decreased enhancement of the bowel wall, a "target" sign, closed loop bowel configuration, bowel wall thickening, increased mesenteric fluid, congestion of mesenteric veins, and a "serrated beak" sign have all been retrospectively described as indicating small bowel ischemia (86,87).

Five studies, representing 399 CT exams, have prospectively examined the diagnostic accuracy of CT in detecting small bowel ischemia (76–78,88,89). These studies have demonstrated a high sensitivity in detecting small bowel ischemia, ranging from 83% to 100%, with a pooled result of 95% sensitivity (95% CI, 88–100%). The demonstrated specificity at this high level of sensitivity ranged from 61% to 100%, with a pooled specificity of 90% (95% CI, 78–100%). When these results are evaluated at the pooled prevalence of small bowel ischemia found in these studies (24%), the positive predictive value of CT in predicting bowel ischemia due to small bowel obstruction was found to be 76% and the negative predictive value 98%.

These results indicate that, at least in the research setting, a patient with a negative CT exam is highly unlikely to be suffering from intestinal ischemia due to bowel obstruction. However, it should be acknowledged that the studies identified did not examine changes in overall patient outcome with CT exam. There is limited evidence that CT exam influences patient management. A single prospective study of 57 patients found that when surgeons were required to state management plans before and after CT examination, 23% of patients had a change in plan due to the CT findings (90).

All of the studies examining CT imaging of small bowel ischemia due to bowel obstruction are limited by verification bias and small individual study sample size. In addition, some trials were limited in that only patients with initial CT findings of small bowel obstruction were enrolled in these trials, possibly selecting for a patient population with increased probability for CT findings (88,89). However, similar results were obtained in trials not limited to this patient population (76–78).

V. What Is the Accuracy of Imaging for Acute Colonic Diverticulitis?

Summary of Evidence: Computed tomography demonstrates a higher sensitivity and specificity in detecting acute colonic diverticulitis than graded compression ultrasound (moderate evidence) (Table 25.4).

The data regarding the relative sensitivity and specificity of CT compared with contrast enema radiography is limited.

Supporting Evidence: The radiographic imaging exam with the longest history of use in the diagnosis of acute colonic diverticulitis is a contrast enema in conjunction with conventional radiography (14). The accuracy of this exam has been examined by two small ($n = 86$ and $n = 38$) prospective trials as a comparison to CT exam (91,92). Sensitivity of contrast enema in detection of acute diverticulitis ranged between 80% and 82%, while the specificity ranged between 80% and 100%. When these test characteristics are applied to a patient population with the prevalence of diverticulitis equivalent to the pooled prevalence in the eligible studies of imaging and diverticular disease (50%), the positive predictive value of contrast enema was found to be 84%, and the negative predictive value 82%. Both of these studies were performed to prospectively compare CT and contrast enema in patients with suspected acute diverticulitis. The study, by Stefansson et al. (92) in 1990, found that CT had a lower sensitivity but higher specificity than contrast enema exam. However, another examination of this topic by Cho et al. (91) determined that CT was more sensitive than contrast enema, but that no difference was found in the imaging modalities' specificities. Both studies were potentially limited due to small sample size and verification bias. In addition, the study by Cho et al. was limited by a failure to blind the image interpreters to the outcome of the other imaging result. Due to this limited, conflicting data, no conclusion can be made regarding the more accurate exam modality for detecting acute diverticulitis. Two more studies looked at CT without direct comparison to radiography

(93,94), and these four studies (91–94) include 412 subjects, and indicate that CT is highly specific, with a pooled specificity of 99% (95% CI, 98–100%). The pooled sensitivity of CT was found to be 89% (95% CI, 78%–100%), resulting in a positive predictive value of 99% and a negative predictive value of 90%. No prospective studies comparing ultrasonography and CT examinations were identified.

Ultrasound examination has been proposed in cases of suspected acute diverticulitis due to its cross-sectional capability, lack of ionizing radiation, and wide availability (15,35). Four eligible prospective trials were identified, consisting of 571 imaging exams (95–98). The pooled sensitivity and specificity were found to be 91% (95% CI, 82%–100%) and 92% (95% CI, 82–100%), respectively, resulting in a positive predictive and negative predictive value of 92% and 91%, respectively. No eligible studies performed a comparison between sonography and other imaging modalities. As with other investigations in this area, all the identified studies were limited by verification bias.

VI. What Is the Accuracy of Computed Tomography in Predicting the Success of Conservative Management in Patients with Suspected Acute Colonic Diverticulitis?

Summary of Evidence: Patients judged to have severe diverticular disease on CT are more likely to require initial surgical management and to secondarily experience relapse, persistence, sigmoid stenosis, and fistula or abscess formation (limited evidence).

Supporting Evidence: A single study by Ambrosetti et al. (99) investigated the accuracy of CT in predicting patient management outcome during the initial episode of diverticulitis (medical versus surgical therapy) and likelihood of relapse of diverticulitis following initially successful medical therapy. This investigation of 542 patients with a positive imaging diagnosis of diverticulitis found that a significantly higher proportion of those judged to have severe diverticulitis on CT examination (26%) went on to require surgical management during the initial hospitalization, compared to 4% of those judged to have mild diverticulitis. In addition, patients considered to have severe diverticulitis by CT exam were more likely to acquire a secondary complication (relapse, persistence, sigmoid stenosis, fistula formation, or abscess persistence) after the initial hospitalization, with secondary complication rates of 36% and 17% for the severe and moderate groups, respectively. This study only enrolled those patients with positive imaging results; therefore, it is unknown how accurately imaging predicts patient outcome in those with negative exams. This study was potentially limited by a lack of blinding and possible verification bias.

Future Research

• The data regarding the effect of imaging on negative appendectomy rate are in conflict. Resolution of this question is critical to determining the effect of imaging on patient outcome.

- While studies have demonstrated that CT has a high accuracy in the detection of ischemia in patients with suspected small bowel obstruction, no investigation has yet determined the impact of CT on overall patient outcome.
- The ability of imaging to differentiate medical from surgical causes of abdominal pain and to influence patient management is not well established.
- Relatively little is known regarding the overall cost and cost-effectiveness of imaging for the set of conditions that make up the acute abdomen.

Take-Home Tables

Table 25.2. Sensitivity and specificity of imaging in patients with suspected acute appendicitis

	Sensitivity (%)	Specificity (%)	Positive predictive value (%)[1]	Negative predictive value (%)[1]
Adults[2]				
Ultrasound	86	81	81	86
CT	94	95	95	95
Pediatric				
Ultrasound[3]	92	97	88	98
CT[4]	95	98	92	99
Ultrasound followed by CT[5]	95	93	77	99

[1] Calculated utilizing a prevalence of appendicitis of 48% and 20%, the mean prevalence of appendicitis in the adult and pediatric trials, respectively.
[2] From Terasawa (39).
[3] Derived from references 51–58 and 64.
[4] From reference 60.
[5] From references 59, 62, and 63.

Table 25.3. Sensitivity and specificity of imaging in patients with suspected small bowel obstruction

Modality	Sensitivity (%)	Specificity (%)	Positive predictive value (%)[1]	Negative predictive value (%)[1]
Detection of obstruction				
Plain film[2]	65	75	85	50
Ultrasound[3]	92	95	98	84
CT[4]	94	78	90	86
Detection of ischemia				
CT	95	90	76	98

[1] Calculated utilizing a prevalence of small bowel obstruction of 68% of those imaged and a prevalence of small bowel ischemia of 25%; these were the pooled prevalence found in the eligible studies.
[2] Adapted from references 38 and 71–73.
[3] Adapted from references 38, 71, and 74.
[4] Adapted from references 71, 72, and 76–80.

Table 25.4. Sensitivity and specificity of imaging in patients with suspected acute colonic diverticulitis

Modality	Sensitivity (%)	Specificity (%)	Positive predictive value (%)[1]	Negative predictive value (%)[1]
Contrast enema[2]	81	85	84	82
Ultrasound[3]	91	92	92	91
CT[4]	89	99	99	90

[1] Calculated utilizing a prevalence of diverticulitis of 50%, a prevalence equal to the pooled prevalence of the eligible studies.
[2] Adapted from references 91 and 92.
[3] Adapted from references 95, 96, 98, and 100.
[4] Adapted from references 91–94.

Imaging Case Studies

Case 1

A 67-year-old man with a history of diabetes and hypertension presented to the ED with a 2-day history of central abdominal pain migrating to the bilateral lower quadrants, nausea, and constipation (Fig. 25.1). In the emergency department he exhibited abdominal tenderness, leukocytosis, and neutrophilia.

A CT scan with intravenous and oral contrast demonstrated an enlarged appendix (11 mm in diameter) with associated periappendicular fat stranding. Following the positive CT examination, the probability of confirmed appendicitis (positive predictive value) rises to 95%, as opposed to the 48% probability found in those who are referred for imaging. The diagnosis of appendicitis was confirmed with pathologic examination of the vermiform appendix removed at surgery.

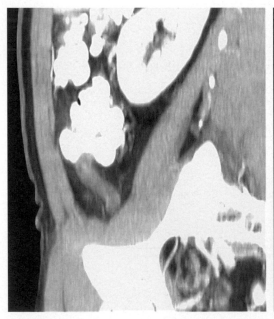 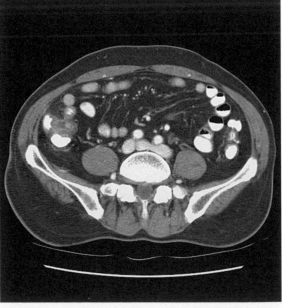

A   B

Figure 25.1. A: Enlarged appendix in sagittal plane. B: Enlarged appendix in transverse plane.

Figure 25.2. Small bowel obstruction.

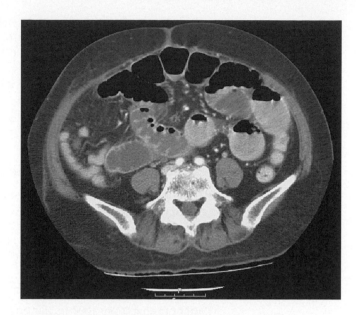

Case 2

A 70-year-old woman presented to the ED with a 2-day history of abdominal pain, nausea, and vomiting. The patient has a history of abdominal surgeries, including repair of an anterior abdominal wall hernia (Fig. 25.2).

An abdominal and pelvic CT examination with intravenous and oral contrast revealed multiple dilated loops of jejunum with decompressed ileum distally. There was no evidence of bowel wall ischemia on the examination. The patient underwent surgical decompression of small bowel obstruction and recovered without complication.

Case 3

A 39-year-old woman presented to the ED with a 3-day history of left lower quadrant abdominal pain, fevers, chills, and vomiting, as well as leukocytosis. The studies in this chapter suggest a clinical suspicion of diverticulitis, as in this case, is accurate approximately 50% of the time (Fig. 25.3).

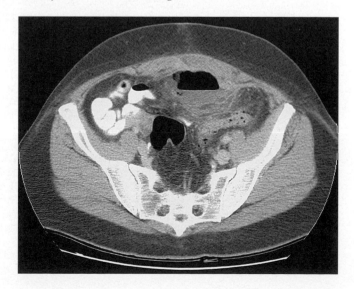

Figure 25.3. Diverticulitis with abscess formation.

Computed tomography revealed multiple diverticula and bowel wall thickening in the sigmoid colon, with fat stranding in the mesocolon, and an extraperitoneal abscess. Under CT guidance a percutaneous drainage catheter was placed into the abscess, with subsequent aspiration of 40cc of purulent material. The patient recovered and was discharged 72 hours after drainage catheter placement.

Suggested Protocols

Appendicitis and Bowel Obstruction Protocol

Patient preparation: 1000mL oral contrast, drink over a 90-minute period. Give rectal contrast if patient is unable to tolerate oral contrast.
Intravenous (IV) contrast: 150cc at 3.0cc/second.
Imaging: venous phase (60-second scan delay), dome of the diaphragm to ischial tuberosities, 2.5-mm detector collimation.

Diverticulitis Protocol

Patient preparation: 1000 to 1500mL rectal contrast instilled via soft rectal tube.
IV contrast: 150cc at 3.0cc/second.
Imaging: venous phase (60-second scan delay), dome of the diaphragm to ischial tuberosities, 2.5-mm detector collimation.

References

1. Tsushima Y, et al. Clin Radiol 2002;57(6):507–513.
2. Urban BA, Fishman EK. Radiographics 2000;20(3):725–749.
3. Ann Emerg Med 1994;23(4):906–922.
4. Martin RF, Rossi RL. Surg Clin North Am 1997;77(6):1227–1243.
5. Adams ID, et al. Br Med J (Clin Res Ed) 1986;293(6550):800–804.
6. Contran R, Kumar V, Collins T, Robbins S. Robbins Pathologic Basis of Disease, 6th ed. Boston: WB Saunders, 1999:1425.
7. Goldman L. Cecil Textbook of Medicine, 21st ed. Philadelphia: WB Saunders, 2000:729–731.
8. Frank JL, et al. Surg Endosc 1998;12(3):274–275.
9. Townisend CM. Sabiston Textbook of Surgery, 16th ed. 919–920.
10. Megibow AJ, et al. Radiology 1991;180(2):313–318.
11. Shih SC, et al. World J Gastroenterol 2003;9(3):603–605.
12. Miller G, et al. Br J Surg 2000;87(9):1240–1247.
13. Fevang BT, et al. Ann Surg 2004;240(2):193–201.
14. Parks TG, et al. Br Med J 1970;2(702):136–138.
15. Ferzoco LB, Raptopoulos V, Silen W. N Engl J Med 1998;338(21):1521–1526.
16. Diner WC, Barnhard HJ. Semin Roentgenol 1973;8(4):415–431.
17. Burkitt DP, Walker AR, Painter NS. JAMA 1974;229(8):1068–1074.
18. Hinchey EJ, Schaal PG, Richards GK. Adv Surg 1978;12:85–109.
19. McCaig LF, Stussman BJ. Adv Data 2002;1–20.
20. Advanced data from Vital and Health Statistics. Hyattsville, MD: National Center for Health Statistics, 2004:340.
21. Powers RD, Guertler AT. Am J Emerg Med 1995;13(3):301–303.
22. Brewer BJ, et al. Am J Surg 1976;131(2):219–223.
23. Lukens TW, Emerman C, Effron D. Ann Emerg Med 1993;22(4):690–696.
24. Jess P, et al. Am J Surg 1982;144(3):338–340.

25. Ann Emerg Med 2000;36(4):406–415.
26. Addiss DG, et al. Am J Epidemiol 1990;132(5):910–925.
27. Al-Omran M, Mamdani M, McLeod RS. Can J Surg 2003;46(4):263–268.
28. Korner H, et al. World J Surg 1997;21(3):313–317.
29. HCUPnet 2002 Statistics [Internet]. Rockville, MD: Agency for Healthcare Research and Quality. [Cited 5/20/05]. Available from: http://hcup.ahrq.gov/HCUPnet.asp
30. Tito SSM. Intestinal obstruction. In: Zuidema GD, ed. Surgery of the Alimentary Tract, 5th ed. New York: WB Saunders, 2001.
31. Pradel JA, et al. Radiology 1997;205(2):503–512.
32. Kircher MF, et al. AJR 2002;178(6):1313–1318.
33. Rhea JT. Emerg Radiol 2000;7(4):237–244.
34. Brengman ML, Otchy DP. Dis Colon Rectum 1998;41(8):1023–1028.
35. Halligan S, Saunders B. Best Pract Res Clin Gastroenterol 2002;16(4):595–610.
36. Gresenz CR, Studdert DM. Ann Emerg Med 2004;43(2):155–162.
37. Flum DR, Koepsell T. Arch Surg 2002;137(7):799–804; discussion 804.
38. Ogata M, Mateer JR, Condon RE. Ann Surg 1996;223(3):237–241.
39. Terasawa T, et al. Ann Intern Med 2004;141:537–546.
40. Whiting P, et al. Ann Intern Med 2004;3(140):189–202.
41. Rao PM, et al. Ann Surg 1999;229(3):344–349.
42. Brandt MM, Wahl WL. Am Surg 2003;69(9):727–731.
43. Horton M, Counter SF, Florence M, Hart M. Am J Surg 2000;179(5):379–381.
44. Weyant MJ, et al. Surgery 2000;128(2):145–152.
45. Balthazar EJ, Rofsky NM, Zucker R. Am J Gastroenterol 1998;93(5):768–771.
46. Franke C, et al. World J Surg 1999;23(2):141–146.
47. Perez J, et al. Am J Surg 2003;185(3):194–197.
48. Lee SL, Walsh AJ, Ho HS. Arch Surg 2001;136(5):556–562.
49. Flum DR, et al. JAMA 2001;286(14):1748–1753.
50. Rao PM, et al. N Engl J Med 1998;338(3):141–146.
51. Rice HE, et al. J Pediatr Surg 1999;34(5):754–758; discussion 758–759.
52. Baldisserotto M, Marchiori E. AJR 2000;175(5):1387–1392.
53. Lessin MS, et al. Am J Surg 1999;177(3):193–196.
54. Hahn HB, et al. Pediatr Radiol 1998;28(3):127–151.
55. Vignault F, et al. Radiology 1990;176(2):501–504.
56. Sivit CJ, et al. Radiology 1992;182(3):723–726.
57. Quillin SP, Siegel MJ. Radiology 1994;191(2):557–560.
58. Schulte B, et al. Eur J Ultrasound 1998;8(3):177–182.
59. Kaiser S, Frenckner B, Jorulf HK. Radiology 2002;223(3):633–638.
60. Lowe LH, et al. Radiology 2001;221(3):755–759.
61. Mullins ME, et al. AJR 2001;176(1):37–41.
62. Teo EL, et al. Singapore Med J 2000;41(8):387–392.
63. Garcia Pena BM, et al. JAMA 1999;282(11):1041–1046.
64. Ramachandran P, et al. J Pediatr Surg 1996;31(1):164–167; discussion 167–169.
65. Pena BM, et al. Pediatrics 2000;106(4):672–676.
66. Applegate KE, et al. Radiology 2001;220(1):103–107.
67. Karakas SP, et al. Pediatr Radiol 2000;30(2):94–98.
68. Martin AE, et al. J Pediatr Surg 2004;39(6):886–890; discussion 886–890.
69. Partrick DA, et al. J Pediatr Surg 2003;38(5):659–662.
70. Bendeck SE, et al. Radiology 2002;225(1):131–136.
71. Suri S, et al. Acta Radiol 1999;40:422–428.
72. Matsuoka H, et al. Am J Surg 2002;183(6):614–617(6):614–617.
73. Frager D, et al. AJR 1994;162:37–41.
74. Czechowski J. Acta Radiol 1996;37:186–189.
75. Schmutz GR, et al. Eur Radiol 1997;7(7):1054–1058.
76. Frager D, et al. AJR 1996;166:67–71.
77. Balthazar EJ, Liebeskind ME, Macari M. Radiology 1997;205:519–522.
78. Obuz F, et al. Eur J Radiol 2003;48:299–304.

79. Peck JJ, Milleson T, Phelan J. Am J Surg 1999;177:375–378.
80. Beall DP, et al. Clin Radiol 2002;57(8):719–724.
81. Seror D, et al. Am J Surg 1993;165(1):121–125; discussion 125–126.
82. Fevang BT, et al. Eur J Surg 2002;168(8–9):475–481.
83. Cox MR, et al. Aust N Z J Surg 1993;63(11):848–852.
84. Deutsch AA, et al. Postgrad Med J 1989;65(765):463–467.
85. Sarr MG, Bulkley GB, Zuidema GD. Am J Surg 1983;145(1):176–182.
86. Balthazar EJ. AJR 1994;163(5):1260–1261.
87. Ha HK, et al. Radiology 1997;204(2):507–512.
88. Zalcman M, et al. AJR 2000;175:1601–1607.
89. Donckier V, et al. Br J Surg 1998;85:1071–1074.
90. Taourel PG, et al. AJR 1995;165:1187–1192.
91. Cho KC, et al. Radiology 1990;176(1):111–115.
92. Stefansson T, et al. Acta Radiol 1997;38(2):313–319.
93. Rao PM, Rhea JT. Radiology 1998;209(3):775–779.
94. Werner A, et al. Eur Radiol 2003;13(12):2596–2603.
95. Verbanck J, et al. J Clin Ultrasound 1989;17(9):661–666.
96. Zielke A, et al. Br J Surg 1997;84(3):385–388.
97. Hollerweger A, et al. AJR 2000;175(4):1155–1160.
98. Schwerk WB, Schwarz S, Rothmund M. Dis Colon Rectum 1992;35(11): 1077–1084.
99. Ambrosetti P, Becker C, Terrier F. Eur Radiol 2002;12:1145–1149.
100. Hollerweger A, et al. Eur Radiol 2001;11(10):1956–1963.

26

Intussusception in Children: Diagnostic Imaging and Treatment

Kimberly E. Applegate

Key Points

- Children with clinically suspected intussusception should undergo enema reduction after surgical consultation. The only absolute contraindications to enema are signs of peritonitis on clinical exam or free air on abdominal radiographs. Air enema has better overall reduction

> rates than liquid enema but the outcome depends on the experience of the radiologist (moderate evidence).
>
> - Barium should not be used due to the poorer outcomes in those children who perforate (moderate evidence).
> - Ultrasound (US) is the primary imaging modality for initial diagnosis outside of the United States and for a growing majority of pediatric radiologists in the U.S. Ultrasound also plays a role in the evaluation of reducibility of intussusception, the presence of a lead point mass, potential incomplete reduction after enema, and of intussusception limited to small bowel (limited evidence).
> - Abdominal radiographs have poor sensitivity for the detection of intussusception but may serve to screen for other diagnoses in the differential diagnosis, such as constipation, and for free peritoneal air. For screening children with a low probability for intussusception, sonography is the preferred screening test (limited evidence).
> - The use of delayed repeat enema for the reduction of intussusception shows promise, but there are few data on the appropriate methods or timing (limited evidence).
> - For recurrence of intussusception, including multiple recurrences, enema is the preferred method for reduction (limited evidence).

Definition and Pathophysiology

Intussusception is an acquired invagination of the bowel into itself, usually involving both small and large bowel, within the peritoneal cavity. The more proximal bowel that herniates into the more distal bowel is called the intussusceptum and bowel that contains it is called the intussuscipiens. It is an emergent condition where delay in diagnosis is not uncommon, and leads to an increased risk of bowel perforation, obstruction, and necrosis. There may be an accompanying pathologic lead point mass in approximately 5% of children (1). Intestinal intussusception may occur along the entire length of the bowel from the duodenum to prolapse of intussuscepted bowel through the rectum. It can also range from classic clinical presentations to asymptomatic transient intussusception seen increasingly on multichannel computed tomography (CT) studies of the abdomen for other indications (2,3). Most cases are idiopathic in that the etiology of the intussusception is due to hypertrophied lymphoid tissue in the terminal ileum, which results in ileocolic intussusception. Some reports have suggested a viral etiology, most commonly adenovirus but also enterovirus, echovirus, and human herpes virus 6 (4). The clinical signs and symptoms of intussusception are often nonspecific and overlap with those of gastroenteritis, malrotation with volvulus, and, in older children, Henoch-Schönlein purpura (HSP). The large majority of clinically symptomatic cases occur in the infant and toddler, with a peak age of 5 to 9 months, although it has been reported on prenatal imaging and may occur in children who present without the typical clinical presentation of vomiting, bloody stools, palpable abdominal mass, and colicky abdominal pain (5). The classic triad of colicky abdominal pain, vomiting, and bloody stools is present in only 7% to 20% of children (6–8).

Epidemiology

Intussusception is the most common cause of small bowel obstruction in children and occurs in at least 56 children per 100,000 per year in the U.S. (9). It is second only to pyloric stenosis as the most common cause of gastrointestinal tract obstruction in children. It occurs in boys more than girls at a ratio of 3:2. Some studies have reported associations with viruses, particularly adenovirus, although the lack of seasonality suggests more than one pathogen (9). Intussusception occurs most commonly in infants beyond the newborn period, with large series reporting 57% to 85% of cases occurring before the age of 1 year (average 67% occur by age 1 year) (5). Delay in diagnosis and treatment is not uncommon, making enema reduction less successful, bowel resection more likely, and death due to bowel ischemia possible (1,5,10,11). There were 323 intussusception-associated deaths in American infants reported to the Centers for Disease Control and Prevention (CDC) between 1979 and 1997. In a review of administrative discharge data of intussusception-associated hospitalizations and deaths in the U.S., Parashar and colleagues (9) noted a peak age of 5 to 7 months with two thirds of patients under age 1 year, no consistent seasonality, hospitalization rates of approximately 56 per 100,000 children, and a general trend toward fewer hospitalizations over the past two decades. The mortality rates also decreased over this time period, from 6.4 per 1,000,000 to 2.3 per 1,000,000 live births. The authors also reported an increased risk of intussusception-related deaths among infants whose mothers were <20 years old, unmarried, nonwhite, and had less than a grade 12 education. The authors concluded that these data suggest that reduced access or delay in seeking care contributed to the risk of death. They did not investigate costs or rates of surgical versus enema reductions.

In another study comparing worldwide data, Meier and colleagues (11) noted that the most important difference between industrialized and developing countries' outcomes was the delay in presentation for treatment and consequent lower rates of enema reduction and higher rates of surgical mortality (18%) from bowel necrosis.

Rotavirus Vaccine

Shortly after the first and only rotavirus vaccine was introduced in the U.S. in 1998 for routine vaccination of infants at ages 2, 4, and 6 months, several reports to the CDC suggested an association between the vaccine and intussusception. This was noted particularly within 2 weeks after vaccination with the first dose. The vaccine was removed from the world market in 1999 (12). Although controversial, subsequent investigations have not found a higher rate of intussusception after rotavirus vaccination (13,14). A new rotavirus vaccine is currently under development (15).

Overall Cost to Society

No data have been identified detailing the total cost to society of intussusception. Three recent surveys have documented practice patterns for the evaluation of intussusception (3,16,17). In centers without pediatric radiologists, the enema is the initial and often only imaging test performed for both diagnosis and treatment. In contrast, at the 2004 Society for Pediatric Radiology (SPR) annual meeting, a survey of pediatric radiologists showed that 57% now use sonography for initial diagnosis prior to enema (16). Overall, the total hospital cost for children with intussusception treated with surgery is approximately four times that of those treated with enema (18–20).

Goals

The goal of initial bowel imaging is early detection of intussusception to enable enema reduction of the intussusception. Additional imaging studies may be performed to further characterize indeterminate results. The ultimate goal that radiologists should strive for is nonoperative reduction for all children with idiopathic intussusception (approximately 95% cases).

Methodology

A Medline search was performed using PubMed (National Library of Medicine, Bethesda, Maryland) for original research publications discussing the diagnostic performance and effectiveness of imaging strategies in intussusception. Clinical predictors of intussusception were also included in the literature search. The search covered the period 1966 to June 2004. The search strategy employed different combinations of the following terms: (1) *intussusception*, (2) *children*, *ages under 18 years*, (3) *diagnosis*, and (4) *therapy* or *surgery* or *etiology*. Additional articles were identified by reviewing the reference lists of relevant papers, identifying appropriate authors, and use of citation indices for MeSH terms. This review was limited to human studies and the English-language literature. The author performed an initial review of the titles and abstracts of the identified articles followed by review of the full text in articles that were relevant.

I. Diagnosis of Intussusception: What Are the Clinical Predictors? Who Should Undergo Imaging?

Summary of Evidence: At this point there are no reliable clinical prediction models that can accurately identify all patients with intussusception (limited evidence). Determination of which children should undergo imaging, and which should not undergo imaging, has not been studied in formal prospective trials.

Supporting Evidence

A. What Are the Clinical Predictors of Intussusception?

Ideally, children with intussusception should be diagnosed early to avoid bowel necrosis and surgery. Yet this goal remains elusive. One report found that only 50% of children were correctly diagnosed at initial presentation to a health care provider (20). The classic triad of colicky abdominal pain (58% to 100% cases), vomiting (up to 85% cases), and bloody stools is present in only 7% to 20% of children (6,8,22). Guaiac-positive stool is present in 75% of children with intussusception (8,23). Kuppermann and colleagues (24) published a cross-sectional study that evaluated the clinical factors that might predict intussusception in 115 children (limited evidence). Using multivariate logistic regression and bootstrap sample analysis, they found that the presence of highly suggestive abdominal radiographs, rectal bleeding, and male sex were independent predictors of intussusception but also noted that these factors were not specific. Harrington and colleagues (6) investigated the positive and negative clinical predictors of intussusception in a prospective cohort study (moderate evidence). They recorded signs and symptoms in 245 children and correlated them with sonographic and enema findings. Significant positive predictive factors for intussusception were the presence of right upper quadrant mass, gross blood in stool, guaiac-positive stool, and the triad of colicky abdominal pain, vomiting, and right upper quadrant mass. They were unable to identify significant negative predictors. Klein and colleagues (25) reviewed clinical history, physical exam, and radiographic findings to develop a prediction model of children with possible intussusception (moderate evidence). Their univariate analysis identified several known factors associated with intussusception, including vomiting, abdominal pain, palpable abdominal mass, guaiac-positive stool, and rectal bleeding. However, they concluded that they were "unable to develop a prediction model that would reliably identify all patients with the diagnosis of intussusception. Previously identified predictors of intussusception remain important in increasing suspicion of this important diagnosis. At this point there is no reliable prediction model that can accurately identify all patients with intussusception."

B. What Are the Clinical Predictors of Reducibility and Bowel Necrosis?

The most important factor that decreases the reduction rate of enema is a longer duration of symptoms. This finding is supported by multiple case series. A significant delay is typically 48 hours, but some reports suggest 24 or 72 hours, as either one of several factors or the single factor predicting unsuccessful enema reduction (5,26). Other factors associated with lower reduction rates include age less than 3 months, dehydration, small bowel obstruction, and intussusception encountered in the rectum (25% reduction rate) (3,21,22,26,27) (limited evidence).

II. Which Imaging Should Be Performed?

Summary of Evidence: Ultrasound has higher accuracy in the diagnosis of intussusception than plain radiographs. Ultrasound also has higher diagnostic accuracy in identifying pathologic lead points than plain radiographs or enema. The role of ultrasound findings in predicting success of reduction is not well known with available literature. Given current evidence, the diagnostic approach should include (1) abdominal radiographs if concern for other diagnoses or for perforation; (2) sonography for diagnosis or exclusion of intussusception; (3) if positive, a surgical consult should be obtained prior to the enema reduction attempt; and (4) air enema reduction (or if no experience with the air technique, liquid enema) (moderate evidence).

Supporting Evidence

A. What Is the Diagnostic Performance of Abdominal Radiographs?

The presence of a curvilinear mass within the course of the colon (the crescent sign), particularly in the transverse colon just beyond the hepatic

Table 26.1. Summary of sensitivity and specificity of diagnostic imaging for intussusception

Test	Sensitivity (%)	Specificity (%)
Abdominal radiographs[1]	45	45
Ultasound[2]	98–100	88–100
Enema[3]	100	100

[1] Based on references 5 and 28.
[2] Based on references 6, 32, 37 and 38.
[3] Approximate levels for ileocolic intussusception (does not include intussusception limited to small bowel) (26).

flexure, is a nearly pathognomonic sign of intussusception. The absence of bowel gas in the ascending colon is one of the most specific sign of intussusception on radiographs (28). However, small bowel or sigmoid colon gas located in the right abdomen on radiographs may mimic ascending colon or cecal gas. Radiographs have low sensitivity and specificity, even when viewed by experienced pediatric radiologists (28,29) (limited evidence). Sargent and colleagues (27) reported a 45% sensitivity in 60 children when evaluated prospectively by pediatric radiologists, using the enema as the reference standard (Table 26.1). Others report similar poor sensitivity in the detection of intussusception (5). In a survey of the SPR 2004 attendees, Daneman (16) found that 79% obtain radiographs, but this practice may not be under the control of radiologists. Only 10% of pediatric radiologists in this survey preferred radiographs for the diagnosis.

B. What Is the Diagnostic Performance of Sonography?

Intussusception can be reliably diagnosed when a donut, target, or pseudokidney sign is seen using linear transducer sonography (30–33). The optimal US technique in this population is well described (31–35). There are no known contraindications or complications resulting from US for this purpose. Ultrasound also plays a role in the evaluation of reducibility of the intussusception, the presence of a pathologic lead point (PLP) mass, and intussusception limited to small bowel, in diagnosing or excluding residual intussusception after enema, and in identifying alternative diagnoses (6,32,34,35) (limited evidence). In a 2004 survey, 57% of North American pediatric radiologists reported the use of sonography to diagnose intussusception as compared to 93% of European pediatric radiologists in a 1999 survey (16,36).

Sonography screening in children has been suggested to reduce cost, radiation exposure, and both patient and parental anxiety/discomfort with enema (35) (limited evidence). Published series from single institutions suggest high accuracy, approaching 100% in experienced hands, with sensitivity of 98% to 100% and specificity of 88% to 100% (6,32,37,38) (limited evidence) (Table 26.1). Eshed and colleagues (39) found similar abilities in sonographic diagnosis of intussusception for staff radiologists as well as senior and junior radiology residents: sensitivity and specificity were 85% and 98% for staff radiologists, 75% and 96% for senior residents, and 83% and 97% for junior residents, respectively. Given that the theoretical cost-effectiveness of sonography is dependent on the prevalence of intussusception, optimization of imaging will require stratification of subjects into different levels of probability of intussusception (40). However, data are lacking for such stratification. Henrikson and colleagues (35) noted a trend of decreased prevalence of intussusception (22%) in those children referred for enema and began sonographic screening (limited evidence). In their small series of 38 children, they were able to avoid 19 enemas in those with negative sonography, resulting in savings in both radiation exposure (an average of 8.2 mGy for negative enemas) and hospital charges. Future cost-effectiveness modeling research is needed to define the population that should undergo sonography.

C. What Are the Sonographic Predictors of Reducibility and Bowel Necrosis?

Del-Pozo and colleagues (41) performed sonography in 145 children with intussusception and found that fluid seen inside the intussusception represented trapped peritoneal fluid and was associated with significantly fewer reductions on enema and bowel ischemia at surgery (42) (limited evidence).

Some US reports have noted that thicker bowel wall was associated with fewer enema reductions (32,43) but others did not find this association (42). Lack of color Doppler signal in the intussuscepted bowel wall suggested bowel ischemia in several small series (44–46). Free intraperitoneal fluid in small or moderate amounts is present in approximately half of children with intussusception and is not a contraindication for enema (33). There are conflicting reports that free peritoneal fluid is associated with fewer reductions (5,22,26,34,47). Some descriptive studies report that the presence of lymph nodes trapped in the intussusception is associated with fewer reductions (34,48). For these US findings, due to the conflicting reports or small series, the evidence is inconclusive.

D. What Are the Pathologic Lead Points?

Approximately 5% to 6% of intussusceptions in children are caused by PLPs, which are due to either focal masses or diffuse bowel wall abnormality. The most common focal PLPs are (in decreasing order of incidence) Meckel's diverticulum, duplication cyst, polyp, and lymphoma (1,5,49) (limited evidence). Diffuse PLPs are most commonly associated with cystic fibrosis or HSP. Although the common teaching remains that focal PLPs are more common in older children, this is somewhat misleading. The relative prevalence of PLP with intussusception is higher in children over the age of 3 years, particularly for lymphoma. However, the absolute number of PLPs in infants versus older children is approximately equal (1).

The detection of lead points by imaging remains problematic, although US is the noninvasive standard of reference 66% of PLPs may be identified on US (50) and 40% of PLPs may be diagnosed by liquid enema (5). Air enema has a lower rate of detection of PLP of 11%–29% (50,51), so that some researchers suggest that US be used afterward to search for PLP (3) (limited evidence).

III. Treatment of Intussusception: How Should the Enema Be Performed?

Summary of Evidence: The air enema is considered superior at reduction, cleaner (based on appearance of peritoneal cavity at surgery when perforation occurs), safer, and faster, with less radiation when compared to

Table 26.2. Summary of published intussusception enema reduction rates and perforation rates

Rates	All studies			Studies with cases >150		
	No. of studies	Mean (SD)	Wt. mean (SD)	No. of studies	Mean (SD)	Wt. mean (SD)
Reduction (%)	71	74.1 (16.8)	87.3 (12)	19	79.6 (12.5)	89.5 (9.3)
Perforation (%)	66	0.8 (1.4)	0.3 (0.7)	18	0.6 (0.8)	0.2 (0.4)

Note: Summary data include a weighted average measure of reduction and perforation rates based on publications with at least 150 pediatric cases. The enema techniques varied and included air versus liquid media, with sonographic or fluoroscopic guidance.
Wt. mean, weighted mean; SD, standard deviation.
Source: Adapted from Daneman and Navarro (26).

liquid enema (23,52–56) (moderate evidence). The recurrence rates for air versus liquid enema reductions do not differ (both are approximately 10%). The rule of threes that is used to guide liquid enema technique is supported by limited evidence. Barium is no longer the liquid contrast medium of choice due to the risk of barium peritonitis, infection, and adhesions when perforation occurs during the enema (23,47,53,57). Neither sedation nor medications increase the enema success rate (limited evidence). Direct comparison of reduction with fluoroscopy versus ultrasound has not been studied (insufficient evidence).

Supporting Evidence: There are multiple investigations of success rates for enema reduction, although most are retrospective. Seventy-one published studies of this question were largely level III (limited evidence) investigations consisting of unselected but often consecutive case series. The average reduction rate for these 71 published studies was 74%. In 19 series with at least 150 children each, retrospective analysis demonstrated reduction rates averaging 80%, range 53% to 96% (26) (Table 26.2). The two largest series from China, using air enema in 6396 and 9028 children, reported reduction rates of 95% and 92% (54,55) (limited evidence). However, while the air enema may be preferred in experienced hands, the liquid enema is also safe and effective. The air enema technique is well described in the literature (54,56,58). Briefly, the enema tip should be placed within the child's rectum and taped in place with abundant tape. The child is placed in a prone position to allow the radiologist or assistant to squeeze the buttocks closed and prevent air from leaking. Air is rapidly insufflated into the colon under fluoroscopic observation. Once the intussusception is encountered, its reduction is followed fluoroscopically until it is completely reduced. Air should flow freely from the cecum into the distal small bowel loops to signify complete reduction. One critical safety issue is to keep air pressure below a maximum limit of 120 mm Hg (although higher pressures occur when the patient performs a Valsalva maneuver) to avoid the risk of perforation (23,47,56).

A. Air vs. Liquid Enema

There are only two randomized controlled trials of the reduction rates of air versus liquid enema (60) (moderate evidence). The 1993 study by Meyer et al. enrolled 101 children and found similar success rates of 76% for air and 63% for liquid enema. However, the trial used sedation and had lower reduction rates than those not using sedation (25). The authors abandoned the use of sedation after this study. The use of sedation may reduce the intraabdominal pressure children create by the Valsalva maneuver and is reported to improve reducibility at enema (47,56). In contrast, Hadidi et al. found significantly higher reduction rates using air (90%) versus barium (70%) in 100 children (61). More recent reports of air reduction show better results than liquid enema reduction (26). The superior air enema results may be due to the level of experience of those who use air reduction techniques as well as the presence of higher intraluminal pressure for air as compared to standard hydrostatic reduction (62,63).

In a 1991 survey of American pediatric radiology chairs, Meyer et al. (17) found that only 24% were using air enema but 64% used barium and 12% water-soluble contrast, as compared to 35% of international pediatric radiologists who used air enema (59). More recently, 65% of American pediatric radiologists now use air enema, 33% use liquid enema (water-soluble contrast or barium), and 3% use liquid enema with sonographic guidance (16). Some pediatric radiologists use air for children older than 3 months, but for younger infants, especially neonates, they prefer liquid contrast due to the greater differential diagnosis in this group (26).

All children should have a surgical consultation prior to enema (1) to assess for peritoneal signs precluding enema, (2) to identify children who cannot be reduced with enema or who are found to have perforation, and (3) for postreduction management. Prior to enema reduction, dehydration should be treated with intravenous fluid resuscitation. Children with evidence of peritonitis, shock, sepsis, or free air on abdominal radiographs are not candidates for enema. Radiologists should achieve enema reduction rates of at least 80% and up to 95% (moderate evidence). Several reports estimate that the rate of spontaneous reduction based on sonographic or enema diagnosis prior to surgery is 10% (1,3,22,43) (limited evidence).

Bratton and colleagues (18) suggest that more experienced radiologists and caregivers at children's hospitals decrease the risk of surgical reduction, length of hospital stay, and cost of care (moderate evidence). Surgical management is performed when the patient is too unstable (shock, dehydration, sepsis) for enema reduction, when the enema is unsuccessful, or when PLP is diagnosed.

B. The Rule of Threes

A general guideline to the liquid enema technique, often taught to radiology residents, is the rule of threes: three attempts of 3 minutes' duration, with the liquid enema bag at 3 feet above the fluoroscopy table. There is little evidence to support this rule, particularly regarding the height of the enema bag (26,64). Many experienced pediatric radiologists alter this general guide in response to the clinical status of the patient and the movement of the intussusceptum mass achieved with the initial enema (22,64). For example, if the intussusception is partially reduced to where it most frequently hangs up, at the ileocecal valve, some radiologists will make further or longer attempts or raise the enema bag above 3 feet. The exam is tailored to the patient and performed in conjunction with the surgeon involved.

C. Radiation Dose

The dose deposited depends on a number of factors, including the type of fluoroscopy equipment, the use of pulsed fluoroscopy, and the fluoroscopy time (1,47). A 1993 study reported a mean effective dose of 55 µSv for enema reduction of an intussusception (65). Experienced pediatric radiologists using air enema averaged 95 seconds of fluoroscopy time to reduce an intussusception and 42 seconds to exclude one in a child without intussusception (56). Air enema radiation doses average one-third to one-half less than the dose for liquid enema (47). A 2003 report showed the average radiation dose saved was estimated at 8.2 mSv (820 mR) (the average dose for negative enema) per patient (35).

D. Alternative Enema Approaches

A number of different approaches have been described to try to improve intussusception reduction on enema that include sedation, anesthesia, use of glucagon, manual palpation, and delayed repeat enema. In the past, sedation, and sometimes anesthesia, were commonly used to improve reduction rates, but case series showed no improvement (17,66,67) (limited evidence). In a 1991 survey Meyer (17) found only 10% of respondents used sedation either always or almost always, as compared to 54% of international pediatric radiologists, and those using sedation reported lower reduction rates (59). Therefore, few pediatric radiologists currently use sedation in the U.S. Glucagon was shown not to improve enema reduction rates in one study (68) and is no longer used (17). The use of manual palpation has been suggested to improve intussusception reduction at enema but has not been systematically studied (47,69). One study by Grasso et al. (69) reported a reduction rate of 76% when manual palpation was used, less than the average of 80% in large series.

E. Fluoroscopy vs. Sonography

In the West, fluoroscopy is almost always used during enema reduction. In the East, and in a few European centers, reports on the use of sonography with either water (70–76) or air (77–79) reduction show reduction rates as high as or higher than those in the West; however, the experience level required for these techniques has not been studied nor has the ability of sonography to detect perforations (limited evidence).

F. Delayed Repeat Enema

In the small percent of children who fail initial enema reduction, delayed repeat enema may avoid the need for surgical reduction. The use of delayed attempts at between 30 minutes and 19 hours after initial attempt have shown promise in increasing the success of enema reductions (80–84) (limited evidence). These four small series showed further reduction rates of 50% to 82% by waiting at least 30 minutes prior to further attempts at enema reduction. Further research to understand optimal timing and technique for delayed repeat enemas is needed. Daneman and Navarro (26), with the largest reported experience to date, suggest a delay of 2 to 4 hours until further research yields more rigorous guidelines. The child must remain clinically stable and be appropriately monitored during this time interval. Delayed enema should not be performed if the initial enema does not move the intussusception at all (26,83).

G. Where Should Patients Be Treated?

Bratton and colleagues (18) performed a retrospective cohort analysis of all children hospitalized with intussusception in the state of Washington from 1987 through 1996 (moderate evidence). They investigated whether the risk of surgical management for these children varied by hospital pediatric caseload, measured by the annual number of pediatric hospital admissions. By reviewing the discharge data of all 507 children, they found an overall surgical reduction rate of 53%, with 20% undergoing bowel resection. Surgical reduction rates varied by pediatric caseload from 36% at hospitals with large pediatric caseloads to 64% at hospitals with low pediatric volumes, resulting in nearly twice the risk of surgical reduction. Children who underwent surgery, versus enema reduction, had similar gender and median age characteristics, but those who had bowel resection were more likely to have coexisting conditions. The median cost of hospital care for these children was $5724 for surgical reduction and $1184 for enema reduction.

H. What Are the Complications of Enema Therapy?

The most important potential complication of enema is bowel perforation. Sixty-six published studies of this question were largely level III (limited evidence) investigations consisting of unselected but often consecutive case series. The mean perforation rate was 0.8% (Table 26.2). In 18 case series with at least 150 children each, perforation rates averaged 0.6%, with a range of 0% to 1.6% (26). There were no statistically significant differences between air and liquid enema perforation rates (Table 26.3). When these averages were weighted to reflect the sample size of each published study, the perforation rates were even lower, at 0.3% for all 66 studies and 0.2% for the larger studies.

Ultimately, however, the risk of perforation depends on each radiologist's patient population and technique. Though determination of clinical predictors of perforation is complicated by a lack of prospective studies, the one acknowledged key factor is symptom length greater than 48 hours. Several reports in both pig models and children suggest that there may be

Table 26.3. Summary comparison of air versus liquid contrast enema reduction and perforation rates

		All studies			Studies with cases >150		
		No. of studies	Mean (SD)	Wt. mean (SD)	No. of studies	Mean (SD)	Wt. mean (SD)
Reduction	Pneumatic	32	82.1 (11.9)	91.4 (5.2)	10	86.4 (6.3)	92.2 (3.3)
(%)	Hydrostatic	39	67.5 (17.6)	69.1 (15.2)	9	72.1 (13.7)	70.0 (14.1)
	p-value		<0.001	<0.001	0.009 < 0.001		
Perforation	Pneumatic	31	1.0 (1.5)	0.3 (0.6)	11	0.8 (0.9)	0.2 (0.4)
(%)	Hydrostatic	35	0.6 (1.4)	0.4 (1.0)	7	0.3 (0.6)	0.2 (0.4)
	p-value		0.30	0.53		0.28	0.99

Note: While the liquid contrast media reduction rates are lower, a number of these studies are older than the newer air enema reports. There was no significant difference in perforation rates.
P values are based on the *t*-test
Source: Adapted from Daneman and Navarro (26).

preexisting focal perforation in the necrotic intussuscipiens or, less commonly, the intussusceptum, that are rarely radiographically apparent as free air (21,23,26,85–88) (moderate evidence). The most common site is at or just proximal to the intussusception in the transverse colon (88). Perforations with air tend to be smaller than those with liquid enema although the overall perforation rates are similar (23,86).

In 1989, Campbell (89) surveyed enema techniques and complications of North American pediatric radiologists. Respondents' combined experience was 14,000 intussusception enemas. Although they did not report enema reduction rates, the combined perforation rate was 0.39% (55/14,000), with only one death. This study remains the basis for the risk of perforation that is explained to parents for consent prior to enema reduction (one in 250 to one in 300) (limited evidence).

Barium is no longer the liquid contrast medium of choice for reduction of intussusception due to the risk of barium peritonitis, infection, and adhesions when perforation occurs during the enema (23,47,53,58) (moderate evidence). While iodinated contrast is now preferred and is considered a safer agent than barium, one should be aware that it may produce fluid and electrolyte shifts if perforation occurs since contrast is absorbed from the peritoneum.

One complication unique to air enema is the tension pneumoperitoneum. In an early report, two deaths occurred from this complication, leading the proponents of air enema to advise having an 18-gauge needle readily available in the fluoroscopy room for emergent decompression (26,47,53). Although theoretically possible, there have been no reports of air embolism.

I. What Are the Surgical Management and Complications?

Depending on the patient population, approximately 20% to 40% of children who undergo surgical reduction of their intussusception require bowel resection [20% (17); 30% to 40% (1)]. If we estimate that 20% of children with intussusception will fail enema reduction and undergo surgical reduction, then only 4% to 8% of all children will require bowel resection. Ideally, only this population and those with pathologic lead points should need surgical intervention.

Short-term complications from laparotomy include infection and bowel perforation. The long-term risk of small bowel obstruction from adhesions is approximately 8% for neonates and 3% to 5% for those children older than 1 month (90).

J. Cost-Effectiveness Analysis

There are no known rigorous economic analyses on diagnosis and treatment strategies for intussusception, although one study evaluated the cost savings of more aggressive enema reduction compared to surgical reduction (20). Stein and colleagues (20) analyzed single institution billing records of 703 children with intussusception to compare government Diagnosis-Related Groups (DRG) reimbursements of hospital care in Australia (limited evidence). In 1993 Australian dollars, the government paid, on average, $727 for enema reduction and $4514 for surgical reduction in hospital care. With the broader indications for enema and the increased use of air, the authors noted decreased use of surgical reduction at their institution—in 1983, 65% children underwent surgical reduction, decreasing to 25% in 1992. Ironically, the authors noted that hospital profit, however, is greater for surgical reductions.

IV. What Is Appropriate Management in Recurrent Cases?

Summary of Evidence: Intussusception recurrence rates average 10% in large series, with a range of 5.4% to 15.4% (1,26,91), regardless of air versus liquid enema technique (moderate evidence). The recurrence rates are less than or equal to 5% when surgical reduction is performed, presumably due to the development of adhesions (92). Repeat enema is both safe and effective in recurrent intussusception (1,47,92,93) as long as the child remains clinically stable (limited evidence). There is insufficient evidence to support any particular approach beyond the performance of the enema and referral to a surgeon for shared decision making with the patient.

Supporting Evidence: Fifty percent of children who develop recurrent intussusception present within 48 hours, although recurrences have been reported up to 18 months later (53) (limited evidence). No clear risk factors are known for why some children have recurrences, although some have focal PLP. In those with PLP, children with diffuse bowel abnormality such as cystic fibrosis, HSP, or celiac disease may be treated with enema reduction more aggressively than those with focal PLPs.

The risk of PLP in children with recurrent intussusception is low. In one large series of 763 children it was 7% (5/69) (53) only slightly higher than the reported 5% to 6% incidence of PLP at first presentation of intussusception (1) (insufficient evidence). No predictive clinical factors have been identified for PLP in these children with recurrent intussusception. Reduction with air enema was possible in 95% of recurrences in the largest reported experience (1,53) (limited evidence).

When there is concern about PLP, sonography may play an important role and may detect 60%–66% of PLPs (1,45,92) (limited evidence). While US will not detect all PLPs, the risk of missing a PLP without other signs or symptoms to guide management is unlikely (49). Ein (92) reviewed 1200 intussusception cases covering 40 years' experience at one institution to analyze this risk. When the enema failed to detect lymphoma as a PLP, Ein noted the presence of clinical signs of illness of greater than 1 week, patient age greater than 3 years, weight loss, and palpable mass in all of these children (limited evidence).

In a randomized, double-blind trial comparing 144 children who received intramuscular corticosteroids versus 137 who received placebo before air enema reduction, Lin and colleagues (4) reported significantly fewer intussusception recurrences at 6 months (moderate evidence). In both groups, the initial reduction rate was 85%. There were no recurrences in the children who received dexamethasone, compared to 5% in the placebo group. They hypothesized that steroids decreased the volume of mesenteric adenopathy and lymphoid hyperplasia in the terminal ileum and thus the risk of recurrence. However, further investigation of the risks and benefits of this intervention is needed.

V. Special Case: Intussusception Limited to the Small Bowel

With the increasing use of multidetector CT scanners, radiologists are reporting the more frequent presence of small, asymptomatic small bowel–small bowel intussusception (2,3,94) (limited evidence). These intussusceptions are typically transient and, since the children are asymptomatic, they are of no known clinical significance.

There is little evidence in the literature regarding the optimal diagnosis and treatment of symptomatic intussusception limited to the small bowel. Most authors agree, however, that the diagnosis is more difficult both clinically and radiologically (1,22,27). Small bowel intussusceptions are unlikely to have associated abdominal mass or rectal bleeding. Treatment is virtually always surgical reduction. Special risk factors for small bowel intussusception include the early postoperative period after either intraperitoneal and retroperitoneal surgery, the presence of long enteric feeding tubes, diffuse PLP (cystic fibrosis or HSP), and small bowel polyps (1,27,95) (limited evidence).

VI. Special Case: Intussusception with a Known Lead Point Mass

The optimal imaging approach to children with intussusception and known PLP is unknown. However, Daneman (16) surveyed the SPR members at their 2004 annual meeting and found that 76% of respondents attempt reduction in these patients. Some surgeons may request enema reduction in these children to partially reduce the intussusception and perhaps decrease the laparotomy incision size (82). There is insufficient evidence to support any particular approach beyond referral to a surgeon for shared decision making with the patient and, if requested, the performance of an enema (26,59,93).

Imaging Case Study

A 9-month-old boy presents to the emergency department with a 1-day history of irritability, vomiting, and intermittent crying (Figs. 26.1 and 26.2).

Future Research

- Investigate the optimal technique and timing of delayed, repeat enema reduction.
- Investigate the role of corticosteroids to decrease the rate of recurrence in a prospective controlled trial.
- Perform cost-effectiveness analyses (CEA) of the role of US in the diagnosis of intussusception. This investigation would include this question: At what disease prevalence or individual case probability is US cost-effective prior to enema?

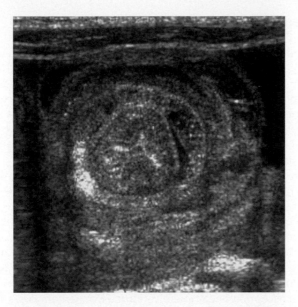

Figure 26.1. Linear sonography of the right middle-lower abdomen demonstrates the target sign of bowel intussusception. There is bowel within bowel and thickened walls of these loops due to edema. No pathologic lead point (PLP) is identified.

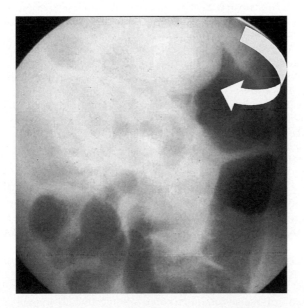

Figure 26.2. The appearance of the intussusception at air enema reduction. The intussusception is encountered at the hepatic flexure, with the baby in a prone position (arrow). Successful reduction should be achieved in at least 80% of such cases.

Suggested Imaging Protocol

- Ultrasound for clinically suspected intussusception: If concern for alternative diagnoses such as constipation, one- to two-view abdominal radiographs (supine or prone, and decubitus) (limited evidence). The abdomen is scanned with a 5 mHz or higher linear transducer using the graded compression technique and a bowel or high contrast application package. All four quadrants of the abdomen must be scanned, typically in transverse planes, beginning with the right upper quadrant, to exclude an intussusception mass.
- Air enema for reduction: Prior to performing the enema, consult the surgeon (moderate evidence). (If the clinician has no experience with air enema or has done few cases, then perform liquid enema with water-soluble contrast using the guide of the rule of threes described above.) The enema tip without a balloon should be placed within the child's rectum and taped in place with abundant tape. With the child prone, the radiologist squeezes the buttocks closed to prevent air leak. Air is rapidly insufflated into the colon under fluoroscopic observation until the intussusception is completely reduced, when air flows freely from the cecum into the distal small bowel loops. Air pressure must remain below a maximum limit of 120 mm Hg to avoid the risk of perforation.
- Repeat enema for recurrences, including multiple recurrences (limited evidence).

References

1. Navarro O, Daneman A. Pediatr Radiol 2004;34:305–312.
2. Strouse PJ, DiPietro MA, Saez F. Pediatr Radiol 2003;33(5):316–320.
3. Kornecki A, Daneman A, Navarro O, Connolly B, Manson D, Alton DJ. Pediatr Radiol 2000;30:58–63.
4. Lin SL, Kong MS, Houng DS. Eur J Pediatr 2000;159(7):551–552.
5. Daneman A, Navarro O. Pediatr Radiol 2003;33:79–85.
6. Harrington L, Connolly B, Hu X, Wesson DE, Babyn P, Schuh S. J Pediatr 1998;132(5):836–839.
7. Lai AH, Phua KB, Teo EL, Jacobsen AS. Ann Acad Med Singapore 2002; 31(1):81–85.
8. Losek JD, Fiete RL. Am J Emerg Med 1991;9(1):1–3.
9. Parashar UD, Holman RC, Cummings KC, et al. Pediatrics 2000;106(6): 1413–1421.
10. Berlin L. AJR 1998;170:1161–1163.
11. Meier DE, Coln CD, Rescorla FJ, OlaOlorun A, Tarpley JL. World J Surg 1996; 20(8):1035–1039; discussion 1040.
12. CDC and Prevention. MMWR 1999;48:1007.
13. Chang HG, Smith PF, Ackelsberg J, Morse DL, Glass RI. Pediatrics 2001;108(1): 54–60.
14. Rennels MB, Parashar UD, Holman RC, Le CT, Chang HG, Glass RI. Pediatr Infect Dis J 1998;17(10):924–925.
15. Dennehy PH, Bresee JS. Infect Dis Clin North Am 2001;15(1):189–207.
16. Daneman A. Personal communication, SPR meeting 2004 unpublished survey.
17. Meyer JS. Pediatr Radiol 1992;22:323–325.
18. Bratton SL, Haberkern CM, Waldhausen JH, Sawin RS, Allison JW. Pediatrics 2001;107(2):299–303.
19. Leonidas JC. AJR 1985;145(4):665–669.
20. Stein JE, Beasley SW, Phelan E. Aust N Z J Surg 1997;67(6):330–331.

21. Beasley S. Pediatr Radiol 2004;34:302–304.
22. Littlewood Teele R, Vogel SA. Pediatr Surg Int 1998;14(3):158–162.
23. Shiels WE II, Kirks DR, Keller GL, et al. AJR 1993;160:931–935.
24. Kuppermann N, O'Dea T, Pinckney L, Hoecker C. Arch Pediatr Adolesc Med 2000;154(3):250–255.
25. Klein EJ, Kapoor D, Shugerman RP. Clin Pediatr (Phila) 2004;43(4):343–347.
26. Daneman A, Navarro O. Pediatr Radiol 2004;34:97–108.
27. Sargent MA, Babyn P, Alton DJ. Pediatr Radiol 1994;24(1):17–20.
28. West KW, Stephens B, Vane DW, Grosfeld JL. Surgery 1987;102(4):704–710.
29. Eklof O, Hartelius H. Pediatr Radiol 1980;9(4):199–206.
30. Bowerman RA, Silver TM, Jaffe MH. Radiology 1982;143:527–529.
31. Lee HC, Yeh HJ, Leu YJ. J Pediatr Gastroenterol Nutr 1989;8(3):343–7.
32. Pracros JP, Tran-Minh VA, Morin de Finfe CH, Deffrenne-Pracros P, Louis D, Basset T. Ann Radiol (Paris) 1987;30(7):525–530.
33. Swischuk LE, Hayden CK, Boulden. Pediatr Radiol 1985;15:388–391.
34. Del-Pozo G, Albillos JC, Tejedor D, et al. RadioGraphics 1999;19:299–319.
35. Henrikson S, Blane CE, Koujok K, Strouse PJ, DiPietro MA, Goodsitt MM. Pediatr Radiol 2003;33:190–193.
36. Schmit P, Rohrschneider WK, Christmann D. Pediatr Radiol 1999;29(10):752–761.
37. Shanbhogue RLK, Hussain SM, Meradji M, Robben SGF, Vernooij JEM, Molenaar JC. J Pediatr Surg 1994;29:324–328.
38. Verschelden P, Filiatrault D, Garel L, et al. Radiology 1992;184:741–744.
39. Eshed I, Gorenstein A, Serour F, Witzling M. Pediatr Radiol 2004;34:134–137.
40. Bhisitkul DM, Listernick R, Shkolnik A, et al. J Pediatr 1992;121(2):182–186.
41. Del-Pozo G, Gonzalez-Spinola J, Gomez-Anson B, et al. Radiology 1996;201:379–383.
42. Britton I, Wilkinson AG. Pediatr Radiol 1999;29(9):705–710.
43. Swischuk LE, John SD, Swischuk PN. Radiology 1994;192:269–271.
44. Lagalla R, Caruso G, Novara V, Derchi LE, Cardinale AE. J Ultrasound Med 1994;13(3):171–174.
45. Lam AH, Firman K. Pediatr Radiol 1992;22(2):112–114.
46. Lim HK, Bae SH, Lee KH, Seo GS, Yoon GS. Radiology 1994;191:781–785.
47. Kirks DR. Radiology 1994;191:622–623.
48. Koumanidou C, Vakaki M, Pitsoulakis G, Kakavakis K, Mirilas P. AJR 2002;178:445–450.
49. Ein SH. J Pediatr Surg 1976;11(2):209–211.
50. Navarro O, Dugougeat F, Kornecki A, Shuckett B, Alton DJ, Daneman A. Pediatr Radiol 2000;30(9):594–603.
51. Miller SF, Landes AB, Dautenhahn LW, et al. Radiology 1995;197:493–496.
52. Beasley SW, Glover J. J Pediatr Surg 1992;27(4):474–475.
53. Daneman A, Alton DJ, Ein S, Wesson D, Superina R, Thorner P. Pediatr Radiol 1995;25:81–88.
54. Gu L, Alton D, Daneman A, et al. AJR 1988;150:1345–1348.
55. Guo JZ, Ma XY, Zhou QH. J Pediatr Surg 1986;21:1201–1203.
56. Shiels WE II, Maves CK, Hedlund GL, Kirks DR. Radiology 1991;181:169–172.
57. Hernanz-Schulman M, Foster C, Maxa R, et al. Pediatr Radiol. 2000;30(6):369–378.
58. Stringer MD, Pablot M, J Brereton. J Surg 1992;79:867–876.
59. Katz ME, Kolm P. Pediatr Radiol 1992;22:318–322.
60. Meyer JS, Dangman BS, Buonomo C, Berlin JA. Radiology 1993;188:507–511.
61. Hadidi AT, El Shal N. Childhood intussusception: a comparative study of non-surgical management. J Pediatr Surg 1999;34(2):304–307.
62. Sargent MA, Wilson BP. Pediatr Radiol 1991;21(5):346–349.
63. Zambuto D, Bramson RT, Blickman JG. Radiology 1995;196:55–58.
64. McAlister WH. Radiology. 1998;206(3):595–598.

65. Thomas RD, Fairhurst JJ, Roberts PJ. Clin Radiol 1993;48(3):189–191.

66. Suzuki M, Hayakawa K, Nishimura K, et al. Radiat Med 1999;17(2):121–124.

67. Touloukian RJ, O'Connell JB, Markowitz RI, Rosenfield N, Seashore JH, Ablow RC. Pediatrics 1987;79(3):432–434.

68. Franken EA, Smith WL, Chernish SM, Campbell JB, Fletcher BD, Goldman HS. Radiology 1983;146:687–689.

69. Grasso SN, Katz ME, Presberg HJ. Radiology 1994;191:777–779.

70. Gonzalez-Spinola J, Del Pozo G, Tejedor D, Blanco A. J Pediatr Surg 1999;34(6): 1016–1020.

71. Khong PL, Peh WC, Lam CH, et al. Radiographics 2000;20(5):E1.

72. Peh WCG, Khong PL, Chan KL, et al. AJR 1996;167:1237–1241.

73. Riebel TW, Nasir R, Weber K. Radiology 1993;188:513–516.

74. Rohrschneider WK, Troger J. Pediatr Radiol 1995;25:530–534.

75. Wang GD, Liu SJ. J Pediatr Surg 1988;23(9):814–818.

76. Woo SK, Kim JS, Suh SJ, Paik TW, Choi SO. Radiology 1992;182:77–80.

77. Gu L, Zhu H, Wang S, Han Y, Wu X, Miao H. Pediatr Radiol 2000;30(5):339–342.

78. Todani T, Sato Y, Watanabe Y, Toki A, Uemura S, Urushihara N Z Kinderchir 1990;45(4):222–226.

79. Yoon CH, Kim HJ, Goo HW. Radiology 2001;218:85–88.

80. Connolly B, Alton DJ, Ein SH, Daneman A. Pediatr Radiol 1995;25:104–107.

81. Gorenstein A, Raucher A, Serour F, Witzling M, Katz R. Radiology 1998; 206:721–724.

82. Navarro OM, Daneman A, Chae A. AJR 2004;182(5):1169–1176.

83. Sandler AD, Ein SH, Connolly B, Daneman A, Filler RM. Pediatr Surg Int 1999; 15(3–4):214–216.

84. Saxton V, Katz M, Phelan E, Beasley SW. J Pediatr Surg 1994;29(5):588–589.

85. Armstrong EA, Dunbar JS, Graviss ER, Martin L, Rosenkrantz J. Radiology 1980;136:77–81.

86. Blane CE, DiPietro MA, White SJ, Klein ME, Coran AG, Wesley JR. J Can Assoc Radiol 1984;35:113–115.

87. Daneman A, Alton DJ, Lobo E, Gravett J, Kim P, Ein SH. Pediatr Radiol 1998; 28(12):913–919.

88. Mercer S, Carpenter B. Can J Surg 1982;25:481–483.

89. Campbell JB. Pediatr Radiol 1989;19:293–296.

90. Janik JS, Ein SH, Filler RM, Shandling B, Simpson JS, Stephens CA. J Pediatr Surg 1981;16:225–229.

91. Champoux AN, Del Beccaro MA, Nazar-Stewart V. Arch Pediatr Adolesc Med 1994;148:474–478.

92. Ein SH. J Pediatr Surg 1975;10:751–755.

93. Katz M, Phelan E, Carlin JB, Beasley SW. AJR 1993;160(2):363–366.

94. Cox TD, Winters WD, Weinberger E. Pediatr Radiol 1996;26:26–32.

95. Hughes UM, Connolly BL, Chait PG, Muraca S. Pediatr Radiol 2000;30(9): 614–617.

Figure 3.2E. Stereotactic biopsy of microcalcifications. Biopsy probe positioned within breast for retrieval of tissues samples from microcalcifications that were targeted with computer assistance from stereotactic images acquired digitally.

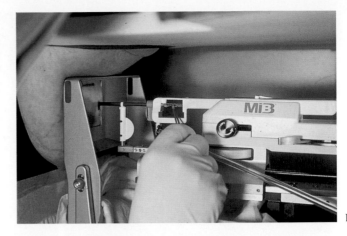

E

B

C

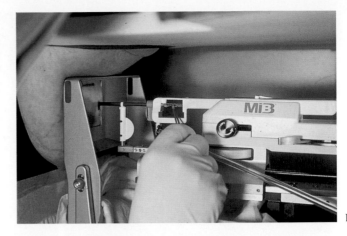

Figure 5.1. False negative CTC. B and C: 3D reconstruction does not reveal a significant lesion. D: Endoscopic view of the transverse colon in the same region reveals a 20 mm sessile lesion. Biopsy confirmed a tubular adenoma.

D

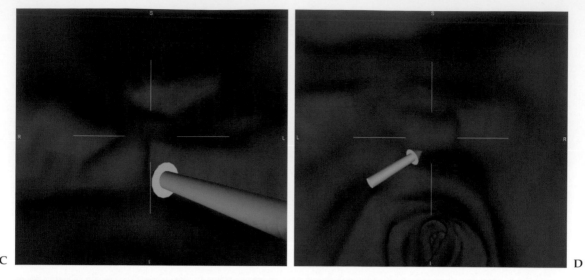

C   D

Figure 5.2. False positive CTC. C and D: 3D reconstruction of region in Figure 5-2A and 5-2B support the presence of a polypoid mass in the splenic flexure. Subsequent colonoscopy was normal.

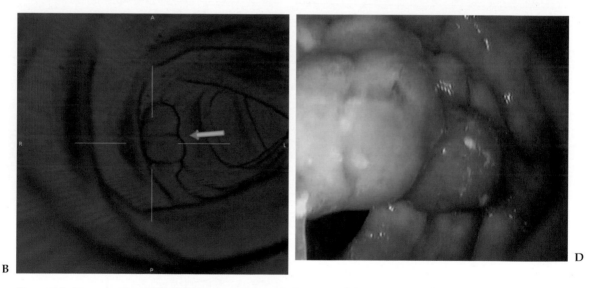

B   D

Figure 5.3. True-positive CTC. B: Digitally subtracted 3D image of the ascending colon provides a lesion projection similar to DCBE. D: Endoscopy reveals a 15 mm polyp. Biopsy confirmed a tubulo-villous adenoma.

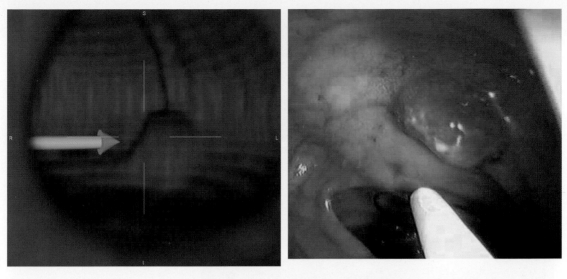

C

D

Figure 5.4. True positive CTC and false negative colonoscopy. C: 3D endoluminal reconstruction supports the findings on axial imaging. D: Colonoscopy performed on the same day as the CTC in a trial protocol was negative. Repeat sigmoidoscopy was advised based on the CTC findings. This revealed a 10 mm invasive carcinoma in the sigmoid colon.

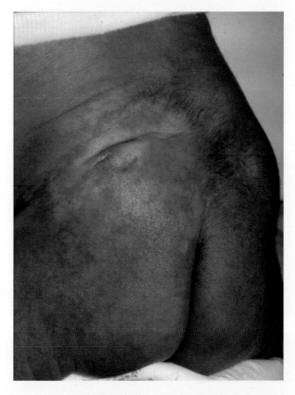

Figure 18.1. Photograph of the lower back reveals skin discoloration, hairy patch, and dorsal lipoma.

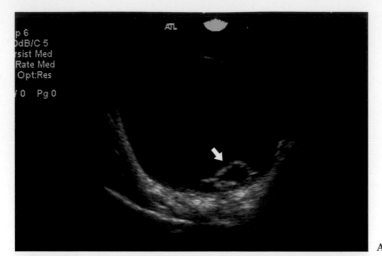

Figure 30.2. Ovarian cancer. Large multiloculated cyst with internal echogenicity and a mural nodule (solid arrow) with vascular flow demonstrated on power Doppler (open arrow).

A

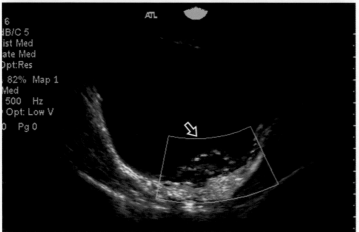

B

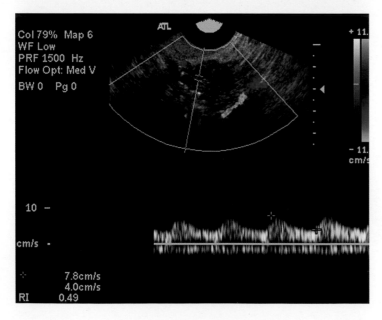

Figure 30.3. Benign ovarian mass. Complex adnexal mass with solid and cystic components. The solid component demonstrates vascular flow with a low resistive index (0.49). Mass was interpreted as an ovarian carcinoma, proved to be a fibroadenoma on resection.

27

Imaging of Biliary Disorders: Cholecystitis, Bile Duct Obstruction, Stones, and Stricture

Jose C. Varghese, Brian C. Lucey, and Jorge A. Soto

VI. What is the best imaging strategy for the diagnosis of choledo-
cholithiasis?
   A. Ultrasonography
   B. Computed tomography
   C. Endoscopic retrograde cholangiopancreatography
   D. Magnetic resonance cholangiopancreatography
   E. Endoscopic ultrasonography
   F. Imaging strategy
VII. What is the best imaging strategy for the evaluation of bile duct
stricture?
   A. Ultrasonography
   B. Computed tomography
   C. Endoscopic retrograde cholangiopancreatography
   D. Magnetic resonance cholangiopancreatography
   E. Endoscopic ultrasonography
   F. Special case: Klatskin tumor
   G. Imaging strategy

Key Points

- Cholescintigraphy is significantly more accurate than ultrasonography in the diagnosis of acute calculous cholecystitis (strong evidence).
- There is no one highly accurate test for the diagnosis of acute acalculous cholecystitis (moderate evidence).
- Cholecystokinin stimulated cholescintigraphy is very helpful in the diagnosis of chronic acalculous cholecystitis, and is predictive of symptom relief after cholecystectomy (strong evidence).
- Magnetic resonance cholangiopancreatography (MRCP) and endoscopic ultrasonography (EUS) are superior to ultrasonography in visualizing the whole of the bile duct, and establishing the level of bile duct obstruction (strong evidence).
- Patients with a high likelihood of choledocholithiasis based on clinical, laboratory, and ultrasonography findings should proceed directly to therapeutic endoscopic retrograde cholangiopancreatography without further cholangiographic studies (strong evidence).
- Magnetic resonance cholangiopancreatography is useful in the diagnosis of bile duct obstruction and in directing further patient management (moderate evidence).
- Endoscopic ultrasound and MRCP have a complementary role in the comprehensive evaluation of patients with bile duct stricture (moderate evidence).

Definition and Pathophysiology

Acute cholecystitis is caused by chemical or bacterial inflammation of the gallbladder leading to mucosal ulceration, wall edema, and fibrinosuppurative serositis. In up to 90% of patients, gallstones are associated and lead to acute calculous cholecystitis (ACC). In the remaining 10% of patients, gallbladder inflammation occurs in the absence of stones and results in acute acalculous cholecystitis (AAC). Repeated episodes of subacute gall-bladder inflammation lead to chronic cholecystitis. Pathologically, the gall-bladder is shrunken and fibrotic with a thickened wall. Gallbladder stones are associated in 95% of these patients leading to chronic calculous chole-cystitis (CCC). In the remaining minority of patients, chronic cholecystitis occurs in the absence of gallstones resulting in chronic acalculous cholecystitis (CAC).

Extrahepatic bile duct obstruction can result from intramural, mural, or extramural lesions of the biliary tract. The major causes of obstruction are stones, tumor, and benign strictures. Of these, choledocholithiasis is by far the commonest cause, accounting for up to 90% of bile duct obstruction. Bile duct strictures can be due to benign or malignant causes. Malignant lesions causing obstruction includes primary neoplasms of the bile ducts such as cholangiocarcinoma, and neoplasms extrinsic to the bile ducts. Most benign strictures of the bile duct are traumatic, infective, or inflam-matory in origin.

Epidemiology

Approximately 25 million (10% to 20%) adults in the United States have gallstones. They occur far more commonly in women than men, with around 40% of women greater than 80 years of age having gallstones. Prevalence is high in fair-skinned people of northern European descent, but is highest in specific races such as the Pima Indians (up to 75%). It is least prevalent in African Americans, unless there is underlying genetic disorders such as sickle cell disease or thalassemia.

Acute cholecystitis typically occurs in women of reproductive age of 30 to 50 years. Chronic cholecystitis also occurs more frequently in women of the same age group. Although traditionally considered a disease of adults, cholecystitis is increasing in incidence in the pediatric population over the last 20 years with 1.3 pediatric cases occurring for every 1000 adult cases. The prevalence is increased in children with chronic hemolysis such as hemolytic anemia. Up to 5% of all cholecystectomies are performed in the pediatric age group for this reason.

Acute acalculous cholecystitis occurs most commonly in hospitalized patients with severe underlying medical and surgical illness. There is no racial predilection. It occurs more commonly in males with a male-to-female ratio of 2–3:1, and occurs at an average age of over 50 years. It is more frequent in the pediatric population compared to adults. In the pedi-atric population, prognosis is good due to earlier diagnosis and treatment with cholecystectomy.

The incidence of biliary obstruction in the United States is approximately 5 cases per 1000 people, with gallstones being by far the commonest cause. However, the vast majority of patients with gallstones are asymptomatic, with only 20% presenting with related symptoms. Malignancy is the second commonest cause of biliary obstruction with cholangiocarcinoma (0.1% to 0.9%), and tumors of the surrounding organs (gallbladder, pan-creas, malignant nodes) being the commonest lesions. Benign strictures of the extrahepatic bile duct are the third commonest cause of bile duct obstruction with traumatic, infective, and inflammatory lesions being the leading causes.

Overall Cost to Society

Due to the high incidence of cholecystitis and the large number of chole-cystectomies performed annually in the U.S., a sizable portion of health care costs is devoted to treating this condition. In addition, 15% of 500,000 cholecystectomies performed in the U.S. each year require common bile duct exploration (75,000), further increasing the surgical costs. The advent of laparoscopic surgery has served to reduce some of these costs, although due to the large volume of cases the health economic burden still remains high.

There is very little information on the cost of managing patients with bile duct obstruction, particularly that due to malignancy. Only the minor-ity of patients undergoes curative surgery. The majority is palliated with stent placement or chemoradiotherapy.

Goals

The goals of imaging in gallbladder disease are (1) to diagnose gallstones, and (2) to identify underlying gallbladder disease (acute or chronic chole-cystitis) that requires treatment. The goals of imaging in patients with sus-pected bile duct obstruction are (1) to confirm the presence of obstruction, (2) to determine the level of obstruction, and (3)to diagnose the cause of obstruction.

Methodology

A search of the Medline/PubMed (National Library of Medicine, Bethesda, Maryland) was performed using a single or combination of key words including *imaging, ultrasonography, computed tomography, magnetic resonance cholangiopancreatography, cholescintigraphy, endoscopic ultrasound, endoscopic retrograde cholangiopancreatography, acute cholecystitis, acalculous cholecystitis, chronic cholecystitis, sphincter of Oddi dysfunction, bile duct obstruction, chole-docholithiasis, neoplasm,* and *stricture.* Reviewing the reference list of rele-vant papers identified additional articles. No time limits were applied for the searches, which were repeated up to several times up to April 16, 2004. Limits included English-language, abstracts, and human subjects. A search of the National Guideline Clearinghouse at www.guideline.gov was also performed.

I. What Is the Best Imaging Strategy for the Diagnosis of Acute Calculous Cholecystitis?

Summary of Evidence: Ultrasonography is useful primarily for the diagno-sis of gallstones, and secondarily in the diagnosis of acute cholecystitis. Its accuracy for diagnosis of cholelithiasis is over 95%, but its accuracy for diagnosis of acute cholecystitis is reduced to around 80%. Cholescintigra-phy is the most accurate test for the diagnosis of acute cholecystitis with an accuracy exceeding 90% (strong evidence). However, in the appropri-ate clinical setting, sonographic findings of gallstones and specific gall-bladder changes are sufficient for management of most patients with suspected ACC. Cholescintigraphy should be performed where doubt exists.

Supporting Evidence: Patients with ACC usually present with the classical triad of right upper quadrant pain, fever, and leukocytosis. Unfortunately, clinical and laboratory findings alone are insufficient for accurate diagnosis (1,2). Therefore, the diagnosis is often heavily dependent on imaging evaluation. Of all the imaging tests available, ultrasonography and cholescintigraphy have proven to be the two most useful tests for this task (3).

A. Ultrasonography

The accuracy for ultrasonography diagnosis of gallbladder stones exceeds 95% (4). However, its ability to diagnose acute cholecystitis is reduced. A meta-analysis by Shea et al. (5) showed ultrasonography to have an overall adjusted sensitivity of only 85%, and a specificity of 80% in the diagnosis of acute cholecystitis.

Despite this, some findings on ultrasonography have been more strongly associated with acute cholecystitis than others: a positive Murphy's sign is reported to have sensitivity as high as 88% (6); and an increased gallbladder wall thickness of >3.5mm has been found to be a reliable and independent predictor of acute cholecystitis (7). In addition, combinations of ultrasonography findings have been found be very predictive of acute cholecystitis. In a study by Ralls et al. (8), a positive Murphy's sign and the presence of gallstones had a positive predictive value of 92%. In the same study, the findings of gallbladder wall thickening and gallstones had a positive predictive value of 95%. However, a single specific finding or several nonspecific findings alone were unreliable for diagnosis of acute cholecystitis (6). Thus, although ultrasonography is reduced in accuracy when broadly applied, in the right clinical setting and taken together with the above-mentioned specific imaging signs, ultrasonography alone is sufficient to direct patient management (9).

B. Cholescintigraphy

In the largest series published by Weissmann et al. (10), cholescintigraphy was found to have a sensitivity of 95% and a specificity of 99% in the diagnosis of acute cholecystitis. Across the board, investigators have consistently found a high sensitivity of over 90% in the diagnosis of acute cholecystitis. However, the specificity of cholescintigraphy has been less consistent and has varied from 73% to 99% (10–13).

When studies directly comparing cholescintigraphy with ultrasonography are evaluated, cholescintigraphy is consistently found to be superior in the diagnosis of ACC (Table 27.1). In a recent study by Alobaidi et al. (14), cholescintigraphy compared to ultrasonography had a sensitivity of 90.9% versus 62%. The results were even more striking in a study by Kalimi et al. (15), in which cholescintigraphy compared to ultrasonography had a sensitivity of 86% versus 48%. Cholescintigraphy is also found to be much more specific than ultrasonography (16). These findings have led some authors to suggest that cholescintigraphy should be the primary diagnostic modality used in patients with suspected acute cholecystitis, with ultrasonography used only for detection of gallbladder stones (5,14,15).

Table 27.1. Accuracy of ultrasonography compared with cholescintigraphy in the diagnosis of acute cholecystitis

Investigator	Cholescintigraphy Sensitivity/specificity (%)		Ultrasonography Sensitivity/specificity (%)	
Zeman et al. (184)	98	82	67	82
Worthen et al. (12)	95	100	67	100
Ralls et al. (185)	86	84	86	90
Freitas et al. (186)	98	90	60	81
Samuels et al. (187)	97	93	97	64
Chatziioannou et al. (188)	92	89	40	89

C. Computed Tomography

Computed tomography (CT) is not routinely used to diagnose ACC due to its poor sensitivity for detection of cholelithiasis (75%) and cholecystitis (17). However, a recent study by Bennett et al. (18) showed an extremely good overall sensitivity, specificity, and accuracy of 91.7%, 99.1%, and 94.3%, respectively, for the CT diagnosis of acute cholecystitis. In practice, CT is more commonly used for detection of complications of acute cholecystitis such as emphysematous cholecystitis, perforation, or abscess formation, rather than for primary diagnosis of acute cholecystitis (19–21).

D. Magnetic Resonance Imaging

Both conventional magnetic resonance imaging (MRI) (22–25) and magnetic resonance cholangiopancreatography (MRCP) (24,26–29) have been evaluated in the diagnosis of ACC and its complications (30). When compared to ultrasonography, some have found MRI to be equivalent (31), some have found it to be superior (32), and others have found mixed results (33). As a primary tool, many workers have found MRI to be extremely accurate in the diagnosis of gallstones, which are seen as low signal intensity lesions surrounded by high signal bile (26,28,29). Similarly, the changes of acute cholecystitis have also been diagnosed with great accuracy (26,28,29). However, the lack of widespread availability of MRI and the relatively high cost prohibits its primary use for now.

E. Imaging Strategy

Based on literature evidence alone, there is no doubt that cholescintigraphy is the most accurate test for the diagnosis of acute cholecystitis. However, due to a combination of reasons including availability, broad imaging capability, and clinician referral pattern, ultrasonography has emerged as the first-line imaging modality for the diagnosis ACC. Almost all patients presenting to the hospital with biliary symptoms undergo an initial ultrasonography examination. An evidence-based algorithm for evaluation of patients with suspected ACC based on clinical suspicion and sonographic findings is given in Figure 27.1. Following such an algorithm should result in a diagnosis of ACC that is sufficiently accurate for clinical management, with the least time and cost burden to the patient.

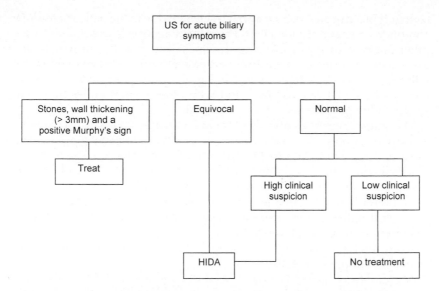

Figure 27.1. An evidence-based algorithm for investigation of suspected acute cholecystitis. All patients with symptoms suggestive of acute cholecystitis should have ultrasonography performed in the first instance. If the three highly specific signs of acute calculous cholecystitis (ACC), that is, gallstones, wall thickening (>3.5 mm), and Murphy's sign, are all present, the patient has a high probability of ACC and should proceed directly to appropriate therapy without further investigations. If the ultrasonography findings are normal and the clinical suspicion is low, the patient should have no further imaging performed. If the ultrasonography findings are normal, but the clinical suspicion is strong, or the patient has equivocal ultra-sonography findings, then the patient should proceed to cholescintigraphy.

II. What Is the Best Imaging Strategy for the Diagnosis of Acute Acalculous Cholecystitis?

Summary of Evidence: There is no ideal test for the diagnosis of AAC (moderate evidence). Ultrasonography, CT, and cholescintigraphy are all moderately accurate, with cholescintigraphy being the most accurate. Occasionally, an empirical trial of percutaneous cholecystostomy may be the only way to make the diagnosis.

Supporting Evidence: There are two well-documented reasons why it is important to promptly diagnose and treat patients with AAC: first, delay in treatment is associated with a high mortality ranging from 10% to 50% (34–37); and second, percutaneous cholecystostomy is effective in ameliorating sepsis (35–40).

A. Ultrasonography

Ultrasonography of the abdomen and pelvis is often the first test requested in the intensive care unit patient with sepsis of unknown etiology (39). Although easy to perform, evidence shows that ultrasonography is insensitive in the diagnosis of AAC (34,40,41), the reasons being that many of the usual indicators of acute cholecystitis are absent or difficult to elicit: gallstones are absent by definition, and the other helpful pointers such as sonographic Murphy's sign may not be elicited due to the patient's medical condition or heavy sedation (34). Thus, the diagnosis is dependent on the other findings such as gallbladder luminal distention (>5 cm transverse), presence of echogenic sludge, wall thickening (>4 mm to 5 mm), subserosal edema, and pericholecystic fluid (34). Unfortunately, these are all nonspecific findings that can also be found with other comorbidities that commonly afflict the intensive care unit patient.

In a study involving critically ill trauma patients, Puc et al. (41) found a sensitivity of only 30%, but a specificity of 93% in the sonographic diagnosis of AAC. They came to the conclusion that despite its convenience as a bedside procedure, ultrasonography was too insensitive to justify its use, and that a more sensitive diagnostic tool was required. However, others have found better sensitivities ranging from 60% to 70%. Apart from the poor sensitivities, reports also show a poor specificity for ultrasonography diagnosis of AAC (40). Overall, the reported accuracy for AAC is not sufficiently high to make ultrasonography definitive in the evaluation of patients with possible AAC.

B. Cholescintigraphy

Due to the above-mentioned reasons, cholescintigraphy has been advocated to increase diagnostic accuracy and avoid unnecessary percutaneous cholecystostomies. The reported sensitivities of cholescintigraphy in the diagnosis of AAC have ranged from 64% to 100%, with a mean of 79% and the specificities from 61% to 100%, with a mean of 87% (Table 27.2). In one direct comparative study, cholescintigraphy was found to be more sensitive than ultrasonography (100% versus 30%) in the diagnosis of AAC, although their specificities were similar (88% versus 93%) (41). Some studies have suggested that ultrasonography and cholescintigraphy are complementary, with each independently improving the overall diagnostic accuracy (42,43).

C. Computed Tomography

Computed tomography of the abdomen and pelvis is sometimes the first test performed in the intensive care unit patient, particularly in the postoperative period when looking for an enteric leak, or when gastrointesti-

Table 27.2. Accuracy of cholescintigraphy in the diagnosis of acute acalculous cholecystitis

Investigator	Sensitivity (%) No. pts./total No. pts.	Specificity (%) No. pts./total No. pts.
Weissmann et al. (189)	14/15 (93)	
Shuman et al. (190)	14/19 (74)	
Ramanna et al. (191)	11/11 (100)	
Mirvis (44)	9/10 (90)	21/34 (62)
Swayne (192)	37/49 (76)	
Flancbaum and Choban (193)	12/16 (75)	29/29 (100)
Kalliafas et al. (194)	9/10 (90)	
Prevot et al. (42)	9/14 (64)	18/18 (100)
Mariat et al. (43)	8/12 (67)	16/16 (100)
Totals	123/156 (79)	84/97 (87)

nal symptoms predominate. When cholecystitis is present, CT can show features that can lead to this diagnosis (44,45). The sensitivity and specificity of CT for the diagnosis of AAC can be as high as 90% to 95%. Thus, CT can be a very useful adjunct for diagnosis of AAC when ultrasonography is equivocal (45).

D. Imaging Strategy

There is as yet no ideal imaging test available for the diagnosis of AAC. Overall, cholescintigraphy has better test characteristics than ultrasonography. However, due to logistical and technical reasons, cholescintigraphy is not often performed or is equivocal in the intensive care unit patient. Although ultrasonography is more practicable, it too is poorly sensitive and specific (20). However, it is almost always performed because the finding of lesions such as gallstones, bile duct obstruction, or extrabiliary source of sepsis would alter patient management.

The management of patients with potential AAC remains difficult and controversial. The best strategy is for the interventional radiologist and the referring physician concerned to evaluate each patient based on the clinical, laboratory, and ultrasonography findings. Ideally, a CT or cholescintigraphy (Fig. 27.2) should be performed before percutaneous cholecystostomy. Sometimes when this is not possible or the imaging results are equivocal, there is no choice but to proceed with a trial of percutaneous catheter drainage (36,46).

III. What Is the Best Imaging Strategy for the Diagnosis of Chronic Calculous Cholecystitis?

Summary of Evidence: In the appropriate setting, ultrasonography is sufficient to make the diagnosis of CCC. Cholecystectomy is curative.

Supporting Evidence: Chronic calculous cholecystitis is the commonest manifestation of gallbladder disease. Patients present with biliary colic, nausea, and flatulent dyspepsia exacerbated by eating fatty foods.

A. Ultrasonography

Ultrasonography is the primary imaging test used in the diagnosis of CCC (47,48), with a sensitivity of 86% and the specificity 90% (49). A contracted thick-walled gallbladder containing stones is the classical appearance (47). In some patients, the gallbladder may be so contracted that it is hard to visualize. Occasionally, associated findings of chronic cholecystitis such as cholesterolosis or adenomyomatosis may be evident.

B. Cholescintigraphy

This examination is performed with the patient fasting for 4 to 24 hours. The diagnosis of chronic cholecystitis is suggested when there is delayed (1 to 4 hours) filling of the gallbladder, either spontaneously or with the help of intravenous morphine (2 mg), given to induce spasm of the sphincter of Oddi. Once the gallbladder is filled, the ejection fraction is measured after intravenous administration of cholecystokinin (Sincalide) at a dose of

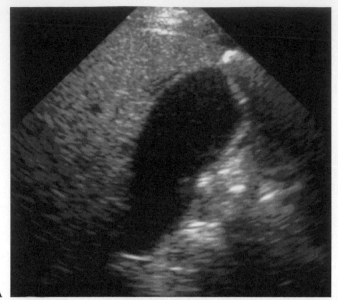

Figure 27.2. A 59–year-old man with a history of abdominal pain, leukocytosis, and abnormal liver function tests. A: Ultrasonography shows a thin layer of fluid around the fundus of the gallbladder. Patient had an associated positive sonographic Murphy's sign. B: Intravenous and oral contrast enhanced CT shows a normal gallbladder. C: Technetium-diisopropyliminodiacetic acid (Tc-DISIDA) cholescintigraphy shows normal intense filling of the gallbladder, ruling out the diagnosis of acute cholecystitis.

A

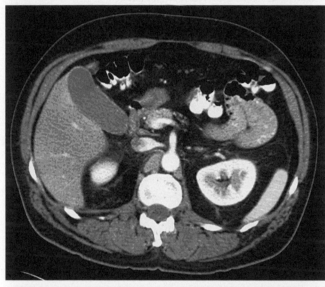

B

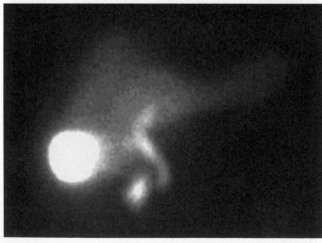

C

0.02 μg per kilogram weight. An ejection fraction of less than 35% after a slow infusion of cholecystokinin given over a period of 30 to 60 minute is considered abnormal (50). Thus, the two findings of delayed gallbladder filling and a poor ejection fraction, in the appropriate clinical setting, are highly suggestive of chronic cholecystitis (51).

C. Imaging Strategy

In a patient with classic clinical and ultrasonography findings of CCC, the generally accepted practice is to perform cholecystectomy without necessarily pursuing further investigations. If there is doubt as to the diagnosis, cholescintigraphy should be performed. Also, if the patient's symptoms are more suggestive of pancreatic or gastrointestinal disease, other tests such as CT and endoscopy may be need before considering cholecystectomy.

IV. What Is the Best Imaging Strategy for the Diagnosis of Chronic Acalculous Cholecystitis?

Summary of Evidence: Cholecystokinin stimulated cholescintigraphy has a pivotal role in the diagnosis of patients with CAC who would benefit from cholecystectomy (strong evidence). The relative roles of quantitative cholescintigraphy versus endoscopic retrograde cholangiopancreatography (ERCP) with manometry in the diagnosis of sphincter of Oddi dysfunction have yet to be established.

Supporting Evidence: In less than 5% of patients, chronic cholecystitis occurs in the absence of gallbladder stones. The identification of these patients is not easy as a number of other biliary disorders can also give rise to similar symptoms. These include sphincter of Oddi dysfunction, ampullary stenosis, occult choledocholithiasis, and extrabiliary diseases such as peptic ulcer. The consequence of performing cholecystectomy in these patients includes the unnecessary risk of such an operation, and persistence of symptoms leading to the postcholecystectomy syndrome. The investigation of these patients includes ultrasonography, cholescintigraphy, MRCP, and ERCP with sphincter of Oddi manometry.

A. Ultrasonography

The gallbladder is usually normal in appearance without gallstones.

B. Cholescintigraphy

In patients with CAC, the gallbladder maintains its normal concentrating function but its contraction and emptying are reduced significantly. This may be due to intrinsic gallbladder disease, partial cystic duct obstruction, or a combination of both. Cholecystokinin cholescintigraphy with calculation of the gallbladder ejection fraction has been found to be a good predictor of pathology and symptom relief after cholecystectomy (51–60). The diagnostic findings are that of delayed (>4 hours) filling of the gallbladder and an ejection fraction less than 35%. However, not all authors have found this test to be specific (61), or to correlate with histologic findings (62). Some have found reduced ejection fractions in control groups (61), and others have found spontaneous resolution of symptoms in patients with an abnormal study (63). However, the overall evidence remains strong that cholecystokinin-stimulated cholescintigraphy is highly predictive for CAC and relief of symptoms after cholecystectomy.

Shaffer et al. (64) demonstrated using quantitative cholescintigraphy, functional obstruction at the ampulla of Vater in a group of patients with the postcholecystectomy syndrome. These workers correctly identified patients with sphincter of Oddi dysfunction before papillotomy and showed functional improvement in the majority of patients following papillotomy. Further more, a recent direct comparison between cholescintigraphy and manometry found that cholescintigraphy was a better predictor of symptom relief after sphincterotomy than clinical symptoms or even manometry (65). However, others have found sensitivities ranging from only 69% to 83%, and specificities ranging from 60% to 88% in the cholangiographic diagnosis of sphincter of Oddi dysfunction (66–70). In a study by Pineau et al. (71), the specificity of cholescintigraphy was as low as 60%, making them question the value of this test in excluding the diagnosis of sphincter of Oddi dysfunction. For these reasons, quantitative cholescintigraphy is not widely used and its clinical utility yet remains to be determined.

C. Endoscopic Retrograde Cholangiopancreatography

Although technically challenging, ERCP with manometry is useful in the diagnosis of sphincter of Oddi dysfunction. At ERCP, pressures can be measured in the lower bile duct and sphincter zones by standard manometric techniques. A resting sphincter pressure of >40 mm Hg is taken to be abnormal and predictive of patients likely to benefit from a therapeutic sphincterotomy (65,72,73).

D. Imaging Strategy

In patients without gallstones and persisting chronic biliary symptoms, cholescintigraphy should be used to select patients with CAC that may benefit from cholecystectomy. In the remaining patients, MRCP is indicated to exclude mechanical lesions of the bile duct. In patients with suspected functional disorders of the bile duct, the relative merits of quantitative cholescintigraphy versus ERCP with manometry have not been fully established. An evidence-based algorithm for imaging of patients with chronic biliary symptoms is given in Figure 27.3.

V. What Is the Best Imaging Strategy for the Evaluation of Bile Duct Obstruction?

Summary of Evidence: Ultrasonography is the initial test for detection of biliary obstruction by identifying intrahepatic or common bile duct dilatation. However, MRCP and EUS are superior to ultrasonography in visualizing the whole of the bile duct, and establishing the level of bile duct obstruction (strong evidence).

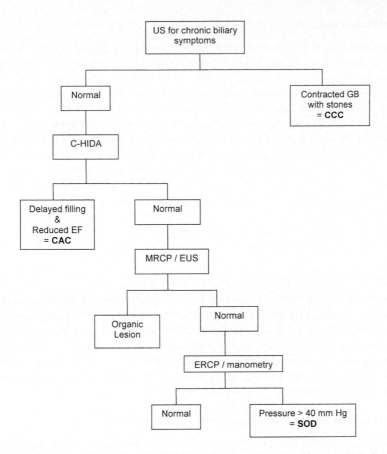

Figure 27.3. An evidence-based algorithm for investigation of suspected chronic biliary disease. US, ultrasonography; C-HIDA, cholecystokinin – hydroxy iminodiacetic acid; SOD, sphincter of Oddi dysfunction; CCC, chronic calculous cholecystitis; CAC, chronic acalculous cholecystitis. All patients with symptoms suggestive of chronic biliary disease should have an initial ultrasonography performed. If a contracted gallbladder with stones is found, the patient should be treated for CCC. If the examination is negative, the patient should then proceed to a cholecystokinin cholescintigraphy. If there is delayed filling of a gallbladder, combined with a reduced ejection fraction, the patient should be treated for CAC. If the examination is negative, an MRCP of EUS should be performed to exclude occult choledocholithiasis or other mechanical cause of symptoms. If this test is negative, the patient should have an ERCP with manometry performed to assess sphincter pressure. If this is elevated, patient should be treated for sphincter of Oddi dysfunction. If the pressure is normal, other causes for patient cholestasis should be sought.

Supporting Evidence: The diagnosis of bile duct obstruction is based on a combination of clinical, laboratory, and imaging findings. The clinical findings of jaundice, pruritus, pale stools, and dark urine, in association with laboratory findings of elevated bilirubin, alkaline phosphatase, and transaminases, are highly suggestive of biliary tract obstruction (74,75). The imaging modalities used for the evaluation of patients with suspected biliary tract obstruction include ultrasonography, CT, MRCP, ERCP, and EUS. The utility of these imaging modalities is based on a number of factors including their diagnostic accuracy, invasiveness, complication rate, availability, ease of use, local expertise, operator preference, and cost.

A. Ultrasonography

Transabdominal ultrasonography is universally accepted as the test of choice for distinguishing hepatocellular disease from mechanical bile duct obstruction, with a sensitivity of 70% to 95%, and a specificity of 80% to 100% (4,76). Thus, together with the high sensitivity for diagnosis of bile duct obstruction, availability, ease-of-use, noninvasiveness, safety, and low cost, ultrasonography has established itself as the first-line imaging modality in the investigation of patients with suspected hepatobiliary disease (4).

Pitfalls in the ultrasonography diagnosis of bile duct obstruction include (1) nonobstructed but dilated common bile duct (CBD) in the elderly or postcholecystectomy patient, giving rise to a false-positive result; (2) bile duct dilatation lagging (as much as 1 week) behind the onset of mechanical obstruction, giving rise to a false-negative result; and (3) obstructive lesion not associated with significant bile duct dilation (as occurs in 10% to 25% of choledocholithiasis), resulting in a false-negative result (4,77).

B. Computed Tomography

Computed tomography is superior to ultrasonography in the diagnosis of bile duct obstruction by revealing intrahepatic and extrahepatic bile duct dilatation (78). It is 96% accurate in determining the presence of biliary obstruction, 90% accurate in determining its level, and 70% accurate in determining its cause (78,79). It is better able to visualize the middle to distal CBD compared to ultrasonography, particularly in the obese patient or those with overlying bowel gas (78).

C. Magnetic Resonance Cholangiopancreatography

With good-quality MRCP, the normal CBD is visualized in up to 98% of patients (80). A recent meta-analysis of 67 MRCP studies performed over a period of 16 years (from January 1987 to March 2003) evaluating a mixture of benign and malignant conditions found an overall sensitivity of 97% for the MRCP detection of the presence of obstruction, and a sensitivity of 98% for the MRCP determination of the level of obstruction (81).

D. Endoscopic Ultrasonography

Endoscopic ultrasonography is rapidly gaining momentum in the evaluation of the extrahepatic biliary system (78,82–86) and other upper gastrointestinal disorders (87). It combines endoscopy with high-frequency (7.5 to 20 MHz) ultrasonography to visualize the whole of the bile duct in up to 96% of patients (78,88). It is able to diagnose the presence of biliary obstruction with a diagnostic accuracy of 98%.

VI. What Is the Best Imaging Strategy for the Diagnosis of Choledocholithiasis?

Summary of Evidence: Ultrasonography is insensitive in the diagnosis of choledocholithiasis. Endoscopic retrograde cholangiopancreatography (ERCP) is no longer indicated for the primary diagnosis of choledocholithiasis but is reserved for its therapeutic role. Both MRCP and EUS are highly accurate alternatives in the diagnosis of choledocholithiasis. Patients with a high likelihood of choledocholithiasis based on clinical, laboratory, and ultrasonography findings should be referred directly for therapeutic ERCP, without further imaging (strong evidence).

Supporting Evidence

A. Ultrasonography

Most of the bile duct stones are found within the middle to distal portion of the CBD (89), a particularly difficult region of the biliary tract to visualize using ultrasonography (4,77,78). There is a further reduction in diagnostic information in patients who are obese. This results in a poor sensitivity for ultrasonography diagnosis of choledocholithiasis, ranging from 18% to 75% depending on the operator experience, the institution where performed, patient population studied, and quality of equipment used (78,90–92). The specificity for diagnosis of choledocholithiasis can be as high as 95% (78), with false positives occurring due to pneumobilia, hematobilia, and overlying gas shadows from adjacent bowel (4,77).

B. Computed Tomography

Bile duct stones are directly visualized or found by using the target or a crescent signs (79). The sensitivity for CT diagnosis of choledocholithiasis is only slightly higher than that for ultrasonography, ranging from 60% to 88%, with a specificity of 84% to 97% (78,93,94). This decreased detection rate is predominantly related to the varying density of gallbladder stones based on their cholesterol and calcium content (94). Up to 20% to 25% of stones are isodense with bile, making them almost impossible to detect.

Computed tomography cholangiography is a relatively new technique that is developed to overcome some of the limitations of CT in the diagnosis of bile duct disease. It provides cholangiographic images by opacification of the bile duct with contrast material administered through the oral or intravenous route. The low-density stones are now seen as filling defects within the contrast opacified bile duct. Improved stone detection rates with sensitivity and specificity of 92% and 92%, respectively, have been reported (93). However, this technique has not gained wide acceptance due to the small but finite incidence of contrast hypersensitivity reactions, poor bile duct opacification in patients with hepatocellular dysfunction/high-grade obstruction, and the availability of other more robust techniques such as MRCP and EUS.

C. Endoscopic Retrograde Cholangiopancreatography

Endoscopic retrograde cholangiopancreatography has a sensitivity of 89% to 90%, and a specificity of 98% to 100% in the diagnosis of choledocholithiasis (95,96). Although long considered the gold-standard test, its accuracy has been questioned (96). More recently, direct studies have shown EUS to be superior to ERCP in the diagnosis of choledocholithiasis (82,96). It is highly likely that as the new technologies of MRCP and EUS mature, one of these will eventually emerge as the new standard of reference. They are already having a significant impact on the practice of ERCP with implications for future development and training (97,98).

Table 27.3. Accuracy of endoscopic ultrasonography in the diagnosis of choledocholithiasis

Investigator	Sensitivity (%)	Specificity (%)	Accuracy (%)
Buscarini et al. (86)	98	99	97
Palazzo et al. (195)	95	98	96
Sugiyama and Atomi (78)	96	100	99
Kohut et al. (196)	93	93	94
Shim et al. (197)	89	100	97
Prat et al. (96)	93	97	95
Canto et al. (121)	84	95	94
Amouyal et al. (198)	97	100	98
Norton and Alderson (108)	88	96	92

D. Magnetic Resonance Cholangiopancreatography

A recent meta-analysis has showed MRCP to have a sensitivity of 92% in the diagnosis of choledocholithiasis (81). The specificities have ranged from 84% to 100%, and the accuracy from 89% to 90% (89,90,93,99,100). In general, false-negative results occur due to small stones (<3 mm to <5 mm) found within nondilated bile ducts, particularly impacted at the ampulla (90,101–103). False-positive results occur due to mistaking of stones for other low signal intensity lesions such as sludge, blood clots, air bubbles, tumor, and ampullary spasm (89,90,102).

E. Endoscopic Ultrasonography

The sensitivity, specificity, and accuracy for EUS in the diagnosis of chole-docholithiasis have ranged from 93% to 98%, 97% to 100%, and 97%, respectively (78,83,86,96,104). A list of sensitivities and specificities for the EUS detection of choledocholithiasis is given in Table 27.3. In particular, EUS is sensitive in detecting small stones (<3 mm), even when situated at the distal bile duct or within a nondilated bile duct (78,82,105,106). In patients with "idiopathic" pancreatitis, EUS was able to diagnose a cause in 77% to 92% patients where their symptoms were caused by small gall-stones missed by conventional imaging (107,108).

F. Imaging Strategy

To help direct therapy, classifications based on clinical, laboratory, and transabdominal ultrasonography findings have been developed to stratify patients according to their likelihood (low, intermediate, and high) of harboring CBD stones at presentation (89,109–117). Calvo et al. (89) validated such a classification by finding bile duct stones at ERCP in 65.3%, 33%, and 0% of their patients with a high, intermediate, and low probability classification, respectively. Even better selection was achieved by Liu et al. (115), who found bile duct stones in over 90% of their patients classified as a high-probability group.

Many studies suggest that patients with a high probability for choledo-cholithiasis should directly undergo diagnostic ERCP with intent to treat (111–115). The needlessness of performing screening tests in such a high-probability group of patients was shown by Sahai et al. (111), who found that a screening MRCP would have prevented ERCP in only less than 4% of their patients. A recent cost-effectiveness study comparing MRCP-, EUS-, and ERCP-based strategies have also shown that outcomes were highly dependent on the pretest probability for choledocholithiasis and that at probabilities of >45%, ERCP alone was the most cost-effective option (112).

In patients with a low or intermediate probability for choledocholithiasis, the literature suggests that a relatively noninvasive screening test such as MRCP or EUS should be used first to select patients with common duct stone for therapeutic ERCP (89,110,118–120). In such a group of patients, Calvo et al. (89) showed that MRCP may replace ERCP without missing pronounced choledocholithiasis. A systematic review of 28 studies with economic evaluation has shown that the preliminary use of MRCP can also reduce cost and improve quality of life outcomes when compared to diagnostic ERCP (118).

The role of EUS has also been validated in a number of studies (119,120). In a study of 55 patients with intermediate probability for choledocholithiasis by Kohut et al. (119), EUS selection for therapeutic ERCP only failed in one of five patients with CBD stones. Canto et al. (121) also found EUS to be a useful test in the low- to intermediate-probability group of patients. Evidence such as this has prompted the National Institutes of Health (NIH) state-of-the-science statement that in patients with a low likelihood of biliary stone disease, diagnostic ERCP should be avoided (120).

The question of whether to use MRCP or EUS as the primary screening tool has not yet been fully settled. They both consistently show diagnostic accuracies of greater than 90% in the diagnosis of choledocholithiasis (80,88,90,110), resulting in the above-mentioned NIH statement declaring MRCP, EUS, and ERCP to be comparable in the diagnosis of choledocholithiasis (120). But MRCP has the advantages of being quick to perform, not requiring sedation, and being completely noninvasive. However, it is relatively expensive and is not yet widely available. Endoscopic ultrasonography is less costly and facilitates interventions that are not possible with MRCP (86,112,122,123). In practice, which of these two tests is used is dictated more by the availability of equipment, local expertise, and physician preference than by strict clinical or economic criteria.

Thus, it would appear that patients with a high pretest probability for choledocholithiasis should directly undergo ERCP for diagnosis and treatment of their probable stones. Performing screening tests such as MRCP or EUS would only serve to add a time and cost burden to the patient. However, in patients with a low or intermediate pretest probability for choledocholithiasis, a test such as MRCP or EUS should be performed to select patients for therapeutic ERCP. Doing so would result in considerable clinical benefit and cost savings by avoiding unnecessary diagnostic ERCP in the vast majority of these patients.

VII. What Is the Best Imaging Strategy for the Evaluation of Bile Duct Stricture?

Summary of Evidence: Ultrasonography is the initial test for diagnosis of biliary obstruction. Magnetic resonance cholangiopancreatography is highly accurate in confirming the presence and level of obstruction, but is slightly inferior in diagnosing the cause of obstruction. However, it is able to provide a sufficiently accurate noninvasive cholangiographic image that is sufficient for directing further management (moderate evidence). Contrast-enhanced CT and MRI are helpful in diagnosis and staging most neoplastic lesions. In the hard-to-diagnose lesion, EUS with fine-needle aspiration is indicated. Thus, MRCP and EUS have complementary roles in the comprehensive evaluation of bile duct stricture (moderate evidence).

Supporting Evidence

A. Ultrasonography

Bile duct strictures can be due to benign or malignant lesions. Ultrasonography is highly accurate in detecting the presence of obstruction, but not accurate in diagnosing the level or cause of obstruction due to its inability to visualize the extrahepatic bile duct consistently (4,124). It is able to diagnose some causes of obstruction such as liver metastasis, porta-hepatis nodes, and pancreatic neoplasms (125). However, infiltrative lesions such as cholangiocarcinoma (77,126) and small neoplasms of the pancreas/ampulla are difficult to diagnose (4). Once the presence of obstruction is established, further cholangiographic evaluation is often required, particularly if therapy is planned (125).

B. Computed Tomography

Oral and intravenous contrast-enhanced CT is moderately well suited to the diagnosis of biliary obstruction (79,127,128). Due to its tomographic capability, CT is able to clearly display neoplastic lesions and the surrounding anatomy, making the accurate diagnosis of cause and level of obstruction possible (77,79,129). The sensitivity, specificity, and accuracy of CT in the diagnosis of malignancy are 77%, 63%, and 83%, respectively (130,131). Computed tomography can also be used to stage neoplasms; in a multimodality study using CT, EUS, and MRI to stage ampullary tumors, CT best predicted arterial vessel invasion, with an accuracy of 85% (131).

The limitations of CT include nonvisualization of very small neoplasms of the pancreas (132) and ampulla (77), and nonvisualization of infiltrative lesions of the bile duct such as cholangiocarcinoma (133). The sensitivity for CT diagnosis of benign strictures such as that arising from inflammatory (e.g., sclerosing cholangitis) and iatrogenic (e.g., surgical trauma) causes is also limited. Often cholangiographic techniques such as ERCP or MRCP are required for diagnosis and full delineation of biliary stricture, particularly if treatment options are being considered.

C. Endoscopic Retrograde Cholangiopancreatography

The role of ERCP in the management of biliary stricture is threefold: first, to distinguish benign from malignant stricture where doubt exists; second, to diagnose ampullary carcinoma as a cause of obstruction; and third, to relieve biliary obstruction using stent placement when indicated (120,134–136). Due to its high spatial resolution and image quality, ERCP is able to distinguish benign from malignant strictures based on their radiographic appearance (77,130,137).

D. Magnetic Resonance Cholangiopancreatography

In patients with a stricture, MRCP is able to diagnose the presence of obstruction with an accuracy of 95% to 100%, and the level of obstruction with an accuracy of 97% to 100% (80,89,131,138,139). Unlike other cholangiographic methods such as ERCP or percutaneous transhepatic cholangiography (PTC), MRCP consistently and fully displays dilated biliary ducts proximal to a tight stricture. This is because MRCP does not require contrast opacification of the obstructed ducts for visualization, while ERCP and PTC can visualize only those ducts that are contrast filled. Thus, in patients with multiple segmentally obstructed intrahepatic biliary ducts, MRCP is often superior to ERCP or PTC in depicting the full extent of the obstruction that is critical in the staging and management of their underlying disease (140,141).

Despite the excellent MRCP accuracy for diagnosis of the presence and level of obstruction, its sensitivity in distinguishing malignant from benign stricture is only 88% (81). This reduced sensitivity is due to a combination of MR signal dropout within a stricture due to lack of fluid, and the lower spatial resolution of MR (142). However, at least in one study involving patients with pancreatic disease, MRCP has been found to be comparable with ERCP in differentiating malignant from benign disease (143). In this prospective controlled study of 111 patients with pancreatic lesions (54 malignant, 57 benign), MRCP compared to ERCP had a sensitivity of 84% versus 70% and a specificity of 97% versus 94%. Performing conventional MRI in the same setting as MRCP has been shown to increase the diagnostic accuracy for differentiating malignant from benign lesions by visualization of mural and extramural components of the disease process (127,139,144,145).

The ability of MR to provide comprehensive staging of pancreaticobiliary neoplasms by adding conventional MRI (146–148) and MR angiography (149) to MRCP in the same setting is also very attractive (128,131,150–152). Thus, MR has the capacity to provide a one-stop imaging package for the compete staging of neoplasms that is suitable for directing therapy (99).

Diffuse stricturing conditions of the biliary tract such as primary sclerosing cholangitis (PSC) and ascending cholangitis can present with characteristic findings of multifocal strictures involving the intra- and extrahepatic biliary ducts with intervening areas of dilatation. In particular, PSC can be accurately diagnosed using MRCP in up to 90% of patients (137,153). Furthermore, Talwalkar et al. (154) suggested that MRCP is comparable to ERCP in the diagnosis of PSC, and is cost-effective when MRCP is used as the primary test. However, in patients with a normal MRCP, ERCP may still be needed to diagnose the subtle ductal changes of early PSC, and in patients with advanced disease and dominant stricture ERCP will be required for therapeutic drainage (99).

E. Endoscopic Ultrasonography

Endoscopic ultrasonography is emerging as a powerful tool in the diagnosis, tissue characterization, and local staging of lesions causing biliary stricture (87,135,155–158). Compared to MRCP for the diagnosis of biliary stricture, at least one study (123) reported EUS to be more specific (100% versus 76%) and to have a much greater positive predictive value (100% versus 25%), although the two had equal sensitivity (67%). However, a second study (130) found the two tests to be comparable, with MRCP compared to EUS having a sensitivity of 85% versus 79%, and a specificity of 71% versus 62%.

Endoscopic ultrasonography is particularly useful in the diagnosis of small tumors causing distal bile duct obstruction; it is able to detect pancreatic carcinoma less than 3 cm in size causing obstruction undiagnosed by conventional imaging modalities (156,159–161), and detect small ampullary tumors with a sensitivity of 100% (131). Due to the clear and detailed imaging provided by EUS, it is a very useful tool in the staging of distal bile duct neoplasms (135,155). In a study of ampullary tumor staging by Cannon et al. (155) comparing EUS with CT and MRI, EUS was found to be significantly superior to the others in the assessment of T stage of tumor (78% versus 24% and 56%, respectively), while these methods were equally sensitive in the detection of lymph node spread (68% versus 59% and 77%, respectively).

In addition to diagnostic imaging, EUS facilitates tissue sampling through EUS-guided fine-needle aspiration (EUS-FNA) (157,158,162–164). The sensitivity of EUS-FNA for diagnosis of malignancy is reported to range from 75% to 90% (165–167), with an accuracy of 85% to 96% (168–171). The main cause of inaccuracies is false-negative findings in the presence of tumor. Performing EUS with EUS-FNA as the first endoscopic procedure in patients suspected of having obstructive jaundice can obviate the need for about 50% of ERCPs, help direct subsequent therapeutic ERCP, and substantially reduce costs (157,162–164).

F. Special Case: Klatskin Tumor

Up to 50% to 60% of cholangiocarcinoma occur at the perihilar region (Klatskin tumor) and pose a particular challenge in diagnosis and treatment (128,152). Accurate staging is important because treatment is based on the extent of bile duct involvement as defined by the Bismuth classification (172), and the extent of extrabiliary spread as diagnosed by CT or MRI (126,128,152). Medically fit patients undergo curative surgery of varying severity based on their tumor staging (126,133,173). Patients unsuitable for surgery due to tumor spread or comorbidity, may be adequately palliated with biliary stenting performed using the endoscopic or percutaneous approach (133). The number of ducts and liver segments drained are also based on the cholangiographic findings (133,140,150,174–176).

Although ERCP has traditionally been used for cholangiography, due to the risk of inducing cholangitis in patients with undrained obstructed bile ducts and the advent of noninvasive imaging its primary role for this application has been questioned. Once an obstructed system has been contaminated, it requires immediate drainage to prevent complications from sepsis (177–179). In patients with unresectable tumor requiring palliative stenting, immediate endoscopic stenting following diagnostic ERCP may be appropriate. However, in the remaining patients where surgery is a consideration, premature intervention may compromise the final clinical outcome (150,175,180,181).

Magnetic resonance cholangiopancreatography provides cholangiographic images that are accurate in staging patients according to the Bismuth classification (131,140,141,148–151) (Fig. 27.4). It is able to depict the length of extrahepatic bile duct involved with disease as well as accurately define its proximal extension, which is important for directing therapy (140,141). If required, the local extent of the tumor can also be

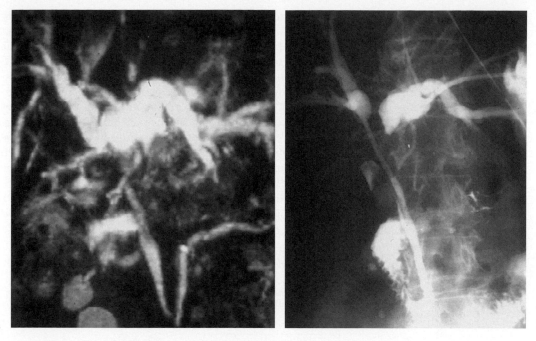

A   B

Figure 27.4. A 72–year-old man with a Klatskin tumor. A: Coronal maximum intensity projection MRCP showing Bismuth type 2 hilar obstruction. B: A percutaneous transhepatic cholangiogram confirms tumor involvement at the confluence with separation of the right and left hepatic ducts.

further evaluated using conventional MRI and MR angiography at the same sitting (126,147–152). This allows for the prospective multidisciplinary planning of ideal treatment option for the patient (99,101,150), may it be percutaneous (140,182,183), endoscopic (174,183), or surgical (126,128,133,173) in approach.

Endoscopic ultrasonography FNA has been used in the evaluation of patients with suspected cholangiocarcinoma (162,163). In a study by Eloubeidi et al. (162), 67% of their patients had no mass identifiable by prior abdominal imaging studies but were found to have lesions measuring less than 2 cm in average size by EUS. They report that the use of EUS-FNA had a positive impact on patient management in 84% of their patients. Similarly, in a study by Fritscher-Ravens et al. (163) of 44 patients with indeterminate hilar strictures, the sensitivity, specificity, and accuracy for distinguishing malignant from benign lesions were 89%, 100%, and 91%, respectively. They found that EUS-FNA was useful for tissue diagnosis of hilar strictures that were indeterminate by other imaging modalities, resulting in a positive change in management in over half of their patients.

G. Imaging Strategy

Patients with suspected biliary stricture should initially undergo imaging using ultrasonography or CT to determine the presence and cause of biliary obstruction. Computed tomography is able to more consistently and comprehensively diagnose the cause of obstruction and define the extent of disease than ultrasonography (128,133). In many patients, particularly in those with extensive metastatic disease, these may be the only imaging tests that are required to effect clinical management (133).

In patients requiring further delineation of disease, or when diagnostic doubt exists, a highly accurate noninvasive test such as MRCP or EUS should be used (128,133). Although MRCP alone is limited at distinguishing malignant from benign stricture (81,130), it is highly accurate at defining the extent of the biliary duct involvement and accurately classifies patients according to the Bismuth classification (140,152). Endoscopic ultrasonography is highly accurate in diagnosing the cause of obstruction, particularly using its ability for FNA (88). Therefore, in patients with hard-to-diagnose stricture of the bile duct, there may be a complementary role for EUS, with MRCP used to define the extent of the stricture and EUS-FNA used to visualize the mass and obtain histologic diagnosis (97,130). An evidence-based algorithm for investigation of patients with suspected bile duct obstruction is given in Figure 27.5.

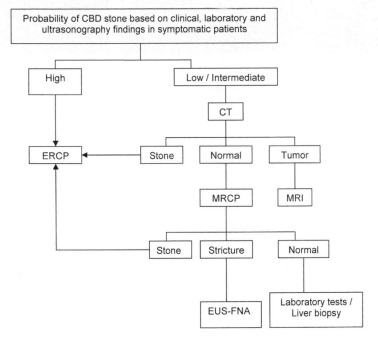

Figure 27.5. An evidence-based algorithm for investigation of suspected biliary obstruction. Patients with suspected bile duct obstruction should be stratified according to the likelihood of having choledocholithiasis based on clinical, laboratory, and ultrasonography findings. Those patients with a high probability of choledocholithiasis should be referred directly for therapeutic ERCP. Patients with a low to intermediate probability of CBD stones should have CT performed to rule out neoplasm or possibly stone. If choledocholithiasis is identified, the patient should be referred for therapeutic ERCP. If a tumor is identified, the investigation may be stopped if the neoplasm is sufficiently staged, or a contrast-enhanced MRI should be performed for complete staging. If CT is normal, an MRCP should be performed to diagnose occult choledocholithiasis or stricture. Patients with choledocholithiasis identified at MRCP should then undergo therapeutic ERCP. Those with a normal bile duct at MRCP should undergo further laboratory investigations to exclude hepatocellular disease as cause of their cholestasis. Patients with a stricture diagnosed at MRCP should undergo EUS-FNA for imaging and histologic diagnosis.

Take-Home Tables

Table 27.4. Suggested parameters for performing computed tomography of the hepatobiliary system

Oral contrast material*	900 mL of 2.2% barium sulfate solution
Intravenous contrast material*	100 to 150 ml of Optiray 320 mg/mL @ 2 to 5 mL/second
Slice thickness	2.5 to 5.0 mm
Reconstruction interval	1.0 to 3.0 mm
Pitch	1 to 6
kVp	120 to 140
mAs	200 to 300

* If CT is performed for the sole purpose of identifying bile duct stones, oral and intravenous contrast material is not administered.

Table 27.5. Suggested parameters for performing magnetic resonance cholangiopancreatography (for GE 1.5–T machine with torso phased array coil)

Sequence	Scout	FSE T2–W	Coronal SSFSE	Axial SSFSE	Thick slab SSFSE
Type	SSFSE	FRFSE-XL	SSFSE	SSFSE	SSFSE
TR	Infinite	2200	Minimum	Minimum	Minimum
TE	96	84	60	60	600
FA			130	130	130
NEX	1	1	1	1	1
2D/3D	2D	2D	2D	2D	2D
ST (mm)	8	7	4	4	60
Gap (mm)	2	2	0	1	0
FOV (mm)	440	350	350	350	260
No. of partitions	20	22	20	20	5
Orientation	Coronal	Axial	Coronal	Axial oblique	Coronal
AT (sec)	17	24	23	24	24
Phase*frequency steps	192*256	160*320	192*256	160*256	256*384
Fat suppression	No	Yes	No	No	Yes
ETL	192	15	n/a	n/a	n/a
BW (kHz)	62.5	31.25	62.5	62.5	62.5
Breath hold	Yes	Yes	Yes	Yes	Yes

SSFSE, single shot fast spin echo; FRFSE, fast recovery fast spin echo; TR, time to repetition; TE, time to echo; FA, flip angle; NEX, number of excitations; ST, slice thickness; FOV, field of view; AT, acquisition time; ETL, echo train length; BW, breath hold.

Future Research

- Comparative studies of MRCP and EUS to determine the most cost-effective test for diagnosis of bile duct stricture.
- Further evaluation of quantitative cholescintigraphy in the diagnosis of biliary dyskinesia.
- Prospective evaluation of the utility of cholecystokinin stimulated cholescintigraphy in patients undergoing percutaneous cholecystostomy.

References

1. Trowbridge RL, Rutkowski NK, Shojania KG. JAMA 2003;289:80–86.
2. Singer AJ, McCracken G, Henry MC, et al. Ann Emerg Med 1996;28:267–272.
3. Bree RL, Ralls PW, Balfe DM, et al. Radiology 2000;215:153–157.

 4. Laing FC. In: Rumak CM, Wilson SR, Charboneau JW, eds. Diagnostic Ultrasonography, 2nd ed. St. Louis: Mosby-Year Book, 1998:175–223.
 5. Shea JA, Berlin JA, Escarce JJ, et al. Arch Intern Med 1994;154:2573–2581.
 6. Laing FC, Federle MP, Jeffery RB, et al. Radiology 1981;140:449–455.
 7. Imhoff M, Raunest J, Ohmann C, et al. World J Surg 1992;16:1160–1165.
 8. Ralls PW, Collette PM, Lapin SA, et al. Radiology 1985;155:767–771.
 9. Adam A, Roddie ME. Baillieres Clin Gastroenterol 1991;5:787–816.
10. Weissmann HS, Badia J, Sugarman LA, et al. Radiology 1981;138:167–175.
11. Ziessman HA. Semin Nucl Med 2003;4:279–296.
12. Worthen NJ, Usler JM, Funamura JL. AJR 1981;137:973–978.
13. Shuman WP, Mack LA, Rudd TG, et al. AJR 1982;139:61–64.
14. Alobaidi M, Gupta R, Jafri SZ, et al. Emerg Radiol 2004;10:256–258.
15. Kalimi R, Gecelter GR, Capliin D, et al. J Am Coll Surg 2001;193:609–613.
16. Lorberhoym M, Simon J, Horne T. J Nucl Med Technol 1999;27:294–297.
17. Paulson EK. Semin Ultrasonography CT MR 2000;21:56–63.
18. Bennett GL, Rusinek H, Lisi V, et al. AJR 2002;178:275–281.
19. Fidler J, Paulson EK, Layfield L. AJR 1996;166:1085–1088.
20. Bennett GL, Balthazar EJ. Radiol Clin North Am 2003;41:1203–1216.
21. Hanbidge AE, Buckler PM, O'Malley ME, et al. Radiographics 2004;24: 1117–1135.
22. Weissleder R, Stark DD, Compton CC, et al. Magn Reson Imaging 1988;6: 345–348.
23. Koenig T, Tamm EP, Kawashima A. Clin Radiol 2004;59:455–458.
24. Adusumilli S, Siegelman ES. Magn Reson Imaging Clin North Am 2002;10: 165–184.
25. Loud PA, Semelka RC, Kettritz U, et al. Magn Reson Imaging 1996;14:349–355.
26. Van Epps K, Regan F. Clin Radiol 1999;54:588–594.
27. Morikawa M, Fukuda T, Aso N, et al. Nippon Rinsho 1998;56:2939–2945.
28. Regan F, Schaefer DC, Smith DP, et al. J Comput Assist Tomogr 1998;22: 638–642.
29. Ito K, Fujita N, Noda Y, et al. Nippon Shokakibyo Gakkai Zasshi 2000;97: 1472–1479.
30. Sood B, Jain M, Khandelwal N, et al. Australas Radiol 2002;46:438–440.
31. Oh KY, Gilfeather M, Kennedy A, et al. Abdom Imaging 2003;28:643–651.
32. Hakansson K, Leander P, Ekberg O, et al. Acta Radiol 2000;41:322–328.
33. Park MS, Yu JS, Kim YH, et al. Radiology 1998;209:781–785.
34. Cornwell EE, Rodriguez A, Mirvis SE, et al. Ann Surg 1989;210:52–55.
35. Owen CC, Bilhartz LE. Semin Gastrointest Dis 2003;14:178–188.
36. Lee MJ, Saini S, Brink JA, et al. AJR 1991;156:1163–1166.
37. Babb RR. J Clin Gastroenterol 1992;15:238–241.
38. Akhan O, Akinci D, Ozmen MN. Eur J Radiol 2002;43:229–236.
39. Lameris JS, van Overhagen H. Baillieres Clin Gastroenterol 1995;9:21–36.
40. Berger H, Forst H, Nattermann U, et al. Rofo 1989;150:694–698.
41. Puc MM, Tran HS, Wry PW, et al. Am Surg 2002;68:65–69.
42. Prevot N, Mariat G, Mahul P, et al. Eur J Nucl Med 1999;26:1317–1325.
43. Mariat G, Mahul P, Prevot N, et al. Intensive Care Med 2000;26:1658–1663.
44. Mirvis SE. AJR 1986;147:1171–1175.
45. Blankenberg F, Wirth R, Jeffery RB, et al. Gastrointest Radiol 1991;196:149–153.
46. Menu Y, Vuillerme MP. Eur Radiol 2002;12:2397–2406.
47. Grossman SJ, Joyce JM. Emerg Med Clin North Am 1991;9:853–874.
48. Marton KI, Doubilet P. Ann Intern Med 1988;109:722–729.
49. Renfrew DL, Witte DL, Berbaum KS, et al. Invest Radiol 1993;28:404–408.
50. Ziessman HA. Radiol Clin North Am 2001;39:997–1006.
51. Khosla R, Singh A, Miedema BW, et al. South Med J 1997;90:1087–1090.
52. Poynter MT, Saba AK, Evans RA, et al. Am Surg 2002;68:382–384.
53. Chen PF, Nimeri A, Pham QH, et al. Surgery 2001;130:578–581.
54. Goncalves RM, Harris JA, Rivera DE. Am Surg 1998;64:493–497.

55. Sorenson MK, Fancher S, Lang NP, et al. Am J Surg 1993;166:672–674.

56. Reed DN Jr, Fernandez M, Hicks RD. Am Surg 1993;59:273–277.

57. Yap L, Wycherley AG, Morphett AD, et al. Gastroenterology 1991;101:786–793.

58. Misra DC Jr, Blossom GB, Fink-Bennett D, et al. Arch Surg 1991;126:957–960.

59. Zech ER, Simmons LB, Kendrick RR, et al. Surg Gynecol Obstet 1991;172:21–24.

60. Kloiber R, Molnar CP, Shaffer EA. AJR 1992;159:509–513.

61. Fink-Bennett D, DeRidder P, Kolozsi WZ, et al. J Nucl Med 1991;32:1695–1699.

62. DeCamp JR, Tabatowski K, Schauwecker DS, et al. Clin Nucl Med 1992;17: 784–786.

63. Mishkind MT, Pruitt RF, Bambini DA, et al. Am Surg 1997;63:769–774.

64. Shaffer EA, McOrmond P, Duggan H. Gastroenterol 1986;79:899–906.

65. Cicala M, Habib FI, Vavassori P, et al. Gut 2002;50:665–668.

66. Oxford JL, Dibos PE, Soudry G. Clin Nucl Med 2000;25:670–675.

67. Thomas PD, Turner JG, Dobbs BE, et al. Gut 2000;46:838–841.

68. Peng NJ, Lai KH, Tsay DG, et al. Nucl Med Commun 1994;15:899–904.

69. Drane WE, Johnson DA. J Nucl Med 1990;9:1462–1468.

70. Fullerton GM, Allan A, Hilditch T, et al. Gut 1988;1397–1401.

71. Pineau BC, Knapple WL, Spicer KM, et al. Am J Gastroenterol 2001;96: 3106–3109.

72. Choudhry U, Ruffolo T, Jamidar P, et al. Gastrointest Endosc 1993;39:492–495.

73. Greene JE, Hogan WJ, Dodds WJ, et al. N Engl J Med 1989;320:82–87.

74. Bilhartz MH, Horton JD. In: Feldman M, ed. Sleisenger and Fordtran's Gastrointestinal and Liver Disease, 6th ed. Philadelphia: WB Saunders, 1998:948–972.

75. Kaplan LM, Isselbacher KJ. In: Fauci AS, Longo DL, Kasper DL, et al., eds. Harrison's Principles of Internal Medicine, 14th ed. New York: McGraw-Hill, 1998:249–255.

76. Hulse PA, Nicholson DA. Br J Hosp Med 1994;52:103–107.

77. Baron RL, Tublin ME, Peterson MS. Radiol Clin North Am 2002;40:1325–1354.

78. Sugiyama M, Atomi Y. Gastrointest Endosc 1997;45:143–146.

79. Brant WE. In: Webb WR, Brant WE, Helms CA, eds. Fundamentals of Body CT, 2nd ed. Philadelphia: WB Saunders, 1998:213–222.

80. Soto JA, Barish MA, Yucel EK, et al. Gastroenterology 1996;110:589–597.

81. Romangnuolo J, Bardou M, Rahme E, et al. Ann Intern Med 2003;139:547–557.

82. Seifert H, Wehrmann T, Hilgers R, et al. Gastrointest Endosc 2004;60:61–67.

83. Napoleon B, Dumortier J, Keriven-Souquet O, et al. Endoscopy 2003;35: 411–415.

84. Yusuf TE, Bhutani MS. J Gastroenterol Hepatol 2004;19:243–250.

85. Ainsworth AP, Rafaelsen SR, Wamberg PA, et al. Scand J Gastroenterol 2004;39: 579–583.

86. Buscarini E, Tansini P, Vallisa D, et al. Gastrointest Endosc 2003;57:510–518.

87. Fickling WE, Wallace MB. J Clin Gastroenterol 2003;36:103–110.

88. Ahmad NA, Shah JN, Kochman ML. Radiol Clin North Am 2002;40:1377–1395.

89. Calvo MM, Bujanda L, Calderon A, et al. Mayo Clin Proc 2002;77:422–428.

90. Varghese JC, Liddell RP, Farrell MA, et al. Clin Radiol 2000;55:25–35.

91. Stott M, Farrands P, Guyer P, et al. J Clin Ultrasonography 1991;19:73–76.

92. Goodman A, Neoptolemos J, Carr-Locke D, et al. Gut 1985;26:125–132.

93. Soto JA, Alvarez O, Munera F, et al. AJR 2000;175:1127–1134.

94. Neitlich JD, Topazian M, Smith RC, et al. Radiology 1997;203:601–603.

95. Frey CF, Burbige EJ, Meinke WB, et al. Am J Surg 1982;144:109–114.

96. Prat F, Amouyal G, Amouyal P, et al. Lancet 1996;347:75–79.

97. Sahel J, Barthet M, Gasmi M. Eur J Gastroenterol Hepatol 2004;16:291–294.

98. Meenan J, Tibble J, Prasad P, et al. Eur J Gastroenterol Hepatol 2004;16:299–303.

99. Fulcher AS, Turner MA. Radiol Clin North Am 2002;40:1363–1376.

100. Soto JA, Barish MA, Alvarez, et al. Radiology 2000;215:737–745.

101. Prasad SR, Sahani D, Saini S. J Clin Gastroenterol 2001;33:362–366.

102. David V, Reinhold C, Hochman M, et al. AJR 1998;170:1055–1059.

103. Zidi SH, Prat F, Le Guen O, et al. Gut 1999;44:118–122.
104. Chak A, Hawes RH, Cooper GS, et al. Gastrointest Endosc 1999;49:599–597.
105. Liu CL, Lo CM, Chan CK, et al. Gastrointest Endosc 2000;51:28–32.
106. Dill JE. Endoscopy 1997;29:646–648.
107. Frossard J, Sosa-Valencia L, Amouyal G, et al. Am J Med 2000;109:196–200.
108. Norton SA, Alderson D. Br J Surg 2000;87:1650–1655.
109. Cotton PB. Am J Surg 1993;165:474–478.
110. Ainsworth AP, Rafaelsen SR, Wamberg PA, et al. Endoscopy 2003;35:1029–1032.
111. Sahai AV, Devonshire D, Yeoh KG, et al. Am J Gasterenterol 2001;96:2074–2080.
112. Arguedas MR, Dupont AW, Wilcox CM. Am J Gastroenterol 2001;96:2892–2899.
113. Nathan T, Kjeldsen J, Schaffalitzky De Muckadell OB. Endoscopy 2004;36:527–534.
114. Menenez N, Marson L, DeBeaux A, et al. Br J Surg 2000;87:1176–1181.
115. Liu T, Consorti E, Kawashima A, et al. Ann Surg 2001;234:33–40.
116. Barkun AN, Barkun JS, Fried GM, et al. Ann Surg 1994;220:32–39.
117. Abboud PA, Malet PF, Berlin JA, et al. Gastrointest Endosc 1996;44:450–459.
118. Kaltenthaler E, Vergel YB, Chilcott J, et al. Health Technol Assess 2004;8:1–89.
119. Kohut M, Nowak A, Nowakowska-Dulawa E, et al. World J Gastroenterol 2003;9:612–614.
120. Cohen S, Bacon BR, Berlin JA, et al. Gastrointest Endosc 2002;56:808–809.
121. Canto MIF, Chak A, Stellato T, et al. Gastrointest Endosc 1998;47:439–448.
122. De Ledingen V, Lecesne R, Raymond JM, et al. Gastrointest Endosc 1999;49:26–31.
123. Scheiman JM, Carlos RC, Barnett JL, et al. Am J Gastroenterol 2001;96:2900–2904.
124. Yoon JH, Gores GJ. Curr Treat Options Gastroenterol 2003;6:105–112.
125. Rubens DJ. Radiol Clin North Am 2004;42:257–278.
126. Khan SA, Davidson BR, Goldin R, et al. Gut 2002;51:1–9.
127. Mortele KJ, Ji H, Ros PR. Gastrointest Endosc 2002;56:206–212.
128. Talamonti MS, Denham W. Radiol Clin North Am 2002;40:1397–1410.
129. Gulliver DJ, Baker ME, Cheng CA, et al. AJR 1992;159:503–507.
130. Rosch T, Meining A, Fruhmorgen S, et al. Gastrointest Endosc 2002;55:870–876.
131. Schwartz LH, Coakley FV, Sun Y, et al. AJR 1998;170:1491–1495.
132. Saisho H, Yamaguchi T. Pancreas 2004;28:273–278.
133. Freeman ML, Sielaff TD. Rev Gastroenterol Disord 2003;3:187–201.
134. Flamm CR, Mark DH, Aronson N. Gastrointest Endosc 2002;56:218–225.
135. Skordilis P, Mouzas IA, Dimoulios PD, et al. BMC Surg 2002;25:1.
136. Hawes RH. Gastrointest Endosc 2002;56:201–205.
137. Fulcher AS, Turner MA, Franklin KJ, et al. Radiology 2000;215:71–80.
138. Varghese JC, Farrell MA, Courtney G, et al. Clin Radiol 1999;54:513–520.
139. Zhong L, Yao QY, Li L, Xu JR. World J Gastroenterol 2003;9:2824–2827.
140. Lopera JE, Soto JA, Munera F. Radiology 2001;220:90–96.
141. Fulcher AS, Turner MA. AJR 1997;169:1501–1505.
142. Mehta SN, Reinhold C, Barkun AN. Gastrointest Endosc Clin North Am 1997;7:247–270.
143. Adamek HE, Albert J, Breer H, et al. Lancet 2000;356:190–193.
144. Awaya H, Ito K, Honjo K, et al. Clin Imaging 1998;22:180–187.
145. Lacomis JM, Baron RL, Oliver JH, et al. Radiology 1997;203:98–104.
146. Kim MJ, Mitchell DG, Ito K, et al. Radiology 2000;214:173–181.
147. Soto JA, Alvarez O, Lopera JE, et al. Radiographics 2000;20:353–366.
148. Guthrie JA, Ward J, Robinson PJ. Radiology 1996;201:347–351.
149. Lee MG, Park KB, Shin YM, et al. World J Surg 2003;27:278–283.
150. Zidi SH, Prat F, Le Guen O, et al. Gut 2000;46:103–106.
151. Yeh TS, Jan YY, Tseng JH, et al. Am J Gastroenterol 2000;95:432–440.
152. Manfredi R, Barbaro B, Masselli G, et al. Semin Liver Dis 2004;24:155–164.
153. Textor HJ, Flacke S, Pauleit D, et al. Endoscopy 2002;34:984–990.

154. Talwalkar JA, Angulo P, Johnson CD, et al. Hepatology 2004;40:39–45.
155. Cannon ME, Carpenter SL, Elta GH, et al. Gastrointest Endosc 1999;50:27–33.
156. Erickson RA, Garza AA. Am J Gastroenterol 2000;95:2248–2254.
157. Erickson RA, Garza AA. Gastrointest Endosc 2001;53:475–484.
158. Lee JH, Salem R, Aslanian H, et al. Am J Gastroenterol 2004;99:1069–1073.
159. Muller MF, Myenberger C, Bertschinger P, et al. Radiology 1994;190:745–751.
160. Nakaizumi A, Uehara H, Iishi H, et al. Dig Dis Sci 1995;40:696–700.
161. Palazzo L, Roseau G, Gayet B, et al. Endoscopy 1993;25:143–150.
162. Eloubeidi MA, Chen VK, Jhala NC, et al. Clin Gastroenterol Hepatol 2004;2: 209–213.
163. Fritscher-Ravens A, Broering DC, Knoefel WT, et al. Am J Gasteroenterol 2004; 99:45–51.
164. Dewitt J, Ghorai S, Kahi C, et al. Gastrointest Endosc 2003;58:542–548.
165. Binmoeller KF, Thul R, Rathod V, et al. Gastrointest Endosc 1998;47:123–129.
166. Faigel DO, Ginsberg GG, Bentz JS, et al. J Clin Oncol 1997;15:1439–1443.
167. Giovannini M, Seitz JF, Monges G, et al. Endoscopy 1995;27:171–177.
168. Chang KJ, Nguyen P, Erickson RA, et al. Gastrointest Endosc 1997;45:387–393.
169. Gress FG, Hawes RH, Savides TJ, et al. Gastrointest Endosc 1997;45:243–250.
170. Suits J, Frazze R, Erickson RA, et al. Arch Surg 1999;134:639–642.
171. Wiersema MJ, Vilmann P, Giovannini M, et al. Gastroenterol 1997;112: 1087–1095.
172. Bismuth H, Corlette MB. Surg Gynecol Obstet 1975;140:170–178.
173. Nordback IH, Coleman J, Venbrux AC, et al. Surgery 1994;115:597–603.
174. Hintze RE, Abou-Rebyeh H, Adler A, et al. Gastrointest Endosc 2001;53:40–46.
175. Chang WH, Kortan P, Harber GB. Gastrointest Endosc 1998;47:354–362.
176. De Palma GD, Galloro G, Siciliano S, et al. Gastrointest Endosc 2001; 53:547–553.
177. Nomura T, Shirai Y, Hatakeyama K. Dig Dis Sci 1999;44:542–546.
178. Freeman ML, Nelson DB, Sherman S, et al. N Engl J Med 1996;335:909–918.
179. Deviere J, Motte S, Dumonceau JM, et al. Endoscopy 1990;22:72–75.
180. Hochwald SN, Burke EC, Jarnagin WR, et al. Arch Surg 1999;134:261–266.
181. Ducreux M, Liguory C, Lefebvre JF, et al. Dig Dis Sci 1992;37:778–783.
182. Lammer J, Hausegger KA, Fluckiger F, et al. Radiology 1996;201:167–172.
183. England RE, Martin DF. Cardiovasc Intervent Radiol 1996;19:381–387.
184. Zeman RK, Burell MI, Cahow CE, et al. Am J Surg 1981;141:446–451.
185. Ralls PW, Colletti PM, Halls JM, et al. Radiology 1982;144: 369–371.
186. Freitas JE, Mirkes SH, Fink-Bennett DM, et al. Clin Nucl Med 1982;8:363–367.
187. Samuels BI, Freitas JE, Bree RL, et al. Radiology 1983;147:2017–2020.
188. Chatziioannou, Moore WH, Ford PV, et al. Surgery 2000;127:6–9.
189. Weissmann HS, Berkowitz D, Fox MS, et al. Radiology 1983;146:177–180.
190. Shuman WP, Rogers JV, Rudd TG, et al. AJR 1984;143:531–534.
191. Ramanna L, Brachman MB, Tanascescu DE, et al. Am J Gastroenterol 1984; 79:650–653.
192. Swayne LC. Radiology 1986;160:33–38.
193. Flancbaum L, Choban PS. Intensive Care Med 1995;21:120–124.
194. Kalliafas S, Ziegler DW, Flancbaum L, et al. Am Surg 1998;64:471–475.
195. Palazzo L, Girollet PP, Salmeron M, et al. Gastrointest Endosc 1995;42:225–231.
196. Kohut M, Nowakowska-Dulawa E, Marek T, et al. Endoscopy 2002;34:299–303.
197. Shim CS, Joo JH, Park CW, et al. Endoscopy 1995;27:428–432.
198. Amouyal P, Amouyal G, Levy P, et al. Gastroenterology 1994;106:1062–1067.

28

Hepatic Disorders: Colorectal Cancer Metastases, Cirrhosis, and Hepatocellular Carcinoma

Brian C. Lucey, Jose Varghese, and Jorge A. Soto

Issues

I. How accurate is imaging in patients with suspected hepatic metastatic disease?
   A. Ultrasonography
   B. Computed tomography
   C. Magnetic resonance imaging
   D. Whole-body positron emission tomography
II. What is the accuracy of imaging in patients with cirrhosis for the detection of hepatocellular carcinoma?
   A. Ultrasonography
   B. Computed tomography
   C. Magnetic resonance Imaging
   D. Whole-body positron emission tomography
III. What is the cost-effectiveness of imaging in patients with suspected hepatocellular carcinoma?

Key Points

- State-of-the-art magnetic resonance imaging (MRI) may be superior to state-of-the-art multidetector computed tomography (CT) for detection of liver metastases from colorectal cancer (insufficient and limited evidence).
- Fluorodeoxyglucose positron emission tomography (FDG-PET) is the most sensitive noninvasive test for detecting liver metastases (limited to moderate evidence).
- Periodic screening with imaging tests of patients with cirrhosis for early detection of hepatocellular carcinoma is beneficial (limited evidence).
- Magnetic resonance imaging may be superior to CT for detecting hepatocellular carcinoma (limited evidence).

Methodology

We performed a search of the Medline/PubMed electronic database (National Library of Medicine, Bethesda, Maryland) using the following keywords: (1) *hepatic metastases*, (2) *colorectal cancer*, (3) *cirrhosis*, (4) *hepatocellular carcinoma*, (5) *CT, computed tomography*, (6) *MR, magnetic resonance*, (7) *US, ultrasonography*, and (8) *PET* or *PET/CT*. No time limits were applied for the searches, which were repeated several times up to September 23, 2004. Limits included English language, abstracts, and human subjects. A search of the National Guideline Clearinghouse at www.guideline.gov was also performed using the following keywords: *hepatic metastases, cirrhosis, hepatocellular carcinoma,* and *imaging.*

Definition and Pathophysiology

Liver Metastases

Hematogenous spread of tumor cells to the liver is a common problem in clinical practice. Although several explanations have been offered, this is likely the result of the dual blood supply through the hepatic artery and portal vein and the relatively common occurrence of primary malignancies of the gastrointestinal tract (such as colon, stomach, and pancreas), for which the liver serves as the first end-capillary bed and can therefore easily trap tumor cells or emboli that have escaped to the bloodstream. As metastases grow and reach a certain size threshold, they become detectable with imaging methods. Other tests that are commonly used to monitor patients with gastrointestinal malignancies and to identify patients who require further evaluation include measurement of serum carcinoembryonic antigen (CEA) and liver function tests. Unfortunately, the sensitivity of CEA assessments is low (50% to 60%) (1,2) and its use in clinical practice is therefore limited. The decision regarding whether or not to perform an imaging test in a patient with possible liver metastases should also take into account the pretest probability of finding disease. An imaging test has the greatest impact when the pretest probability is intermediate (20% to 50%) (3). This means that patients with very low or very high likelihood of harboring metastases may not need any specific imaging test of the liver, if the indication is that of detecting possible lesions.

Cirrhosis and Hepatocellular Carcinoma

Cirrhosis is characterized by irreversible scarring of the liver that can lead to liver failure and death. Causes include excessive alcohol use, chronic viral hepatitis, including chronic hepatitis B (HBV) and hepatitis C (HCV), autoimmune disease, hemochromatosis, and drugs, among many others. These entities may result in inflammation of the liver, which may lead to fibrosis. Fibrosis results in the loss of liver parenchyma and impairs liver function. Cirrhosis is characterized by the formation of nodules within the liver. These nodules represent attempts by the liver to regenerate. These nodules may be large or small, resulting in macronodular or micronodular cirrhosis. These nodules may in turn undergo dysplasia and become dysplastic nodules that in turn may develop into hepatocellular carcinoma (HCC).

The pathophysiology of HCC is related to underlying liver dysfunction, and cirrhosis is a predisposing condition. In adults, infectious and autoimmune hepatitis, alcoholic cirrhosis, and hemochromatosis are strongly associated with HCC. Although children are less likely to have chronic liver disease, congenital liver disorders increase the chance of developing HCC. Hepatitis B carries a 100-fold increase in the risk for developing HCC. Hepatitis B is a DNA virus whose mechanism for tumor genesis involves integrating into the hosts DNA. The mechanism of tumor genesis with hepatitis C is less well defined but is thought most likely to result from chronic inflammation. Although HCC is frequently indolent, it may undergo hemorrhage or necrosis. Vascular invasion, particularly of the portal veins, may occur. Invasion into the biliary system is less common. Occasionally, HCC may result in rupture and hemoperitoneum.

The annual risk of developing HCC among persons with cirrhosis is between 1% and 6%. Most patients with HCC die within 1 year after diagnosis. Survival is dependent on tumor size at the time of diagnosis and on associated diseases at the time of diagnosis. Patients with cirrhosis have a shorter survival. Surgical cure is possible in less than 5% of patients.

Despite the overall dismal prognosis of HCC, when diagnosed early it is a potentially curable cancer. Treatment is most likely to be successful when the number of foci of HCC in the cirrhotic liver and the size of the lesions is small. This implies that early detection is essential. Traditionally, either liver transplant or surgical resection has been the only treatment modality available to provide a cure for HCC. The results of surgery for HCC are poor and many patients with HCC and cirrhosis are not surgical candidates. More recently, with the advent of percutaneous treatment options including thermal therapy and alcohol injection, there is renewed interest in treating HCC in cirrhotic patients. These treatments show promise with success rates very much dependent on tumor size and number. With radiofrequency ablation (RFA), tumors less than 3 cm in size have an excellent chance of cure and tumors between 3 and 5 cm are often treated successfully. But RFA is less successful in attempting cure in tumors greater than 5 cm. The success rates are higher with smaller lesions and in patients with few lesions.

As a result of the close association between cirrhosis and HCC and the relative success of early treatment of HCC, enormous efforts are made to identify the early development of HCC in the cirrhosis population. Hematologic tests for HCC are limited to α-fetoprotein (AFP), a protein that may be elevated in patients with HCC. This is of limited value in the detection of HCC, with reported sensitivity for detection of HCC varying between 48% and 65% (4,5). This leaves imaging as the test of choice for detecting the early development of HCC in patients with cirrhosis. As with the detection of hepatic metastatic disease, there are multiple imaging modalities available to detect HCC in the cirrhotic liver. These include sonography, CT, MRI, and PET. There is extensive literature available detailing the sensitivity and specificity of these imaging modalities for detecting HCC in cirrhotic patients. In evaluating these studies, direct comparison is often difficult given the wide differences in the study designs.

Epidemiology

Liver Metastases

In most cases, a liver metastasis is a poor prognostic sign and usually indicates incurable disease. One exception may be that of metastases from colorectal carcinoma. Colorectal cancer is the third most common cancer found in men and women in the United States. The American Cancer Society estimates that there were about 106,370 new cases of colon cancer and 40,570 new cases of rectal cancer in 2004 in the United States. Combined, they will cause about 56,730 deaths. The death rate from colorectal cancer has been going down for the past 15 years. One reason is that there are fewer cases. Also, they are being found earlier, and treatments have improved. The liver is a common site of metastatic spread of colorectal cancer, and therefore early detection of liver metastases is critical for guiding decisions regarding therapy.

Liver metastases develop in nearly 40% of patients who undergo "curative" resection for colorectal cancer. Several randomized studies have shown that aggressive therapy with wide resections of liver metastases from colorectal carcinoma leads to improved survival when compared to control groups receiving other forms of standard therapy. Not uncommonly, the liver is the only site of distant spread of the tumor in patients with colorectal carcinoma. Survival rates of up to 20% to 40% have been reported after wide resections of liver metastases from colorectal carcinoma (6–8). As imaging-guided interstitial therapies of liver tumors (including metastases), such as radiofrequency ablation, cryoablation, microwave ablation, and laser photocoagulation, increase in popularity, the need for accurate imaging of the liver will also increase. In a decision analysis study, Gazelle et al. (9) concluded that an aggressive approach with resection of six or sometimes more metastases from colorectal cancer has a positive impact in patient outcome, as measured by the dollar/quality-adjusted life year (QALY) index. Thus, in the patient with newly diagnosed colorectal carcinoma, a thorough evaluation of the liver to rule out metastases is mandatory prior to bowel resection with curative intent.

Cirrhosis

Cirrhosis is the seventh leading cause of disease-related death in the United States. It is twice as common in men as in women. The disease kills approximately 25,000 people a year in the U.S. and is the third most common cause of death in adults between the ages of 45 and 65.

Hepatocellular carcinoma is relatively uncommon in the U.S. The reported prevalence is four cases per 100,000 population or 2% of all malignancies. Approximately 5000 to 10,000 cases per year are seen. Worldwide, HCC is the fourth most common cancer. It is more common in Asia and Africa than in the U.S. The highest incidence of HCC is in Japan, and other high-incidence regions include sub-Saharan Africa. The incidence of HCC continues to rapidly increase in the U.S. These findings are consistent with a true increase in HCC and could be explained by consequences of HCV acquired earlier in life during the 1960s and 1970s. In the U.S., chronic hepatitis B and C account for about 30% to 40% of HCC.

Goals of Imaging

In patients with colorectal cancer imaging studies are acquired periodically in order to detect development of recurrent disease and to assess tumor burden and response to therapy. In the cirrhotic patient, the main goal of imaging is detection of developing complications, the most important of which is HCC. Many imaging modalities currently available have been used for detecting liver metastases, with variable success. Regardless of the technique used, the ability to detect a focal space-occupying lesion in the liver depends on the size of the tumor, the spatial and contrast resolution of the imaging method, the difference in contrast and perfusion between the tumor and background liver parenchyma, and the adequacy of the method used for displaying the images after acquired (10). All these factors affect the performance parameters of the various imaging techniques. A test is useful if sensitivity remains high at an acceptable specificity level. In a meta-analysis that studied the detection rate of liver metastases from gastrointestinal malignancies with multiple modalities, Kinkel et al. (3) suggest that, in order to be useful in clinical practice, the minimum acceptable specificity of imaging methods in this context should be 85%. Lower specificities would lead to excessive and unnecessary interventions such as biopsies, excessive complementary imaging tests, and follow-up examinations. When assessing cost-effectiveness of the imaging methods, other factors need to be considered: availability, cost, risks (such as radiation and use of toxic contrast agents), and potential benefit of tumor detection (i.e., likelihood of achieving long-term remission or cure with appropriate therapy).

Overall Cost to Society

On an individual level, cirrhosis results in impaired quality of life and indirect costs involving decreased productivity and lost days from work. The Centers for Disease Control and Prevention conservatively estimates U.S. expenditures in excess of $600 million annually on patients with HCC. In 2002, in the U.S., a total of 15,654 patients were discharged from hospitals with the diagnosis of HCC and 2522 patients died in the hospital with HCC. The mean length of hospital stay was 7.2 days with a mean cost of $32,193. This resulted in a total cost of $501,998,078.

I. How Accurate Is Imaging in Patients with Suspected Hepatic Metastatic Disease?

Summary of Evidence: Computed tomography (CT) and magnetic resonance imaging (MRI) are the most widely used techniques for evaluating the liver in the initial staging and follow-up of cancer patients. For detecting liver metastases, carefully performed CT and MRI studies with state-of-the-art equipment and interpretation by experienced radiologists afford similarly good results. Some studies showed a slight advantage for MRI (11,12) (moderate evidence). Others, including a multiinstitutional study of 365 patients (13) (moderate evidence), have not. Computed tomography is usually preferred because it is more widely available and because it is a well-established technique for surveying the extrahepatic abdominal organs and tissues (such as the peritoneum and lymph nodes). However, MRI has an advantage in the characterization of focal lesions. Thus, MRI is commonly used as a problem-solving tool or for initial staging of a tumor. It is also preferred for patients who cannot receive intravenous iodinated contrast material. Finally, concerns about the risk of radiation from repeated exposure to CT examinations make MRI a valuable alternative for children or young adults with malignancies. As mentioned previously, a comparison of the performance of CT vs. MRI for this and other indications needs to be reassessed periodically, considering the rapid evolution of both technologies and the increase in therapeutic options available.

Kinkel et al. (3) reviewed a total of 111 studies that included over 3000 patients. At a specificity of at least 85%, the weighted sensitivities were ultrasonography (US) 55%, CT 72%, MRI 76%, and positron emission tomography (PET) 90% (moderate evidence). These data, however, need to be validated in prospective trials before broad conclusions can be drawn. Intraoperative ultrasonography (IOUS) has higher sensitivity than transabdominal ultrasonography, CT, and MRI (14,15). The role of FDG-PET and PET-CT will continue to expand, but cost constraints will limit their use to patients in whom the possible impact is greatest.

Supporting Evidence: The most widely used imaging techniques today include US, CT, MRI, and, more recently, PET. There is extensive literature available regarding the relative merits and limitations of each of these modalities for detecting metastases of primary tumors from various organs. When analyzing the multiple studies published on this topic, several limitations are evident: insufficient definition of inclusion and exclusion criteria, incomplete reporting of methods used, and lack of a uniform standard of reference. Although the best standard of reference available is findings at laparotomy with bimanual palpation or intraoperative ultrasonography, this was used as the gold standard in only a minority of studies (14,16,17). As indicated by van Erkel et al. (18), use of a suboptimal standard of reference results in underreporting of lesions and overestimation of detection rate. Another confounding factor is the varying method for reporting sensitivity numbers: per patient (detection of at least one lesion per patient) and per lesion (detection of all lesions per patient). Thus, it is important to continually scrutinize the results of all available current studies as evolving and improving technology can make results of prior studies redundant. Following is a review of the available data regarding the benefits and limitations of the various imaging techniques commonly used for evaluating the liver in patients with colorectal cancer and other gastrointestinal primary malignancies.

A. Ultrasonography

Ultrasonography has the advantage of being widely available throughout the world, inexpensive, and essentially risk-free. The reported sensitivity of US for detecting liver metastases varies between 60% and 90% (3).

Unfortunately, many of the published studies were performed in the 1980s (19,20) (limited evidence) and were largely limited to reporting sensitivity results on a per patient basis. More recently, the advent of US contrast agents has led several investigators to evaluate the use of US with current equipment. For detecting liver metastases, the sensitivity and specificity of US improve substantially with the addition of microbubble contrast agents. Microbubbles are essentially blood pool agents that augment the Doppler and harmonic US signal. In addition, some of these agents have a hepatosplenic specific late phase, which enables visualization of tumor foci in the liver that were otherwise undetectable (21). In a multicenter study, Albrecht et al. (22) found that the addition of a microbubble contrast agent increased the per patient sensitivity of US from 94% to 98% (not significant), while the per lesion sensitivity increased from 71% to 87% (highly significant, $p < .05$).

Intraoperative ultrasonography has higher sensitivity than transabdominal US, CT, and MRI (14,15). Conlon et al. (14) compared MRI with IOUS in 80 patients with colorectal cancer metastases who underwent hepatic resection and found that IOUS findings added important information in 37 patients and changed the surgical approach in 14 patients. They concluded that IOUS provides valuable information prior to hepatic resection of colorectal cancer metastases.

B. Computed Tomography

Multiple factors pertaining to technique need to be considered when planning CT scans of patients with suspected metastatic disease and when examining reports that deal with this topic. The typical colorectal cancer metastasis is hypoattenuating and hypovascular relative to liver parenchyma. Thus, detectability is maximized by administering intravenous contrast material and by acquiring the CT images during the time of peak enhancement of the liver parenchyma. This typically occurs during the portal venous dominant phase, which occurs approximately 60 to 80 seconds after the initiation of contrast injection. Ideally, hepatic parenchyma attenuation should increase by at least 50 Hounsfield units after the administration of intravenous contrast material. The addition of images acquired prior to the administration of intravenous contrast material or in the arterial-dominant or delayed phases of contrast enhancement are not routinely necessary when the indication for the scan is suspected hypovascular metastases. These are necessary when evaluating the cirrhotic liver, when attempting to characterize a focal lesion, or when the primary tumor is one that is known to be associated with hypervascular metastases, such as neuroendocrine and carcinoid tumors, thyroid cancer, melanoma, breast cancer, or renal cell carcinoma (Fig. 28.1).

Although specific protocols vary among institutions, most use a total load of 37 to 50g of iodine (23). Although as little as 30g have been used, detection of hypovascular focal lesions may be limited with this approach (24). In the patient with colorectal cancer who is being scanned to decide among the several therapeutic options available, the risk of overlooking a potentially resectable small liver metastasis needs to be outweighed vs. the benefit of limiting the amount of contrast material injected.

In a carefully performed study, Valls et al. (25) used contrast-enhanced helical CT to detect liver metastases in 157 patients with colorectal

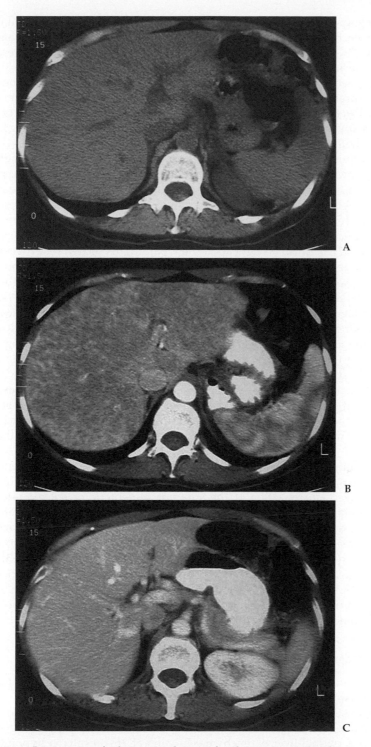

Figure 28.1. Importance of adequate technique for detecting computed tomography (CT) of metastatic disease to the liver. Noncontrast (A), arterial phase (B), and
portal venous phase (C) CT images of a 57–year-old patient with breast cancer and
abnormal results of liver function tests. There are multiple foci of hypervascular
metastatic deposits seen exclusively in the arterial phase image (B). The appearance
of the liver is near normal on the noncontrast (A) and portal venous phase (C)
images.

carcinoma. Using intraoperative palpation and US as the standard of reference, helical CT correctly depicted 247 (85.2%) of 290 metastases and had a 96.1% positive predictive value (moderate evidence). Surgical resection of the liver metastases was attempted in 112 patients and the authors achieved a 4-year survival rate of 58.6%. In their study, all false-negative interpretations occurred in lesions less than 1.5 cm in diameter. Other studies that also used surgical findings and IOUS as the standard of reference found similar high sensitivity and specificity (16), for detecting lesions as small as 4 mm in diameter.

Although with the multirow detector helical CT (MDCT) scanners that are now available it is possible to acquire CT images in multiple phases after administration of intravenous contrast material, it has not been convincingly demonstrated that detection of hypovascular metastases such as those from colorectal carcinoma is improved significantly by scanning in any phase other than the peak portal venous phase (16,26,27). The advent of MDCT has also brought about new paradigms related to CT technique. Although scanning with slice thickness of less than 1 mm and often with isotropic voxels is tempting, there is debate as to what is the limit in thickness that achieves the performance that is adequate for demonstrating small metastatic lesions in clinical practice. Some studies have shown that scanning with a slice thickness of less than 5 mm does not result in a significant improvement in sensitivity for detecting small lesions (28). Other investigators have obtained better results using thinner collimation (29). However, detection of even small lesions in the patient with cancer is important, since approximately 12% of lesions less than 1 cm in diameter will prove to be metastatic in nature (30). The possible added benefit of images acquired with isotropic voxels remains to be determined and will undoubtedly be the focus of multiple studies in the near future.

Another CT technique that continues to be used at some institutions is CT during arterial portography (CTAP). This is an invasive technique that requires catheterization of the superior mesenteric or splenic artery for direct injection of contrast into the territory drained by the portal vein. This direct delivery of contrast into the porto-mesenteric circulation achieves the greatest degree of hepatic parenchymal enhancement and maximizes lesion detection with CT, with a sensitivity that exceeds 90% (17,31). The technique, however, is invasive and has a false-positive rate as high as 25% (17,31). This has led to decreased enthusiasm for this technique and its replacement with noninvasive CT and MRI methods using state-of-the-art equipment (32,33).

C. Magnetic Resonance Imaging

Magnetic resonance imaging of the liver for detecting metastases requires the acquisition of multiple sequences and administration of intravenous contrast material. Although the appearance of metastatic lesions on MRI is variable, the T1 and T2 relaxation times of metastases are prolonged relative to normal liver parenchyma. In general, this results in hypointensity on T1-weighted sequences and hyperintensity on T2-weighted images (Fig. 28.2). T2-weighted MRI is also useful for characterizing focal lesions and differentiating nonsolid benign lesions such as cysts and hemangiomas

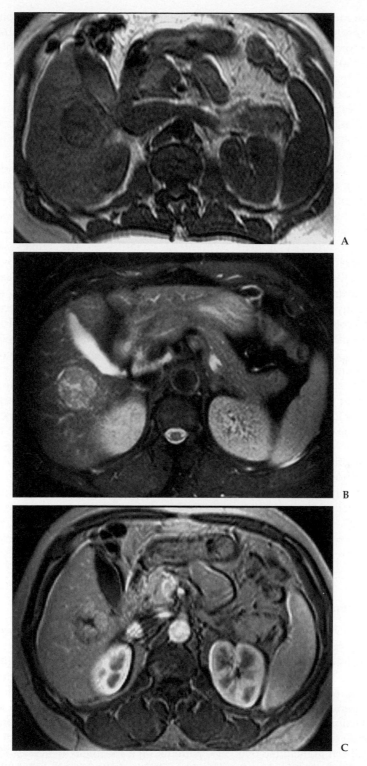

Figure 28.2. Typical appearance of hepatic metastasis on magnetic resonance imaging (MRI). T1-weighted (A), T2-weighted (B), and late arterial phase (C) MRI acquired in a patient with known colon cancer demonstrate a large metastatic deposit in the right hepatic lobe. The lesion is hypointense (relative to liver parenchyma) on the T1-weighted image, slightly hyperintense on the T2-weighted image, and demonstrates moderate enhancement after administration of gadolinium-DTPA.

from metastases. In multiecho T2-weighted scans, metastases become less intense when the echo time (TE) is increased from <120 msec to 160 msec or more. Conversely, cysts and hemangiomas typically remain hyperintense as the TE increases. For lesions with equivocal behavior, MRI can be used to measure the T2 value; the T2 of malignant tumors is approximately 90 msec, while that of hemangiomas and cysts exceeds 130 msec (34,35). However, metastases with liquefactive necrosis or cystic neoplasms may remain hyperintense on heavily T2-weighted images. Metastases can have a perilesional halo of high signal, indicating viable tumor, or demonstrate a doughnut or target appearance (36,37).

For detection of liver metastases, a three-phase technique after administration of gadolinium is recommended; these phases are the arterial-dominant phase, the portal venous phase, and the hepatic venous or interstitial phase. Similar to CT, the detection of colorectal cancer metastases using MRI is maximized during the portal venous phase. In this phase, the lesions typically appear hypointense relative to the enhanced liver parenchyma and may exhibit variable degrees of enhancement (Fig. 28.2). In addition to lesion detection, this protocol also allows characterization of coexisting nonmetastatic focal lesions. This is important for staging recently detected malignant tumors, and has implications in determining the type of therapy to be offered. The reported sensitivity of MRI using multiple combinations of the sequences available varies between 65% and 95% (3,33,38–41), with a mean of approximately 76% (3) (moderate evidence).

The administration of organ-specific contrast agents increases the lesion-to-liver contrast-to-noise ratio (CNR), thereby improving the conspicuity and detection rate of metastatic lesions. These include hepatobiliary agents such as mangafodipir trisodium (MnDPDP) (40) and gadobenate dimeglumine (Gd-BOPTA), and reticuloendothelial agents such as superparamagnetic iron oxide (SPIO) particles (41). The available data regarding the need for these liver-specific agents is controversial, with some studies showing improved results (17,42) while others do not (3,43,44). In addition to a lack of consensus regarding the benefits associated with their use, these agents are generally considered costly and not widely available. Thus, a broad use of liver-specific contrast material for detecting liver metastases is not recommended at this time.

D. Whole-Body Positron Emission Tomography

Whole body PET performed with fluorine-18-fluorodeoxyglucose (18F-FDG) has also been used successfully for detecting extracolonic spread of colorectal carcinoma, including liver metastases. Although published studies have included small groups of patients, early results are encouraging, with sensitivity and specificity exceeding 80% (45,46). Kinkel et al. (3) performed a meta-analysis study comparing the data available for detection of liver metastases from gastrointestinal tract neoplasms with noninvasive tests: US, CT, MRI, and PET. They reviewed a total of 111 studies that included over 3000 patients. At a specificity of at least 85%, the weighted sensitivities were US 55%, CT 72%, MRI 76%, and PET 90%. The strength of these data is moderate and they need to be validated in randomized trials before broad conclusions can be drawn.

II. What Is the Accuracy of Imaging in Patients with Cirrhosis for the Detection of Hepatocellular Carcinoma?

Summary of Evidence: Screening for HCC in patients with cirrhosis is not easy. No one imaging modality dominates over the others. All imaging modalities have advantages and disadvantages with no one modality offering both high sensitivity and specificity. The results of these individual studies often depend on the date of the study. This is primarily because of the rapid change in technology available in all imaging modalities. A reasonable consensus for screening includes biannual measurement of the AFP level. Annual sonography is the imaging modality most commonly used, as it is cheap, portable, and most widely available. If the AFP value increases and the sonogram does not show evidence of an HCC, either CT or MRI should be performed.

Although MRI at present has marginally higher specificity than CT, the recent improvement in CT technology may change this soon (Fig. 28.3). Published sensitivities for MRI range from 48% to 87% (47–50). The CT sensitivities for these studies range from 47% to 71% without the use of computed tomography hepatic arteriography (CTHA) or CTAP. These reports conclude that MRI is certainly as sensitive and perhaps a little more so than CT. The use of superparamagnetic iron oxide (SPIO) has increased the sensitivity of MRI.

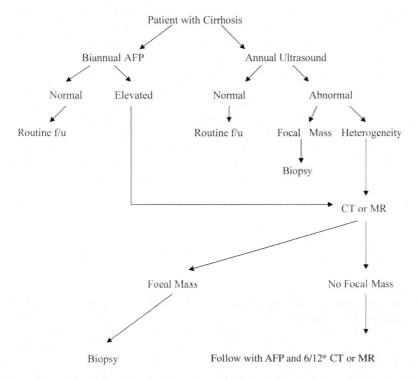

Figure 28.3. Algorithm for imaging to detect HCC in a patient with cirrhosis. AFP, α-fetoprotein; f/u, follow-up. *6/12 means six months.

The sensitivity of sonography for detecting HCC has been reported between 59% and 90% (51–55), with lower sensitivity for smaller lesions (55). Ultrasound may also lead to a high percentage of false-positive studies. Overall, there is little evidence to support the use of PET imaging in the detection of HCC. The value of PET in this patient population lies in detecting distant metastases, and PET may be useful in monitoring the response to treatment.

Supporting Evidence

A. Ultrasonography

The 59% to 90% sensitivity of sonography cited above varies with lesion size, with the sensitivity for detecting lesions 2 cm or less approaching 60%, with larger lesions having higher sensitivity (55). The sensitivity for detecting HCC also depends on patient selection. Screening a population at risk for developing HCC (i.e., chronic hepatitis carriers) is often performed differently from screening a population with documented cirrhosis. As a result, lesions missed by sonography in cirrhotic patients may be picked up by CT or AFP measurement, thus masking the false-negative cases that may be attributable to sonography (52). One major difficulty with sonography in the detection of HCC is the high percentage of false-positive studies. This is particularly difficult in the cirrhotic patient population as the risk of developing HCC is higher and therefore any focal geographic area of heterogeneity is concerning for HCC. This may lead to frequent percutaneous biopsy to obtain a definitive diagnosis with the attendant morbidity and mortality. Despite the difficulties of sonography, given the widespread availability, portability, and safety of the modality, sonography remains the imaging modality of choice for screening for HCC in cirrhotic patients. The time interval between sonograms remains controversial. There is no consensus as to when to perform repeat imaging; however, authors have suggested that annual or biannual interval imaging with sonography is the most effective approach to detecting HCC.

There is great interest in the use of intravenous contrast agents for enhancing the value of sonography to detect and characterize liver lesions. There are many reports describing the value of these agents in patients with HCC (56–59). There is no doubt that these microbubbles demonstrate increased vascularity in HCC when used, increasing the color flow within HCC from 33% to 92% in one study (57); however, there is little published evidence to support the value of these agents in identifying HCC from degenerative nodules in patients with cirrhosis. Increased flow may be detected in other hepatic lesions also and not just in HCC after injection of the microbubbles. One potential use for the microbubbles is in the evaluation of patients following RFA. The results for contrast-enhanced sonography for detecting tumor recurrence post-RFA have been reported to be similar to those for CT (60).

B. Computed Tomography

Computed tomography has benefited even more than sonography from recent advances in technology. With the move from incremental CT to single-detector CT to multidetector CT, the ability to detect HCC in the cirrhotic liver has improved. This difference in technology is the most important consideration when attempting to compare the results of studies performed to evaluate CT in the detection of HCC. This improvement allows for thinner slice collimation and improved image quality. Another technical parameter to consider is the use of dual-phase imaging. The liver has a dual blood supply from both the hepatic artery and portal vein. In normal livers, approximately three quarters of the blood supply comes from the portal system. In contrast, HCC depends more on the hepatic artery for blood supply. Therefore, ideally, imaging to detect HCC should include images obtained in the hepatic arterial phase, usually commencing at 30 seconds after contrast administration. With the advent of multidetector CT, imaging in dual phase became possible and this improved detection of HCC.

When examining the reports available for detecting HCC in cirrhotic patients, it is important to differentiate between identifying patients with HCC and identifying lesions that represent HCC. This fact may change the sensitivity of an imaging modality greatly. The effect of this is clearly demonstrated in a study by Peterson et al. (61) evaluating patients pre–liver transplant for HCC, in which CT had a prospective sensitivity to detect patients with HCC of 59%. This fell to 37% when attempting to detect HCC on a lesion-by-lesion basis.

Reported sensitivity for detecting HCC by CT varies greatly. Most recent reports yield sensitivities between 68% and 88% (5,62). These reports generally refer to the percentage of patients in whom an HCC is found. Figures for detecting individual lesions are much lower. The value of some of these reports is always in some doubt, however, given the previously described rapid change in CT technology today. In an effort to improve detection of HCC using CT, CTAP is occasionally used. This involves placing a catheter into the splenic or superior mesenteric artery and directly injecting contrast. Computed tomography hepatic arteriography (CTHA) has also been used, in which a catheter is placed directly into the hepatic artery. These techniques have yielded high sensitivities when used together. Makita et al. (63) found the sensitivity of CTAP alone to be 85.5%, CTHA alone to be 88.1%, and combined to be 95%. Specificity, however, suffers and the combined specificity reported by that group was only 54%. Similar findings have been reported by others (64,65) with sensitivities ranging from 82% to 97%, although the high number of false-positive studies with these techniques leads most authors to conclude that they have minimal role in the evaluation for HCC in cirrhotic patients, particularly given the relatively invasive nature of the procedures.

C. Magnetic Resonance Imaging

The MRI sequences used in the evaluation of the cirrhotic liver are the same as those used for the detection of liver metastases. The use of intravenous gadolinium is required in all cases. As with CT, the difficulty with MRI lies in differentiating early HCC from dysplastic nodules. As nodules change from regenerative to dysplastic to malignant, the T1 signal characteristics become more hypointense and the T2 signal characteristics become more hyperintense. As one moves along this spectrum, the primary blood supply of the mass changes from predominantly portal to predominantly hepatic arterial. As a result, HCC generally demonstrates early enhancement in the arterial phase following gadolinium injection. In the same manner as CT, MRI technology is advancing rapidly. Some of the difficulties with MRI include respiratory and peristalsis motion artifact. With newer, faster sequences, these are becoming less of a problem. This therefore leaves us to decide which imaging modality is best for detecting HCC in a cirrhotic liver.

There are many reports published using MRI to detect HCC and many of these compare directly with CT. The results of many of the studies performed in the 1990s are extremely variable. Sensitivity in these studies for MRI in detecting HCC lies between 44% and 75% (66–71). Although all these studies compared MRI with CT, the results of some support CT as the imaging modality of choice (66,67), others support MRI as the imaging modality of choice (69,71), and yet others suggest that the imaging modalities have equal capability in detecting HCC (68,70), with one report stating that intraarterial CT is an improvement over both CT and MRI using intravenous contrast (68). The reasons for such discrepancy are multiple, but certainly the lack of consistency in study design contributes to the variability. The results also vary considerably depending on the size of the HCC identified.

The figures published comparing CT to MRI since 2000 make interesting reading. Although there is not yet a clear advantage of MRI over CT, more studies give MRI a slight edge over CT. Published sensitivities for MRI range from 48% to 87% (47–50). Sensitivities for CT in these studies range from 47% to 71% without the use of CTHA or CTAP. These reports conclude that MRI is certainly as sensitive and perhaps a little more so than CT. The use of SPIO has increased the sensitivity of MRI. Its use by Kwak et al. (50) when combined with gadolinium-enhanced imaging increased the sensitivity of MRI from 87% to 95%, which surpassed the sensitivity of CTHA and CTAP combined. Other authors have reported similar advantages of using SPIO (49,72), including increased sensitivity compared to CT imaging.

D. Whole-Body Positron Emission Tomography

Although PET has been around as an imaging modality for many years, it is only recently that the modality has been used with any frequency in the clinical setting. The studies available for detecting HCC using PET are few in number and generally have few patients evaluated. Three studies looking directly at the value of PET imaging in HCC all had 20 or fewer patients (73–75). In these studies, the sensitivity of PET for detecting HCC was low, varying from 20% to 55%. Well-differentiated HCCs are not identified using PET imaging. Moderately differentiated or poorly differentiated HCC may be identified. Tumors greater than 5cm and tumors associated with elevated AFP levels are also more likely to be identified using PET. One advantage to the use of PET imaging in patients with HCC is the ability to detect extrahepatic metastases. This is especially important in the workup of patients with cirrhosis for liver transplant. In a larger study evaluating PET in HCC with 91 patients (76), PET had a clinical impact on the management of 28% of patients. This included not only detecting unsuspected metastases but also monitoring the response to therapy. Several other studies have evaluated PET in detecting HCC in patients with hepatitis C and cirrhosis prior to transplant (77–79). These show poor sensitivity for PET ranging from 0% to 30%.

III. What is the Cost-Effectiveness of Imaging in Patients with Suspected Hepatocellular Carcinoma?

Summary of Evidence: A study concluded that screening all patients with cirrhosis is of limited value given the high cost, and the benefit in terms of patient survival is poor. However, targeted screening in high-risk patients with HCC and imaging may yet be of value.

Supporting Evidence: There are a number of reports on the cost-effectiveness of screening for HCC. The results of some of these studies conclude that there is little value to be gained from screening (80–82). One such report by Bolondi et al. (80) evaluated 324 patients with cirrhosis for HCC using sonography and AFP every 6 months. In all, 1800 sonographic examinations and AFP titrations were obtained at a cost of $219,600 per patient. The cost of diagnosing each of the successfully treated HCC was $24,400. The authors concluded that screening all patients with cirrhosis is of limited value given the high cost, and the benefit in terms of patient survival is poor. Targeted screening may yet be of value according to this group. Two similar studies reach similar conclusions (81,82). Sarasin et al. (81) compared screening patients with cirrhosis for HCC with imaging for HCC only when clinically suspected. The cost for each year of life gained ranged between $48,000 and $284,000 in the screening group. The cost of each year of life gained in the group with predicted cirrhosis-related survival rate above 80% at 5 years ranged between $26,000 and $55,000. This suggests that screening to identify asymptomatic tumors provides a negligible benefit in life expectancy, yet targeted screening may increase life expectancy by 3 to 9 months at a lower cost. A meta-analysis type study by Yuen and Lai (82) concluded that AFP with sonography remains the screening modality of choice given that they are convenient, accessible, and noninvasive. They also concluded that screening for HCC in countries with a low prevalence of HCC was not cost-effective but targeted screening of high-risk patients in countries with a higher incidence of HCC makes screening for HCC more cost-effective.

As with the studies based purely on detection of HCC, there is little consensus on the most cost-effective imaging modality to use to detect HCC. While acknowledging that screening for HCC may not be cost-effective at all, if one is to perform imaging, which modality is most cost-effective is open to debate. In a retrospective study, Gambarin-Gelwan et al. (83) compared AFP with sonography and with CT. They found that sensitivity and specificity of sonography and CT were similar and that sonography was preferable given the lower cost. A similar study by Lin et al. (84) compared AFP and sonography annually, biannually, biannual AFP with annual sonography, and biannual AFP with annual CT. They found that biannual AFP with annual sonography gave the most QALY gain while still maintaining a cost-effectiveness ratio <$50,000 per QALY. In addition, they found the cost-effectiveness ratio of biannual AFP with annual CT to be

$51,750 per QALY. This compares to the $33,083 per QALY for sonography. The authors suggest that CT screening may be becoming cost-effective. This is supported by other work that evaluated the cost-effectiveness of no screening, AFP alone, and imaging with sonography, CT, and MRI all performed in conjunction with AFP levels (85). This study was performed in a patient population with high risk for developing HCC as all patients had cirrhosis secondary to hepatitis C. The results found that compared to no screening, sonography had a cost of $26,689 per QALY; CT had a cost of $25,232 per QALY and MRI had a cost of $118,000 per QALY. These figures would certainly support the value of CT for screening; however, this study did involve the so-called targeted screening described by the previous authors.

Take-Home Tables and Figure

Table 28.1. Performance of various tests for diagnosis of liver metastases from colorectal cancer

Test	Sensitivity (%)	References	Strength of evidence
CT	71–91	10,16,25,27–29,40,86	Moderate
MRI	72	11,12,32,38–40	Moderate
MRI with organ-specific contrast	87–90	17,31,33,38,40–44	Moderate
US	54–77	3,19,20	Moderate
PET and PET/CT	88	41,45,46	Weak to moderate

Table 28.2. Sensitivity of various imaging tests for detecting hepatocellular carcinoma

Imaging modality	Sensitivity (%)
US	59–90
US with intravenous contrast	92
CT	47–88
CTAP	85
CTHA	88
CTAP + CTHA	95
MRI	44–87
MRI + SPIO	95
PET	0–55
AFP	48–65

AFP, α-fetoprotein; CTAP, CT during arterial portography; CTHA, computed tomography hepatic arteriography; SPIO, superparamagnetic iron oxide.

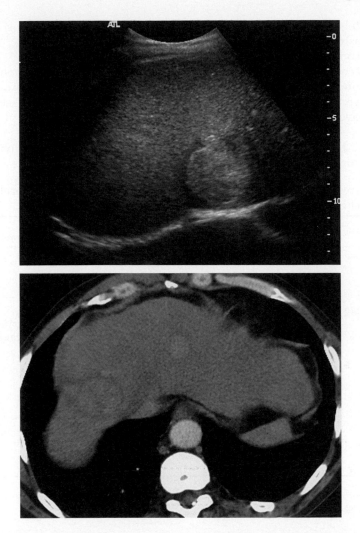

Figure 28.4. A: Sonographic image showing large hyperechoic mass in the liver in a 67–year-old man with chronic hepatitis C. B: CT image showing arterial enhancement of multiple masses, which proved to be hepatocellular carcinoma (HCC) following biopsy.

Imaging Technique Protocols

Abdominal Computed Tomography for Detection of Hepatocellular Carcinoma Using Multirow Detector Computed Tomography

Slice thickness: 2 to 3 mm
Scan parameters: 120–140 kVp; 180–220 mAs
Number of acquisitions: 3
Area of coverage first acquisition: top of diaphragm through the liver
Area of coverage second acquisition: top of diaphragm to inferior pubic ramus
Area of coverage third acquisition: top of diaphragm to inferior pubic ramus

Breath hold: full inspiration or full expiration
Reconstruction algorithm: standard
Oral contrast: 800 cc 2 hours prior to imaging
Intravenous (IV) contrast: first acquisition performed without IV contrast;
    second acquisition 120 to 150 cc nonionic contrast injected at 3 to 4 cc/sec;
    30-second prescan delay; third acquisition obtained with a 60-second
    delay

Liver Magnetic Resonance Imaging for Detection of Metastases or Hepatocellular Carcinoma (Minimum Sequences)

Table 28.3. Liver magnetic resonance imaging for detection of metastases or hepatocellular carcinoma (minimum sequences)

Sequence	TR	TE	Flip angle	Slice thickness (mm)	Matrix	Fat suppression	Breath hold
T1 gradient-echo axial in and out of phase	200	4.6/2.3	80	7	192 × 256	No	Yes
T2 dual echo, fast spin-echo	2350	40/140	90	6	256 × 512	Yes	No, respiratory triggered
Precontrast T1 fat-suppressed gradient-echo	200	4.6	80	7	192 × 256	Yes	Yes
Dynamic gadolinium 20 cc IV	3.5	1.7	10	2	192 × 256	Yes	Yes
Precontrast T1 fat-suppressed gradient-echo	200	4.6	80	7	192 × 256	Yes	Yes

Future Research

1. A randomized, multicenter, trial comparing the performance of state-of-the-art CT, MRI and PET-CT for detecting colorectal cancer metastases is highly desirable at this time.
2. Need to develop an imaging modality that will differentiate dysplastic nodules from HCC.
3. Need to identify HCC earlier. Study design similar to the one shown for colorectal cancer metastases above is recommended—relates to entry 1, above.
4. The role of PET and PET-CT in these populations of patients should continue to be explored.
5. Molecular imaging and tagging HCC cells will be the future of screening; CT and MRI are operating at the limits of their sensitivity and specificity.

References

1. Ohlsson B, Tranberg KG, Lundstedt C, Ekberg H, Helderestrom E. Eur J Surg 1993;159:275–281.

2. Moertel CG, Fleming TR, Macdonald JS, Haller DG, Laurie JA, Tangen C. JAMA 1993;270:943–947.
3. Kinkel K, Lu Y, Both M, Warren RS, Thoeni RF. Radiology 2002;224:748–756.
4. Maringhini A, Cottone M, Sciarrino E, et al. Dig Dis Sci 1988;33(1):47–51.
5. Chalasani N, Horlander JC Sr, Said A, et al. Am J Gastroenterol 1999;94(10): 2988–2993.
6. Scheele J, Stang R, Altendorf-Hofmann A, Paul M. World J Surg 1995;19: 1959–1971.
7. Fong Y, Cohen AM, Fortner JG, et al. J Clin Oncol 1997;15:938–946.
8. Fusai G, Davidson BR. Management of colorectal liver metastases. Colorectal Dis 2003;5:2–23.
9. Gazelle GS, Hunin MG, Kuntz KM, et al. Ann Surg 2003;237:544–555.
10. Pijl MEJ, Wasser MNJM, Joekes EC, van de Velde CJH, Bloem JL. Radiology 2003;227:747–751.
11. Semelka RC, Shoenut JP, Asher SM, et al. J Magn Reson Imaging 1994;4:319–323.
12. Semelka RC, Worawattanakul S, Kelekis NL, et al. J Magn Reson Imaging 1997; 7:1040–1047.
13. Zerhouni EA, Rutter C, Hamilton SR, et al. Radiology 1996;200:443–451.
14. Conlon R, Jacobs M, Dasgupta D, Lodge JP. Eur J Ultrasound 2003;6:211–216.
15. Hartley JE, Kumar H, Drew PJ, et al. Dis Colon Rectum 2000;43:320–324.
16. Soyer P, Poccard M, Boudiaf M, et al. Radiology 2004;231:413–420.
17. Strotzer M, Gmeinwieser J, Schmidt J, et al. Acta Radiol 1997;38:986–992.
18. van Erkel AR, Pijl MEJ, van den Berg-Husymans AA, Wasser MNJM, van de Velde CJH, Bloem JL. Radiology 2002;224:4040–4094.
19. Tempero MA, Williams CA, Anderson JC. J Clin Oncol 1986;4:1074–1078.
20. Grace RH, Hale M, Mackie G, Marks CG, Bloomberg TJ, Walker WJ. Br J Surg 1987;74:480–481.
21. Hohmann J, Albrecht T, Oldenburg A, Skrok J, Wolf KJ. Abdomin Imagin 2004;29.
22. Albrecht T, Blomkey MJK, Burns PN, et al. Radiology 2003;227;361–370.
23. Silverman PM, Kohan L, Ducic I. AJR 1998;170:149–152.
24. Freeny PC, Gardner JC, vonIngersleben G, Heyano S, Nghiem HV, Winter TC. Radiology 1995;197:89–93.
25. Valls C, Andia E, Sanchez A, et al. Radiology 2001;218:55–60.
26. Miller FH, Butler RS, Hoff FL, Fitzgerald SW, Nemcek AA, Gore RM. AJR 1998; 171:643–649.
27. Scott DJ, Guthrie JA, Arnold P, et al. Clin Radiol 2001;56:235–242.
28. Haider MA, Amitai MM, Rappaport DC. Radiology 2002;225:137–142.
29. Weg N, Scheer MR, Gabor MP. Radiology 1998;209:417–426.
30. Schwartz LH, Gandras EJ, Colangelo SM, Ercolani MC, Panicek DM. Radiology 1999;210:71–74.
31. Soyer P, Levesque M, Caudron C, Elias D, Zeitoun G, Roche A. J Comput Assist Tomogr 1993;17:67–74.
32. Kondo H, Kanematsu M, Hoshi H, et al. AJR 2000;174:947–954.
33. Seneterre E, Taourel P, Bouvier Y, et al. Radiology 1996;200:785–792.
34. McFarland EG, Mayo SW, Saini S, Hahn PF, Goldberg MA, Lee MJ. Radiology 1994;193:43–47.
35. Tello R, Fenlon HM, Gagliano T, de Carvalho VLS, Yucel EK. AJR 2001;176: 870–884.
36. Wittenberg J, Stark DD, Forman BH, et al. AJR 1988;151:79–84.
37. Outwater E, Tomaszewski JE, Daly JM, Kressel HY. Radiology 1991;180:327–332.
38. Yamashita Y, Tank Y, Namimoto T, Mitsuzaki K, Takahashi M. Radiology 1998; 207:331–337.
39. Kanematsu M, Hoshi H, Murakami T, et al. Radiology 1999;211:363–371.
40. Bartolozzi C, Donati F, Cioni D, et al. Eur Radiol 2004;14:14–20.
41. Vogl TJ, Schwarz W, Blume S, et al. Eur Radiol 2003;13:262–272.

42. Ward J, Naik KS, Guthrie JA, Wilson D, Robinson PJ. Radiology 1999;210: 459–466.
43. Said B, McCart JA, Libutti SK, Choyke PL. Magn Reson Imaging 2000;18: 305–309.
44. Matsuo M, Kanematsu M, Itoh K, et al. AJR 2001;177:637–643.
45. Kantorova I, Lipska L, Belohlavek O, Visokai V, Trubac M, Schneiderova M. J Nucl Med 2003;44:1784–1788.
46. Abdel-Nabi H, Doerr RJ, Lamonica DM, et al. Radiology 1998;206:755–760.
47. Noguchi Y, Murakami T, Kim T, et al. J Comput Assist Tomogr 2002 Nov-Dec; 26(6):981–987.
48. Noguchi Y, Murakami T, Kim T, et al. AJR 2003;180(2):455–460.
49. Hori M, Murakami T, Kim T, et al. J Comput Assist Tomogr 2002;26(5):701–710.
50. Kwak HS, Lee JM, Kim CS. Eur Radiol 2004;14(3):447–457.
51. Shinagawa T, Ohto M, Kimura K, et al. Gastroenterology 1984;86(3):495–502.
52. Okazaki N, Yoshida T, Yoshino M, Matue H. Clin Oncol 1984;10(3):241–246.
53. Ikeda K, Saitoh S, Koida I, et al. Hepatology 1994;20(1 pt 1):82–7.
54. Tanaka S, Kitamura T, Ohshima A, et al. Cancer 1986;58(2):344–347.
55. Okano H, Shiraki K, Inoue H, et al. Anticancer Res 2001;21(4B):2979–2982.
56. Angeli E, Carpanelli R, Crespi G, Zanello A, Sironi S, Del Maschio A. Radiol Med (Torino) 1994;87(5 suppl 1):24–31.
57. Maruyama H, Matsutani S, Sato G, et al. Abdom Imaging 2000;25(2):164–171.
58. Khong PL, Chau MT, Fan ST, Leong LL. Australas Radiol 1999;43(2):156–159.
59. Choi BI, Kim AY, Lee JY, et al. J Ultrasound Med 2002;21(1):77–84.
60. Shimizu M, Iijima H, Horibe T, et al. Hepatol Res 2004;29(4):235–242.
61. Peterson MS, Baron RL, Marsh JW Jr, Oliver JH 3rd, Confer SR, Hunt LE. Radiology 2000;217(3):743–749.
62. Bhattacharjya S, Bhattacharjya T, Quaglia A, et al. Dig Surg 2004;21(2):152–159.
63. Makita O, Yamashita Y, Arakawa A, et al. Acta Radiol 2000;41(5):464–469.
64. Matsuo M, Kanematsu M, Inaba Y, et al. Clin Radiol 2001;56(2):138–145.
65. Jang HJ, Lim JH, Lee SJ, Park CK, Park HS, Do YS. Radiology 2000;215(2): 373–380.
66. Hori M, Murakami T, Oi H, et al. Acta Radiol 1998;39(2):144–151.
67. Kanematsu M, Hoshi H, Murakami T, et al. AJR 1997;169(6):1507–1515.
68. Murakami T, Kim T, Oi H, et al. Acta Radiol 1995;36(4):372–376.
69. Oi H, Murakami T, Kim T, Matsushita M, Kishimoto H, Nakamura H. AJR 1996;166(2):369–374.
70. Kim T, Murakami T, Oi H, et al. J Comput Assist Tomogr 1995;19(6):948–954.
71. Yamashita Y, Mitsuzaki K, Yi T, et al. Radiology 1996;200(1):79–84.
72. Lee JM, Kim IH, Kwak HS, Youk JH, Han YM, Kim CS. Korean J Radiol 2003; 4(1):1–8.
73. Trojan J, Schroeder O, Raedle J, et al. Am J Gastroenterol 1999;94(11):3314–3319.
74. Khan MA, Combs CS, Brunt EM, et al. J Hepatol 2000;32(5):792–797.
75. Verhoef C, Valkema R, de Man RA, Krenning EP, Yzermans JN. Liver 2002; 22(1):51–56.
76. Wudel LJ Jr, Delbeke D, Morris D, et al. Am Surg 2003;69(2):117–124.
77. Liangpunsakul S, Agarwal D, Horlander JC, Kieff B, Chalasani N. Transplant Proc 2003;35(8):2995–2997.
78. Schroder O, Trojan J, Zeuzem S, Baum RP. Nuklearmedizin 1998;37(8):279–285.
79. Teefey SA, Hildeboldt CC, Dehdashti F, et al. Radiology 2003;226(2):533–542.
80. Bolondi L, Gaiani S, Casali A, Serra C, Piscaglia F. Radiol Med (Torino) 1997; 94(1–2):4–7.
81. Sarasin FP, Giostra E, Hadengue A. Am J Med 1996;101(4):422–434.
82. Yuen MF, Lai CL. Ann Oncol 2003;14(10):1463–1467.
83. Gambarin-Gelwan M, Wolf DC, Shapiro R, Schwartz ME, Min AD. Am J Gastroenterol 2000;95(6):1535–1538.
84. Lin OS, Keeffe EB, Sanders GD, Owens DK. C. Aliment Pharmacol Ther 2004;19(11):1159–1172.

85. Arguedas MR, Chen VK, Eloubeidi MA, Fallon MB. Am J Gastroenterol 2003;
    98(3):679–690.
86. Lopez Hanninen E, Vogl TJ, Felfe R, et al. Radiology 2000;216:403–409.

29

Imaging of Nephrolithiasis, Urinary Tract Infections, and Their Complications

Julia R. Fielding and Raj S. Pruthi

Key Points

Nephrolithiasis

- Non–contrast-enhanced helical computed tomography (CT) with 5-mm slice thickness is the test of choice for the patient with a suspected obstructing ureteral stone. In the absence of an available CT scanner, intravenous urography (IVU) or a combination of plain film and ultrasonography (US) should be performed (moderate evidence).
- Plain film should be used to follow the descent of stones along the ureter (moderate evidence).
- For the pregnant patient with a suspected renal stone, there is insufficient evidence to determine whether IVU or CT is the appropriate test when US is not diagnostic (insufficient evidence).

Urinary Tract Infection

- Uncomplicated urinary tract infections (UTIs) in women, those without systemic signs or symptoms, do not require imaging (moderate evidence).
- Complicated UTIs in women, those that occur in combination with pregnancy or with symptoms that extend beyond 10 days and evolve to include fever, chills, and flank pain may require imaging to exclude renal abscess. It is unclear what clinical finding should prompt imaging and whether CT or US should be performed (insufficient evidence).
- Uncomplicated, isolated UTIs in men are uncommon. It is unclear when US or cystoscopy should be performed to exclude associated infection of the testis or epididymis and bladder cancer, respectively (insufficient evidence).
- Because of the high likelihood of vesicoureteral reflux in children with UTIs, US and voiding cystourethrogram (VCUG) should be performed in children with a UTI (moderate evidence). At most academic institutions in the United States, both US and VCUG are performed in boys and girls to exclude hydronephrosis, significant renal scars, and vesicoureteral reflux. Nuclear medicine cystogram may be substituted for VCUG; however, the currently used low-dose fluoroscopy units and higher spatial resolution make VCUG the more commonly used test.
- Patients with neurogenic bladders often have colonized the urine with pathogens. They may demonstrate few signs and symptoms when developing a complicated infection. It is unclear when and what type of imaging should be performed (insufficient evidence).

Definition and Pathophysiology

Urolithiasis is the presence of stones within the urinary tract. Some patients with stones in the kidney live out their lives without incident. Many patients suffer from hematuria as the stones grow and move within the renal pelves and experience severe flank pain when the stone(s) become lodged in the ureter. The most common renal stones in the United States are calcium based and are formed at the tip of the papilla when excess calcium is excreted into the urine. Less common stone varieties include those made of uric acid, struvite (ammonium/magnesium/phosphate), cystine, and xanthine.

Urinary tract infection occurs when urine stasis or an altered local resistance allows a bacterial pathogen to grow in the bladder. Patients complain of pain and usually have a urinalysis positive for the presence of white blood cells (>100,000 organisms/1 mL of urine) and bacterial organisms. On occasion, the infectious process will ascend the ureter to involve the intrarenal collecting system and renal cortex leading to pyelonephritis and renal abscess. With certain organisms, such as tuberculosis, the bacteria may be hematogenously seeded into the renal cortex and the infectious process descends into the bladder.

Epidemiology

Nephrolithiasis is a common problem of people living in temperate climates. It is estimated that at least 5% of female and 12% of the male population will have at least one episode of renal colic due to stone disease by the age of 70 years (1). In the U.S., the majority of stone disease cases are seen in the southeastern part of the country where diet, genetic predisposition, and certain occupations all may predispose to stone formation. Nephrolithiasis is three times more common in males. The peak age for onset of renal stone disease is age 20 to 30, but stone formation is often a lifelong problem. Stone disease is rare in children.

Urinary Tract Infection

Because of the short female urethra, it is much easier for bacteria to ascend into the bladder and therefore the vast preponderance of infections occur in females, particularly in children and women of childbearing age. During any given year, 11% of women report having had a UTI and more than half of all women has at least one such infection during their lifetime (2). After the age of 50, the number of infections in males and females is nearly equal, likely because the bladder outlet obstruction due to enlargement of the prostate in males leads to urine stasis.

Overall Cost to Society

Nephrolithiasis

Because nephrolithiasis is such a common process, the cumulative expense of imaging and clinical evaluations is quite high. In 1995 Clark et al. (3) estimated the annual cost of nephrolithiasis in the U.S. to be $1.23 billion, with the cost of outpatient evaluation at $278 million.

Urinary Tract Infection

Again, because UTIs are extremely common, the cost of diagnosis and treatment is very high. Each year in the U.S., uncomplicated acute cystitis is responsible for 3.6 million office visits, accounting for direct costs of $1.6 billion (4,5). The majority of patients are treated based on symptomatology and the results of a urine dipstick detecting the presence of nitrite of leukocyte esterase. Only a small percentage of these patients will undergo imaging as part of the workup, usually when structural abnormalities of the urinary tract are suspected or the patient fails treatment and develops signs of an upper tract infection.

Goals

The goal of imaging in the case of nephrolithiasis is twofold: first, to determine the presence or absence of an obstructing ureteral stone; and second, to contribute to treatment planning. In a patient who chronically forms stones, imaging can also be used to follow renal stone burden. Imaging of UTIs is undertaken to identify complications, specifically renal abscess. In children with UTIs, imaging is undertaken to exclude vesicoureteral reflux or renal scarring.

Methodology

A Medline search was performed using PubMed (National Library of Medicine, Bethesda, Maryland) for original research publications relating the diagnostic performance and accuracy for imaging of nephrolithiasis and UTIs. Clinical indicators of urinary tract disease including hematuria and flank pain were also included. The search covered the period 1966 to March 2004. The search strategy employed different combinations of the following terms: (1) *nephrolithiasis*, (2) *renal abscess*, (3) *UTI*, and (4) *radiography* or *imaging* or *computed tomography* or *intravenous urography* or *ultrasound*. This search was limited to the English language and human studies. Using the Limits feature of PubMed and the above terms, the database was also searched specifically for clinical trials and meta-analyses. After review of the abstracts of the search results, we reviewed the entire text of relevant articles. In addition, additional pertinent publications were gleaned from a review of the reference lists.

I. What Is the Appropriate Test for Suspicion of Obstructing Ureteral Stone?

Summary of Evidence: Patients with clinical signs and symptoms of renal obstruction should undergo unenhanced helical CT of the abdomen and pelvis. The accuracy of this test has been shown to be higher than that of IVU and a combination of US and plain film in level II (moderate evidence) studies. In addition, CT is quick to perform and interpret and does not require the administration of intravenous contrast medium. Findings on the CT scan can be used by the referring physician to determine treatment. The drawbacks of the technique include cost and a relatively high dose of ionizing radiation (30–40 mSv). When CT is not available either IVU or a combination of plain film and sonography may be used.

Supporting Evidence: For many years, IVU served as the test of choice for identification of obstructing ureteral stones. Following administration of intravenous contrast medium, delayed renal enhancement and excretion and a filling defect within the ureter were diagnostic findings. Because this test dates to the beginning of modern radiology, no prospective studies were performed to determine its accuracy. It was one of the few imaging tests available. In recent years, level II and III (moderate and limited evidence) studies have revealed an accuracy between 85% and 90% (6,7). Unfortunately, the IVU, while accurate, often requires several hours to perform. In addition, the excretion of contrast into the dilated ureter tends to increase the patient's already severe pain.

An alternative imaging scenario used commonly in Europe and the Far East combines a plain film with an ultrasound examination. In a level II (moderate evidence) study comparing IVU and US in the identification of ureteral stones, both modalities revealed 44 stones for a sensitivity of 64% (8). More recently, unenhanced helical CT has become the preeminent test for the diagnosis of renal colic in the U.S. In one of the largest published series, 210 patients with a confirmed diagnosis for flank pain underwent helical CT (9); 100 stones were recovered and 30 patients were found to have a source for pain beyond the urinary tract. There were three false negatives and four false positives for stone disease. These data yield a sensitivity of 97%, specificity of 96%, and accuracy of 97% for the diagnosis of obstructing ureteral stone. Of note, all stones are radiodense on CT with the exception of the urinary concretions formed by HIV patients taking protease inhibitors (10,11). Similar level II (moderate evidence) clinical studies have been performed by multiple groups with reported diagnostic accuracies ranging from 0.90 to 0.97, high interobserver reliability, and accurate depiction of stone size (12–15). Level II (moderate evidence) and level III (limited evidence) studies have also shown that stone size, shape, and location can be used to determine whether the stone will pass spontaneously or is likely to require intervention (12,14). Stones that are 5 mm or less in size, of regular shape, are located in the distal two thirds of the ureter, and are present on one or two consecutive CT images 5 mm in thickness are most likely to pass spontaneously. These same studies also demonstrate an alternative source for flank pain in 15% of cases, including ovarian masses, appendicitis, and diverticulitis.

In a level II (moderate evidence) study comparing the combination of plain film and sonography with unenhanced CT in 181 patients with flank pain, CT was found to have a greater sensitivity (92% vs. 77%), negative predictive value (87% vs. 68%), and overall accuracy (94% vs. 83%) for identification of flank pain (16). Sourtzis et al. (6) reported similar results in a level III (limited evidence) study. When CT was compared with both IVU and sonography in 64 patients with recovered ureteral stones, sensitivities were 94%, 52%, and 19%, respectively (7).

II. How Should Stones Be Followed After Treatment?

Summary of Evidence: Because plain film has the highest spatial resolution of any imaging modality, has good contrast sensitivity, is inexpensive, and delivers minimal radiation dose, it is at present the best way to follow the passage of a stone down the ureter over time.

Supporting Evidence: Level II and III (moderate and limited evidence) studies report that 60% of ureteral stones are visible on plain radiography (17,18). The low detection rate is likely due to overlying fecal material and the presence of some radiolucent stones, such as those composed of uric acid. Despite the relatively low detection rate, the use of repeat CT studies is likely not justified because of the cumulative radiation dose. An exception may be made when following the results of lithotripsy and the detection of small intrarenal stone fragments is of importance.

III. Special Case: The Pregnant Patient

Summary of Evidence: There is no compelling published evidence that IVU, plain film, and sonography or helical CT is the preferred test. In dealing with the pregnant patient, fetal age and estimated radiation dose is of paramount importance. Pregnant patients routinely have right hydronephrosis as the enlarging uterus turns slightly to the right, compressing the ureter.

Computed tomography, the most accurate test, delivers approximately 16 mSv to the fetus. Two plain films obtained prior to and after administration of intravenous contrast material deliver significantly less radiation but may be more difficult to interpret because of the overlying bony fetal parts and lateral deviation of the ureters. Dilation of the left ureter is thought to be less common, and the presence of left hydronephrosis with flank pain or hematuria is often enough clinical evidence for clinicians to begin treatment for stone disease.

IV. When Is Imaging Required in the Adult Female with a Urinary Tract Infection?

Summary of Evidence: Level II (moderate evidence) studies have revealed that IVU and US are of little value in males or females in the diagnosis of uncomplicated UTIs in which symptoms are confined to the pelvis. In evaluating recurrent UTIs, IVU may be of some use, particularly when a structural abnormality of the urinary tract is suspected. There is no compelling evidence to determine when and how imaging of complicated UTIs should be performed. Complicated infections include those in which symptoms exceed 10 days, there is coexisting pregnancy, or symptoms evolve to include fever, chills, and flank pain.

Supporting Evidence: In a study of 328 patients referred for imaging of the urinary tract performed by Lewis-Jones et al. (19) in the United Kingdom, the small subset with a positive urine culture and UTI (n = 33) had no abnormalities detected using either IVU or US. In a similar study performed by Little et al. (20), 200 consecutive patients were evaluated for a variety of complaints using IVU. In the subset of patients with recurrent UTI (n = 60) five patients (8%) had abnormalities including at least one case of carcinoma.

Urinary tract infection is the most common medical complication of pregnancy. Although pregnant women are at no greater risk for developing an uncomplicated UTI, the compression of the bladder and uterus on the ureters is thought to lead to a higher incidence of reflux and pyelonephritis. For asymptomatic patients, treatment is usually antibiotics on an outpatient basis. The exception would be group B streptococcus, which usually requires inpatient intravenous antibiotic treatment because of its association with neonatal sepsis (21).

There is no compelling evidence to suggest when CT or US should be performed when a renal abscess is suspected. Opinion articles, level IV (insufficient evidence), suggest that development of the appropriate clinical symptomatology despite treatment with antibiotics for 10 days should prompt imaging (22,23).

V. When Is Imaging Required in the Adult Male with a Urinary Tract Infection?

Summary of Evidence: There is no compelling evidence to indicate the role of imaging in men with UTIs. Isolated UTIs are uncommon. Associated disorders such as orchitis, epididymitis, and prostate enlargement can be detected using US. It is possible that IVU and other contrast studies may be of use when stones or strictures of the ureter are suspected; however, there is no compelling evidence to support this (20).

VI. When is Imaging Required in the Child with a Urinary Tract Infection?

Summary of Evidence: During the first 6 years of life, 8% of all girls and 2% of all boys will have a symptomatic UTI (24). The diagnosis is confirmed by the presence of bacterial organisms and white blood cells in the urine. Diagnosis of pyelonephritis in small children who cannot communicate the location of pain remains a challenge. In a study of 919 girls undergoing a first imaging evaluation for UTI, Gelfand et al. (25) found that vesicoureteral reflux was extremely uncommon in girls with a fever less than 38.5°C and greater than 10 years of age. Because UTIs can be associated with vesicoureteral reflux, the standard imaging algorithm consists of a voiding fluoroscopic or nuclear cystourethrogram and a renal US.

Supporting Evidence: Level II (moderate evidence) suggests that the current model of VCUG and US is appropriate. Kass et al. (26) examined 453 children with UTI using ultrasound and VCUG; 152 had normal renal US, of whom 101 also had normal VCUG. Vesicoureteral reflux was identified on VCUG in 23 (23%) of patients with normal sonography. Similar results were obtained by Goldman et al. (27), who studied 45 male neonates presenting with a first UTI. Both investigators suggested that US and VCUG should be routinely performed. Power Doppler may improve the sensitivity of US. In a level II (moderate evidence) study of 19 children with pyelonephritis as diagnosed by clinical symptomatology and contrast-enhanced CT, power Doppler US identified 89% of cases (28). For patient convenience and because of the high loss to follow-up, most institutions perform a US and VCUG on the same day. Despite its lower radiation dose, nuclear cystogram has fallen out of favor in many areas of the U.S. because referring urologists require a clear assessment of ureteral anatomy and because new fluoroscopic equipment allows acquisition of 7 frames/sec, decreasing the amount of radiation received by the child by 75% compared with standard adult fluoroscopic technique.

   Nuclear cystogram using technetium-99m (Tc-99m)-labeled dimercaptosuccinic acid (DMSA) may be of particular value in girls, for whom urethral obstruction is not an issue or for follow-up of well-documented vesicoureteral reflux. Level II, moderate evidence, studies have shown an increase in the incidence (25–45%) of vesicoureteral reflux in siblings afflicted with the disease (29,30). For this reason, siblings under 10 years of age are often tested for reflux. Laboratory studies have shown that sensitivity of Tc-99m DMSA for diagnosis of pyelonephritis in a piglet model is approximately 90% (31,32). In a large retrospective level II (moderate evidence) study of inpatients and outpatients, Desphande and Jones (33) found renal scarring present on DMSA scans in 2% of the outpatients and 33% of inpatients, indicating that clinical findings of severe disease may be important in deciding on this imaging algorithm. There is no compelling evidence describing the imaging findings of CT or magnetic resonance imaging (MRI) in the diagnosis of pyelonephritis in adults or children. Case series of CT scans often describe a striated nephrogram or diminished regions of uptake in the affected kidney. Magnetic resonance imaging, while avoiding patient radiation exposure, also lacks specific findings to indicate renal infection.

In a recent laboratory study, Majd et al. (34) compared Tc-99m single photon emission computed tomography (SPECT), helical CT, MRI, and power Doppler US for diagnosis of pyelonephritis in a piglet model. They found that Tc-99m SPECT, CT, and MRI were equally sensitive (87–92%) and specific (88–94%) for the diagnosis of pyelonephritis in 38 kidneys with 102 zones of disease. Power Doppler US performed at a lower level, with sensitivity of 57% and specificity of 82%. A level III (limited evidence) study performed on 37 children with fever-producing UTIs by Lonergan et al. (35) showed abnormality consisting of diminished perfusion in 38 kidneys using MRI. Determination of whether CT or MRI, with their respective drawbacks of radiation exposure and sedation, should be added to the routine diagnostic imaging algorithm of pyelonephritis awaits further scientific work.

VII. Special Case: The Neurogenic Bladder

Summary of Evidence: The neurogenic bladder fails to fill and empty on a regular basis due to neuropathy. This may be due to a congenital anomaly such as myelomeningocele, trauma to the spinal cord or pelvic nerves, or ischemic neuropathy such as occurs in diabetes mellitus. Because of stasis, the urine of many of these patients is colonized by bacterial pathogens. Asymptomatic UTIs are rarely treated. The difficulty arises when a complicated infection occurs. Because of the neuropathy, affected patients may not feel pain or distention of the bladder, and the immune system may not respond adequately leading to minimal symptoms.

Supporting Evidence: There is no compelling evidence to determine when such patients require imaging. Expert opinion (level IV, insufficient evidence) suggests that patients who develop fevers undergo a urologic workup including Gram stain and culture of the urine to determine correct antibiotic usage. Failure to respond to antibiotics within a short period of time should prompt the use of US or CT (36,37).

Take-Home Table

Table 29.1. Diagnostic performance for CT, US, and IVU in detection of ureteral stones

Lead author	Year of publication	N	Stones +	Test	Sensitivity	Specificity
Catalano	2002	181	82	CT	0.92	0.96
				US/plain radiography	0.77	0.96
Boulay	1999	51	49	CT	1.0	0.96
Sheley	1999	180	87	CT	0.86	0.91
Sourtzis	1999	36	36	CT	1.0	1.0
				IVU	0.66	1.0
Yilmaz	1998	97	64	CT	0.94	0.97
				US	0.19	0.97
				IVU	0.52	0.94
Smith	1996	210	100	CT	0.97	0.96

Future Research

- Clinical prediction rules for development of pyelonephritis in pregnant women and those patients with a neurogenic bladder.
- Imaging diagnosis of pyelonephritis and its sequelae in children, particularly using sonographic and MRI contrast agents.

Imaging Case Studies

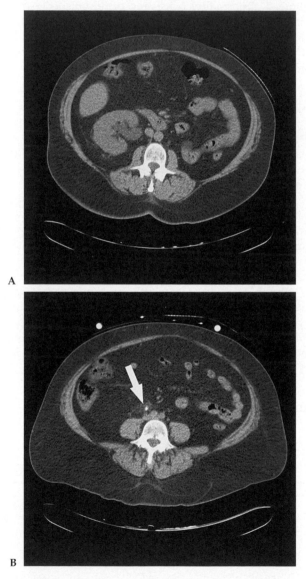

Figure 29.1. Imaging case study for nephrolithiasis. Woman with right flank pain underwent non–contrast-enhanced helical computed tomography (CT) that revealed a solitary right kidney with hydronephrosis (A) and an obstructing ureteral stone at the level of the mid-ureter (B) (arrow).

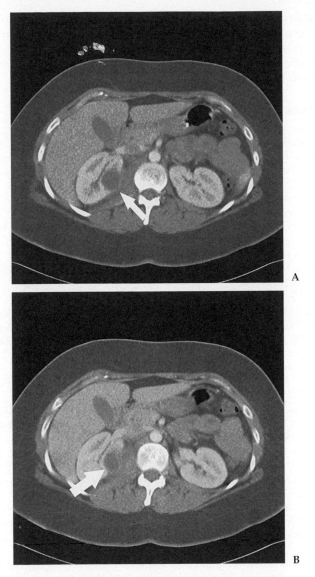

Figure 29.2. Imaging case study for urinary tract infection (UTI). Woman with UTI unresponsive to antibiotics for days and with interval development of flank pain and fever. An ovoid right renal mass is hypodense to the adjacent renal parenchyma on a contrast-enhanced CT scan (A) (arrow). There is rim enhancement of the developing renal abscess and stranding of the adjacent fat (B) (arrow).

Suggested Computed Tomography Imaging Protocols

Suspected obstructing ureteral stone: non–contrast-enhanced helical CT performed with 120 kV and the milliamperes (mA) approximately equal to the patient's weight in pounds (to minimize radiation dose). Data acquisition thickness and table speed vary with scanner type; reconstructed images should be 5 mm in thickness. Viewing the images using cine mode facilitates stone detection.

Suspected renal abscess: CT following administration of intravenous contrast agent, 120 kV and mA approximately equal to the patient's weight in pounds (to minimize radiation dose). Data acquisition thickness and table speed vary with scanner type; reconstructed images should be 5 to 10 mm in thickness.

References

1. Sierakowski R, Finlayson B, Landes RR, et al. Invest Urol 1978;15:438–441.
2. Foxman B, Barlow R, D'Arcy H, Gillespie B, Sobel JD. Ann Epidemiol 2000; 10:509–515.
3. Clark JY, Thompson IM, Optenber SA. J Urol 1995;154:2020–2024.
4. Schappert SM. Ambulatory care visits to physician offices, hospital outpatient departments, and emergency departments: United States, 1997. Vital and Health Statistics. Series 13. No. 143. Atlanta: National Center for Health Statistics, November 1999. DHHS publication no. (PHS) 2000–1714.
5. Foxman B. Am J Public Health 1990;80:331–333.
6. Sourtzis S, Thibeau JF, Damry N, Raslan A, Vandendris M, Bellemans M. AJR 1999;172:1491–1494.
7. Yilmaz S, Sindel T, Arslan G, et al. Eur Radiol 1998;8(2):212–217.
8. Sinclair D, Wilson S, Toi A, Greenspan L. Ann Emerg Med 1989;18(5):556–559.
9. Smith RC, Verga M, McCarthy S, Rosenfield AT. AJR 1996;166:97–101.
10. Blake SP, McNicholas MM, Raptopoulos V. AJR 1998;171(3):717–720.
11. Schwartz BF, Schenkman N, Armenakas NA, Stoller ML. J Urol 1999; 161(4):1085–1087.
12. Fielding JR, Silverman SG, Samuel S, Zou KH, Loughlin KR. AJR 1998;171: 1051–1053.
13. Sheley RC, Semonsen KG, Quinn SF. Am J Emerg Med 1999;17(3):279–282.
14. Boulay I, Holtz P, Foley WD, White B, Begun FP. AJR 1999;172:1485–1490.
15. Olcott EW, Sommer FG, Napel S. Radiology 1997;207:19–25.
16. Catalano O, Nunziata A, Altei F, Siani A. AJR 2002;178:379–387.
17. Assi Z, Platt JF, Francis IR, Cohan RH, Korobkin M. AJR 2000;175:333–337.
18. Levine JA, Neitlich J, Verga M, Dalrymple N, Smith RC. Radiology 1997; 204(1):27–31.
19. Lewis-Jones HG, Lamb HR, Hughes PL. Br J Radiol 1989;62:977–980.
20. Little MA, Stafford Johnson DB, O'Callaghan JP, Walshe JJ. Nephrol Dial Transplant 2000;15:200–204.
21. Zinner SH, Kass EH. N Engl J Med 1971;285(15):820–824.
22. Ribeiro RM, Rossi P, Guidi HGC, Pinotti JA. Int Urogynecol J 2002;13:198–203.
23. Bjerklund Johansen TE. Curr Opin Urol 2002;12:39–43.
24. Marild S, Jodal U. Acta Paediatr 1998;87(5):549–552.
25. Gelfand MF, Koch Bl, Cordero GG, Salmanzadeh A, Garside PS. Pediatr Radiol 2000;30:121–124.
26. Kass EJ, Kernen KM, Carey JM. BJU Int 2000;86(1):94–96.
27. Goldman M, Lahat E, Strauss S, et al. Pediatrics 2000;105(6):1232–1235.
28. Dacher J, Pfister C, Monroc M, Eurin D, Le Dosseur P. AJR 1996;166:1451–1455.
29. Jerkins GF, Noe HN. J Urol 1982;128:774–778.
30. Connolly LP, Treves St, Connolly SA, et al. J Urol 1997;157:2287–2290.
31. Parkhouse HG, Godley ML, Cooper J, Risdon RA, Ranslay PG. Nucl Med Commun 1989;10:63–70.
32. Rushton HG, Majd M, Chandra R, Yim D. J Urol 1988;140;1169–1174.
33. Deshpande PV, Jones KV. Arch Dis Child 2001;84:324–327.
34. Majd M, Nussbaum Blask AR, et al. Radiology 2001;218:101–108.
35. Lonergan GJ, Pennington DJ, Morrison JC, Haws RM, Grimley MS, Kao TC. Radiology 1998;207:377–384.
36. Sasaki K, Yoshimura N, Chancellor MB. Urol Clin North Am 2003;30:1–12.
37. Rubenstein JN, Schaeffer AJ. Infect Dis Clin North Am 2003;17:333–351.

30

Current Issues in Gynecology: Screening for Ovarian Cancer in the Average Risk Population and Diagnostic Evaluation of Postmenopausal Bleeding

Ruth C. Carlos

Issues

I. Ovarian cancer screening: what is the role of biochemical markers such as CA 125?

II. Ovarian cancer screening: what is the diagnostic performance (accuracy) of imaging?

III. Ovarian cancer screening: what is the role of imaging?
   A. Screening with gray-scale ultrasound only
   B. Screening with ultrasound and color Doppler imaging
   C. Multimodality approach using CA 125 and ultrasound

IV. Postmenopausal bleeding evaluation: when should a woman with postmenopausal bleeding be referred for additional evaluation?

V. Postmenopausal bleeding evaluation: what is the accuracy of imaging tests?
   A. Transvaginal ultrasonography
   B. Saline-infused hysterosonography
   C. Hysteroscopy

VI. Postmenopausal bleeding evaluation: what is the role of imaging?

VII. How should women on tamoxifen therapy be evaluated?

Key Points

- Current data do not support ovarian cancer screening women who are at average risk, with any screening regimen (moderate evidence).
- Transvaginal ultrasound (TVUS) is preferred as the initial test in evaluating women with postmenopausal bleeding who are not on tamoxifen (moderate evidence).
- Histologic sampling is necessary in women with postmenopausal bleeding and a positive TVUS (moderate evidence).
- Hysteroscopy and curettage is the preferred diagnostic test, over Pipelle endometrial biopsy, to detect polyps and other benign lesions (limited evidence).

> ▪ In women with postmenopausal bleeding and tamoxifen use, hysteroscopy and curettage is preferred as the initial diagnostic test (limited evidence).

Definition and Pathophysiology

Ovarian cancer is a heterogeneous group of malignancies that arises from the various cell types that comprise the organ (1). Epithelial tumors represent the most common histology (90%) of ovarian tumors. Other histologies include (1) low malignant or borderline ovarian tumors, (2) sex cord stromal tumors, (3) germ cell tumors, (4) primary peritoneal carcinoma, and (5) metastatic tumors of the ovary. The etiology of ovarian cancer is poorly understood; however, its epidemiology and risk factors have been well described.

Endometrial cancer is also a heterogeneous disease with two apparent subtypes. The majority of women with endometrial cancer have a well-differentiated carcinoma with grade 1 or 2 endometrioid histology and well-defined risk factors. A minority of cases are diagnosed with poorly differentiated tumors (grade 3 endometrioid, clear cell, and papillary serous carcinoma), which occur spontaneously in postmenopausal women.

Epidemiology

Ovarian Cancer

Ovarian cancer is estimated to have caused over 25,000 new cancers in women in 2004 and is the most frequent cause of death from a gynecologic cancer (2). Ovarian cancers typically present few symptoms before having reached a large size or having disseminated. The vast majority of patients are diagnosed with metastatic disease. Therefore, survival rates remain poor despite marked advances in surgery and chemotherapeutics. Women with metastatic disease have a less than 30% chance of surviving 5 years after diagnosis. In contrast, women diagnosed with stage I ovarian cancer (with cancer confined to the ovaries) have a greater than 90% chance of 5-year survival (3). Baseline lifetime risk for developing ovarian cancer is estimated at 1.4% to 1.8% (3,4). The most significant risk factor for ovarian cancer is positive family history, increasing the baseline risk five- to sevenfold. Identification of *BRCA1* or *BRCA2* gene mutations increases the estimated risk to approximately 30% to 40% (5,6). Approximately 90% of all familial ovarian cancers are attributable to these two mutations with the remaining 10% accounted for by mutations at other loci (7,8).

Increasing parity has a protective effect against ovarian cancer. A review of 12 case-control studies demonstrated that having a single term pregnancy reduces the risk of ovarian cancer by half with progressive risk reduction with each additional pregnancy (9). The findings above were supported by additional findings from the Nurses Cohort study, where each pregnancy reduced the risk of ovarian cancer by approximately 15% (10). The linkage between infertility and increased risk of ovarian cancer is not as well established. After adjusting for confounding variables, a weak association [odds ratio (OR), 1.21; 95% confidence interval (CI), 0.83–1.77] between infertility and ovarian cancer was demonstrated in a large Australian population (11). Further, there appear to be subgroups of infertile women who are at higher risk for ovarian cancer, specifically nulliparous women and women with unexplained infertility (12). Although early menarche and late menopause have been implicated as risk factors for ovarian cancer, Whittemore et al. (9) and Hankinson et al. (10) independently demonstrated nonsignificant effects of early menarche and of late menopause on ovarian cancer risk. Oral contraceptive pill (OCP) use as a protective factor has been demonstrated in a United Kingdom–based study involving over 15,000 women, where OCP use for more than 8 years reduced the risk of ovarian cancer (OR, 0.4); these findings were confirmed in a large Australian case-control study.

In screening for ovarian cancer, as in all cancers, important time points to note are the lead time required to alter the natural history of the disease with intervention in order to increase survival, and the duration of marker-positive preclinical disease when disease can be detected using current tests at a stage sufficiently early to successfully intervene. Both of these time points have not been defined in the natural history of ovarian cancer.

Endometrial Cancer

The American Cancer Society estimated that cancer of the uterine corpus, of which endometrial cancer is the most common, caused greater than 40,000 new cancer cases and approximately 7000 deaths in 2004 (2). The absolute risk of endometrial cancer in patients without hormone replacement therapy (HRT) who present with postmenopausal bleeding ranges from 5.7% to 11.5% (13–15). Menopause, as defined by the World Health Organization, is the permanent cessation of menstruation resulting from the loss of ovarian follicular activity (16). In general, postmenopausal bleeding (PMB) represents an episode of bleeding occurring 12 months or more after the last period (17). Abnormal bleeding occurring during HRT can be difficult to define and depends on the type of HRT. Breakthrough bleeding or heavy/prolonged bleeding after the progestogen phase while on sequential HRT may be considered abnormal. Any bleeding occurring after the first 6 months of treatment or after amenorrhea has been established while on continuous combined HRT may be considered abnormal (18).

The primary genetic risk factor for endometrial cancer is hereditary nonpolyposis colorectal cancer, where endometrial cancer is the most commonly associated extracolonic cancer. The lifetime risk for developing endometrial cancer in this population has been estimated at 42% to 60% (19,20). In these women, endometrial cancer occurs prior to menopause, distinct from the sporadic type of endometrial cancer that occurs primarily in postmenopausal women (21).

The major reproductive risk factors increasing endometrial cancer risk are late menopause and early menarche, while increasing parity decreases risk with an approximately 30% reduction in risk with first birth compared to an approximately 15% reduction with each subsequent birth (22–26).

The use of OCP decreases the risk significantly. At premenopausal ages, the risk is reduced by approximately 10% per year of use (27,28), but this declines with increasing age. Obesity greatly increases the risk (29). Unopposed estrogen therapy for menopausal symptoms increases the risk of endometrial cancer approximately 120% at doses commonly used in the United States when used for 5 years (29). The addition of progesterone markedly decreases the risk of endometrial cancer with continuous combined estrogen-progesterone therapy associated with essentially no increased risk. Women on tamoxifen are at a three to six times higher risk for endometrial cancer (30–33).

Overall Cost to Society

Ovarian Cancer

The average present value of the 15-year costs attributable to ovarian cancer is $21,285 for local-stage disease and $32,126 for distant-stage disease in 1990 dollars, using data derived from Medicare claims data linked with Surveillance, Epidemiology, and End Results (SEER) cancer registry data (34). Long-term costs attributable to ovarian cancer were $64,000 as measured in a health maintenance organization (35).

Endometrial Cancer

Unlike ovarian cancer, the symptom most associated with endometrial cancer, namely PMB, accounts for the majority of societal cost. It accounts for 5% of all office gynecologic visits, but indicates endometrial cancer only 10% of the time (36). Data do not exist on the total monetary cost of evaluation of PMB and subsequent staging and treatment of detected endometrial cancer.

Goals

Screening in Ovarian Cancer

The relationship between stage at diagnosis and survival has provided the rationale for screening. The focus of screening in ovarian cancer rests on the identification of disease at a stage early enough to allow intervention to change survival. However, the ability of current techniques, namely the cancer antigen 125 (CA 125) tumor marker and ultrasonography (US), for detecting ovarian cancer at this early stage has not been fully established.

Evaluation in Postmenopausal Bleeding

Postmenopausal bleeding is a common clinical complaint; however, the optimal algorithm for its evaluation has not been fully elucidated. One of the goals of this chapter is to review the evidence for diagnostic testing in PMB.

Methodology

A Medline search was performed using PubMed (National Library of Medicine, Bethesda, Maryland) for original research publications discussing the diagnostic performance and effectiveness of screening strategies in ovarian cancer screening. The search covered the years 1966 to 2003 and included the following search terms: (1) *ovarian cancer screening*, (2) *CA 125*, (3) *ovarian cancer* and *ultrasound*, and (4) *ovarian cancer* and *imaging*. Additional articles were identified by reviewing the reference lists of relevant papers. This review was limited to human studies and the English-language literature.

A separate Medline search was performed using PubMed for original research publications discussing the diagnostic performance and effectiveness of diagnostic strategies in PMB. The search covered the years 1966 to 2003 and included the following search terms: (1) *postmenopausal bleeding*,

(2) *endometrial cancer*, (3) *endometrial cancer* and *ultrasound*, (4) *endometrial cancer* and *hysteroscopy*, and (5) *endometrial biopsy*. Additional articles were identified by reviewing the reference lists of relevant publications. This review was limited to human studies and the English-language literature.

I. Ovarian Cancer Screening: What Is the Role of Biochemical Markers Such as CA 125?

Summary of Evidence: CA 125 represents the most extensively studied biochemical marker used as a screening test for ovarian cancer. Elevated levels of CA 125 ($\geq$35 U/mL) have a high sensitivity for ovarian cancer at stage II or greater, with only low to moderate (approximately 50%) sensitivity in early-stage disease (moderate evidence). Longitudinal trends in CA 125 levels appear to be more predictive of developing ovarian cancer than a fixed upper limit, as increasing levels of CA 125 were associated with malignancy, whereas stable, though elevated levels of CA 125 were associated with benign disease (Limited evidence).

Supporting Evidence: Although other tumor markers have been recently developed, this review focuses on the use of CA 125, the most frequently used tumor marker. This tumor marker has been developed predominantly using samples from women with clinically detected disease, rather than from women with preclinical disease. Nevertheless, elevated CA 125 (>35 U/mL) was demonstrated in 83% of women with epithelial ovarian cancer. As has been previously mentioned, reported sensitivity of elevated CA 125 for detecting ovarian cancer exceeds 90% in the women with greater than stage I disease, but drops to 50% in women with stage I disease (37,38). A study of 59 serum samples obtained 5 years before the diagnosis of ovarian cancer found that 25% had elevated levels of CA 125, suggesting the potential use of CA 125 for screening for preclinical disease.

The use of trends in serial CA 125 values may be more predictive than a fixed cut-off. Skates et al. (39,40) observed that CA 125 levels tended to rise in women with malignancy but remained the same or decreased in women without malignancy. Incorporating trends in serial CA 125 levels increases the sensitivity of the screening regimen as women with normal but rising CA 125 levels are identified at increased risk of malignancy; identifying women with elevated though stable CA 125 at lesser risk of malignancy increases the specificity (40).

II. Ovarian Cancer Screening: What Is the Diagnostic Performance (Accuracy) of Imaging?

Summary of Evidence: The diagnostic performance of gray-scale US imaging in screening for ovarian cancer in the general population has variable sensitivity ranging from 85% to 97% with lesser specificity of 56% to 97% (limited evidence). Color Doppler has more variability in its accuracy for detecting ovarian cancer with much weaker supporting evidence, such that there is insufficient evidence to warrant use of color Doppler alone as a screening tool.

Supporting Evidence: Real-time TVUS represents the current state of the art in imaging ovarian changes associated with ovarian cancer. Increased ovarian volume (greater than 10 mL in postmenopausal women) and alterations in normal ovarian morphology have been associated with malignancy (41). Specifically, complex ovarian cysts with multilocularity, wall or septal thickening, internal echogenicity, mural nodules, papillary projections, or solid components are have been used as imaging markers for ovarian cancer (42–45). Typically, repeat imaging at 4 to 6 weeks to verify stability of abnormal findings is recommended to decrease false positives. The sensitivity of morphologic analysis with US in predicting malignancy in ovarian tumors has been shown to be 85% to 97%, whereas its specificity ranges from 56% to 95% (44,46–49).

Gray-scale imaging of the ovaries can be augmented with duplex and color Doppler imaging to detect low resistance flow induced by tumoral neovascularity. In general, lower mean pulsatility indices have been previously demonstrated to be associated with malignancy compared to benign lesions. Resistive indices less than 0.4 to 0.8 (50–56) and pulsatility indices less than 1.0 are generally considered to be suspicious for malignancy (50,51,53–59). Despite these reports, the duplex Doppler parameters consistently differentiating ovarian malignancies from benign lesions have not been established. A comparison of different studies shows that no standard has been established concerning which Doppler index to use or what cutoff value is most appropriate. Doppler US has yielded variable results in distinguishing benign from malignant masses, with a sensitivity of 50% to 100% and a specificity of 46% to 100% (44,45,47,48,52,57,60,61). Different results are partly due to varying threshold values and corresponding trade-offs between sensitivity and specificity.

Jeng et al. (62) demonstrated that in 740 benign masses, all tumors had a resistive index of greater than 0.4, with 354 having no intratumoral blood flow. In the same study, five of six cases of borderline ovarian malignancies had resistive indices of 0.5 to 0.6, with the sixth case without intratumoral flow, while 52 of the 55 malignancies had resistive indices less than 0.4. Jeng et al. and others have demonstrated that color Doppler improves performance characteristics of gray-scale US (52,62,63). However, there appears to be little support for the use of color duplex Doppler imaging alone as a screening tool for detecting malignant ovarian masses.

Use of prediction rules and neural networks incorporating US imaging characteristics has been reported. To improve the sensitivity and specificity of gray-scale imaging, Timmerman et al. (64) incorporated patient characteristics such as age, menopausal status, and CA 125 level with specific US characteristics of the ovarian mass to derive a risk of malignancy index. The characteristics most predictive of malignancy were postmenopausal status, CA 125 level, the presence of one or more papillary growths, and a color score indicating tumor vascularity and blood flow. The optimized prediction model had a sensitivity of 95.9% and a specificity of 87.1%. Others have also derived morphologic indices by weighting specific US characteristics. However, the application of these indices or prediction rules can be difficult, as there is no consensus on the number and type of characteristics to include in the model (42,43,45,64–66). Furthermore, at least one investigator has demonstrated no significant difference in clinician estimate of probability of malignancy and estimate of malignancy made with a prediction model, using a standardized set of cases (66).

The use of magnetic resonance imaging or computed tomography has not been tested as a screening test (insufficient evidence).

III. Ovarian Cancer Screening: What Is the Role of Imaging?

Summary of Evidence: There is marked heterogeneity in the available evidence for screening in the asymptomatic population with limited to moderate evidence. The specificities from the above studies range from 91% to 98.9%, although the low incidence of ovarian cancer in the general population precluded sufficient assessment of sensitivity. Only one study reported survival, which was increased to 73 months in the screening group, compared to 42 months. Limited evidence supports the use of imaging alone as a screening tool. Even through the evidence is more robust for the use of initial CA 125 level followed by TVUS if CA 125 is elevated, current evidence does not support population-based screening for ovarian cancer in the general population regardless of screening algorithm (limited evidence).

Supporting Evidence: To present the best available evidence for ovarian cancer screening in the general population, only prospective studies with clear enrollment criteria are included in this review. If multiple publications using the same population were identified, only the most recent publication reporting the longest term follow-up was included.

A. Screening with Gray-Scale Ultrasound Only

Campbell et al. (67) evaluated 5479 self-referred women without symptoms of ovarian cancer using serial transabdominal US conducted annually, with subsequent referral for laparoscopy, laparotomy, or both if positive. Participants without a family history of ovarian cancer were enrolled if they were 45 years and older. All participants with a family history of ovarian cancer (4%) were included regardless of age. A total of 326 women screened positive. Of the nine women who were eventually diagnosed with ovarian cancer, five had stage I cancers. Despite a 97.7% specificity of the screening regimen, individual US characteristics were insufficient to differentiate benign from malignant lesions.

Tabor et al. (68) conducted a population-based randomized control trial of ovarian cancer screening using TVUS in women 45 to 65 years old. A total of 950 participants were randomized into either no screening (400 women) or one-time screening with TVUS (450 women). Women with abnormal ovarian morphology on TVUS were referred to laparotomy. A total of nine women were referred for operative evaluation, none of whom had ovarian cancer. Overall specificity for the screening arm was 98%.

Van Nagell et al. (41) performed annual TVUS screening on a total of 14,469 women—11,170 asymptomatic women 50 years and over without a family history of ovarian cancer and 3299 asymptomatic women 25 years and older with a family history of ovarian cancer received a TVUS at enrollment. Women with a normal TVUS received a follow-up TVUS at 12 months after enrollment. Ultrasound was repeated in women with an abnormal initial TVUS at 4 to 6 weeks. If the TVUS was persistently abnormal, women received CA 125, color Doppler sonography, and referral for surgery. The TVUS was classified as abnormal if ovarian volume exceeded $10\,cm^3$ in postmenopausal women ($20\,cm^3$ in premenopausal women) or a papillary or complex tissue projection was identified in a cystic ovarian mass. A total of 180 women with persistently abnormal TVUS received salpingo-oophorectomy with or without hysterectomy. Seventeen women eventually were diagnosed with ovarian cancer, 11 of which were stage I cancers. Specificity of the screening algorithm was 98.9%. But TVUS did not reliably distinguish between benign and malignant tumors.

B. Screening with Ultrasound and Color Doppler Imaging

Vuento et al. (69) enrolled 1364 asymptomatic women of ages 56 to 61 years using gray-scale TVUS (96%) or transabdominal US (4%) and color Doppler imaging. Repeat imaging was performed 1 to 3 months later in women with an abnormal US, with referral to exploratory laparotomy in women with persistently abnormal US. The US examination was classified as abnormal if ovarian volume equaled or exceeded $8\,cm^3$, ovarian echogenicity was inhomogeneous, or pulsatility index of the ovarian artery or tumor vessel did not exceed 1.0. Women who had a normal screening US were followed using the Finnish Cancer Registry to identify women who subsequently developed ovarian cancer. Eighteen women had persistent sonographic abnormalities; only three women had an abnormal pulsatility index. Of these 18 women, only one ovarian cancer (stage I) was identified. Specificity of the screening algorithm was 98%.

C. Multimodality Approach Using CA 125 and Ultrasound

Einhorn et al. (70) evaluated 5550 women 40 years and older randomly identified through the Stockholm Population registry. Elevated CA 125 was defined as greater than $35\,U/mL$ in the first 3455 women enrolled. The threshold for CA 125 was subsequently lowered to $30\,U/mL$ for the latter 2095. A total of 175 women with elevated CA 125 with age-matched controls were subjected to additional workup with serial CA 125 every 3 months and transabdominal US and pelvic examination every 6 months. Of the 175 women with elevated CA 125, six were found to have ovarian cancer, only two of which were stage I. Of the remainder of women with normal CA 125, three women with ovarian cancer were identified through the Swedish Cancer Registry, only one of which was stage I. In women 50 years and older, the specificity of CA 125 was 98.5% using $35\,U/mL$ as a threshold, and 97% using $30\,U/mL$. In women under 50 years old, specificity for CA 125 using $35\,U/mL$ and $30\,U/mL$ were 94.5% and 91%, respectively.

Jacobs et al. (39) randomized 21,955 postmenopausal women 45 years and older who were asymptomatic to screening or follow-up without screening. The screening regimen consisted of CA 125 and ultrasound if CA 125 was $30\,U/mL$ or greater. The screening regimen was performed annually for 3 years. Transabdominal US was used for the first screen and TVUS for the second and third screens. Women with elevated CA 125 and an abnormal US were referred for surgical evaluation. Follow-up for women who screened negative for ovarian cancer and women in the control group was performed through the National Health Service Central Register. A total of 29 patients were referred for surgical evaluation after detection of elevated CA 125 and abnormal ultrasounds, six of whom had an ovarian cancer. Through the Central Register, an additional 10 women in the screening group and 20 women in the control group were identified with ovarian cancer. The median survival time of women with a diagnosed cancer in the screened group was 72.9 months compared to 41.8 months in the control group.

IV. Postmenopausal Bleeding Evaluation: When Should a Woman with Postmenopausal Bleeding Be Referred for Additional Evaluation?

Summary of Evidence: Although there is limited evidence supporting mandatory evaluation of PMB, clinician or patient concern regarding the risk of endometrial cancer warrants additional testing.

Supporting Evidence: As will be discussed in Section VI below, the risk for endometrial cancer varies widely in different populations. Although PMB previously represented an absolute indication for further evaluation, given the variable risk of endometrial cancer, the following considerations guide the need for additional workup:

1. Increased prevalence of irregular bleeding in women with HRT: Other causes of abnormal bleeding in this population includes skipped doses, especially progestogens, poor gastrointestinal absorption for oral preparations, drug interactions, coagulation disorders, or other gynecologic abnormalities such as cervical polyps.

2. Paucity of evidence on the clinical significance of bleeding patterns, where a single episode of bleeding should be of equal concern as persistent bleeding or if the magnitude of bleeding should precipitate evaluation.

3. Patient preference for additional evaluation can guide referral.

There is no evidence supporting mandatory referral, but rather the above points may be considered prior to additional testing. Despite this lack of evidence, the risk of endometrial cancer in women not on HRT with PMB or women on HRT with abnormal bleeding is sufficient to warrant further testing (71).

V. Postmenopausal Bleeding Evaluation: What Is the Accuracy of Imaging Tests?

Summary of Evidence: In women with postmenopausal bleeding, TVUS is the most sensitive test (moderate evidence), detecting more abnormalities than saline-infused hysterosonography (moderate evidence) or hysteroscopy (moderate evidence).

Supporting Evidence

A. Transvaginal Ultrasonography

The best evidence available for the test performance of TVUS in postmenopausal bleeding results from two recent meta-analysis studies. In symptomatic postmenopausal women not on tamoxifen therapy, Smith-Bindman et al. (72), using a double wall measurement of 5mm as an upper threshold, demonstrated that the sensitivity for endometrial disease detection reached 92% and for endometrial cancer detection reached 96%. Transvaginal US performed equally well in identifying endometrial disease in women using HRT and women not on HRT. The TVUS false positive rate was 8% in women not on HRT and 23% in women on HRT. Decreasing the threshold for endometrial thickness increases sensitivity (98% using a

3-mm cutoff) with a false-positive rate of 38%. The meta-analysis conducted by Gupta et al. (73) identified 1243 cases of endometrial carcinoma among 8890 patients reported in the literature, giving a pretest probability of 14.0%. Using double wall thickness of 5 mm as a cutoff yielded a sensitivity of 97% with a specificity of 45%.

B. Saline-Infused Hysterosonography

De Kroon et al. (74) conducted a meta-analysis to evaluate the diagnostic accuracy of saline contrast hysterosonography in the evaluation of the uterine cavity abnormalities in pre- and postmenopausal women with symptoms of abnormal uterine bleeding.

The main outcome measure was the test performance in detection of any endometrial abnormality in the evaluation of the uterine cavity in cases of abnormal uterine bleeding. The authors did not segregate test results (i.e., they did not separate findings of endometrial cancer from benign etiologies of bleeding). The gold standard used was variable, but inclusion criteria maximized the gold standard by hysteroscopy or avoidance of verification bias in the selection of studies. Pooled sensitivity and specificity were 95% and 88%, respectively. Heterogeneity in sensitivity was not influenced by menopausal status, but specificity was. Baseline prevalence of any uterine abnormality was 56%, much higher than the generally accepted prevalence of endometrial cancer. Pooled likelihood ratio for a positive saline-infused hysterosonogram was 8.23 with an increase in posttest probability to 91%. For a negative test, the likelihood ratio was 0.06, with reduction in posttest probability to 7%.

C. Hysteroscopy

Meta-analysis of observational studies by Clark et al. (75) evaluated 65 primary studies including 26,346 women and assessed the diagnostic accuracy of hysteroscopy in detecting endometrial cancer and hyperplasia. The review included summarized studies including both premenopausal and postmenopausal women. The diagnostic reference standard was endometrial histologic findings. The authors presented pooled sensitivity and specificity across the population. In the detection of endometrial cancer, the variations in sensitivity were much greater than the variations in specificity. Weighted by the number of cases, the overall sensitivity was 86.4% and specificity was 99.2%. Diagnostic accuracy was lower for endometrial disease than for endometrial cancer, with weighted overall sensitivity of 78.0% and specificity of 95.8%. The authors noted that heterogeneity in test performance for detection of endometrial cancer was not explained by menopausal status; however, performance for detection of endometrial disease increased in postmenopausal women. Other measures of the clinical impact of hysteroscopy, namely likelihood ratios and changes in posttest probability, were segregated by menopausal status. For endometrial cancer, pretest probability (prevalence in women with postmenopausal bleeding) increased from 3.9% to 61% with a positive hysteroscopy (positive likelihood ratio 38.3) and decreased to 0.5% with a negative hysteroscopy (negative likelihood ratio 0.13). For endometrial disease, pretest probability (prevalence in women with postmenopausal bleeding) increased from 10.6% to 71% with a positive hysteroscopy (positive likelihood ratio 20.4) and decreased to 1.6% with a negative hysteroscopy (negative likelihood ratio 0.14).

VI. Postmenopausal Bleeding Evaluation: What Is the Role of Imaging?

Summary of Evidence: Transvaginal US is recommended as the best initial test for postmenopausal bleeding, as a negative test effectively excludes an underlying endometrial abnormality (moderate evidence). Hysteroscopy is recommended as a complementary test to a positive TVUS (moderate evidence). There is insufficient evidence for the routine use of saline-infused hysterosonography unless hysteroscopy is unavailable or more difficult to obtain due resource or expertise limitations.

Supporting Evidence: The high sensitivity of TVUS makes it an excellent noninvasive test for determining which women with vaginal bleeding do not require endometrial biopsy. The specificity is low, and thus US is not very accurate in predicting endometrial disease (72,73). Therefore, an abnormal TVUS result in a woman with vaginal bleeding needs to be followed by a histologic biopsy.

Hysteroscopy is highly accurate and thereby clinically useful in diagnosing endometrial cancer in women with abnormal uterine bleeding. However, its high accuracy relates to diagnosing cancer rather than excluding it (74). Therefore, this test is more useful as a diagnostic tool complementary to a test such as TVUS, which has a high sensitivity and low specificity.

VII. How Should Women on Tamoxifen Therapy Be Evaluated?

Summary of Evidence: There is insufficient evidence for routine imaging in asymptomatic women on tamoxifen. Symptomatic women should be evaluated with hysteroscopy and biopsy (limited evidence) as the initial algorithm as tamoxifen causes increased false positives with TVUS (moderate evidence).

Supporting Evidence: Long-term use of tamoxifen increases risk of endometrial cancer, as previously mentioned. Furthermore, differentiating potential cancers from other tamoxifen-induced endometrial changes is challenging using any diagnostic test. The evidence does not support the use of investigating asymptomatic women on tamoxifen (76–82). Assigning an absolute upper limit in endometrial thickness detected by TVUS in the setting of tamoxifen administration is difficult as tamoxifen, even in the absence of pathology, causes endometrial thickening, thus increasing false positives using the standard upper limit of 5 mm employed in the postmenopausal woman (83,84). At least one investigator has proposed increasing the limit to 9 mm, although further studies are required to support this limit. Clearly, the use of TVUS in patients with abnormal bleeding while on tamoxifen is less accurate. As physician and patient concern should be taken into account in the evaluation of abnormal bleeding, hysteroscopy combined with biopsy as the initial test may be more appropriate in this high-risk group (17).

Take-Home Tables and Figure

Table 30.1. Summary of screening regimens in ovarian cancer detection

Screening regimen	Study type	Subjects (cancers)	Specificity
Gray-scale transvaginal ultrasound (TVUS)			
Campbell	Observational	5,479 (9)	98%
Tabor	RCT	950 (0)	98%
Van Nagell	Observational	14,469 (17)	99%
Gray-scale and Doppler TVUS			
Vuento	Observational	1,364 (1)	98%
CA 125 + gray-scale TVUS			
Einhorn	Observational	5,500 (7)	99%
Jacobs	RCT	21,955 (36)	97%

Note: Due to the extremely low prevalence of ovarian cancer in the screening population, none of the studies presented reliable information on sensitivity.
RCT, randomized controlled trial.

Table 30.2. Summary of imaging techniques in the evaluation of postmenopausal bleeding

Imaging technique	HRT use	Endometrial disease detection			Endometrial cancer detection		
		Sensitivity	Specificity	PLR (NLR)	Sensitivity	Specificity	PLR (NLR)
Transvaginal ultrasound							
Smith-Bindman,	Yes	95%	92%	11.9 (0.12)			
5-mm threshold	No	91%	77%	4.0 (0.5)			
	Pooled				96%	61%	nr
Gupta, 5-mm threshold	Pooled	nr	nr	nr	97%	45%	2.17 (0.15)
Saline-infused sonography							
de Kroon	Pooled	95%	88%	8.23 (0.06)			
Hysteroscopy							
Clark	Pooled	78%	96%	20.4 (0.14)	86%	99%	38.3 (0.13)

PLR, positive likelihood ratio; NLR, negative likelihood ratio; nr, not reported.

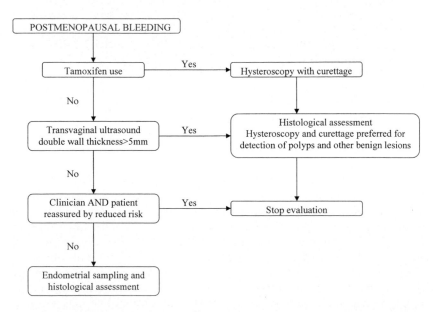

Figure 30.1. Algorithm for evaluating women with postmenopausal bleeding.

Imaging Case Studies

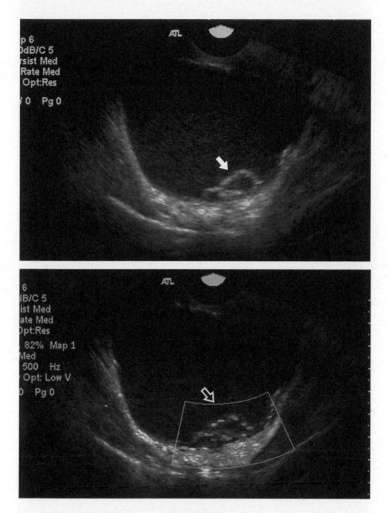

Figure 30.2. Ovarian cancer. Large multiloculated cyst with internal echogenicity and a mural nodule (solid arrow) with vascular flow demonstrated on power Doppler (open arrow). (See color insert)

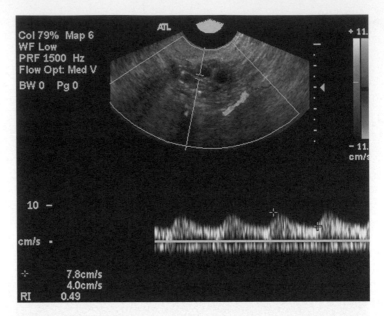

Figure 30.3. Benign ovarian mass. Complex adnexal mass with solid and cystic components. The solid component demonstrates vascular flow with a low resistive index (0.49). Mass was interpreted as an ovarian carcinoma, proved to be a fibroadenoma on resection. (See color insert)

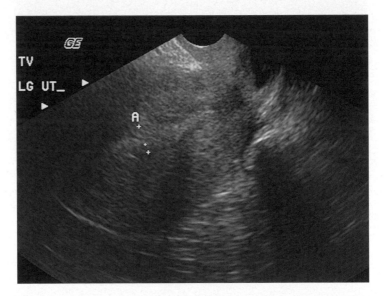

Figure 30.4. Proliferative endometrium. Thickening of the endometrium (10 mm) detected on transvaginal ultrasound in a postmenopausal woman on hormone replacement therapy. Repeat evaluation demonstrated similar thickening. Pathologic samples from intraoperative hysteroscopy and biopsy demonstrated proliferative endometrium, without evidence of endometrial cancer.

Protocol: Transvaginal Ultrasound

Sonography should be performed using a 5- to 10-MHz transducer, and the patient's bladder should be empty for sufficient resolution of the endometrial cavity, uterine morphology, and adnexal morphology. Imaging of the uterus should be performed in short axis and long axis relative to the uterus. Sagittal and transverse imaging of the adnexa should be performed.

Future Research

- Longitudinal analysis of population-based cohort for ovarian cancer screening.
- Randomized trial of different algorithms for ovarian cancer screening.
- High-quality cohort studies comparing saline-infused hysterosonography to a rigorous standard of reference.
- Analysis of a higher threshold for endometrial thickening in women on tamoxifen.

References

1. Chen VW, Ruiz B, Killeen JL, Cote TR, Wu XC, Correa CN. Cancer 2003;97(10 suppl):2631–2642.
2. Cancer Facts and Figures 2004. Available at http://www.cancer.org.
3. Holschneider CH, Berek JS. Semin Surg Oncol 2000;19(1):3–10.
4. Edmondson RJ, Monaghan JM. Int J Gynecol Cancer 2001;11(6):423–429.
5. Rubin SC, Blackwood MA, Bandera C, et al. Am J Obstet Gynecol 1998; 178(4):670–677.
6. Boyd J, Rubin SC. Gynecol Oncol 1997;64(2):196–206.
7. Boyd J. In: Rubin S, Sutton G, eds. Ovarian Cancer. Philadelphia: Lippincott Williams & Wilkins, 2001:3–17.
8. Marra G, Boland C. J Natl Cancer Inst 1995;87:1114–1125.
9. Whittemore AS, Harris R, Itnyre J, et al. Am J Epidemiol 1992;136:1184–1203.
10. Hankinson SE, Colditz GA, Hunter DJ, et al. Cancer 1995;76:284–290.
11. Purdie D, Green A, Bain C, et al. Int J Cancer 1995;62:678–684.
12 Mosgaard BJ, Lidegaard O, Kjaer SK, Schou G, Andersen AN. Fertil Steril 1997; 67:1005–1012.
13. Ferrazzi E, Torri V, Trio D, Zannoni E, Filiberto S, Dordoni D. Ultrasound Obstet Gynecol 1996;7:315–321.
14. Gredmark T, Kvint S, Havel G, Mattsson LA. Br J Obstet Gynaecol 1995; 102:133–136.
15. Lidor A, Ismajovich B, Confino E, David MP. Acta Obstet Gynecol Scand 1986; 65:41–43.
16. Research on the Menopause in the 1990s Report of a WHO Scientific Group. World Health Organization, WHO Technical Report Series No. 866, 1996.
17. Investigation of post-menopausal bleeding: a national clinical guideline. Scottish Intercollegiate Guidelines Network 2002. Available at http://www.guideline.gov/summary/summary.aspx?doc_id=3456.
18. Spencer CP, Cooper AJ, Whitehead MI. BMJ 1997;315:37–42.
19. Dunlop MG, Farrington SM, Carothers AD, et al. Hum Mol Genet 1997;6: 105–110.
20. Aarnio M, Sankila R, Pukkala E, et al. Int J Cancer 1999;81:214–218.
21. Vasen HF, Wijnen JT, Menko FH, et al. Gastroenterology 1996;110:1020–1027.

22. Pettersson B, Adami HO, Bergstrom R, Johansson EDB. Acta Obstet Gynecol Scand 1986;65:247–255.

23. Kvale G, Heuch I, Ursin G. Cancer Res 1988;48:6217–6221.

24. Brinton LA, Berman ML, Mortel R, et al. Am J Obstet Gynecol 1992;167:1317–1325.

25. Albrektsen G, Heuch I, Tretli S, Kvale G. Int J Cancer 1995;61:485–490.

26. Lambe M, Wuu J, Weiderpass E, Hsieh CC. Cancer Causes Control 1999;10:43–49.

27. Henderson BE, Casagrande JT, Pike MC, Mack T, Rosario I, Duke A. Br J Cancer 1983;47:749–756.

28. Cancer and Steroid Hormone Study. N Engl J Med 1987;316:650–655.

29. Pike MC, Peters RK, Cozen W, et al. J Natl Cancer Inst 1997;89:1110–1116.

30. Rutqvist LE, Johansson H, Signomklao T, Johansson U, Fornander T, Wilking N. J Natl Cancer Inst 1995;87:645–651.

31. Fisher B, Costantino JP, Wickerham DL, et al. J Natl Cancer Inst 1998;90:1371–1388.

32. Fornander T, Rutqvist LE, Cedermark B, et al. Lancet 1989;1:117–120.

33. Curtis RE, Boice JD Jr, Shriner DA, Hankey BF, Fraumeni JF Jr. J Natl Cancer Inst 1996;88:832–834.

34. Etzioni R, Urban N, Baker M. J Clin Epidemiol 1996;49:95–103.

35. Fireman B, Quesenberry C, Somkin C, et al. Health Care Finance Rev 1997;18:51–76.

36. Develioglu OH, Bilgin T, Yalcin OT, Ozalp S. Arch Gynecol Obstet 2003;268(3):175–180.

37. Fritsche HA, Bast RC. Clin Chem 1998;44:1379–1380.

38. Jacobs IJ, Menon U. Mol Cell Proteomics 2004;3(4):355–366.

39. Jacobs IJ, Skates SJ, Macdonald N, et al. Lancet 1999;353:1207–1210.

40. Skates SJ, Pauler DK, Jacobs IJ. J Am Stat Assoc 2001;96:429–439.

41. van Nagell JR Jr, DePriest PD, Reedy MB, et al. Gynecol Oncol 2000;77:350–356.

42. Sassone AM, Timor-Tritsch IE, Artner A, Westhoff C, Warren WB. Obstet Gynecol 1991;78:70–76.

43. Lerner JP, Timor-Tritsch IE, Federman A, Abramovich G. Am J Obstet Gynecol 1994;170:81–85.

44. Reles A, Wein U, Lichtenegger W. J Clin Ultrasound 1997;25:217–225.

45. Ferrazzi E, Zanetta G, Dordoni D, Berlanda N, Mezzopane R, Lissoni AA. Ultrasound Obstet Gynecol 1997;10:192–197.

46. Leibman AJ, Kruse B, McSweeney MB. AJR 1988;151:89–92.

47. Hata K, Hata T, Manabe A, Sugimura K, Kitao M. Obstet Gynecol 1992;80:922–926.

48. Kurjak A, Predanic M. J Ultrasound Med 1992;11:631–638.

49. Franchi M, Beretta P, Ghezzi F, Zanaboni F, Goddi A, Salvatore S. Acta Obstet Gynecol Scand 1995;74:734–739.

50. Hamper UM, Sheth S, Abbas FM, Rosenshein NB, Aronson D, Kurman RJ. AJR 1993;160:1225–1228.

51. Stein SM, Laifer-Narin S, Johnson MB, et al. AJR 1995;164:381–386.

52. Bromley B, Goodman H, Benacerraf BR. Obstet Gynecol 1994;83:434–437.

53. Brown DL, Frates MC, Laing FC, et al. Radiology 1994;190:333–336.

54. Carter J, Saltzman A, Hartenbach E, Fowler J, Carson L, Twiggs LB. Obstet Gynecol 1994;83:125–130.

55. Jain KA. Radiology 1994;191:63–67.

56. Levine D, Feldstein VA, Babcook CJ, Filly RA. AJR 1994;162:1355–1359.

57. Salem S, White LM, Lai J. AJR 1994;163:1147–1150.

58. Weiner Z, Thaler I, Levron J, Lewit N, Itskovitz-Eldor J. Fertil Steril 1993;59:743–749.

59. Rehn M, Lohmann K, Rempen A. Am J Obstet Gynecol 1996;175:97–104.

60. Timor-Tritsch LE, Lerner JP, Monteagudo A, Santos R. Am J Obstet Gynecol 1993;168:909–913.

61. Schneider VL, Schneider A, Reed KL, Hatch KD. Obstet Gynecol 1993;81: 983–988.
62. Jeng CJ, Lin SY, Wang KL, Yang YC, Wang KG. Ultrasound Med Biol 1994;20;180.
63. Fleischer AC, Cullinan JA, Kepple DM, Williams LL. J Ultrasound Med 1993; 12:705–712.
64. Timmerman D, Bourne TH, Tailor A, et al. Am J Obstet Gynecol 1999;181:57–65.
65. Ueland FR, DePriest PD, Pavlik EJ, Kryscio RJ, van Nagell JR Jr. Gynecol Oncol 2003;91:46–50.
66. Mol B, Boll D, DeKanter M, et al. Gynecol Oncol 2001;80:162–167.
67. Campbell S, Bhan V, Royston P, Whitehead MI, Collins WP. Br Med J 1989; 299:1363–1367.
68. Tabor A, Jensen FR, Bock JE, Hogdall CK. J Med Screen 1994;1:215–219.
69. Vuento MH, Pirhonen JP, Makinen JI, Laippala PJ, Gronroos M, Salmi TA. Cancer 1995;76:1214–1218.
70. Einhorn N, Sjovall K, Knapp RC, et al. Obstet Gynecol 1992;80:14–18.
71. Department of Health. Referral guidelines for suspected cancer. London: Department of Health, 2000. Available at url:http:// www.doh.gov.uk/cancer/referral.htm.
72. Smith-Bindman R, Kerlikowske K, Feldstein VA, et al. JAMA 1998;280: 1510–1517.
73. Gupta JK, Chien PF, Voit D, Clark TJ, Khan KS. Acta Obstet Gynecol Scand 2002; 81(9):799–816.
74. de Kroon CD, de Bock GH, Dieben SW, Jansen FW. BJOG 2003;110(10):938–947.
75. Clark TJ, Voit D, Gupta JK, Hyde C, Song F, Khan KS. JAMA 2002; 288(13):1610–1621.
76. Timmerman D, Deprest J, Bourne T, Van den Berghe I, Collins WP, Vergote I. Am J Obstet Gynecol 1998;179:62–70.
77. Cecchini S, Ciatto S, Bonardi R, et al. Tumori 1998;84:21–23.
78. Tepper R, Beyth Y, Altaras MM, et al. Gynecol Oncol 997;64:386–391.
79. Love CD, Muir BB, Scrimgeour JB, Leonard RC, Dillon P, Dixon JM. J Clin Oncol 1999;17:2050–2054.
80. Berliere M, Charles A, Galant C, Donnez J. Obstet Gynecol 1998;91:40–44.
81. Gerber B, Krause A, Muller H, et al. J Clin Oncol 2000;18:3464–3470.
82. Barakat RR, Gilewski TA, Almadrones L, et al. J Clin Oncol 2000;18:3459–3463.
83. Bornstein J, Auslender R, Pascal B, Gutterman E, Isakov D, Abramovici H. Reprod Med 1994;39:674–678.
84. Mourits MJ, Van der Zee AG, Willemse PH, Ten Hoor KA, Hollema H, De Vries EG. Gynecol Oncol 1999;73:21–26.

Index